# Practical Case Studies in Urology

# Practical Case Studies in Urology

Editor: Kane Palmer

AMERICAN
MEDICAL PUBLISHERS
www.americanmedicalpublishers.com

AMERICAN
MEDICAL PUBLISHERS
www.americanmedicalpublishers.com

**Cataloging-in-Publication Data**

Practical case studies in urology / edited by Kane Palmer.
p. cm.
Includes bibliographical references and index.
ISBN 979-8-88740-657-2
1. Urology. 2. Urinary organs--Diseases. 3. Urinary organs--Diseases--Treatment.
4. Urinary organs--Diseases--Diagnosis. I. Palmer, Kane.
RC900 .C55 2023
616.6--dc23



American Medical Publishers,
41 Flatbush Avenue,
1st Floor, New York,
NY 11217, USA

ISBN 979-8-88740-657-2 (Hardback)

# Contents

# Preface

Over the recent decade, advancements and applications have progressed exponentially. This has led to the increased interest in this field and projects are being conducted to enhance knowledge. The main objective of this book is to present some of the critical challenges and provide insights into possible solutions. This book will answer the varied questions that arise in the field and also provide an increased scope for furthering studies.

Urology is a medical specialty that focuses on the diagnosis and treatment of diseases and disorders related to the urinary tract and the male reproductive system. It encompasses the surgical as well as non-surgical treatment of urological diseases. The various diseases and diagnostic procedures which fall within this field are urinary tract infections, kidney stones and benign prostatic hyperplasia. Urinary tract infections are bacterial infections that can affect any part of the urinary system, including the bladder, urethra, ureters and kidneys. Kidney stones are hard deposits that form in the kidneys and can cause severe pain and other urinary symptoms. The book aims to shed light on some of the unexplored aspects of urology and the recent researches in this field. It includes contributions of medical experts which will provide innovative insights into this field. This book is a resource guide for experts as well as students.

I hope that this book, with its visionary approach, will be a valuable addition and will promote interest among readers. Each of the authors has provided their extraordinary competence in their specific fields by providing different perspectives as they come from diverse nations and regions. I thank them for their contributions.

**Editor**

# 1

# Renal Oncocytoma and Retroperitoneal Ancient Schwannoma: A Benign Mimic of Metastatic Renal Cell Carcinoma

**Tyler J. Maiers,[1,2] Daniel C. Wang,[1,2] Ali H. Houjaij,[1,2] and Oussama M. Darwish[1,2]**

[1] *Western New York Healthcare System-Buffalo Veterans Affairs Medical Center, 3495 Bailey Ave, Buffalo, NY 14215, USA*
[2] *Department of Urology, Jacobs School of Medicine and Biomedical Sciences, University at Buffalo, Buffalo General Medical Center, Suite B280, 100 High Street, Buffalo, NY 14203, USA*

Correspondence should be addressed to Tyler J. Maiers; tmaiers@buffalo.edu

Academic Editor: Fumitaka Koga

Renal oncocytomas and retroperitoneal schwannomas are rare and typically benign tumors with characteristic histopathologic features. Ideal management of both renal oncocytoma and retroperitoneal schwannoma is surgical resection. We present a rare case of a 63-year-old man with multifocal renal oncocytoma and retroperitoneal ancient schwannoma which, preoperatively, masqueraded as metastatic renal cell carcinoma. Both tumors were successfully resected surgically. Immunochemistry and histopathology confirmed each diagnosis.

## 1. Introduction

Renal oncocytoma is a rare tumor accounting for approximately 4% of all solid renal masses [1]. While the majority of oncocytomas are benign, there have been several case reports of malignant behavior and metastasis [2, 3]. Oncocytomas are composed of oncocytes, which are uniform, round, or polygonal neoplastic cells exhibiting a granular eosinophilic cytoplasm. Long-term outcomes in patients with oncocytomas are highly favorable, with previous reports indicating a disease-specific survival of up to 100% [4].

Similarly, primary tumors of the retroperitoneum are uncommon. Schwannomas are thought to occur in approximately 4% of all primary retroperitoneal tumors [5]. Schwannomas originate in peripheral nerve fibers and are typically found in the head, neck, or flexor surfaces of the extremities. Although malignant schwannomas have been reported in the literature [6], the vast majority are benign in nature. The term "ancient" schwannoma is reserved for schwannomas exhibiting signs of degeneration including hemorrhage, cyst formation, hyalinization, and calcification [7].

To the best of our knowledge, the present study reports the first case of multifocal renal oncocytoma and retroperitoneal ancient schwannoma. The patient was treated with open right radical nephrectomy and retroperitoneal lymph node dissection. The clinical, radiographic, and pathologic findings of this case are discussed in detail.

## 2. Case Presentation

A 63-year-old man with chronic kidney disease presented with elevated baseline creatinine. He had no urologic symptoms and no history of flank pain or hematuria. Family history was notable for renal malignancy in the patient's grandmother. The physical examination was unremarkable, with no palpable flank mass or tenderness. Laboratory studies were notable for a creatinine of 2.02 (eGFR = 34 ml/min), up from a baseline of 1.60 (eGFR = 42 ml/min). Renal ultrasound revealed a 12 x 15 cm predominantly solid mass in the right kidney with internal cystic changes and central flow. In the left kidney renal ultrasound revealed a solid-appearing mass in the upper pole measuring 6.5 x 6 x 5.5 cm, a hypoechoic structure measuring 4.8 x 4.1 x 4.6 cm in the lower pole, and an adjacent 6.1 x 5.8 x 6.4 cm solid left lower pole renal mass with a small amount of central flow. Computed Tomography (CT) revealed a 14 x 13 x 16 cm right renal mass almost completely replacing the interpolar region, with significant mass effect on the right kidney (Figures 1 and 2). Adjacent tissue nodularity in the perinephric fat was concerning for satellite nodules or metastatic disease

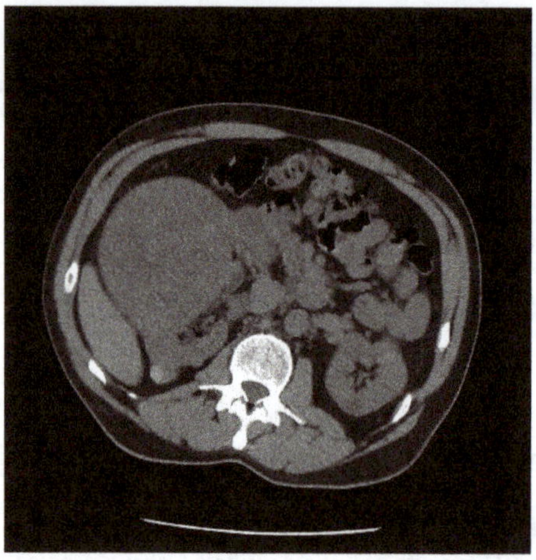

FIGURE 1: Computed tomography without contrast revealed a large right renal mass with significant mass effect on the right kidney. Adjacent soft tissue nodularities were concerning for satellite nodules or metastatic disease.

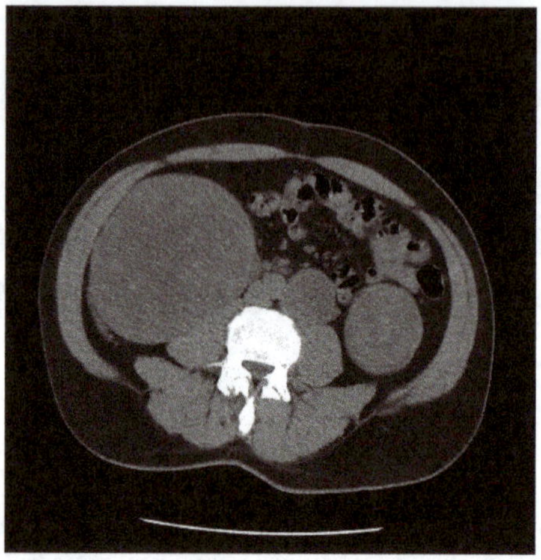

FIGURE 3: Computed tomography without contrast demonstrating left paraaortic mass, left interpolar renal mass, and large right renal mass.

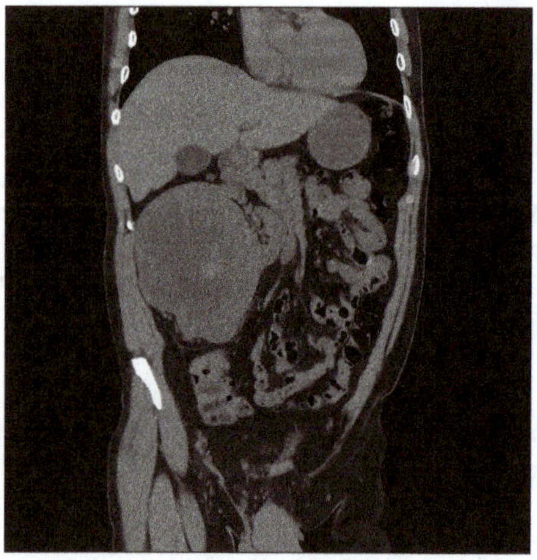

FIGURE 2: Computed tomography without contrast demonstrating a large heterogeneous right renal mass.

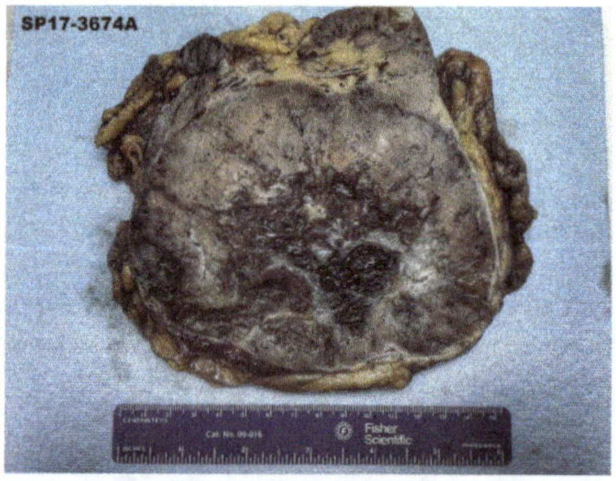


FIGURE 4: Gross specimen of right kidney containing maroon-colored mass with gray-white central scar.

(Figure 1). Right retroperitoneal adenopathy measuring 2.4 x 2.7 cm at the level of the renal hilum was identified. In addition, multiple 2-3 cm hyper- and isodense indeterminate soft tissue lesions were identified in the right kidney. The left kidney was notable for multiple solid renal masses measuring 6.3 cm at the upper pole and 4.6 cm at the interpolar region (Figure 3). A left paraaortic soft tissue mass measuring 4.6 x 4.6 cm with associated calcification was concerning for adenopathy (Figure 3). Whole body positron emission tomography (PET)/CT imaging was obtained to evaluate for metastatic disease. PET/CT revealed bilateral metabolically active solid renal masses concerning for malignancy and metabolic activity in a left paraaortic soft tissue mass concerning for lymphadenopathy. Magnetic resonance imaging (MRI) revealed no evidence of inferior vena cava thrombus.

The patient was discussed in a multidisciplinary oncology meeting and the decision was made to proceed with surgical extirpation of the right kidney and the paraaortic mass. We performed an open right radical nephrectomy with right retroperitoneal lymph node dissection and excision of left paraaortic mass.

Grossly, the right kidney contained a spherical, encapsulated, and homogenous maroon-colored mass with a gray-white lobulated central scar (Figure 4). Two additional smaller masses with similar gross appearance but without central scar were also present. Histologic examination revealed nests of round and polygonal cells with granular, eosinophilic cytoplasm (Figure 5) consistent with oncocytoma. Immunohistochemical staining of the right renal mass with colloidal iron, CD117, CK7, RCC, and CD10 was performed. The tumor cells were positive for CD117, CK7 (Figure 6), and weakly positive for CD10. The tumor cells were negative for Hale colloidal iron and RCC.

Cross sections of the left paraaortic mass revealed a smooth, encapsulated mass with a pearly and glistening tan-white surface (Figure 7). Histologic examination revealed multiple regions of cystic degeneration, positive staining for S100, and Antoni A and Antoni B areas. The final pathologic diagnoses were renal oncocytoma and left paraaortic ancient, benign schwannoma.

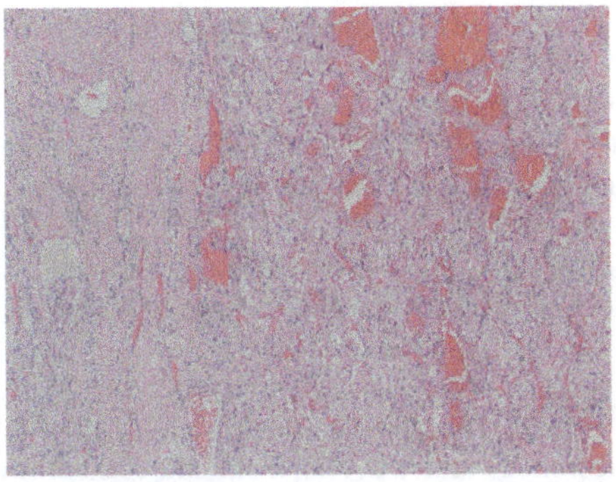

FIGURE 5: Microscopic (100x) H & E stained tumor revealing nests of round and polygonal cells with granular, eosinophilic cytoplasm classic for oncocytoma.

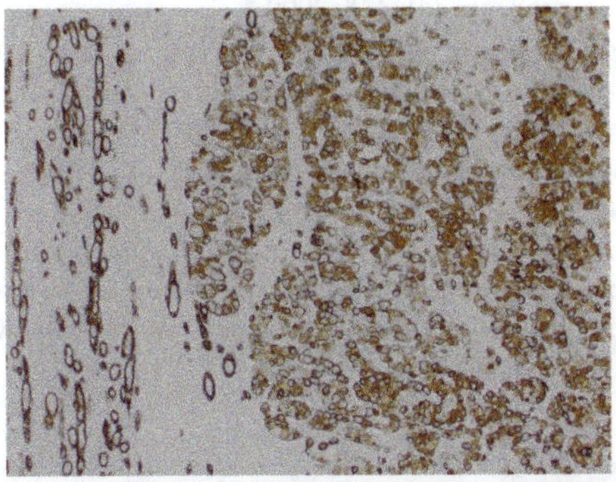

FIGURE 6: Microscopic (40x) renal tumor cells demonstrated positive staining for CK7.

## 3. Discussion

Renal oncocytoma is a benign tumor that is often thought to represent renal cell carcinoma during the preoperative workup due to similar enhancement on imaging. Distinguishing between the two is critically important yet consistently challenging for the practicing urologist. The similar rate of growth, age at presentation, and peak incidence during the seventh decade further complicate the task of distinguishing the two from one another. This case demonstrates the inherent difficulty in distinguishing preoperatively the difference between metastatic renal cell carcinoma and a combination of rare, typically benign tumors of the kidney and retroperitoneum.

The gross appearance of an oncocytoma is described as a homogeneous tan or mahogany mass with a pseudocapsule and central scar. Microscopically, oncocytomas are characterized by nests of round and polygonal, highly eosinophilic cells with granular cytoplasm secondary to a high concentration of mitochondria [2]. Oncocytomas are found more commonly in men than women (1.2:1), and multifocal oncocytomas are identified in up to 13% of patients with oncocytoma [2]. Cytogenetic abnormalities used to identify an oncocytoma include a diploid karyotype, loss of chromosomes 1, loss of Y, or various rearrangements of 11q13 [8]. Immunohistochemical characteristics used to identify oncocytoma include positive

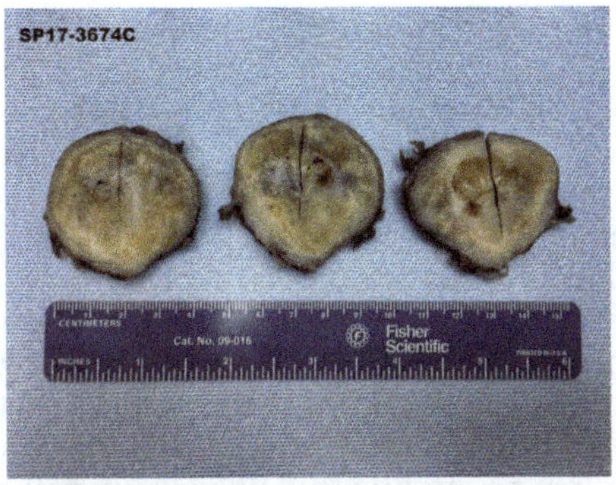


FIGURE 7: Cross sections of retroperitoneal ancient schwannoma with glistening tan-white surface.

staining for CK7, CD117, negative staining for vimentin, and negative or luminal staining for Hale colloidal iron [8]. The eosinophilic variant of chromophobe renal cell carcinoma represents perhaps the most histologically similar variant to oncocytoma. Specific cutoffs for distinguishing between oncocytoma and the eosinophilic variant of chromophobe renal cell carcinoma on the basis of CK7 positivity are highly variable and not well agreed upon in the literature [8]. Despite the inherent difficulty in confirming a diagnosis, distinguishing between these two entities is critical as the incidence of coexisting renal cell carcinoma and oncocytoma in patients with multiple renal tumors is approximately 10% [9]. When multiple renal tumors are present as in the patient described in this case, the urologist must maintain a high index of suspicion for coexisting renal cell carcinoma.

A number of subtle imaging findings have been described in an attempt to differentiate oncocytoma from renal cell carcinoma on CT and MRI. On CT, oncocytomas typically have a high peak Hounsfield unit attenuation in the nephrogenic phase as opposed to the corticomedullary phase most often seen in renal cell carcinomas. A form of segmental enhancement inversion on CT has been proposed as a unique method to distinguish between small oncocytomas and renal cell carcinoma [10]. A later study comparing segmental enhancement inversion on MRI, among a variety of other features, found no reliable characteristics to use in distinguishing between renal oncocytoma and chromophobe renal cell carcinoma [11]. Unfortunately for the practicing urologist, distinguishing the two entities radiographically remains challenging.

In this case, the identification of a solid retroperitoneal mass was concerning preoperatively for metastatic disease. The retroperitoneum can host a wide range of benign and malignant neoplasms. Schwannomas are composed of Schwann cells arising from a peripheral nerve sheath. Characteristic findings include S100 positivity and distinct regions of hypercellularity and hypocellularity, termed Antoni A and Antoni B regions, respectively. Ancient schwannoma is an uncommon variant used to describe a schwannoma with degenerative changes mimicking a malignant tumor including hemorrhage, cystic necrosis, calcification, and hyalinization [7]. The specimen obtained in this case contained multiple regions of cystic degeneration consistent with the ancient schwannoma variant. Complete surgical excision of a schwannoma is recommended and portends a good prognosis [7]. Approximately 11.7% of all schwannomas excised with a wide surgical margin are found to recur, with higher rates of recurrence reported following partial excision or enucleation [12].

Renal mass biopsy was discussed extensively at a multidisciplinary oncology conference before deciding upon the ultimate treatment strategy in this case. The large right renal tumor exhibited significant mass effect on the right kidney and replaced nearly the entire interpolar region with localized extension into perinephric fat. Definitive surgical management was thus considered optimal irrespective of biopsy results. Furthermore, the right renal mass was considered the most likely candidate to represent primary tumor in the setting of possible metastatic disease. The left renal masses, by comparison, were significantly smaller in size with fewer concerning features. Preoperatively, there was concern for a single metastatic site to the retroperitoneum. In the setting of perceived oligometastatic disease in a patient with ECOG performance status of 1, we elected to pursue a cytoreductive nephrectomy via surgical extirpation of the right kidney and excision of the left paraaortic mass.

Despite an extensive preoperative workup highly concerning for metastatic renal cell carcinoma, this patient was found to have separate, benign lesions with a favorable overall prognosis. To the best of our knowledge, this is the first described case of combined multifocal renal oncocytoma and retroperitoneal ancient schwannoma masquerading as metastatic renal cell carcinoma. Due to the possibility of a hybrid tumor on the left consisting of chromophobe renal cell carcinoma and oncocytoma, planned follow-up includes CT imaging every six months to assess for interval growth. Follow-up CT imaging at six months revealed no interval growth and no evidence of metastasis.

## Consent

Written informed consent was obtained.

## References

[1] M. N. Morra and S. Das, "Renal oncocytoma: a review of histogenesis, histopathology, diagnosis and treatment," *The Journal of Urology*, vol. 150, no. 2, pp. 295–302, 1993.

[2] B. Perez-Ordonez, G. Hamed, S. Campbell et al., "Renal oncocytoma: a clinicopathologic study of 70 cases," *The American Journal of Surgical Pathology*, vol. 21, no. 8, pp. 871–883, 1997.

[3] S. E. Wobker, C. G. Przybycin, K. Sircar, and J. I. Epstein, "Renal oncocytoma with vascular invasion: a series of 22 cases," *Human Pathology*, vol. 58, pp. 1–6, 2016.

[4] M. A. Benatiya, G. Rais, M. Tahri et al., "Renal oncocytoma: experience of clinical urology A, urology department, CHU IbnSina, Rabat, Morocco and literature review," *Pan African Medical Journal*, vol. 12, no. 1, article no 84, 2012.

[5] M. Dede, G. Yagci, M. C. Yenen et al., "Retroperitoneal benign schwannoma: report of three cases and analysis of clinico-radiologic findings," *The Tohoku Journal of Experimental Medicine*, vol. 200, no. 2, pp. 93–97, 2003.

[6] A. Bohlok, M. El Khoury, A. Bormans et al., "Schwannoma of the colon and rectum: a systematic literature review," *World Journal of Surgical Oncology*, vol. 16, no. 1, article no 125, 2018.

[7] S. Çalişkan, G. Gümrükçü, and C. Kaya, "Retroperitoneal ancient schwannoma: a case report," *Reviews in Urology*, vol. 17, no. 3, pp. 190–193, 2015.

[8] S. E. Wobker and S. R. Williamson, "Modern pathologic diagnosis of renal oncocytoma," *Journal of Kidney Cancer and VHL*, vol. 4, no. 4, pp. 1–12, 2017.

[9] C. B. Dechet, D. G. Bostwick, M. L. Blute, S. C. Bryant, and H. Zincke, "Renal oncocytoma: multifocality, bilateralism, meatachronous tumor development and coexistent renal cell carcinoma," *The Journal of Urology*, vol. 162, no. 1, pp. 40–42, 1999.

[10] J. I. Kim, J. Y. Cho, K. C. Moon, H. J. Lee, and S. H. Kim, "Segmental enhancement inversion at biphasic multidetector CT: characteristic finding of small renal oncocytoma," *Radiology*, vol. 252, no. 2, pp. 441–448, 2009.

[11] A. B. Rosenkrantz, N. Hindman, E. F. Fitzgerald, B. E. Niver, J. Melamed, and J. S. Babb, "MRI features of renal oncocytoma and chromophobe renal cell carcinoma," *American Journal of Roentgenology*, vol. 195, no. 6, pp. W421–W427, 2010.

[12] S. Kuriakose, S. Vikram, S. Salih, S. Balasubramanian, N. Mangalasseri Pareekutty, and S. Nayanar, "Unique surgical issues in the management of a giant retroperitoneal schwannoma and brief review of literature," *Case Reports in Medicine*, vol. 2014, 2014.

# 2

# A Fatal Case of Life-Threatening Interstitial Pneumonitis Induced by Everolimus for Metastatic Renal Cell Carcinoma: A Comment about the Increased Risk of Interstitial Lung Disease in Japanese

**Yasukiyo Murakami, Tetsuo Fujita, Yoji Wakatabe, and Masatsugu Iwamura**

*Department of Urology, Kitasato University School of Medicine, Japan*

Correspondence should be addressed to Yasukiyo Murakami; yaskiyomura@yahoo.co.jp

Academic Editor: Sandhya Srinivas

We describe an 81-year-old woman with metastatic renal cell carcinoma who did not recover from life-threatening interstitial pneumonitis induced by everolimus therapy. She received everolimus due to disease progression after sunitinib, but 2 months after starting everolimus treatment, she visited the emergency department after developing a sudden fever and dyspnea. Chest CT revealed diffuse ground-glass opacities, thickening of the interlobular septa, and consolidation throughout both lung fields. The diagnosis was surmised to be everolimus-induced interstitial pneumonitis. Everolimus administration was stopped and 3 courses of steroid pulse therapy were administered, along with intensive care, but the patient died due to rapid respiratory failure.

## 1. Introduction

The mTOR (mammalian target of rapamycin) inhibitors for the treatment of advanced renal cell carcinoma have expanded the available treatment options with molecular-targeted drug therapies. Among mTOR inhibitors, everolimus is positioned as a sequential therapy agent [1]. Interstitial lung disease (ILD) is listed as an adverse event that requires caution, but severe ILD resistant to appropriate treatment is rare. We observed a case of life-threatening interstitial pneumonitis induced by everolimus in a patient with metastatic renal cell carcinoma and reported our findings.

## 2. Case Presentation

The patient was an 81-year-old woman with metastatic renal cell carcinoma. Due to a clinical suspicion of renal cell carcinoma, patient initially underwent right radical nephrectomy. The histopathological diagnosis was pT2 clear cell carcinoma. After a 10-year disease-free interval, distal pancreatectomy and splenectomy were performed for pancreatic mass lesion recurrence. Two years later, recurrence at the site of the pancreatectomy was diagnosed by an abdominal CT scan, and then further surgical resection of the recurrent tumor was performed. However, a recurrent mass lesion was found at the head of the pancreas a year after surgical resection of the recurrent tumor. As surgical resection was not indication for treatment due to postoperative adhesions, sorafenib (800 mg/day) was initiated. The lesion persisted in a stable disease condition, but 16 months after starting the sorafenib therapy, the metastatic lesion at the head of pancreas became a progressive disease, so the regimen was switched to sunitinib (37.5 mg/day). However, 4 months later, a CT scan showed disease progression with the appearance of liver metastatic lesions, so everolimus (10 mg/day) was initiated. In evaluation prior to everolimus, there were no findings of respiratory dysfunction. Arterial blood gas analysis revealed a pH of 7.333, $PaCO2$ 40.0mmHg, bicarbonate 20.8 mmol/L, and $PaO2$ 10.5 mmHg on 97.5% $FiO2$. Laboratory data also showed normal CRP levels. No apparent changes, including interstitial opacities, were observed on the chest CT taken 1

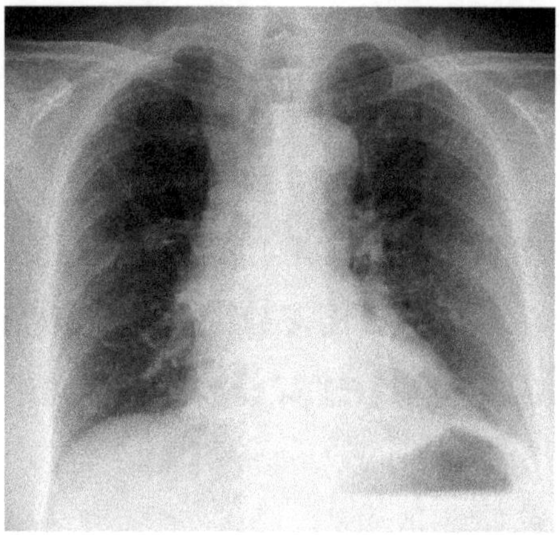

FIGURE 1: Chest X-ray one and a half months after the initiation of everolimus treatment, showing no infiltrative shadows in both lung fields.

month after starting everolimus administration. At one and a half months after everolimus induction, the patient showed no remarkable respiratory symptom and no remarkable change was seen in the patient's chest X-ray (Figure 1). Two months after starting everolimus administration, the patient presented to the emergency department after developing a sudden fever and dyspnea. Her peripheral capillary oxygen saturation level was 93% (under inhalation of O2 3 L), and blood gas analysis revealed decompensated alkalosis. The results of the general blood biochemistry tests were normal apart from an elevated C-reactive protein level of 13.93 mg/dl. Her blood serum KL6 level was elevated at 1929 IU/ml, as was her surfactant protein A (SP-A) and surfactant protein D (SP-D) levels, to 103.0 and 513.0 IU/ml, respectively. Her serum $\beta$D-glucan level was within the normal range. Linear, reticular shadows were found in both lung fields during chest radiography (Figure 2(a)), and a chest CT revealed diffuse ground-glass opacities, thickening of the interlobular septa, and consolidation throughout both lung fields. Mild pericardial effusion was found, but there is no findings of suspecting cardiogenic pulmonary edema, which indicate acute respiratory distress syndrome (Figure 2(b)). The diagnosis was surmised to be everolimus-induced interstitial pneumonitis. The patient was immediately treated with oxygen and steroid pulse therapies (methylprednisolone 1 g/day for 3 days) by a respiratory specialist, and everolimus administration was promptly stopped. The patient's respiratory status continued to rapidly worsen, however. The patient received ventilation on day 3 of hospitalization at the intensive care unit. The possibility of pneumonitis caused by infection, including fungal infection, was ruled out after subsequent culture tests returned negative. Accordingly, a respiratory specialist concluded the diagnosis as everolimus-induced interstitial lung disease. The patient had two more courses of steroid pulse therapy but showed no improvement in her respiratory status. The patient died on day 49 of hospitalization due to rapid respiratory failure.

## 3. Discussion

Everolimus is an oral mTOR inhibitor widely used for metastatic renal cell carcinoma, which is presented as a subsequent therapy option in accordance with the National Comprehensive Cancer Network guidelines [1]. Noninfectious pneumonitis, including ILD, is one of the most important adverse events that require attention during everolimus treatment. This adverse event is considered a class effect of rapamycin derivatives [2].

Reports indicate that the incidence of noninfectious pneumonitis with the use of everolimus ranges from 13.5% to 27% [3–6]. In an international randomized phase III RECORD1 trial for the treatment of metastatic renal cancer, noninfectious pneumonitis developed in 14% of all patients, while grade 3/4 complications occurred in 4% of patients [6]. Another blinded prospective study including 274 patients with metastatic renal cancer who received everolimus found that clinical noninfectious pneumonitis was suspected for 13.5% patients, but no life-threatening severe pneumonitis was observed [7]. It is reported that the incidence of this type of pneumonitis has a racial difference and Japanese patients have a higher incidence of noninfectious pneumonitis [8, 9]. In the Japanese subgroup analysis of the RECORD-1 Trial, the prevalence of noninfectious pneumonitis was higher than in the overall population (Japanese vs. overall: 27% vs. 13.5%, respectively) [10]. The reason for the higher incidence of noninfectious pneumonitis in Japanese patients is still not fully understood. However, differences in genetic sensitivity may have a role in the adverse reaction [11]. Indeed, in the treatment of nonsmall cell lung cancer, Japanese patients are known to have a higher incidence of severe drug-induced ILD caused by the tyrosine kinase inhibitor gefitinib [12]. Individual cancer type and aggressiveness may also affect the incidence of adverse reactions in addition to racial difference, because the incidence of respiratory-related adverse events has been reported to be extremely low in patients with renal angiomyolipoma treated with everolimus therapy [5]. These results suggest that, other than race, identifying the risk factors for drug-induced ILD will help prevent disease development. During gefitinib administration, preexisting pulmonary fibrosis with a performance status ≥2 has been identified as a risk factor for developing ILD in Japanese cohort [13]. However, the risk factors for everolimus-induced ILD are not detected due to the small sample size (Table 1). Therefore, close respiratory follow-up will be needed for patients with renal cell carcinoma using Everolimus. Moreover, further multiinstitutional investigation is warranted to determine the risk factor of everolimus-induced ILD.

It is recommended that treatment for everolimus-induced ILD is in line with the severity of the condition [17]. If the radiological findings are positive in an otherwise asymptomatic condition, treatment could be continued without cessation of everolimus therapy, because even severe cases respond well to steroid therapy [18]. The respiratory status of the present patient did not improve even after 3 courses of steroid pulse therapy, and the patient ultimately died from respiratory failure caused by ILD. As far as we could find, this is the relatively rare reported case of fatal everolimus-induced

TABLE 1: Comparison of previous studies regarding interstitial lung disease associated with TKI or mTOR inhibitor in Japanese patients with renal cell carcinoma and lung cancer.

| Series | Type of cancer | Type of drug | n | % of ILD All grades | Grade 3/4 | Grade 5 |
|---|---|---|---|---|---|---|
| Mizuno et al. [3] | RCC | mTOR inhibitor (Everolimus) | 11 | 63.6 | 36.3 | 0 |
| Mikami et al. [14] | RCC | mTOR inhibitor (Everolimus) | 16 | 31 | 0 | 0 |
| Akamatsu et al. [15] | NSCLC | TKI (Gefetinib) | 201 | 5 | 2.5 | 1 |
| Nakagawa et al. [16] | NSCLC | TKI (Erlotinib) | 3488 | 4.5 | 2.6 | 1.6 |
| Ando et al. [13] | NSCLC | TKI (Gefetinib) | 1976 | 3.5 | 1.9 | 1.6 |

RCC, renal cell carcinoma; NSCLC, nonsmall cell lung carcinoma; ILD, interstitial lung disease; mTOR, mammalian target of rapamycin; TKI, tyrosine kinase inhibitor.

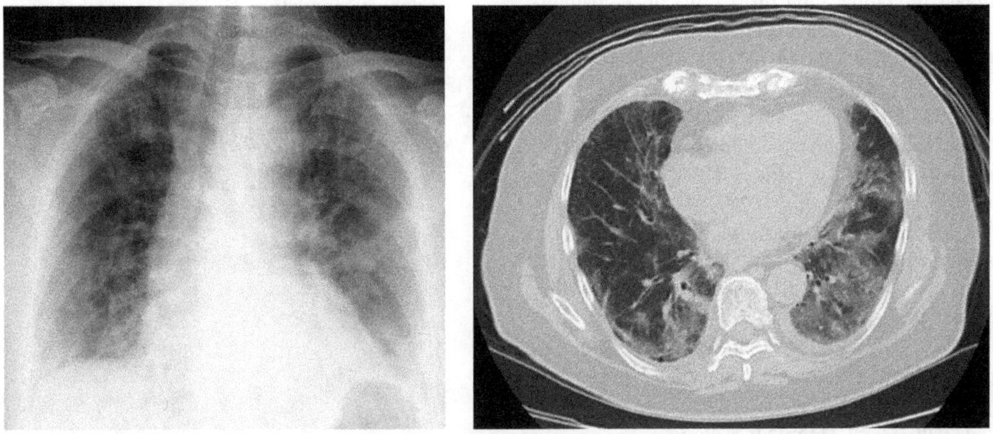

(a) (b)

FIGURE 2: (a) Chest X-ray two months after starting everolimus administration, showing diffuse infiltrative shadows in both lung fields. (b) Chest CT scan two months after starting everolimus administration, showing ground-glass attenuation with diffuse alveolar consolidation in both lung fields.

ILD. KL-6, surfactant protein (SP)-A, SP-D, are reported to be sensitive markers for interstitial lung diseases (ILD) [16]. Of these markers, KL-6 is useful for making a differential diagnosis between interstitial pneumonia and other kinds of pneumonia. KL-6 is a mucinous high-molecular weight glycoprotein that is expressed on type II pneumocytes, which is highly sensitive and specific and correlates with the ground-glass opacities on the chest CT. This marker is also considered useful for detecting everolimus-induced ILD because KL-6 demonstrated a stronger correlation with fibrotic lesions than the other markers [19]. In a report that investigated 7 patients with metastatic renal cell carcinoma who developed ILD after administration of everolimus, all of the patients had an elevated KL-6 level [3]. In the current case, the KL-6 level increased to 1929 IU/ml immediately after the onset of ILD and the KL-6 levels continued to increase despite steroid therapy, reaching 2490 IU/ml immediately before the patient died. KL-6 is also recognized as being useful for assessing the disease activity of interstitial pneumonia. Reports on idiopathic ILD indicated that patients with ILD who had KL-6 levels of ≥1000 IU/ml had a poorer prognosis than those with KL-6 levels of <1000 IU/ml [20]. This study suggests the potential usefulness of KL-6 as a prognostic factor.

Everolimus-induced ILD is manageable in almost cases, but our case suggests that ILD during everolimus treatment still requires attention. Further investigation on follow-up examinations of KL-6 levels and everolimus-induced ILD prognostic factors is necessary.

## 4. Conclusion

We observed a case of severe interstitial pneumonitis in a patient who was receiving everolimus therapy for advanced renal cell carcinoma that resulted in a serious outcome, and we reported our findings along with the potential to use KL-6 levels during follow-up examinations as prognostic factor for everolimus-induced ILD.

## References

[1] R. J. Motzer, E. Jonasch, N. Agarwal et al., "Kidney Cancer, Version 2.2017, NCCN Clinical Practice Guidelines in Oncology," *Journal of the National Comprehensive Cancer Network*, vol. 15, no. 6, pp. 804–834, 2017.

[2] J. P. Maroto, G. Hudes, J. P. Dutcher et al., "Drug-related pneumonitis in patients with advanced renal cell carcinoma treated with temsirolimus," *Journal of Clinical Oncology*, vol. 29, no. 13, pp. 1750–1756, 2011.

[3] R. Mizuno, K. Asano, S. Mikami, H. Nagata, G. Kaneko, and M. Oya, "Patterns of interstitial lung disease during everolimus treatment in patients with metastatic renal cell carcinoma," *Japanese Journal of Clinical Oncology*, vol. 42, no. 5, Article ID hys033, pp. 442–446, 2012.

[4] P. Ivanyi, T. Fuehner, M. Adam et al., "Interstitial lung disease during targeted therapy in metastatic renal cell carcinoma: a case series from three centres," *Medical Oncology*, vol. 31, no. 9, p. 147, 2014.

[5] A. E. C. A. B. Willemsen, J. C. Grutters, W. R. Gerritsen, N. P. Van Erp, C. M. L. Van Herpen, and J. Tol, "mTOR inhibitor-induced interstitial lung disease in cancer patients: Comprehensive review and a practical management algorithm," *International Journal of Cancer*, vol. 138, no. 10, pp. 2312–2321, 2016.

[6] R. J. Motzer, B. Escudier, S. Oudard et al., "Efficacy of everolimus in advanced renal cell carcinoma: a double-blind, randomised, placebo-controlled phase III trial," *The Lancet*, vol. 372, no. 9637, pp. 449–456, 2017.

[7] D. A. White, P. Camus, M. Endo et al., "Noninfectious pneumonitis after everolimus therapy for advanced renal cell carcinoma," *American Journal of Respiratory and Critical Care Medicine*, vol. 182, no. 3, pp. 396–403, 2010.

[8] S. Kudoh, H. Kato, Y. Nishiwaki et al., "Interstitial lung disease in Japanese patients with lung cancer: A cohort and nested case-control study," *American Journal of Respiratory and Critical Care Medicine*, vol. 177, no. 12, pp. 1348–1357, 2008.

[9] M. Schwaiblmair, W. Behr, T. Haeckel, B. Märkl, W. Foerg, and T. Berghaus, "Drug induced interstitial lung disease," *The Open Respiratory Medicine Journal*, vol. 6, no. 1, pp. 63–74, 2012.

[10] T. Tsukamoto, N. Shinohara, N. Tsuchiya et al., "Phase III trial of everolimus in metastatic renal cell carcinoma: Subgroup analysis of Japanese patients from RECORD-1," *Japanese Journal of Clinical Oncology*, vol. 41, no. 1, Article ID hyq166, pp. 17–24, 2011.

[11] I. Sekine, N. Yamamoto, K. Nishio, and N. Saijo, "Emerging ethnic differences in lung cancer therapy," *British Journal of Cancer*, vol. 99, no. 11, pp. 1757–1762, 2008.

[12] P. Camus, S. Kudoh, and M. Ebina, "Interstitial lung disease associated with drug therapy," *British Journal of Cancer*, vol. 91, 2, pp. S18–S23, 2004.

[13] M. Ando, I. Okamoto, N. Yamamoto et al., "Predictive factors for interstitial lung disease, antitumor response, and survival in non-small-cell lung cancer patients treated with gefitinib," *Journal of Clinical Oncology*, vol. 24, no. 16, pp. 2549–2556, 2006.

[14] K. Mikami, F. Hongo, and T. Miki, "Management of side effects of everolimus treatment for metastatic renal cell carcinoma," *Hinyokika Kiyo*, vol. 58, no. 11, pp. 647–650, 2012.

[15] H. Akamatsu, A. Inoue, T. Mitsudomi et al., "Interstitial lung disease associated with gefitinib in Japanese patients with EGFR-mutated non-small-cell lung cancer: Combined analysis of two phase III trials (NEJ 002 and WJTOG 3405)," *Japanese Journal of Clinical Oncology*, vol. 43, no. 6, pp. 664–668, 2013.

[16] K. Nakagawa, S. Kudoh, Y. Ohe et al., "Postmarketing Surveillance Study of Erlotinib in Japanese Patients with Non-Small-Cell Lung Cancer (NSCLC): An Interim Analysis of 3488 Patients (POLARSTAR)," *Journal of Thoracic Oncology*, vol. 7, no. 8, pp. 1296–1303, 2012.

[17] F. Joly, J.-C. Eymard, L. Albiges et al., "A prospective observational study on the evaluation of everolimus-related adverse events in metastatic renal cell carcinoma after first-line anti-vascular endothelial growth factor therapy: the AFINITE study in France," *Supportive Care in Cancer*, vol. 25, no. 7, pp. 2055–2062, 2017.

[18] C. Porta, S. Osanto, A. Ravaud et al., "Management of adverse events associated with the use of everolimus in patients with advanced renal cell carcinoma," *European Journal of Cancer*, vol. 47, no. 3, pp. 1298-1298, 2011.

[19] K. Sakamoto, H. Taniguchi, Y. Kondoh et al., "Serum KL-6 in fibrotic NSIP: Correlations with physiologic and radiologic parameters," *Respiratory Medicine*, vol. 104, no. 1, pp. 127–133, 2010.

[20] A. Yokoyama, K. Kondo, M. Nakajima et al., "Prognostic value of circulating KL-6 in idiopathic pulmonary fibrosis," *Respirology*, vol. 11, no. 2, pp. 164–168, 2006.

3

# Retrocaval Ureter: Report of Two Cases

**Henry Atawurah,[1] Patrick Opoku Manu Maison,[1] Mohammed Owusu-Ansah,[2] and Alvin Asante-Asamani[3]**

[1]*Department of Surgery, School of Medical Sciences, College of Health and Allied Sciences, University of Cape Coast, Cape Coast, Ghana*
[2]*Department of Radiology, Cape Coast Teaching Hospital, Cape Coast, Ghana*
[3]*Department of Surgery, Cape Coast Teaching Hospital, Cape Coast, Ghana*

Correspondence should be addressed to Patrick Opoku Manu Maison; kwamemaison@yahoo.co.uk

Academic Editor: Imran Morhason-Bello

Retrocaval ureter (RCU) is a rare congenital anomaly in which the ureter passes posterior to the inferior vena cava (IVC). A little over 200 cases have been reported worldwide since Hochstetter's first report in 1893. We present two cases of retrocaval ureter which were successfully managed at the Cape Coast Teaching Hospital in Ghana. *Case 1.* A 55-year-old woman presented with a history of dull right flank pain of 2 years duration. Physical examination and basic laboratory investigations performed on her were normal. Abdominal ultrasound showed right hydronephrosis and a retrograde right ureteropyelogram (RPG) showed right hydroureteronephrosis with an "S" shaped proximal ureter. A diagnosis of retrocaval ureter was made and confirmed at surgery. *Case 2.* A 25-year-old man presented with dull intermittent right flank pain of 1 year duration. Clinical examination and laboratory investigation were normal. Abdominal ultrasound showed right hydronephrosis and a CT urogram made a diagnosis of retrocaval ureter which was confirmed at surgery. *Conclusion.* Retrocaval ureter is a rare congenital anomaly that is now increasingly being reported. Surgical treatment of symptomatic cases successfully relieves symptoms.

## 1. Introduction

Retrocaval ureter (RCU) is a rare congenital anomaly in which the ureter passes posterior to the inferior vena cava (IVC) [1]. This anomaly occurs between the $4^{th}$ and $8^{th}$ weeks of intrauterine development and is due to abnormal formation of infrarenal IVC from anteriorly located subcardinal vein instead of supracardinal vein which are located posteriorly [2]. In normal circumstances, the infrarenal IVC originates from dorsally located supracardinal vein, but when it develops from ventrally located subcardinal vein, the ureter is trapped posteriorly leading to pre-ureteral vena cava [2].

This rare anomaly, first described in 1893 by Hochstetter in a cadaver [3] and the first clinical diagnosis in 1940 by Harrill [4], has an incidence of 0.06–0.17% worldwide [5]. Very few cases have been reported from Sub-Saharan Africa including four from Nigeria and two from Ghana [6, 7]. Though it no longer attracts the curiosity witnessed in the 1940s, it is still worth reporting on it especially in the case of successful surgical correction.

We present two cases of retrocaval ureter which were successfully managed at the Cape Coast Teaching Hospital in Ghana. This is the second case report from Ghana.

*1.1. Case 1.* A 55-year-old woman presented with a history of dull right flank pain of 2 years duration. She was otherwise well and clinical examination of the abdomen was normal. Laboratory evaluation including urinalysis, full blood count, urea, creatinine and electrolytes were within normal limits. Abdominal ultrasound showed right hydronephrosis and a retrograde right ureteropyelogram (RPG) (Figure 1) showed right hydroureteronephrosis with an "S" shaped or "fish hook" deformity of the proximal ureter, which terminated abruptly. A diagnosis of retrocaval ureter was made and the findings at operation were that of right retrocaval ureter, proximal dilated ureteral segment and a normal distal segment lying between the aorta and IVC. The redundant retrocaval segment was mobilized and excised, and end-to-end anastomosis was achieved over a JJ stent. The patient's symptoms resolved at follow-up.

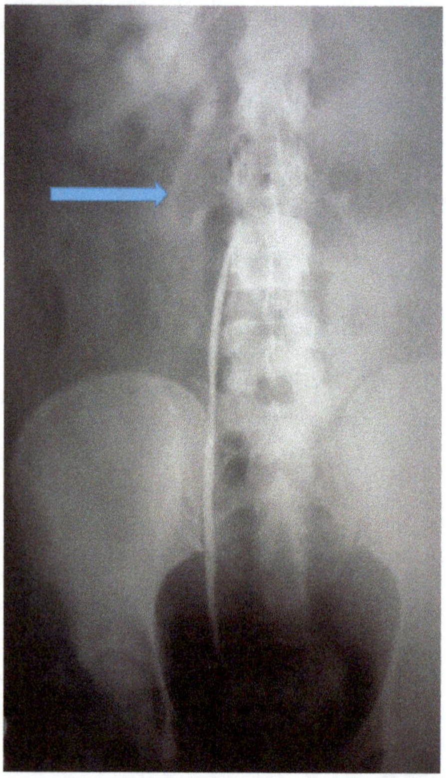

FIGURE 1: Retrograde ureteropyelogram showing an "S" shaped or "fish hook" deformity of the proximal ureter (Bold arrow).

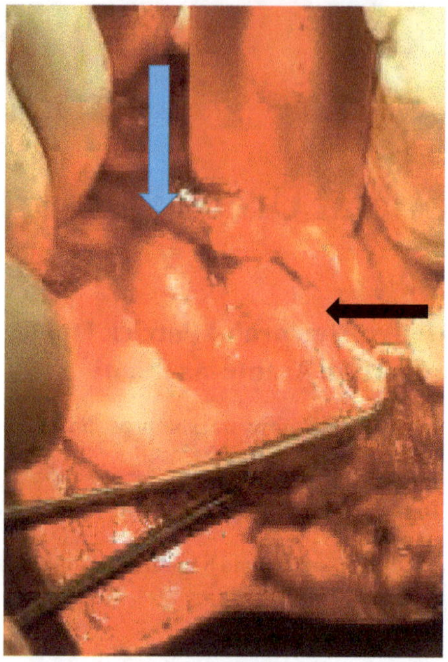

FIGURE 2: Operative photograph showing the right proximal ureter (blue arrow) coursing behind the inferior vena cava (black arrow).

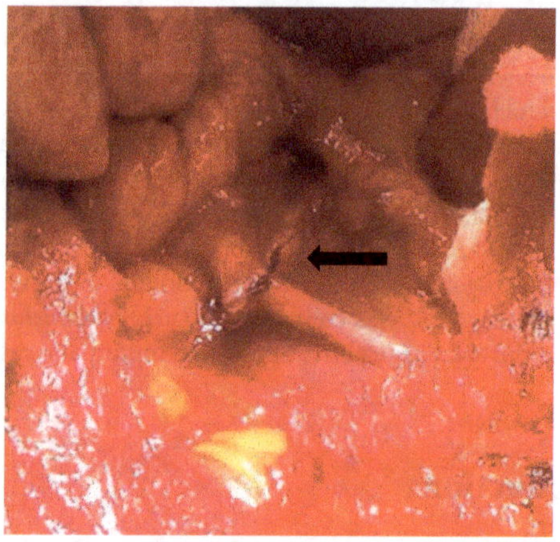

FIGURE 3: Excision with end to end ureteral anastomosis done over a JJ stent (arrow).

*1.2. Case 2.* A 25-year-old man presented with a history of dull intermittent right flank pain of 1 year duration. He had no history of fever, dysuria, haematuria or weight loss. Clinical examination of the abdomen was within normal limits. Laboratory evaluation was normal. Abdominal ultrasound showed right hydronephrosis with proximally dilated ureter. A CT urogram to delineate the ureter made a diagnosis of retrocaval ureter with proximally dilated ureter which was confirmed at surgery (Figure 2). Excision of the retrocaval segment with end to end ureteral anastomosis over a stent was done (Figure 3). The patient's symptoms resolved at follow-up.

## 2. Discussion

Retrocaval ureter is a rare congenital anomaly that is caused by an abnormal formation of infrarenal IVC from anteriorly located subcardinal vein instead of supracardinal vein which are located posteriorly [2]. It entraps a segment of the proximal ureter, resulting in the ureter wrapping around the IVC. Therefore, it is also known as circumcaval ureter or preureteral vena cava [8]. This anomaly is rare with an incidence of 0.06–0.17% worldwide [5]. A little over 200 cases have been reported worldwide since Hochstetter's first report in 1893 [3]. There are very few reported cases from Sub-Saharan Africa but Ahmed et al. who managed four patients between 2010 and 2017 in Nigeria believe that the condition is probably under-reported [6]. In Ghana, Kyei et al. reported on two patients with retrocaval ureter in 2011 [7].

It is three times more common in males than in females [9, 10]. It usually occurs on the right side but can be on the left side in patients with situs inversus, duplication of IVC or persistent left subcardinal vein [11, 12]. Although congenital, it usually becomes symptomatic in the third or fourth decade of life due to hydronephrosis from compression of the ureteral segment by the IVC against the psoas muscle, ureteral kinking or from an adynamic retrocaval ureteral segment [2, 13]. The symptoms include flank or abdominal pain and haematuria. Urinary infection, stone formation, and renal dysfunction may complicate the ureteral obstruction. Some patients may present with symptoms earlier than the third or fourth decade of life and it may also be asymptomatic; discovered only during imaging or surgery for unrelated conditions or at autopsy [14]. In this series, one patient was a male in the third decade and presented with right flank pains. However, the other patient was a female in her sixth decade. Retrocaval ureter may be associated with other anomalies mainly in the urogenital and cardiovascular systems. Some of the associated anomalies include duplication of IVC, situs inversus, imperforate anus, oesophageal atresia, myelomeningocele, renal agenesis, horse shoe kidney, ureteral duplication, congenital absence of vas deference, hypospadias, intestinal malrotation, VACTERL and Turner's branchial arch [15].

There are two types of RCU. The more common form, Type I, is a low-loop of the proximal ureter. The obstruction is typically at the edge of the iliopsoas muscle, at which point the ureter deviates cephalad before passing behind the vena cava. This results in a proximal ureteral dilation and hydronephrosis, demonstrating a fishhook, reverse-J, or S-shaped ureteral curve as observed on the retrograde ureteropyelogram of the first patient in this series. The less common Type II is a high-loop of the ureteropelvic junction. The proximal ureter passes behind the vena cava at a higher level, with the renal pelvis and upper ureter lying almost horizontal before encircling the vena cava [1]. It has a lesser degree of hydronephrosis or none and demonstrates a sickle shaped smooth curve on IVU [1]. The two patients in this series had type I RCU.

RCU is usually diagnosed with an intravenous urogram (IVU), retrograde pyeloureterogram (RGP) or computerized tomography (CT) scan [16]. Spiral CT scan is considered the investigation of choice compared to IVU because it can outline both the ureter and IVC [17]. Magnetic Resonance Imaging (MRI) may be preferable to CT scan as it can delineate the course of the ureter and IVC with no exposure to radiation as compared to IVU or CT scan [5]. Nuclear renal scan is useful to evaluate degree of the obstruction and renal function [18].

Repair usually involves open or laparoscopic resection of the redundant retrocaval ureteral segment, anteposition, and ureteroureteral or ureteropelvic anastomosis [19].

## 3. Conclusion

Retrocaval ureter is a rare congenital anomaly that is now increasingly being reported. The low clinical incidence may be due to a number of asymptomatic cases that are not diagnosed in the patient's lifetime. Surgical treatment of symptomatic cases successfully relieves symptoms.

## References

[1] E. M. Bateson and D. Atkinson, "Circumcaval ureter: a new classification," *Clinical Radiology*, vol. 20, no. 2, pp. 173–177, 1969.

[2] K. H. Huang, S. C. Chang, C. Y. Huang, Y. S. Pu, and J. C. Huang, "Retrocaval ureter: report of 12 cases and literature review," *JTUA*, vol. 16, no. 4, pp. 163–167, 2005.

[3] F. Hochstetter, "Contribution to the developmental history of the venous system of the amniotes III," *Sucker Morphology Jahrbücher*, vol. 20, pp. 543–548, 1893.

[4] H. C. Harrill, "Retrocaval ureter: report or a case with operative correction of the defect," *The Journal of Urology*, vol. 44, no. 4, pp. 450–457, 1940.

[5] M. C. Uthappa, D. Anthony, and C. Allen, "Case report: retrocaval ureter: MR appearances," *The British Journal of Radiology*, vol. 75, no. 890, pp. 177–179, 2002.

[6] M. Ahmed, A. Alhassan, M. A. Sadiq, A. T. Lawal, A. Bello, and H. Y. Maitama, "Variable presentation of retrocaval ureter: report of four cases and review of literature," *Nigerian Postgraduate Medical Journal*, vol. 24, no. 2, pp. 126–197, 2017.

[7] M. Y. Kyei, E. D. Yeboah, G. O. Klufio et al., "Retrocaval ureter: two case reports," *Ghana Medical Journal*, vol. 45, no. 4, pp. 177–808, 2011.

[8] V. S. Gosavi, N. N. Hombalkar, P. D. Dhandore, N. B. Mody, and S. S. Bankar, "Retrocaval ureter: an innocent bystander," *Journal of Clinical and Diagnostic Research*, vol. 8, no. 5, pp. ND05–ND06, 2014.

[9] J. E. Heslin and C. Mamonas, "Retrocaval ureter: report of four cases and review of literature," *Journal of Urology*, vol. 65, no. 2, pp. 212–222, 1951.

[10] J. S. Pandya, P. P. Shilotri, and R. R. Satoskar, "Circumcaval ureter," *Journal of Postgraduate Medicine*, vol. 44, no. 1, pp. 19–20, 1998.

[11] E. Liu, X. Sun, H. Guo et al., "Retroperitoneoscopicureteroplasty for retrocaval ureter: report of nine cases and literature review," *Scandinavian Journal of Urology*, vol. 50, no. 4, pp. 319–322, 2016.

[12] G. Q. Ding, L. W. Xu, X. D. Li et al., "Pure transperitoneal laparoscopic correction of retrocaval ureter," *Chinese Medical Journal*, vol. 125, no. 13, pp. 2382–2385, 2012.

[13] N. Hyseni, S. Llullaku, M. Berisha, A. Shefkiu, S. Grajqevci, and H. Jashari, "Case presentation of preureteral vena cava and review of the literature," *Open Journal of Urology*, vol. 3, no. 5, pp. 206–209, 2013.

[14] A. Yarmohammadi, M. MohamadzadehRezaei, B. Feizzadeh, and H. Ahmadnia, "Retrocaval ureter: a study of 13 cases," *Urology Journal*, vol. 3, no. 3, pp. 175–178, 2006.

[15] P. Perimenis, K. Gyftopoulos, A. Athanasopoulos, V. Pastromas, and G. Barbalias, "Retrocaval ureter and associated abnormalities," *International Urology and Nephrology*, vol. 33, no. 1, pp. 19–22, 2002.

[16] J. E. Bass, M. D. Redwine, L. A. Kramer, P. T. Huynh, and J. H. Harris Jr., "Spectrum of congenital anomalies of the inferior vena cava: crosssectional imaging findings," *Radiographics*, vol. 20, no. 3, pp. 639–652, 2000.

[17] D. K. Gupta, V. Singh, and R. J. Sinha, "Retrocaval ureter with contralateral renal agenesis with renal failure: a rare, reversible surgical cause of renal failure," *UroToday International Journal*, vol. 5, no. 3, 2012.

[18] R. Méndez Gallart, D. Vela Nieto, M. Gómez Tellado, M. Montero Sánchez, E. País Piñeiro, and A. J. Candal, "Retrocaval ureter in children: surgical approach based on the obstructive pattern in the diuretic renogram with 99mTc DTPA," *Actas Urologicas Espanolas*, vol. 22, no. 9, pp. 789–792, 1998.

[19] I. Y. Seo, T. H. Oh, and S. H. Jeon, "Transperitoneal laparoscopic ureteroureterostomy with excision of the compressed ureter for retrocaval ureter and review of literature," *Investigative and Clinical Urology*, vol. 60, no. 2, pp. 108–113, 2019.

4

# Robot-Assisted Infratrigonal Vesicovaginal Fistula Repair

**João Pádua Manzano,[1,2] Fábio da Silva Crochik,[3] Felipe Guimarães Pugliesi,[3] Renato Vasconcelos Souza de Almeida,[3] Petronio Augusto de Souza Melo,[2] and Ricardo Luís Vita Nunes[4]**

[1] *Surgery Department at Federal University of São Paulo, São Paulo, Brazil*
[2] *São Paulo's Military Hospital, Brazilian Army, São Paulo, Brazil*
[3] *Division of Urology, Men's Health Centre, Hospital Brigadeiro, Sao Paulo, SP, Brazil*
[4] *Benign Prostate Hyperplasia Department in Brazilian Urology Society, Urology Department in Sao Paulo's Military Hospital, Brazilian Army, São Paulo, Brazil*

Correspondence should be addressed to Renato Vasconcelos Souza de Almeida; renato.vsa@gmail.com

Academic Editor: David Duchene

*Background.* Although relatively rare, vesicovaginal fistula is the most common genitourinary fistula, causing a significant decrease in patients' quality of life. Location of fistula is major supratrigonal, with some cases located in the trigone and rarely below it. Disease treatment is surgical, and repair can be performed by several techniques, including robot-assisted. *Case Presentation.* We present a case of a patient who developed an infratrigonal vesicovaginal fistula after treatment of a cervical cancer. The patient was submitted to robotic repair of the vesicovaginal fistula. *Conclusion.* The use of robot-assisted laparoscopy is expanding over all areas of urology and its applicability to repair vesicovaginal fistulas brings good results.

## 1. Introduction

Vesicovaginal fistula (VVF) is the most common fistula between the female genital tract and the urinary tract, and it is characterized by drainage of urine through the vagina, with a significant reduction in patients' quality of life [1]. It is presented by urinary flow through the vagina, unrelated to urination, and the volume of loss is directly related to the diameter of the fistula [2, 3]. In low-resourced countries, it often occurs as a result of prolonged obstructed labour due to the ischemia, as the bladder becomes compressed between the foetus and the pubic symphysis. Meanwhile, the VVFs that are seen in well-resourced countries commonly develop following iatrogenic injury, with over 60% following a hysterectomy. In a study of the English National Health Service, one in every 788 hysterectomies is associated with urogenital fistulae [4], occurring about 1 to 6 weeks after hysterectomy, and when recurrent, about 3 months after the first repair [5–8]. In addition, other risk factors also favor the appearance of genitourinary fistulas, such as pelvic surgeries, radiation, infection, and neoplasias affecting the pelvic floor [9, 10]. The most common location of the fistulas is supratrigonal, with fewer cases of trigonal and infratrigonal fistulas [11–13].

Investigation of the disease should always contain a detailed pelvic evaluation, with specular examination of the vagina and cystoscopy [10]. The vaginal tamponade test with infusion of intravesical methylene blue can also be performed but only serves to identify the presence of the fistula, without assessing size, position, number, and complexity [9]. Other exams such as cystography and micturition urethrocystography may help in the evaluation of the fistula. Another important point is always to evaluate the upper urinary tract, since concomitant ureteral lesions are present in about 12% of the cases, and computed tomography with intravenous contrast or even a pyelography may be performed during cystoscopy [14].

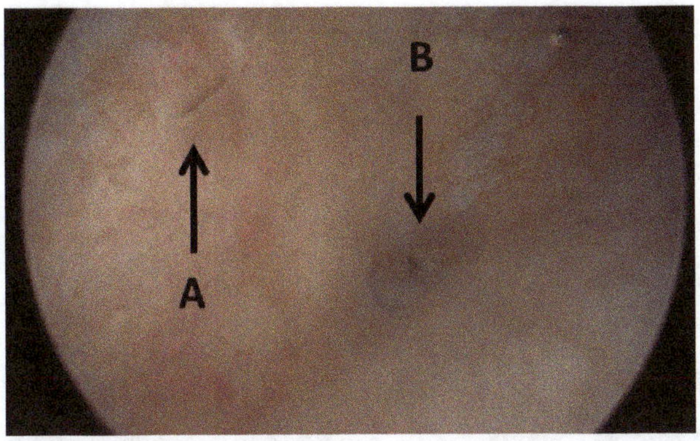


FIGURE 1: Cystoscopy performed before surgery. A: left ureteral meatus; B: fistulous orifice.

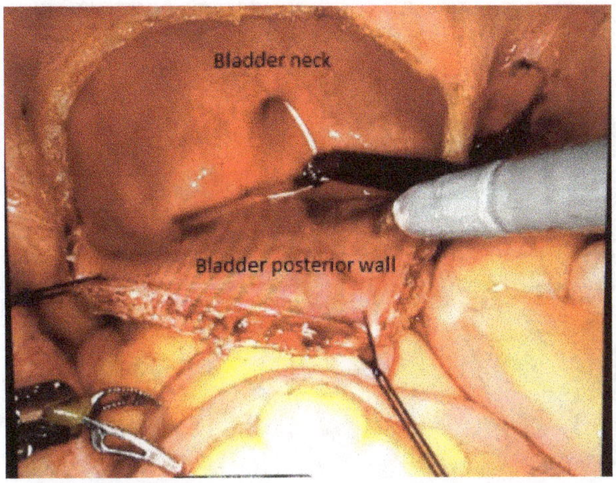


FIGURE 2: Transperitoneal view of open bladder: a white ureteral catheter positioned through urethra into left ureteral meatus.

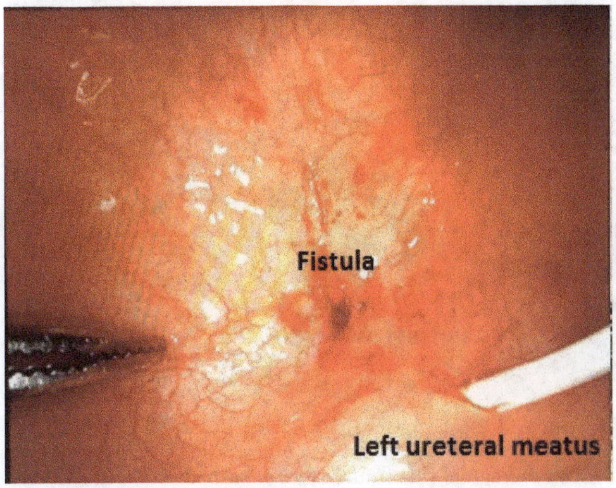


FIGURE 3: Fistula identification: in the transperitoneal view infratrigonal fistula is identified above the ureteral meatus.

## 2. Case Report

L.O., a 58-year-old female married white patient, with previous history of subtotal hysterectomy in 2012 due to endometriosis, was diagnosed in 2016 with invasive endocervical adenocarcinoma, being treated with colpectomy and brachytherapy. During follow-up, progression of the disease was detected, with metastases in the liver, the peritoneum, and the vaginal dome. In 2017, she was submitted to the excision of the peritoneal implants, the hepatic lesion, the omentum, the vaginal dome, the tuba, and the left ovary. Pathological analysis confirmed metastatic lesions in the vaginal dome and peritoneum, without neoplasia in the other resected tissues. She was submitted to adjuvant chemotherapy with carboplatin and paclitaxel weekly and bevacizumab every 21 days. About 2 weeks after the last surgery she complained of moderate amount of continuous urinary loss through the vagina and the use of 3 to 4 PADs per day. Despite the continuous loss, she continued to urinate through the urethra. Urinary urgency episodes were also reported, with no response to oxybutynin and mirabegron. Recurrent urinary tract infection was not present. A complete evaluation was performed with specular examination, urethrocystography, and contrasted computed tomography, with no lesions identified. Cystoscopy was then performed and revealed a 3mm diameter infratrigonal fistulous lesion, right under the left meatus (Figure 1).

Patient underwent robot-assisted repair of the vesicovaginal fistula, with transperitoneal access. First, the patient was positioned in lithotomy and a cystoscopy was performed, identifying the fistulous orifice right under the left ureteral meatus. An ureteral catheter was placed thought the urethra in the left ureter. The position was then changed to a steep Trendelemburg and 5 ports were inserted: one 12mm optic port (3cm above the umbilicus and 1cm left of the middle line), three 8mm robotic ports (at the umbilicus level, symmetrically placed 2 ports on left and right pararectal line, and one more port placed up from the iliac crest on the left side), and one 5mm assistant port (placed up from the iliac crest of the right side). After the ports were placed, the robot was docked and the laparoscopy initiated. Right at the beginning of the laparoscopy, a lot of adherences were visualized, needing a careful adhesiolysis of the bowel from the surrounding structures. With the bladder well dissected, a transversal cystotomy was performed, to expose the vesical side of the fistula (Figures 2 and 3). The fistula was dissected with a good margin of healthy tissue until vaginal side (Figure 4). The synthesis was initiated with a barbed 3-0 continuous suture (V-Loc™), closing the vagina. The vesical side was closed in 2 layers, using the same suture (Figure 5). In the end of procedure, a 4.7mm ureteral stent and an 18Fr bladder catheter were placed (Figure 6). The bladder was also closed with the 3-0 barbed suture (V-Loc™). Total operative time was 87 minutes, estimated blood loss was less than 50mL, and the length of hospitalization was 30 hours. Bladder catheter remained for 2 weeks and the ureteral stent for 4 weeks. After the withdrawal of bladder catheter, patient remained well, without further complaints and no longer losing urine.

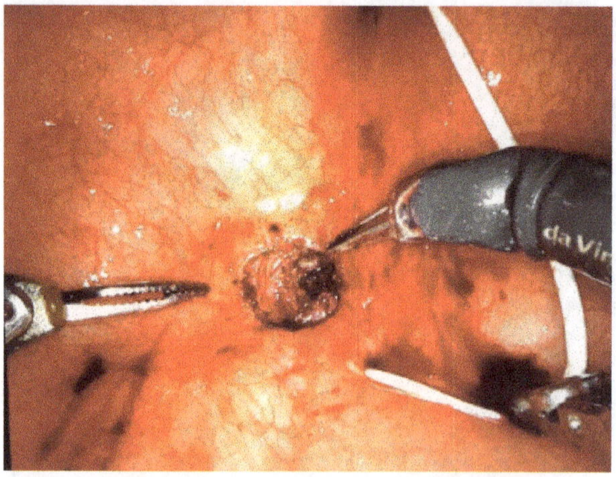


FIGURE 4: Fistula dissection is performed by separating vaginal and bladder sides.

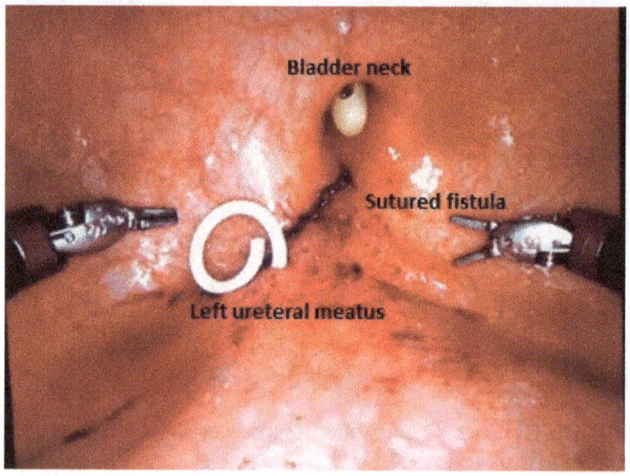


FIGURE 6: Final appearance of the treated fistula after suture of bladder.

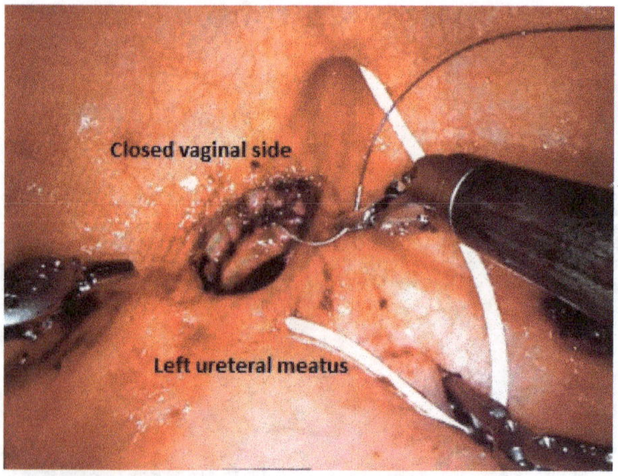


FIGURE 5: Vaginal side sutured by 3-0 barbed suture in 2 layers.

## 3. Discussion

There are several ways to treat vesicovaginal fistulas, including conservative treatment with 8% of success [15]. Given this poor result of nonoperative treatment, surgery is the main way of treatment. The most important principle in repair is to provide a tension-free, watertight closure, and the surgical route should be the one that provides the best possible chance of closure on the first attempt [16]. There are different ways of repairing a vesicovaginal fistula including vaginal, abdominal, and laparoscopic/ robotic approaches [17]. The route depends partly on the characteristics of the fistula but also on the experience of the surgeon. Two conventional approaches for VVF repair are transabdominal repair for supratrigonal VVF and transvaginal approach for low lying fistulae [18]. An ideal time for repair is still debatable. Irrespective of the approach used the principle of VVF repair remains the same, i.e., the separation of bladder and vagina, closure of the fistula in 2 separate layers preferably perpendicular to each other, tissue interposition, and urinary drainage [19].

The first fistula treated by open abdominal access was described in 1803 [20]. In the 1990s, with evolution of technology and the aim of reducing surgical morbidity, laparoscopic approach was described for the first time [21]. Despite the minor trauma, the laparoscopic technique did not initially have as many supporters probably due to the technical difficulty of dissection of vesicovaginal fistula and intracorporeal suture. Given this difficulty, Melamud et al. described for the first time in 2005 the robotic correction of a vesicovaginal fistula, showing good results and less difficulty in dissection and suturing with the articulated arms [22]. Since that moment the robotic technique is increasing, with good results even in complex cases [23].

In a comparative study between open and robot-assisted repair of recurrent supratrigonal VVF, Gupta et al. demonstrated similar efficacy but significantly lower morbidity in terms of blood loss and postoperative hospital stay with the robot-assisted approach [24]. The advantages of using the robotic system for this surgery are evident from the outset as it needs reconstruction deep inside the pelvis [25]. However, data on the use of robotic-assisted approach in managing VVF is still limited.

As reported in the literature, the operative times vary between 95 minutes and 305 minutes. This heterogeneity arises from varying surgeon experience and variability in timings itself as few authors reporting only the console time. The blood loss is usually insignificant varying between minimal and 120 ml. The length of hospitalization is usually short, in consistence with the prevalent advantages of minimally invasive approach. The mean follow-up period is also variable between 3 months and 28.3 months after surgery [26]. The data we report are compatible with literature.

Several reports describe the repair of supratrigonal fistulas but there are few descriptions of infratrigonal repairs with robot-assisted technique, as the location of fistula favors transvaginal repair. Furthermore, as the patient had a previous omentectomy, no tissue was interposed between the two layers of the suture. Various interposition flaps have been described in the literature, including omental flaps, peritoneal flaps, and amniotic allograft interposition tissue flaps. An interposition flap for VVF works on two theoretical principles: it functions as a barrier and it introduces vascular and theoretically lymphatic vessels that improve tissue growth and maturation. Omentum is the most common flap described in literature. In the absence of endogenous tissue, the use of biological sealants has also been reported (e.g., Fibrin glue) with the aim of avoiding fistula relapse and showing good results [22, 26]. Our case shows the possibility of performing robot-assisted transabdominal repair of infratrigonal fistulas without interposed tissue, with no more urine loss complaints after one year of follow-up.

## References


[1] M. Bangser, "Obstetric fistula and stigma," *The Lancet*, vol. 367, no. 9509, pp. 535-536, 2006.

[2] P. M. Tebeu, J. N. Fomulu, S. Khaddaj, L. De Bernis, T. Delvaux, and C. H. Rochat, "Risk factors for obstetric fistula: A clinical review," *International Urogynecology Journal*, vol. 23, no. 4, pp. 387–394, 2012.

[3] M. L. Tancer, "Observations on prevention and management of vesicovaginal fistula after total hysterectomy," *Surgery, Gynecology and Obstetrics*, vol. 175, no. 6, pp. 501–506, 1992.

[4] P. Hilton and D. A. Cromwell, "The risk of vesicovaginal and urethrovaginal fistula after hysterectomy performed in the English National Health Service-a retrospective cohort study examining patterns of care between 2000 and 2008," *BJOG: An International Journal of Obstetrics & Gynaecology*, vol. 119, no. 12, pp. 1447–1454, 2012.

[5] P. Hilton and A. Ward, "Epidemiological and surgical aspects of urogenital fistulae: A review of 25 years' experience in southeast Nigeria," *International Urogynecology Journal and Pelvic Floor Dysfunction*, vol. 9, no. 4, pp. 189–194, 1998.

[6] K. Thomas and G. Williams, "Medicolegal aspects of vesicovaginal fistulae," *BJU International*, vol. 86, no. 3, pp. 354–359, 2000.

[7] P. Hilton, "Vesico-vaginal fistula: New perspectives," *Current Opinion in Obstetrics and Gynecology*, vol. 13, no. 5, pp. 513–520, 2001.

[8] J. R. Miklos, C. Sobolewski, and V. Lucente, "Laparoscopic management of recurrent vesicovaginal fistula," *International Urogynecology Journal*, vol. 10, no. 2, pp. 116-117, 1999.

[9] N. V. Raghavaiah, "Double dye test to diagnose various types of vaginal fistulas," *The Journal of Urology*, vol. 112, no. 6, pp. 811-812, 1974.

[10] J. F. Redman, "Female urologic diagnostic techniques," *Urologic Clinics of North America*, vol. 17, no. 1, pp. 5–8, 1990.

[11] A. B. Diallo, T. M. Oury Diallo, I. Bah et al., "Vesicovaginal fistulas: anatomical clinical and surgical aspects in the conakry university hospital center," *Open Journal of Urology*, vol. 5, no. 12, pp. 224–230, 2015.

[12] P. H. Daru, J. A. Karshima, S. Mikah, and D. Nyango, "The burden of vesico-vaginal fistula in north central nigeria," *Journal of the West African College of Surgeons*, vol. 1, no. 2, pp. 50–62, 2010.

[13] A. Cardoso, R. Soares, T. Correia et al., "Abordagem terapêutica de fístulas vésico-vaginais análise retrospectiva e revisão temática," *Acta Urológica*, vol. 26, no. 1, pp. 19–25, 2009.

[14] W. E. Goodwin and P. T. Scardino, "Vesicovaginal and ureterovaginal fistulas: A summary of 25 years of experience," *The Journal of Urology*, vol. 123, no. 3, pp. 370–374, 1980.

[15] B. Bodner-Adler, E. Hanzal, E. Pablik, H. Koelbl, K. Bodner, and A. G. Passi, "Management of vesicovaginal fistulas (VVFs) in women following benign gynaecologic surgery: A systematic review and meta-analysis," *PLoS ONE*, vol. 12, no. 2, p. e0171554, 2017.

[16] E. M. Mellano and C. M. Tarnay, "Management of genitourinary fistula," *Current Opinion in Obstetrics and Gynecology*, vol. 26, no. 5, pp. 415–423, 2014.

[17] R. A. Lee, R. E. Symmonds, and T. J. Williams, "Current status of genitourinary fistula," *Obstetrics & Gynecology*, vol. 72, no. 3, pp. 313–319, 1988.

[18] C. F. Tenggardjaja and H. B. Goldman, "Advances in minimally invasive repair of vesicovaginal fistulas," *Current Urology Reports*, vol. 14, no. 3, pp. 253–261, 2013.

[19] D. V. Matei, V. Zanagnolo, M. D. Vartolomei et al., "Robot-assisted vesico-vaginal fistula repair: Our technique and review of the literature," *Urologia Internationalis*, vol. 99, no. 2, pp. 137–142, 2017.

[20] L. Von Dittel, "Abdominale blasenscheidenfistel-operation," *Wein Klin Wochenschr*, vol. 6, pp. 449–452, 1893.

[21] P. von Theobald, P. Hamel, and W. Febbraro, "Laparoscopic repair of a vesicovaginal fistula using an omental J flap," *British Journal of Obstetrics and Gynaecology*, vol. 105, no. 11, pp. 1216–1218, 1998.

[22] O. Melamud, L. Eichel, B. Turbow, and A. Shanberg, "Laparoscopic vesicovaginal fistula repair with robotic reconstruction," *Urology*, vol. 65, no. 1, pp. 163–166, 2005.

[23] A. K. Hemal, S. B. Kolla, and P. Wadhwa, "Robotic reconstruction for recurrent supratrigonal vesicovaginal fistulas," *The Journal of Urology*, vol. 180, no. 3, pp. 981–985, 2008.

[24] N. P. Gupta, S. Mishra, A. K. Hemal, A. Mishra, A. Seth, and P. N. Dogra, "Comparative analysis of outcome between open and robotic surgical repair of recurrent supra-trigonal vesico-vaginal fistula," *Journal of Endourology*, vol. 24, no. 11, pp. 1779–1782, 2010.

[25] G. S. Bora, S. Singh, R. S. Mavuduru et al., "Robot-assisted vesicovaginal fistula repair: a safe and feasible technique," *International Urogynecology Journal*, vol. 28, no. 6, pp. 957–962, 2017.

[26] A. P. Sharma, R. M. Mavuduru, G. S. Bora, S. K. Devana, S. K. Singh, and A. K. Mandal, "Robot-assisted vesico-vaginal fistula repair: a compilation," *Urology*, vol. 119, pp. 1–4, 2018.

5

# Unusual Suspect: A Case Report of Tubulocystic Renal Cell Carcinoma with Features of Cystic Renal Oncocytoma

**Jacob D. McFadden,[1] Isabell A. Sesterhenn,[2] and Sean Q. Kern[3]**

[1]*Department of Urology, Walter Reed National Military Medical Center, 8901 Wisconsin Avenue, Bethesda, MD, USA*
[2]*Joint Pathology Center, 606 Stephen Sitter Ave, Silver Spring, MD, USA*
[3]*Department of Urology, Fort Belvoir Army Medical Center, 9300 DeWitt Loop, Fort Belvoir, VA, USA*

Correspondence should be addressed to Jacob D. McFadden; jakemcfadden17@gmail.com

Academic Editor: Tun-Chieh Chen

Tubulocystic renal cell carcinoma is an uncommon subtype of renal cell carcinoma that was only recently acknowledged by the World Health Organization. There is a relatively small collection of literature dedicated to the features and clinical course of this lesion. Despite its rarity, this diagnosis should remain in the differential for all cystic renal masses. We present a case report of tubulocystic renal cell carcinoma (TC-RCC) with remarkable similarity to cystic renal oncocytoma, highlighting the diagnostic challenges associated with this unusual renal malignancy.

## 1. Introduction

Tubulocystic renal cell carcinoma is a relatively new and unusual variant of renal cell carcinoma that can pose diagnostic challenges. In 2004, Amin et al. first reported a case series in which he described 31 tumors considered "tubulocystic carcinoma," though the tumor was not included in the World Health Organization classification of Genitourinary Tumors that year [1, 2]. Tubulocystic renal cell carcinoma (TC-RCC) became a distinct entity acknowledged first by the American Joint Committee on Cancer in 2010; it was then included in the Vancouver Classification of Renal Cancer in 2012 and was officially added into the 2016 World Health Organization modified classification of RCC as a newly recognized renal tumor [3, 4].

Characterization of the tumor accelerated after formalizing its classification and has been underscored in earlier literature reviews. The tumor demonstrates a male: female ratio of approximately 7: 1 and a left-sided predominance and is seen in patients in the 5th and 6th decades of life. Unique risk factors for this type of RCC have not been identified. Patients most commonly are asymptomatic on presentation, though hematuria, distention, and abdominal pain are sometimes reported [5]. On imaging, TC-RCC shows a combination of high echogenicity on ultrasound, a cystic or indeterminate appearance on contrast-enhanced CT, and a cystic pattern on MRI; the cysts associated with TC-RCC have been classified from Bosniak I to Bosniak IV [6, 7].

Grossly, the tumors have an average size of 4 cm (with maximum reported size of 17.5cm [8]) and a white-gray color and have variably been described to have a cut surface reminiscent of "bubble wrap," "sponge," or "Swiss cheese," owing to the cystic components of the tumor. Microscopically, the tumor is lined with cuboidal or columnar cells and will often demonstrate hobnail cells in a fibrotic stroma with numerous small tubules and cysts. The tumor cells typically have prominent nucleoli and few mitotic figures [1, 5, 8–10]. TC-RCC tumor cells typically stain positive for CK8, CK18, CK19, parvalbumin, CD10, P504S, AMACR, and vimentin. HMWK and CD117 are typically negative [11].

The differential for cystic masses of the kidney is broad and includes papillary RCC, fumarate hydratase-deficient RCC, collecting duct carcinoma, clear cell renal cell carcinoma with prominent cysts, multilocular cystic renal cell carcinoma, cystic nephroma or mixed epithelial and stromal tumors, synovial sarcoma, and cystic renal oncocytoma, in addition to TC-RCC [8, 12]. Notably, TC-RCC has been found coexisting in tumor specimens that also harbor renal

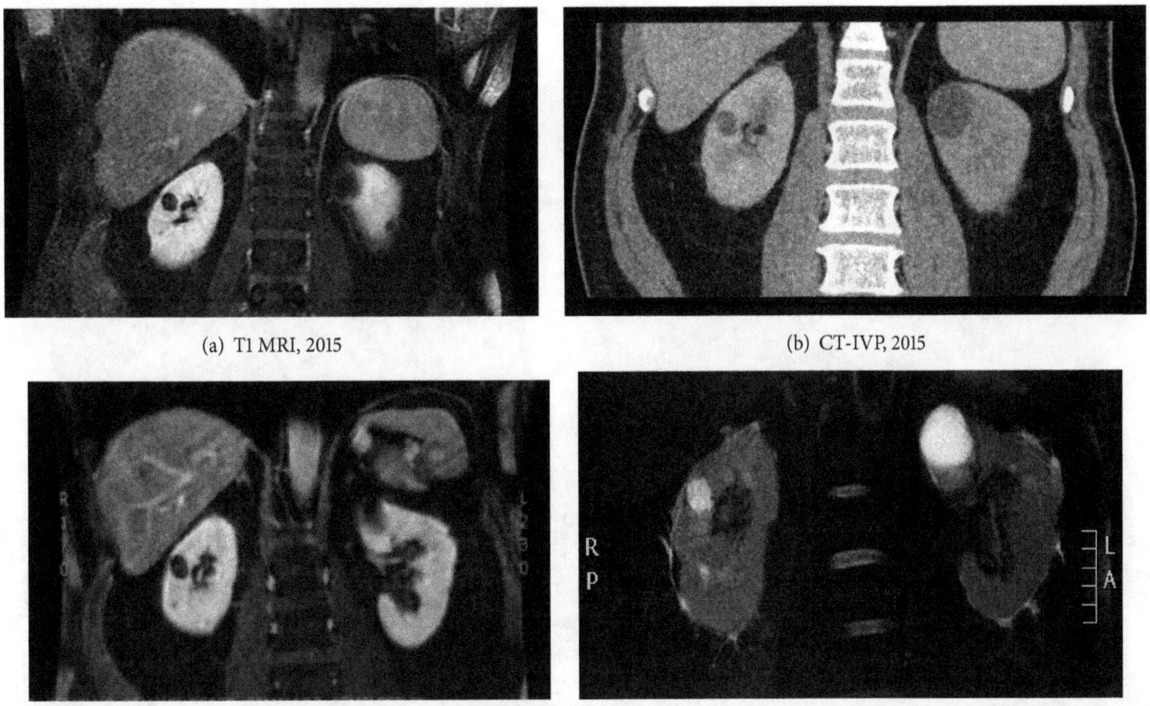


(a) T1 MRI, 2015

(b) CT-IVP, 2015

(c) T1 MRI, 2018

(d) T2 MRI, 2018

FIGURE 1

papillary carcinoma and other forms of renal cell carcinoma [13]. Of that differential, cystic renal oncocytoma can be particularly challenging to distinguish from TC-RCC based on its clinical and histopathologic features.

We present a case of tubulocystic renal cell carcinoma with similarity to cystic renal oncocytoma (CRO), in the setting of bilateral cystic disease, highlighting the diagnostic challenges of this relatively new and uncommon condition.

## 2. Case Report

The patient is a 59-year-old male who presented with interval increase in size of an endophytic right interpolar Bosniak III renal cyst on surveillance imaging. The Bosniak III cyst had developed in the setting of mild bilateral cystic disease identified on previous imaging (Figures 1(a)–1(d)). His medical history was notable for hypertension, hyperlipidemia, type II diabetes, and gout, and a baseline GFR of 77 mL/min; he was on appropriate medications for his comorbidities. The patient did not have a family history of genitourinary malignancy, including no family history of renal cancers; there was also no history of skin or uterine leiomyomas. He endorsed a 22-pack-year history of smoking and denied history of toxic environmental exposures. The patient elected to discontinue his active surveillance and proceed with surgical extirpation of the Bosniak III cyst. He was asymptomatic with a normal lab profile at the time of surgery.

He underwent an uncomplicated robot-assisted right partial nephrectomy for his 1.9 × 2.0 × 1.6cm renal mass. He recovered well during the postoperative period.

## 3. Histopathologic Report

The pathologic analysis of his cystic lesion confirmed negative margins. Tissue analysis was remarkable for a well-circumscribed renal mass consisting of cysts, which varied in size from small, more closely packed tubules to larger simple cysts, separated by fibrous stroma, with some areas demonstrating papillary architecture. The cysts were predominantly lined by a single layer and occasionally by multiple layers of cells with variable amounts of eosinophilic cytoplasm resembling oncocytic cells (Figures 2(a)–2(c)). In areas, the tumor cells had a hobnail appearance and focally they contained intracytoplasmic vacuoles. Nucleoli were prominent (grade 3), typical of tubulocystic carcinoma. Ovarian-type stroma seen in cystic nephromas, seen almost exclusively in women, was absent. By immunohistochemistry, the tumor cells were focally positive for CK7 and 34-beta-E12 and diffusely positive for AMACR and vimentin. Fumarate hydratase loss was not detected. The cells were weakly positive for RCC, but negative for S100 protein and c-kit. The proliferative activity in the Ki-67 stain was low (Figures 2(c)–2(g)).

The differential diagnosis generated by the histopathology report included an unusual variant of oncocytoma and the rare tubulocystic renal cell carcinoma. The diagnosis of TC-RCC was supported by the diffuse and strong reaction for vimentin and the lack of CD117.

Given the information collected, the mass was classified as a pT1a renal cell carcinoma. Established National Comprehensive Cancer Network (NCCN) and American Urological Association (AUA) guidelines were used to generate the patient's short-term follow-up plan: a repeat clinic visit 6

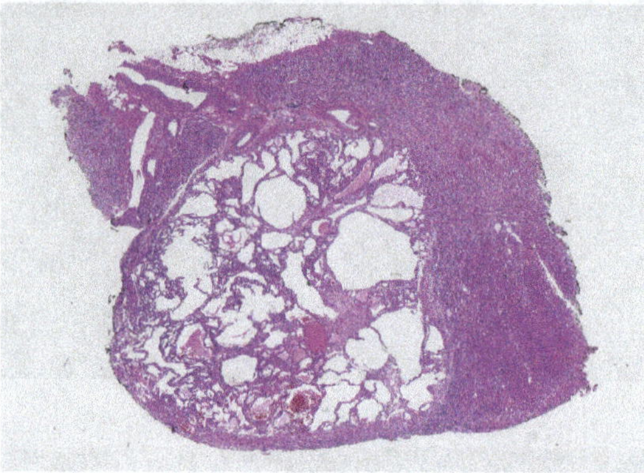

(a) H&E, 3x

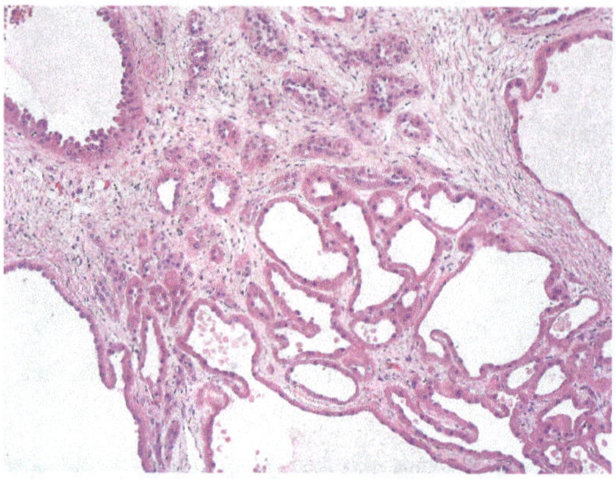

(b) Cysts of variable size lined by single and, focally multiple, layers of tumor cells in loose stroma, with hobnailing around the cysts; H&E, 10x

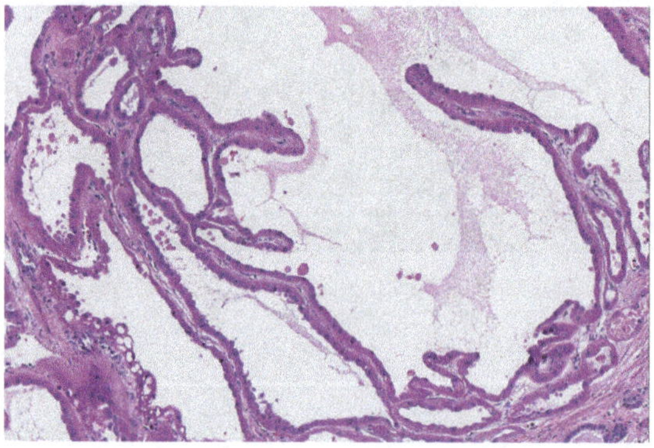

(c) Scattered papillary architecture in cystic background; H&E, 15x

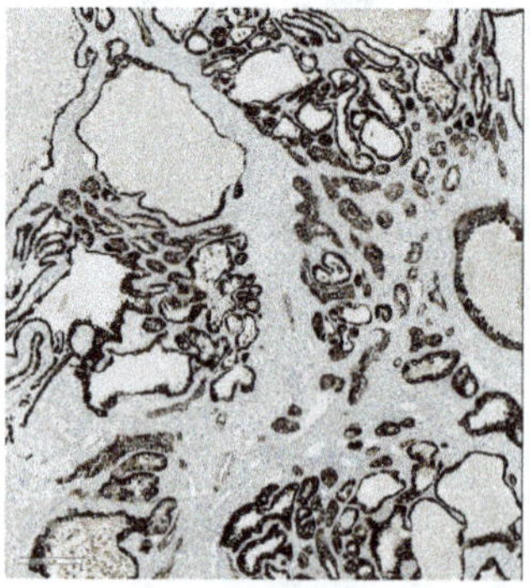

(d) AMACR; 8x

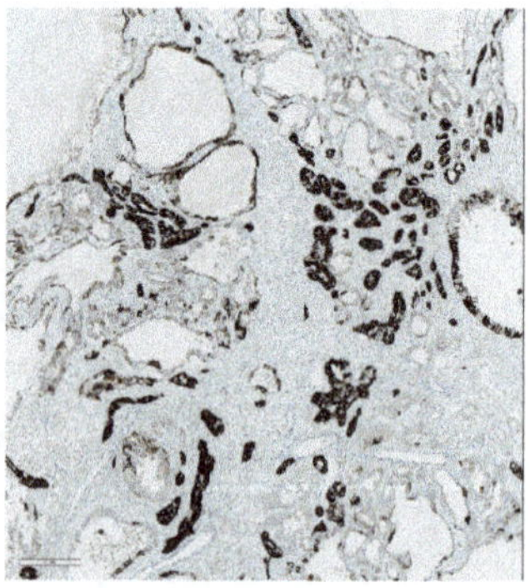

(e) CK7; 8x

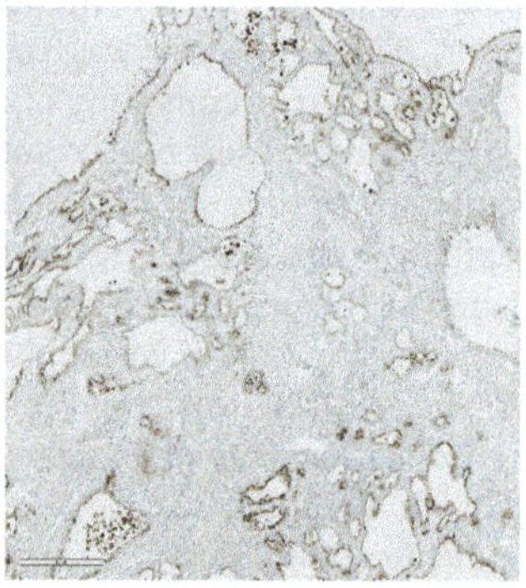

(f) RCC; 8x

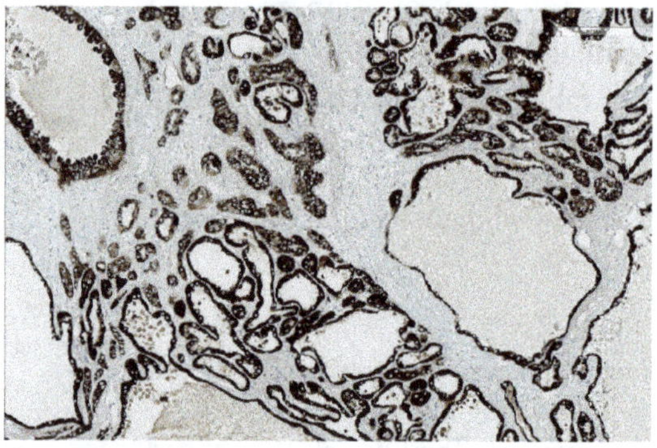

(g) AMACR positive staining in same field as diffuse CK7 positivity; 10x

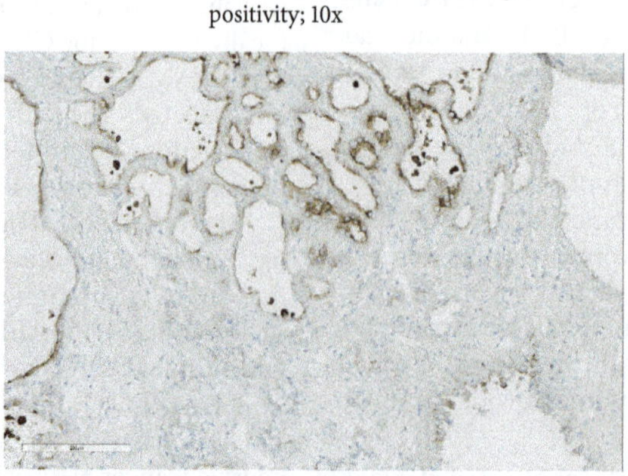

(h) RCC weakly and focally positive; 20x

Figure 2

months from the date of surgery, with repeat imaging and labs at that time [14].

## 4. Discussion

Oncocytoma is a common, benign renal mass that is well known for its ability to mimic malignant lesions of the kidney, especially on clinical and imaging criteria. The treatment for these lesions is often surgical removal, as they can grow quickly and are difficult to distinguish from renal cell carcinoma on active surveillance. Once removed, the challenge of oncocytoma can persist, as they have well-described histologic similarities to malignant lesions, most notably to eosinophilic chromophobe renal cell carcinoma [15]. Immunohistochemistry is paramount for these cases and can be the separating factor in deciding whether a lesion is benign or malignant.

Approximately 3-7% of renal oncocytomas will demonstrate a tubulocystic histologic pattern [11, 16]. In these situations, the distinction between cystic renal oncocytoma (CRO) and tubulocystic renal cell carcinoma can be nuanced. Skenderi et al. compared the morphologic features and IHC profile of 24 cystic renal oncocytomas and 15 TC-RCCs, noting a handful of key differences. Grossly, CRO will often have more solid components and a less prominent "bubble wrap" appearance. On microscopy, CRO will have tumor islands, unlike TC-RCC. Additionally, TC-RCC shows higher grade nucleoli, mitotic figures, and necrosis—all features not typically observed in CROs [11].

TC-RCC will typically stain negative for CD117, but positive for CD10, AMACR, and CK7. Diffuse vimentin positivity and high Ki-67 proliferative indices (>15%) can also help identify TC-RCC, especially when differentiating from cystic renal oncocytoma [11, 17]. In this case, the lack of CD117 and the strongly positive reaction for vimentin clinched the diagnosis of TC-RCC.

Unlike renal oncocytoma, TC-RCC is uncommon and malignant. Most lesions are small and indolent, though progression and/or metastasis have been reported [5, 8]. Per AUA guidelines, partial nephrectomy is the preferred option for cT1a renal masses in most situations. Because of the paucity of data on TC-RCC, treatment strategies for these advanced cases remain experimental and unproven. Sunitinib and everolimus both have been trialed in the treatment of metastatic TC-RCC [8]. Despite the recent classification of this tumor and its infrequency, strides have been made to define the lesion. Yang et al. used gene expression microarray analysis to demonstrate a unique molecular signature of TC-RCC, as compared with other renal tumors and normal renal tissue. Their data revealed that TC-RCC is closely related to papillary renal cell carcinoma, with further analysis placing it between low- and high-grade papillary RCC. They also discovered that TC-RCC shows trisomy 17 but does not demonstrate trisomy 7, unlike papillary RCC, which typically has both trisomy 7 and 17 [9]. Onsukoya et al. also used gene expression profiles to distinguish TC-RCC from collecting duct carcinoma [18]. A detailed molecular analysis provided by Lawrie et al. demonstrated noncoding RNA and mutational profiles that confirmed a distinct genetic signature for this tumor type. These in-depth analyses have added greatly to the characterization and understanding of this renal cancer subtype.

It is clear that despite an increasing collection of literature, more studies will be required to further characterize TC-RCC and optimize treatment and surveillance strategies for this lesion moving forward. It is unclear whether renal cystic disease is a risk factor for TC-RCC or higher Bosniak scores more frequently harbor TC-RCCs (TC-RCC has been reported in both Bosniak I and II cysts) [6, 8]. In this case report, the distinction between cystic renal oncocytoma and TC-RCC was only made with careful immunohistologic qualification. The radiologic, gross, and histologic features of this lesion can easily be confused with tumors both benign (CRO, cystic nephroma) and aggressively malignant (collecting duct carcinoma), highlighting the diagnostic challenges that can be associated with the uncommon tubulocystic renal cell carcinoma.

## Disclosure

The views expressed in this manuscript are those of the author and do not reflect the official policy of the Department of Army/Navy/Air Force, Department of Defense, or US Government.

## Acknowledgments

This work was presented in poster format at the 66th Annual James C. Kimbrough Urological Meeting (January 2019, Kona, HI).

## References

[1] M. B. Amin, G. T. MacLennan, R. Gupta et al., "Tubulocystic carcinoma of the kidney: clinicopathologic analysis of 31 cases of a distinctive rare subtype of renal cell carcinoma," *The American Journal of Surgical Pathology*, vol. 33, no. 3, pp. 384–392, 2009.

[2] J. N. Eble, G. Sauter, J. I. Epstein, and I. A. Sesterhenn, "World health organization classification of tumours," in *Pathology and Genetics of Tumours of the Urinary System And Male Genital Organs*, IARC Press, Lyon, France, 2004.

[3] J. R. Srigley, B. Delahunt, J. N. Eble et al., "ISUP renal tumor panel. the international society of urological pathology (ISUP) vancouver classification of renal neoplasia," *The American Journal of Surgical Pathology*, vol. 37, pp. 1469–1489, 2013.

[4] H. Moch, A. L. Cubilla, P. A. Humphrey, V. E. Reuter, and T. M. Ulbright, "The 2016 WHO classification of tumours of the urinary system and male genital organs—part A: renal, penile, and testicular tumours," *European Urology*, vol. 70, no. 1, pp. 93–105, 2016.

[5] J. S. Bhullar, N. Varshney, A. K. Bhullar, and V. K. Mittal, "A new type of renal cancer – tubulocystic carcinoma of the kidney: a review of the literature," *International Journal of Surgical Pathology*, vol. 22, no. 4, pp. 297–302, 2013.

[6] F. Cornelis, O. Hélénon, J. M. Correas et al., "Tubulocystic renal cell carcinoma: a new radiological entity," *European Radiology*, vol. 26, no. 4, pp. 1108–1115, 2016.

[7] Y. Ishibashi, T. Koie, N. Fujita et al., "Tubulocystic renal cell carcinoma in the left kidney: a case report," *Journal of Medical Case Reports*, vol. 8, no. 265, 2014.

[8] I. Banerjee, S. S. Yadav, V. Tomar, S. Yadav, and S. Talreja, "Tubulocystic renal cell carcinoma: a great imitator," *Reviews in Urology*, vol. 18, no. 2, pp. 118–121, 2016.

[9] X. J. Yang, M. Zhou, Hes O. et al., "Tubulocystic carcinoma of the kidney. Clinicopathologic and molecular characterization," *The American Journal of Surgical Pathology*, vol. 32, no. 2, pp. 177–187, 2008.

[10] J. S. Bhullar, S. Bindroo, N. Varshney, and V. Mittal, "Tubulocystic renal cell carcinoma: a rare renal tumor," *Journal of Kidney Cancer and VHL*, vol. 1, no. 5, pp. 56–62, 2014.

[11] F. Skenderi, M. Ulamec, S. Vranic et al., "Cystic renal oncocytoma and tubulocystic renal cell carcinoma," *Applied Immunohistochemistry & Molecular Morphology*, vol. 24, no. 2, pp. 112–119, 2016.

[12] H. Moch, "Cystic renal tumors: new entities and novel concepts," *Advances in Anatomic Pathology*, vol. 17, no. 3, pp. 209–214, 2010.

[13] C. Brennan, J. R. Srigley, C. Whelan, J. Cooper, and B. Delahunt, "Type 2 and clear cell papillary renal cell carcinoma, and tubulocystic carcinoma: A unifying concept," *Anticancer Reseach*, vol. 30, no. 2, pp. 641–644, 2010.

[14] S. M. Donat, M. Diaz, J. T. Bishoff et al., "Follow-up for clinically localized renal neoplasms: AUA guideline," *The Journal of Urology*, vol. 190, no. 2, pp. 407–416, 2013.

[15] A. J. Wein, L. R. Kavoussi, A. Partin, and C. A. Peters, "Campbell-Walsh Urology," in *Chapter 56: Benign Renal Tumors*, V. Margulis, J. A. Karam, and C. G. Wood, Eds., Elsevier, 11th edition, 2016.

[16] K. Trpkov, A. Yilmaz, D. Uzer et al., "Renal oncocytoma revisited: a clinicopathological study of 109 cases with emphasis on problematic diagnostic features," *Histopathology*, vol. 57, no. 6, pp. 893–906, 2010.

[17] B. A. Alexiev and C. B. Drachenberg, "Tubulocystic carcinoma of the kidney: a histologic, immunohistochemical, and ultrastructural study," *Virchows Archiv*, vol. 462, no. 5, pp. 575–581, 2013.

[18] A. O. Osunkoya, A. N. Young, W. Wang, G. J. Netto, and J. I. Epstein, "Comparison of gene expression profiles in tubulocystic carcinoma and collecting duct carcinoma of the kidney," *The American Journal of Surgical Pathology*, vol. 33, no. 7, pp. 1103–1106, 2009.

# 6

# Alfa-Fetoprotein-Producing Female Primary Urethral Adenocarcinoma with Neuroendocrine Differentiation

**Takao Natsuyama,[1,2] Yozo Mitsui,[1,3] Masato Uetani,[1] Shigeyuki Ohta,[1] Masafumi Inoue,[4] and Koichiro Akakura[2]**

[1] *Department of Urology, Chiba-Nishi General Hospital, 270-2251 Chiba, Japan*
[2] *Department of Urology, Japan Community Health Care Organization, Tokyo Shinjuku Medical Center, Tokyo, Japan*
[3] *Department of Urology, Toho University Faculty of Medicine, 143-8540 Tokyo, Japan*
[4] *Department of Pathology, Japan Community Health Care Organization, Tokyo Shinjuku Medical Center, Tokyo, Japan*

Correspondence should be addressed to Yozo Mitsui; yozo_321@yahoo.co.jp

Academic Editor: Giorgio Carmignani

We report an extremely rare case of an alpha-fetoprotein- (AFP-) producing female primary urethral adenocarcinoma with neuroendocrine differentiation (NED). The patient was a 65-year-old woman with a 2-year history of urinary frequency and voiding difficulty. Enhanced computed tomography showed an approximately 3.0×5.0-cm mass around the proximal urethra and bladder neck. Of examined tumor markers, serum AFP was elevated (48.3 ng/mL), while others including carcinoembryonic antigen were within a normal range. Transurethral resection of the tumor led to a diagnosis of carcinosarcoma of the urethra, with a radical cystourethrectomy and ileal conduit formation subsequently performed. The pathological assessment was poorly differentiated adenocarcinoma in the urethra. Immunostaining showed tumor cells strongly positive for AFP. In addition, some cancer cells were positive for CD56, chromogranin A, and synaptophysin, indicating focal NED. The tumor was finally diagnosed as an AFP-producing urethral adenocarcinoma with NED. Serum AFP was immediately normalized after surgery and no sign of tumor recurrence has been noted 2 years postoperatively.

## 1. Introduction

Tumor markers can provide valuable information regarding specific features as well as tumor burden and thus contribute to accurate disease diagnosis and prediction of therapeutic response. Elevated levels of carcinoembryonic antigen (CEA) and carbohydrate antigen (CA) 19-9 in serum are sometimes found in patients with urethral carcinoma [1]. However, elevation of serum alpha-fetoprotein (AFP) is extremely rare in association with this disease [2]. Furthermore, neuroendocrine differentiation (NED) is occasionally observed in various types of malignancy, including that of the genitourinary tract such as prostate cancer during an advanced disease stage [3], whereas the phenomenon is uncommon in cases of urethral cancer. Here, we present an extremely rare case of AFP-producing female primary urethral adenocarcinoma with NED.

## 2. Case Presentation

A 65-year-old Japanese woman came to our hospital because of increased urinary frequency and dysuria over a 2-year period. Abdominal ultrasonography and cystoscopy findings revealed a broad based non-papillary tumor with a diameter of approximately 3.0 cm around the neck of the urinary bladder, with urine cytology findings positive for malignancy. Enhance computed tomography revealed a 3.0×5.0-cm mass with a heterogeneous contrasting effect between the urethra and bladder neck (Figure 1), though no distant metastasis was found. Additional examinations showed a serum AFP level of 48.3 ng/mL (normal <10.0 ng/mL), while CEA, CA19-9, and prostate specific antigen (PSA) levels were within normal ranges. Transurethral resection of the tumor between the urethra and bladder neck did not lead to a definitive diagnosis, but the possibility of carcinosarcoma of the urethra was indicated. Based on these findings, we diagnosed

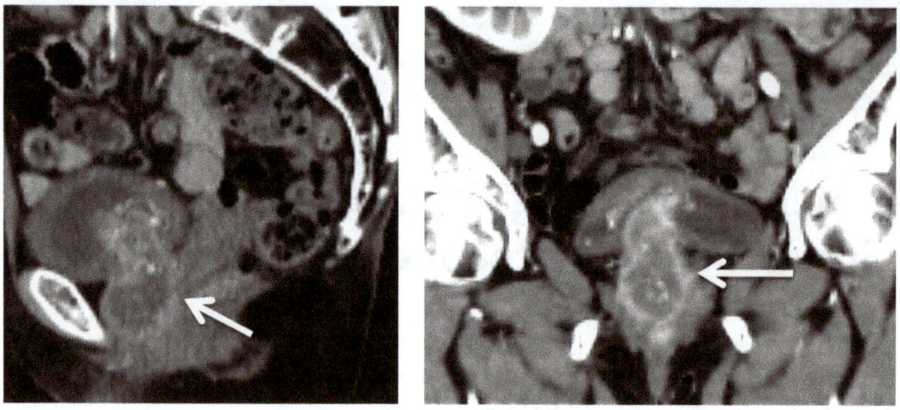

(a) (b)

FIGURE 1: Abdominal enhanced computed tomography images showing a 3.0×5.0 cm mass with a heterogeneous contrasting effect between the urethra and bladder neck. (a) Sagittal section (arrow indicates tumor). (b) Coronal section (arrow indicates tumor).

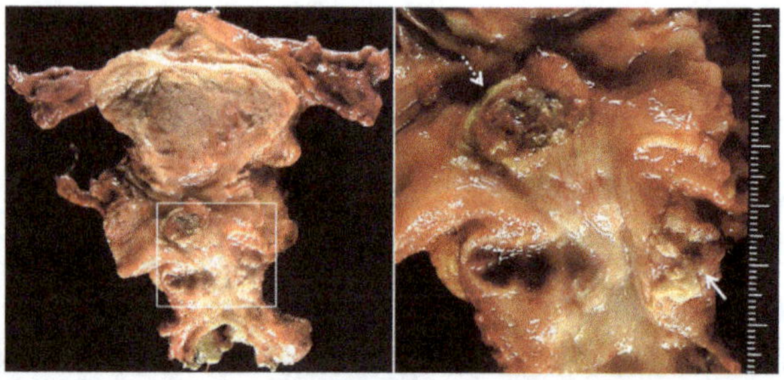

FIGURE 2: Macroscopic view of excised specimen. On the left is the full specimen and on the right is an enlarged image showing the tumor. The excised specimen had two ulcerated cancer lesions, one (3.0×1.8 mm in diameter, dotted arrow) around the trigon of the urinary bladder and the other (2.5×3.0 mm in diameter, arrow) on the proximal urethra.

urethral cancer, clinical stage T3N0M0, and performed a radical cystourethrectomy procedure along with ileal conduit formation. Lymphadenectomy was not performed in this case.

The total operation time was 8 hours 28 minutes and blood loss was 1081 mL. As shown in Figure 2, the excised specimen contained two ulcerated cancer lesions, one around the trigon of the urinary bladder and the other on the proximal urethra. Pathological assessment of the resected specimen revealed a poorly differentiated adenocarcinoma with various characteristics, such as clear cytoplasm and an NE tumor appearance (Figure 3). Immunohistochemistry was performed, which showed cells stained positive for AFP (Figure 4(a)), and negative for CEA, CA19-9, PSA, and p63. In addition, some cancer cells were positive for the NE markers CD56 (Figure 4(b)), chromogranin A (Figure 4(c)), and synaptophysin (Figure 4(d)). As these characteristics of the tumors were common to the two lesions, we considered that they were originally continuous lesion before transurethral resection. Finally, the morphologic and immunohistochemical findings confirmed a diagnosis of AFP-producing primary urethral adenocarcinoma with focal NED (the final tumor stage was pT3).

There were no peri-operative complications and the patient was discharged 37 days after surgery without adjuvant treatment. Serum AFP was immediately normalized after surgery and no signs of tumor recurrence including re-elevation of serum AFP have been noted 2 years postoperatively.

## 3. Discussion

We describe here the first known case of AFP-producing female primary urethral adenocarcinoma with neuroendocrine components. To the best of our knowledge, only a single case of urethral cancer with elevated AFP in serum has been reported thus far [2], while the phenomenon of NED has scarcely been reported to occur in patients with a primary urethral carcinoma. Thus, the present case is extremely unusual, as the patient showed both rare features concurrently.

Primary urethral carcinoma is a rare disease that accounts for less than 1% of cases of malignancy, with 5-year survival rates ranging from 40% to 60% [4, 5]. The ratio of female to male has been reported to be 2:3 and the most common histologic subtype among women is adenocarcinoma [6]. An adenocarcinoma can occur in a variety of tissues and organs, including the lungs, colorectum, and prostate, as well as others, and may occasionally be accompanied by NED [3, 7–9]. Interestingly, it has been reported that this phenomenon occurs only rarely, even in female patients with an adenocarcinoma in the urethral diverticulum [10]. Some adenocarcinomas with a diverticular form can arise from the proximal portion of the female paraurethral duct or gland, each of which expresses numerous endocrine cells [11, 12]; thus it is not surprising that cancer arising from these ducts exhibit focal NED. Furthermore, the proximal portion of the female paraurethral duct sometimes shows positive staining for PSA because it is embryologically homologous to the male prostate gland [12]. However, the existence

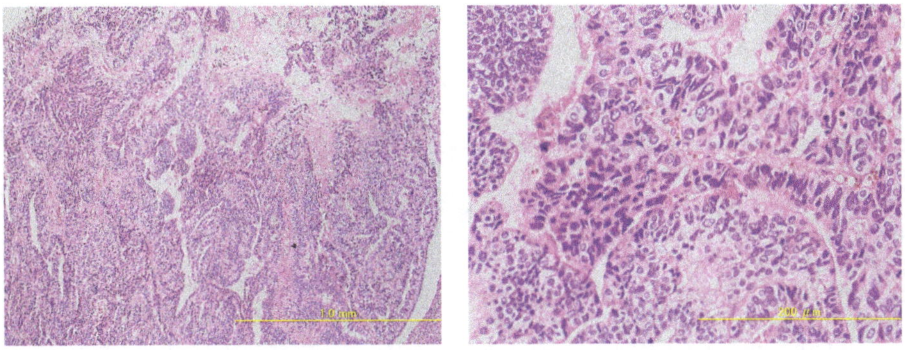

(a) (b)

FIGURE 3: Histopathological findings. The diagnosis was urethral adenocarcinoma with various characteristics. (a) Hematoxylin and eosin stain, ×40. (b) Hematoxylin and eosin stain, ×200.

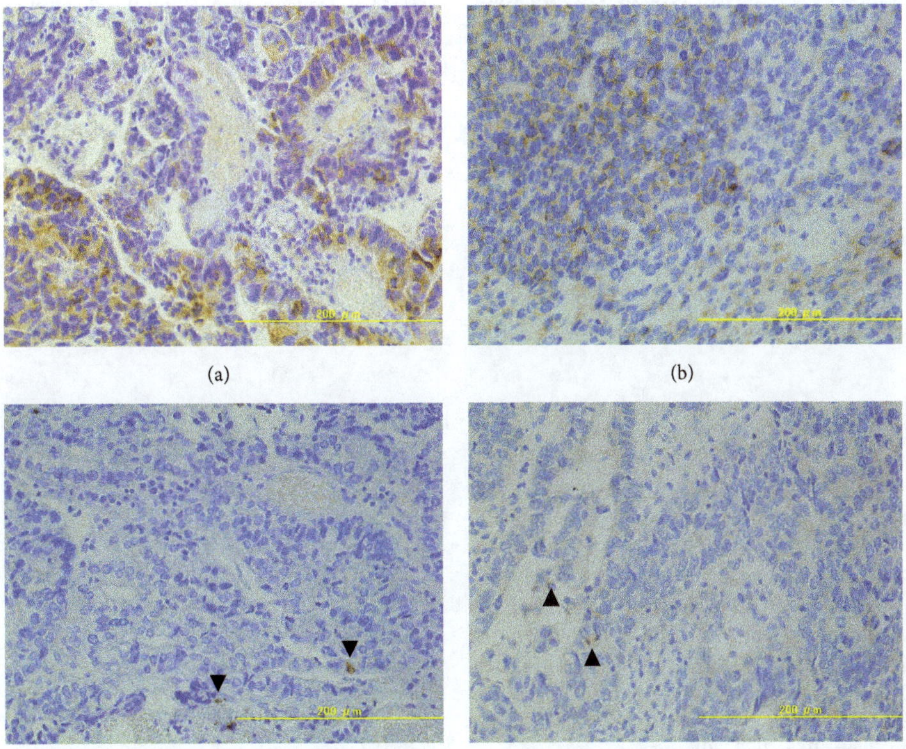

(a) (b) (c) (d)

FIGURE 4: Immunohistochemical findings. (a) Tumor cells strongly positive stained for AFP (×200). (b) Positive staining for CD56 (×200). (c, d) Several cells were immunohistochemically positive for (c) chromogranin A (×200, arrowheads) and (d) synaptophysin (×200, arrowheads).

of distinct subsets of paraurethral ducts showing negative staining for PSA is assumed. On the basis of such reported findings, Kato et al. presented diagnostic criteria, in which the phenomenon of NED is considered to indicate a female urethral adenocarcinoma with a diverticular form originating from the proximal portion, while positive for PSA staining is excluded from those criteria [11]. Although the present case was a primary urethral adenocarcinoma that did not contain diverticular components, focal NED was observed in cancer tissues with negative staining for PSA. A previous study suggested that a female primary urethral adenocarcinoma can arise from more than one tissue of origin [13]. Therefore, we considered that the cancer cells in our case may have been, at least in part, derived from the proximal portion of the paraurethral duct.

AFP is a protein normally produced by the liver and yolk sac of a developing fetus, and widely used as a serum biomarker for hepatocellular carcinomas and yolk sac tumors. In addition to those tumors, several types of malignancy, including lung, ovarian, and gastrointestinal cancer, are known to occasionally produce AFP [7–9], though an elevated level in serum is extremely rare in cases of urethral cancer. To date, the mechanisms underlying AFP production by these tumor cells has not been well elucidated.

Interestingly, cancer with NED has been reported to be occasionally accompanied by an elevated serum AFP level, which is thought to be a marker of tumor cell dedifferentiation [7, 9, 14]. In addition, it is important to note that the urethra is embryologically derived from a cloaca containing AFP. On the basis of these reports, we speculated that some of the tumor cells in the present case had dedifferentiated and acquired an embryonic-like stemness, thus were subsequently capable of producing AFP.

When the serum level of AFP is found to be elevated, it is important to exclude the possibility of carcinoma metastasis to the liver or non-neoplastic liver injury. In the present case, laboratory examination results showed normal liver function, and CT imaging revealed no definite liver findings of metastasis or hepatobiliary lesions. In addition, immunohistochemical analysis showed that tumor cells were positive for AFP and the serum AFP level quickly returned to a normal range after surgery. Together, those results strongly suggested that AFP in our patient was produced by urethral cancer cells and the level in serum was correlated with tumor burden. In general, female urethral carcinoma is diagnosed as an aggressive disease in an advanced stage [6]. In addition, both NED phenomenon and AFP secretion are features indicating an aggressive malignant potential, as well as high propensity for metastasis to other organs [3, 7–10]. Thus, cancer patients with theses features require careful follow-up. We believe that monitoring the serum level of AFP can contribute to early detection of tumor recurrence and metastasis in such cases.

## References


[1] T. Koizumi, S. Bando, K. Kanda, and T. Inai, "Two cases of primary female urethral cancer," *The Japanese Journal of Urology*, vol. 98, no. 6, pp. 790–794, 2007.

[2] Y. Mimura, H. Mizusawa, T. Saito, and N. Hirabayashi, "A case of alpha-fetoprotein-producing female urethral adenocarcinoma," *Acta Urologica Japonica*, vol. 59, no. 6, pp. 373–376, 2013.

[3] Y. Mitsui, N. Arichi, M. Hiraki, Y. Harada, H. Yasumoto, and H. Shiina, "Tissue chromogranin a expression during prostate cancer progression: Prediction of chemosensitivity," *Urology Journal*, vol. 12, no. 3, pp. 2165–2172, 2015.

[4] M. A. Swartz, M. P. Porter, D. W. Lin, and N. S. Weiss, "Incidence of primary urethral carcinoma in the United States," *Urology*, vol. 68, no. 6, pp. 1164–1168, 2006.

[5] O. Visser, J. Adolfsson, S. Rossi et al., "Incidence and survival of rare urogenital cancers in Europe," *European Journal of Cancer*, vol. 48, no. 4, pp. 456–464, 2012.

[6] C. C. Peyton, M. Azizi, J. Chipollini et al., "Survival Outcomes Associated With Female Primary Urethral Carcinoma: Review of a Single Institutional Experience," *Clinical Genitourinary Cancer*, vol. 16, no. 5, pp. e1003–e1013, 2018.

[7] M. Kitada, K. Ozawa, K. Sato et al., "Alpha-fetoprotein-producing primary lung carcinoma: a case report," *World Journal of Surgical Oncology*, vol. 9, p. 47, 2011.

[8] H.-H. Lin, C.-C. Chang, S.-H. Yang et al., "Elevated serum alpha-fetoprotein in poorly differentiated adenocarcinoma with neuroendocrine differentiation of the ascending colon: a case report," *World Journal of Surgical Oncology*, vol. 14, no. 1, article 84, 2016.

[9] T. Li, T. Liu, M. Wang, and M. Zhang, "A-fetoprotein producing hepatoid gastric adenocarcinoma with neuroendocrine differentiation: a case report," *Medicine*, vol. 97, no. 37, Article ID e12359, 2018.

[10] A. H. M. M. Islam, H. Kato, M. Hayama, S. Kobayashi, H. Ota, and O. Nishizawa, "Adenocarcinoma of female paraurethral duct showing neuroendocrine differentiation," *Urology*, vol. 58, no. 6, p. 1058, 2001.

[11] H. Kato, S. Kobayashi, A. M. Islam, and O. Nishizawa, "Female para-urethral adenocarcinoma: Histological and immunohistochemical study," *International Journal of Urology*, vol. 12, no. 1, pp. 117–119, 2005.

[12] S. Ogihara and H. Kato, "Endocrine cell distribution and expression of tissue-associated antigens in human female paraurethral duct: Possible clue to the origin of urethral diverticular cancer," *International Journal of Urology*, vol. 7, no. 1, pp. 10–15, 2000.

[13] M. K. Dodson, W. A. Cliby, P. P. Pettavel, G. L. Keeney, and K. C. Podratz, "Female urethral adenocarcinoma: evidence for more than one tissue of origin?" *Gynecologic Oncology*, vol. 59, no. 3, pp. 352–357, 1995.

[14] T. Shah, R. Srirajaskanthan, M. Bhogal et al., "$\alpha$-Fetoprotein and human chorionic gonadotrophin-$\beta$ as prognostic markers in neuroendocrine tumour patients," *British Journal of Cancer* vol. 99, no. 1, pp. 72–77, 2008.

# Management of an Extremely Low Birth Weight Infant with Bilateral Renal Obstruction Caused by *Candida albicans* Fungus Balls

**Fabian Brüning ,[1] Axel Hegele,[1] Günter Klaus,[2] Rolf F. Maier,[3] and Rainer Hofmann[1]**

[1]*Department of Urology and Pediatric Urology, University Hospital, Philipps-University Marburg, Baldingerstr. 1, 35043 Marburg, Germany*
[2]*KfH Pediatric Kidney Center and Department of Pediatrics, University Hospital, Philipps-University Marburg, Baldingerstr. 1, 35043 Marburg, Germany*
[3]*Children's Hospital, Philipps-University Marburg, Baldingerstr. 1, 35043 Marburg, Germany*

Correspondence should be addressed to Fabian Brüning; bruening@med.uni-marburg.de

Academic Editor: Fumitaka Koga

We report an extremely low birth weight infant with anuria caused by bilateral *Candida albicans* fungus balls it was treated with a combination of antifungal therapy, irrigation and pyelotomy. This lead to a recovery of renal function, after a follow-up of 77 month no more Candida was cultured from urine.

## 1. Introduction

Candida infections in very/extremely low birth weight infants are frequent (up to 16.7% among very low-birth-weight infants (birth weight <1,500 g) and up to 20% among extremely low-birth-weight infants (birth weight <1,000 g)) [1]; renal obstruction caused by fungus balls are rare [2].

Treatment varies from conservative strategies with single or combined antifungal therapies, to drainage with percutaneous nephrostomy with or without local irrigation or open/endoscopic surgical removal of fungal balls [3].

Here a case is reported on the use of a combination of antifungal therapy, urokinase irrigation and pyelotomy of an extremely low birth weight infant with bilateral ureteral obstruction caused by bilateral Candida fungus balls following *Candida septicaemia*.

## 2. Case Report

The male infant was born at an external hospital by ceasarean section at 25 weeks of gestation with a birth weight of 770 g. A broad spectrum of antibacterial and antifungal drugs was administered for recurrent bacterial and fungal infections including septicaemia and meningitis leading to repeated respiratory insufficiencies with the need for artificial ventilation.

On day 58, he again suffered from sepsis and *Candida albicans* was cultured from urine (susceptible for Fluconazole) and blood specimen. Systemic intravenous antifungal treatment with Fluconazole (6 mg/kg every day without a loading dose) was initiated. Nevertheless acute renal failure developed with anuria (serum creatinine 2.02 mg/dl, blood urea nitrogen 18 mg/dl).

For further treatment, the infant was transferred to our neonatal intensive care unit with the diagnosis of acute renal failure secondary to Candida urinary tract infection.

Renal and bladder ultrasonography revealed bilateral dilatation of the collecting systems with echogenic contents within the renal pelvis bilaterally. This was more pronounced on the right side where the content filled the whole renal pelvis including the proximal ureter. Renal parenchyma revealed hyperechogenic, the bladder was empty (Figure 1).

The infant received mechanical ventilation and inotropic support. After stabilization of ventilation and circulation renal replacement therapy by peritoneal dialysis was started via a Tenckhoff catheter.

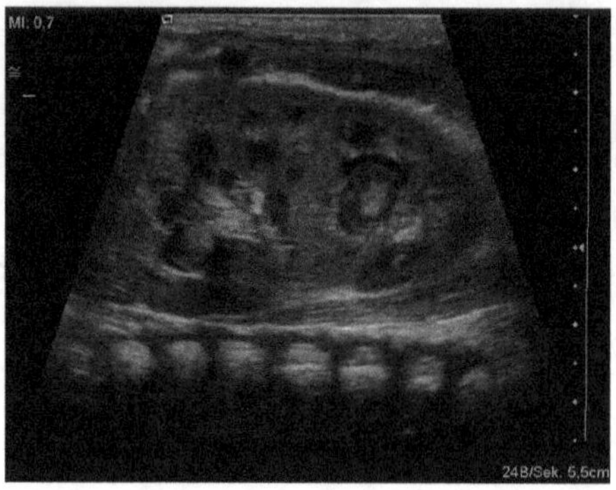

FIGURE 1: Left kidney with hydronephrosis and fungus balls in the collecting system.

We changed antifungal treatment to Caspofungin because of a persistence of Candida in urine culture with resistance to Fluconacole. Because of the obstructive effect of the fungus balls an open bilateral pyelotomy was performed. On the right side complete removal of the fungus balls was achieved, whereas on the left side residuals in the upper calices remained due to complex anatomical conditions. On both sides we placed 6 F percutaneous nephrostomy tubes. As early as during this surgery diuresis started again.

Blood urea nitrogen and creatinine levels returned to normal ranges after 7 days with normal diuresis after initial polyuria and peritoneal dialysis was stopped.

From the removed fungal balls *Candida albicans* and *Enterobacter cloacae* was proven. *Enterobacter cloacae* was also detected in blood cultures so that antibiotic therapy with vancomycin and meropenem was started.

Antegrade pyelograpy was performed on day 13 after surgery; it showed residuals of fungus balls in the left renal pelvis as a central filling defect and a normal filling of the collecting system on the right side. The right ureter did not show up; on the left side it occurred wormed with passage of contrast media into the bladder.

Because of persisting Candida in the urine culture of the left nephrostomy we started local irrigation with Amphotericin-B solution (50 mcg/ml in saline) for 14 days in addition to the intravenous therapy with caspofungin.

In addition, we started on both sides with local irrigation of urokinase solution (15,000 IU/ml 2x/d) to dissolve local adherence due to inflammatory tissue responses on the right side and to dissolve the residues of fungus balls on the left side.

A next antegrade pyelography was performed 7 days after starting the local irrigation therapy and showed a passage of contrast media on both sides into the bladder. The right ureter was thin, the left ureter looked still wormed and segmentally dilated. On the left side residues of fungus balls were still detectable (Figure 2).

After collecting sterile urine cultures after 14 days of irrigation therapy we removed both nephrostomy catheters and the Tenckhoff-catheter. The systemic caspofungin therapy was stopped 28 days after it has been started. No serious side effects associated with this treatment were observed.

Repeated urine cultures continued to yield *Candida albicans*. Therefore oral Fluconazol therapy was continued until month 56. Thereafter no *Candida albicans* were cultured from urine even after stop of the antifungal treatment. At the last follow up at 77 month of life, renal function was stable with serum creatinine of 0.39 mg/dl, leading to an normal estimated creatinine clearance (134 ml/min $*1.73$ m$^2$).

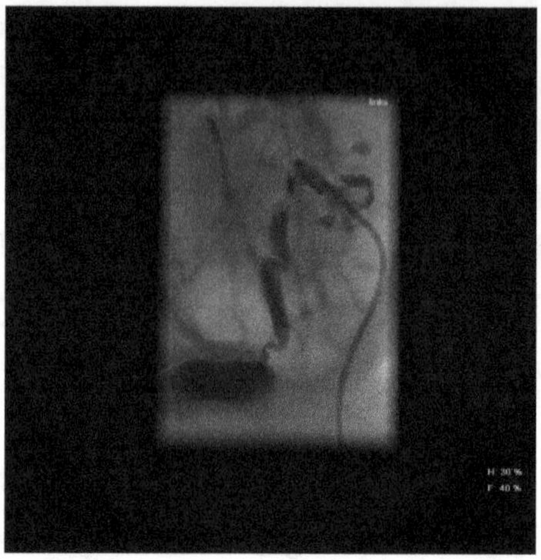

FIGURE 2: Antegrade pyelography, left ureter wormed and segmentally dilated, residues of fungus balls in the collecting system.

## 3. Discussion

Candida colonisation has been reported in up to 34% of all infants treated on neonatal intensive care units followed by septicaemia in 7.7% of the cases [4]; urinary tract involvement has been reported in up to 70% of all infants with Candida sepsis [5].

With decreasing birth weight the rate of septicaemia caused by Candida species increases.

*Candida* species are the 3$^{rd}$ most common organism isolated in late-onset sepsis in very low birth weight infants. It is the most common cause of urinary tract infection in neonatal intensive care units [6].

Renal involvement in infants with Candida sepsis presents as parenchymal infiltration and/or fungus balls in the collecting system.

Although urinary candidiasis is a common finding in very low birth weight infants, renal obstruction caused by fungus balls is very rare [2].

Diagnosis of dilatation and fungus balls is done by ultrasound. It shows hyperechogenic material in the collecting system without posterior shadowing [7].

Diagnosis of obstruction can be difficult [8]. In our case anuria and rapidly progressive renal failure suggested complete obstruction so that a combination of systemic and local antifungal drugs, pyelotomy and urokinase irrigation was used to treat an extremely low birth weight infant. Pyelotomy was justified by anatomical circumstances due to the extremely low birth weight.

In the literature, treatment varies from conservative strategies with single or combined antifungal therapies to drainage with percutaneous nephrostomy with or without local irrigation or open/endoscopic surgical removal of fungal balls.

Treatment depends on the presence of complete or incomplete obstruction of the pelviureteric junction [3, 8].

In case of partial obstruction conservative treatment with systemic antifungal medication may be sufficient [8]. Fluconazole is the drug of first choice [9], but treatment should be guided by drug susceptibility of the fungi in urine culture. There is no consensus on the appropriate duration of treatment [10].

In presence of upper urinary tract obstruction systemic antifungal therapy may not be sufficient. Therefore, drainage procedures are indicated with percutaneous nephrostomy being the procedure of choice [8]. This can be a difficult procedure because of the small renal pelvis and the small size of the neonate. In such situations surgical removal of fungus balls with open procedures may be required [11, 12], like in our case.

Sufficient drainage may be enough to clear fungal balls, but mostly systemic antifungal medication is needed additionally. If this is not successful, local irrigation therapy through nephrostomy with fluconazole or amphotericine B was described in some cases to be effective. When local irrigation fails, a fibrinolytic agent (streptokinase or urokinase) has been used successfully in few cases to clear obstructing fungus balls [8].

There is currently no consensus avaible for the treatment of extremely low birth weight infants with obstructive fungus balls.

Clinicians should know the various treatment options, a helpful algorithm for management of these rare cases is given by Bisht and van der Voort [8]. However, treatment still remains an individual decision in each case.

## 4. Conclusion

Candida infections in infants and extremely low birth weight infants are frequent; renal obstruction caused by fungus balls is rare.

In our case the combination of systemic antifungal therapy, urokinase irrigation and pyelotomy lead to a complete recovery of renal function and to a partial removal of the fungal balls with small residuals.

After a follow-up of 77 month no more *Candida albicans* was cultured from urine.

The renal function was preserved and was normal with an estimated creatinin clearance of 134 ml/min $*1.73\ m^2$.

## References

[1] R. L. Chapman, "Prevention and treatment of candida infections in neonates," *Seminars in Perinatology*, vol. 31, no. 1, pp. 39–46, 2007.

[2] K. Bryant, C. Maxfield, and G Rabalais, "Renal candidiasis in neonates with candiduria," *The Pediatric Infectious Disease Journal*, vol. 18, no. 11, pp. 959–963, 1999.

[3] J. V. Schilperoort, L. L. de Wall, H. J. R. van der Horst, J. A. E. van Wijk, J. I. M. L. Verbeke, and A. Bokenkamp, "Anuria in a solitary kidney with candida bezoars managed conservatively," *European Journal of Pediatrics*, vol. 173, no. 12, pp. 1623–1625, 2014.

[4] J. E. Baley, R. M. Kligman, and A. A. Fanaroff, "Disseminated fungal infections in very low birth weight infants: clinical manifestationsand epidemiology," *Pediatrics*, vol. 73, no. 2, pp. 144–152, 1984.

[5] M. Wald, K. Lawrenz, V. Kretzer et al., "A very low birth weigth infant with Candida nephritis with fungal balls. Full recovery after pyelotomy and antifungal combination therapy," *European Journal of Pediatrics*, vol. 162, no. 9, pp. 642–643, 2003.

[6] M. Narendrababu, S. Ramesh, B. V. Raghunath, and B. C. Gowrishankar, "Successful management of a renal fungal ball in a pretermature neonate: a case report and review of literature," *Journal of Indian Association of Pediatric Surgeons*, vol. 18, no. 3, pp. 121–123, 2013.

[7] C. Kintanar, B. C. Cramer, W. D. Reid, and W. L. Andrews, "Neontal renal candidiasis: sonographic diagnosis," *American Journal of Roentgenology*, vol. 147, no. 4, pp. 801–805, 1986.

[8] V. Bisht and J. van der Voort, "Clinical practice," *European Journal of Pediatrics*, vol. 170, no. 10, pp. 1227–1235, 2011.

[9] L. L. De Wall, M. M. C. van den Heijkant, A. Bökenkamp, C. F. Kuijper, H. J. R. van der Horst, and T. P. V. M. de Jong, "Therapeutic approach to candida bezoar in children," *Journal of Pediatric Urology*, vol. 11, no. 2, pp. 81.e1–81.e7, 2015.

[10] M. G. Karlowicz, "Candidal renal and urinary tract infection in neonates," *Seminars in Perinatology*, vol. 27, no. 5, pp. 393–400, 2003.

[11] V. K. Rehan and D. C. Davidson, "Neonatal renal candidal bezoar," *Archives of Disease in Childhood*, vol. 67, no. 1 Spec No, pp. 63–64, 1992.

[12] B. Rikken, N. G. Hartwig, and J. Hoek, "Renal candida infection in infants and neonates: report of four cases. Review of literature and treatment proposal," *Current Urology*, vol. 1, no. 3, pp. 113–120, 2007.

8

# Polycythemia with Renal Cell Carcinoma and Normal Erythropoietin Level

**Jonathan Kopel**[1] **Pranav Sharma,**[2] **Irfan Warriach,**[3] **and Sriman Swarup**[4]

[1]*Texas Tech University Health Sciences Center, School of Medicine, Lubbock, TX, USA*
[2]*Department of Urology, Texas Tech University Health Sciences Center, Lubbock, TX, USA*
[3]*Department of Pathology, Texas Tech University Health Sciences Center, Lubbock, TX, USA*
[4]*Department of Hematology and Oncology, Texas Tech University Health Sciences Center, Lubbock, TX, USA*

Correspondence should be addressed to Jonathan Kopel; jonathan.kopel@ttuhsc.edu

Academic Editor: Fumitaka Koga

A 61-year-old obese Caucasian male with past medical history of smoking, hypertension, chronic obstructive pulmonary disease (COPD), and sleep apnea presented to the hematology clinic with polycythemia. Despite the newly-diagnosed polycythemia, the patient denied any significant symptoms or history of blood clots. Further evaluation with computerized tomography (CT) and ultrasound showed a large renal mass suspicious for renal cell carcinoma of the right kidney. An incidental abdominal aortic aneurysm (AAA) measuring was also appreciated on imaging. Subsequent histological sections of the tumor showed cell renal cell carcinoma. Though previously reported, the concomitant finding of an AAA with renal cell carcinoma with a normal erythropoietin levels is surprising. Given the surgical complications associated with concomitant conditions with renal cell carcinoma, further investigation into paraneoplastic syndromes secondary to renal cell carcinoma remains open to investigation.

## 1. Introduction

Despite being the 14$^{th}$ most common cause of cancer, renal cell carcinoma accounts for 85% of all renal neoplasms [1]. Although the cancer classically presents with a palpable mass, hematuria, and flank pain, over 10–40% of renal cell carcinoma patients exhibit paraneoplastic syndromes, particularly hypercalcemia, hypertension, and polycythemia [2–4]. As many urologists concede, renal cell carcinomas are medicine's "great masqueraders" affecting multiple organs from a primary cancer [4]. Current studies suggest that unregulated secretion of signaling molecules and antigen mimicking from tumor cells are the primary culprits producing organ damage associated with paraneoplastic syndrome [4, 5]. Paraneoplastic syndromes also influence the severity and metastasis of primary tumors [4]. For example, patients with hypercalcemia secondary to renal cell carcinoma are associated with higher-stage lesions and bone metastasis while those with hypertension acquire low-grade tumors of clear-cell histology [4]. A rising number of care reports describe several unique paraneoplastic syndromes associated with renal cell carcinoma ranging, including intractable coughs, limbic encephalitis, and bullous pemphigoid [6–8]. In general, patients with concurrent renal cell carcinoma and paraneoplastic syndromes have worse outcomes after undergoing nephrectomy compared with incidentally found tumors. Furthermore, the mechanisms underlying the synergistic actions of renal cell carcinomas and paraneoplastic syndromes remains elusive [9]. Therefore, renal cell carcinomas provide a unique opportunity to investigate the mechanisms and clinical manifestations cancer has upon organ system function and integrity. In this case report, we report polycythemia secondary to renal cell carcinoma with normal erythropoietin (EPO) and an incidental abdominal aortic aneurysm (AAA). Specifically, the finding of normal EPO levels in the presence of a paraneoplastic syndrome is both surprising and unique given the large amount of literature demonstrating elevated EPO levels with renal cell carcinoma [10]. In the following case report, we hope to contribute to the diversity and complexity associated with concomitant conditions secondary to renal cell carcinoma while providing a plausible mechanism of action.

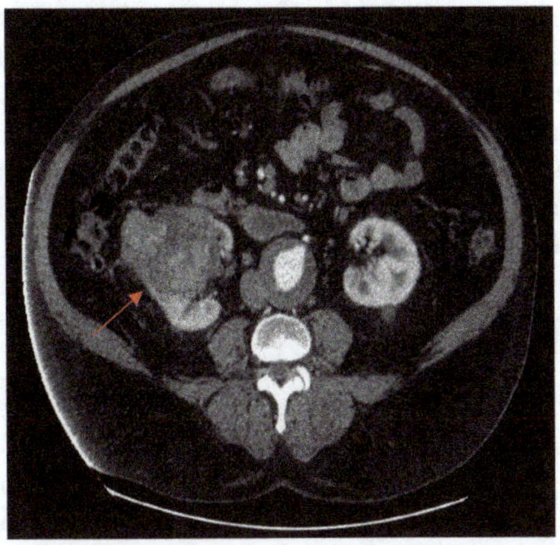

Figure 1: Right lower pole, anterior renal mass.

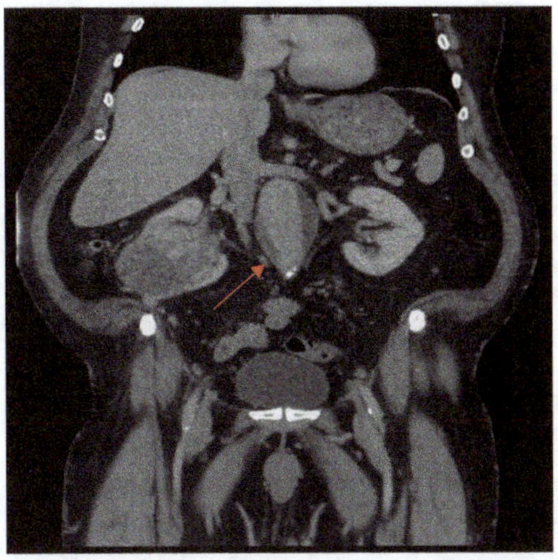

Figure 2: Abdominal aortic aneurysm (AAA).

## 2. Case Report

A 61-year-old obese Caucasian male with past medical history of smoking, hypertension, chronic obstructive pulmonary disease (COPD), and sleep apnea presented in consultation to the hematology clinic with newly-diagnosed polycythemia with an elevated hemoglobin level (22.4 g/dL), elevated hematocrit (66.9%), and high partial thromboplastic time (40.9 sec). The polycythemia with high hemoglobin and hematocrit levels were first discovered during a preoperative work-up for a planned elective rotator cuff surgery. Due to concern for increased clot formation during elective surgery, the patient was referred to the hematology clinic for further evaluation and treatment.

Despite the newly-diagnosed polycythemia, the patient denied any significant symptoms or history of blood clots. Further evaluation by the hematologist was conducted using a renal ultrasound as well as cross-sectional imaging of the abdomen and pelvis with computerized tomography (CT) scan to determine the underlying cause of the polycythemia in this patient. The ultrasound and CT scan imaging showed a large 10 cm right lower pole, anterior renal mass suspicious for renal cell carcinoma of the right kidney, as shown in Figure 1. The patient's renal cell carcinoma was diagnosed as a T2N0M0 according to the Tumor, Nodes, and Metastasis staging system, which evaluates a renal cell carcinoma according to its size/infiltration to surrounding anatomical structures, lymph node enlargement, or metastasis to surrounding organs [11]. A paraneoplastic syndrome was suspected to account for the patient's polycythemia and elevated hemoglobin. An incidental AAA measuring 6 cm in the juxtarenal position with normal bilateral iliac arteries was also appreciated on imaging, as shown in Figure 2.

For definitive diagnosis and treatment of the patient's suspected right lower pole, anterior renal mass as well as treatment of the patient's polycythemia secondary to a suspected paraneoplastic syndrome, open right radical nephrectomy was recommended. Additionally, given the current size of the juxtarenal AAA with >50% risk of rupture, open repair of the AAA with Dacron tube graft was also recommended in the same operative setting.

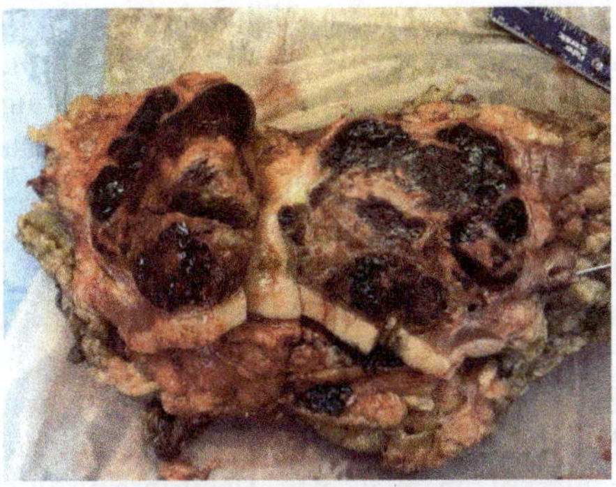

Figure 3: Renal carcinoma confined to capsule.

Subsequently, an open repair of the juxtarenal AAA with a 24 mm Dacron tube graft with open right radical nephrectomy was successfully performed on the patient several days later through a large, midline abdominal incision with minimal blood loss (50 ml). There were no immediate perioperative or postoperative complications, and the patient recovered well after the surgery and was discharged home on postoperative day 5. The patient's preoperative hemoglobin and erythropoietin level was 18.3 g/dL and 8.5 IU/L respectively, which normalized to a hemoglobin level of 13.1 g/dL within 2-3 days after the surgery. Subsequent measurements months after the surgery measured hemoglobin to be 12.0 g/dL. The patient's blood pressure pre- and postoperatively was measured to be 145/85 mmHg to consistently 120/70 mmHg. No further treatment or surgical interventions were required. The tumor was confined by renal capsule, limited to the kidney situated 1 mm away from the renal pelvis, as shown in Figure 3. Histological sections of the tumor showed predominantly hemorrhagic and infarcted tumor with only a small focus of viable tumor. The sections showed tumor cells with abundant clear cytoplasm and inconspicuous nucleoli consistent with a clear cell renal cell carcinoma Fuhrman grade 1, as shown in Figure 4. The patient was followed for a year and half after the surgery with significant improvement on physical exam and normalized hemoglobin, blood pressure, and EPO values.

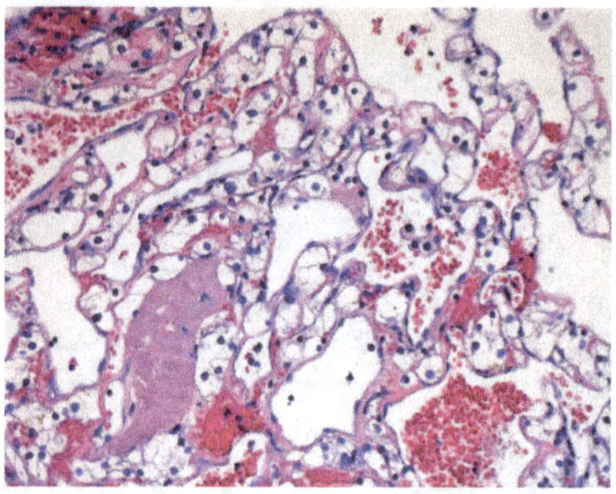

FIGURE 4: Microscopy image of resected tumor showing clear cell renal cell carcinoma.

## 3. Discussion

In this case report, the patient exhibited two of the three most common paraneoplastic syndromes associated with renal cell carcinoma: polycythemia and hypertension. Although several mechanisms have been proposed to explain hypertension in renal cell carcinoma patients, current studies suggest that the vasoactive peptides endothelin-1, urotensin-II, and adrenomedullin are likely to be involved [12–18]. Furthermore, polycythemia also contributes to hypertension through the upregulation of hypoxia inducible factor-1 (HIF-1) from renal cancer and epithelial cells increasing EPO production [19–21]. Under physiological states, tissue hypoxia stimulates peritubular fibroblast in the renal cortical labyrinth producing EPO, which stimulates the bone marrow to produce red blood cells [22]. In many renal cell carcinomas, EPO receptors in the renal proximal tubule are overexpressed hastening tumor growth through increased angiogenesis [22]. Furthermore, increased EPO receptor expression is correlated with a worse prognosis in renal carcinoma patients [23, 24]. Despite elevated EPO receptor and serum levels, a significant proportion of renal cell carcinoma patients exhibit anemia and polycythemia, which may result from EPO hyporesponsiveness, iron deficiency, and chronic inflammation [10].

Among renal cell carcinoma patients, 66% have elevated EPO levels despite only 8% having polycythemia [4]. Furthermore, 20% of renal cell carcinoma patients have hypercalcemia while 40% have hypertension [4]. In this light, the finding of renal cell carcinoma and normal EPO levels was both surprising and unique. In this patient, a significant proportion of the renal cell carcinoma was necrotic upon examination, which possibly decreased the number of EPO secreting cells and lowered serum EPO levels. The normal EPO level is likely to involve in the renal cell carcinoma, contralateral kidney, and the patient's medical comorbidities. One study suggests that renal cell carcinoma cells may produce an inactive form of EPO, which may explain the lack of erythrocytosis in renal cell carcinoma patients with elevated EPO levels [25]. However, the contralateral kidney of the patient was unaffected and had the ability to compensate for the loss of EPO. A retrospective analysis of partial or complete nephrectomies showed that the contralateral kidney successfully maintained renal function and hemodynamics for several years after surgical resection [26]. Therefore, it is likely the contralateral kidney may compensate for reduced EPO production and other hemodynamic factors necessary for maintaining proper homeostasis. A recent study also found male gender and tumor size were positively correlated with an increase in contralateral kidney volume after a complete nephrectomy [27]. Therefore, the complete nephrectomy puts an increases metabolic requirement for the contralateral kidney to maintain the proper homeostasis through secretion of EPO and other humoral factors.

Furthermore, the patient's concurrent COPD, sleep apnea, and smoking history should increase EPO levels through hypoxic stimulation. Measurements of EPO levels in COPD found higher levels of EPO levels under anemic conditions [28, 29]. However, chronic COPD exacerbations can produce low EPO levels through systemic inflammatory processes mediated by proinflammatory cytokines, such as interleukin-1 (IL-1) and tumor necrosis factor-$\alpha$ (TNF-$\alpha$) [29–31]. Sleep apnea can stimulate EPO production in the contralateral side through hypoxic stimulation. Interestingly, sleep apnea is associated with increased renal cell carcinoma tumor growth through vascularization processes mediated by vascular endothelial growth factor (VEGF) [32]. The patient's sleep apnea in this case may explain the significant tumor growth and necrotic tissue present in the gross pathology examination. Although no study has systematically examined the mechanism underlying renal cell carcinoma and low EPO levels, the patient's history of COPD, smoking, and sleep apnea and the presence of a functioning contralateral kidney provide a mechanism through which EPO levels are maintained during and after the removal of a renal cells carcinoma.

Further investigation is required to elucidate the mechanism underlying a decrease in EPO level in the presence of both renal cell carcinoma and chronic respiratory syndromes. In either case, surgical removal of the renal cell carcinoma and repair of surrounding vasculature successfully resolve most complications [33–35]. Specifically, it is unknown whether serum EPO levels correlate with the severity of renal cell carcinoma evaluated through the TNM. Given the rising interest and reports of surgical complications of concomitant conditions with renal cell carcinoma, more investigation into the mechanism, occurrence, and additional risk factors posed by these paraneoplastic syndromes secondary to renal cell carcinoma remains open to investigation [34, 36, 37].

## References

[1] J. Ferlay, H.-R. Shin, F. Bray, D. Forman, C. Mathers, and D. M. Parkin, "Estimates of worldwide burden of cancer in 2008: globocan 2008," *International Journal of Cancer*, vol. 127, no. 12, pp. 2893–2917, 2010.

[2] J. J. Hsieh, M. P. Purdue, S. Signoretti et al., "Renal cell carcinoma," *Nature Reviews Disease Primers*, vol. 3, no. 1, 2017.

[3] W.-H. Chow, L. M. Dong, and S.S. Devesa, "Epidemiology and risk factors for kidney cancer," *Nature Reviews Urology*, vol. 7, no. 5, pp. 245–257, 2010.

[4] G. S. Palapettu, B. Kristo, and J. Rajfer, "Paraneoplastic syndromes in urologic malignancy: the many faces of renal cell carcinoma," *Reviews in Urology*, vol. 4, no. 4, pp. 163–170, 2002.

[5] D. Tarin, "Update on clinical and mechanistic aspects of paraneoplastic syndromes," *Cancer and Metastasis Reviews*, vol. 32, no. 3-4, pp. 707–721, 2013.

[6] J. W. Harrison, R. Cherukuri, and D. Buchan, "Renal cell carcinoma presenting with paraneoplastic hallucinations and cognitive decline from limbic encephalitis," *Journal of General Internal Medicine*, vol. 30, no. 7, pp. 1037–1040, 2015.

[7] T. Klein, S. Rotterdam, J. Noldus, and A. Hinkel, "Bullous pemphigoid is a rare paraneoplastic syndrome in patients with renal cell carcinoma," *Scandinavian Journal of Urology and Nephrology*, vol. 43, no. 4, pp. 334–336, 2009.

[8] S. Sullivan, "Paraneoplastic cough and renal cell carcinoma," *Canadian Respiratory Journal*, vol. 2016, pp. 1–3, 2016.

[9] D. M. Moreira, B. Gershman, C. M. Lohse et al., "Paraneoplastic syndromes are associated with adverse prognosis among patients with renal cell carcinoma undergoing nephrectomy," *World Journal of Urology*, vol. 34, no. 10, pp. 1465–1472, 2016.

[10] C. Morais, D. W. Johnson, D. A. Vesey, and G. C. Gobe, "Functional significance of erythropoietin in renal cell carcinoma," *BMC Cancer*, vol. 13, no. 1, 2013.

[11] V. Ficarra, A. Galfano, M. Mancini, G. Martignoni, and W. Artibani, "TNM staging system for renal-cell carcinoma: current status and future perspectives," *The Lancet Oncology*, vol. 8, no. 6, pp. 554–558, 2007.

[12] M. Stojanovic, B. Goldner, and D. Ivkovic, "Renal cell carcinoma and arterial hypertension," *Clinical and Experimental Nephrology*, vol. 13, no. 4, pp. 295–299, 2009.

[13] M. Murai and M. Oya, "Renal cell carcinoma: etiology, incidence and epidemiology," *Current Opinion in Urology*, vol. 14, no. 4, pp. 229–233, 2004.

[14] K. Takahashi, K. Totsune, and O. Murakami, "Expression of three vasoactive peptides, urotensin-II, adrenomedullin, and endothelin-1, in a human renal cell carcinoma cell line VMRC-RCW," *Clinical and Experimental Nephrology*, vol. 5, no. 4, pp. 246–249, 2001.

[15] R. M. Touyz and E. L. Schiffrin, "Role of endothelin in human hypertension," *Canadian Journal of Physiology and Pharmacology*, vol. 81, no. 6, pp. 533–541, 2003.

[16] M. Iglarz and E. L. Schiffrin, "Role of endothelin-1 in hypertension," *Current Hypertension Reports*, vol. 5, no. 2, pp. 144–148, 2003.

[17] E. L. Schiffrin, "Vascular endothelin in hypertension," *Vascular Pharmacology*, vol. 43, no. 1, pp. 19–29, 2005.

[18] C. Feldstein and C. Romero, "Role of endothelins in hypertension," *American Journal of Therapeutics*, vol. 14, no. 2, pp. 147–153, 2007.

[19] M. Krieg, R. Haas, H. Brauch, T. Acker, I. Flamme, and K. H. Plate, "Up-regulation of hypoxia-inducible factors HIF-1$\alpha$ and HIF-2$\alpha$ under normoxic conditions in renal carcinoma cells by von Hippel-Lindau tumor suppressor gene loss of function," *Oncogene*, vol. 19, no. 48, pp. 5435–5443, 2000.

[20] H. F. Bunn and R. O. Poyton, "Oxygen sensing and molecular adaptation to hypoxia," *Physiological Reviews*, vol. 76, no. 3, pp. 839–885, 1996.

[21] G. L. Semenza, "Regulation of mammalian $O_2$ homeostasis by hypoxia-inducible factor 1," *Annual Review of Cell and Developmental Biology*, vol. 15, no. 1, pp. 551–578, 1999.

[22] C. Westenfelder and R. L. Baranowski, "Erythropoietin stimulates proliferation of human renal carcinoma cells," *Kidney International*, vol. 58, no. 2, pp. 647–657, 2000.

[23] K. Ito, H. Yoshii, T. Asano et al., "Impact of increased erythropoietin receptor expression and elevated serum erythropoietin levels on clinicopathological features and prognosis in renal cell carcinoma," *Experimental and Therapeutic Medicine*, vol. 3, no. 6, pp. 937–944, 2012.

[24] B. Ljungberg, T. Rasmuson, and K. Grankvist, "Erythropoietin in renai celi carcinoma: evaluation of its usefulness as a tumor marker," *European Urology*, vol. 21, no. 2, pp. 160–163, 1992.

[25] D. Shouval and J. B. Sherwood, "Production of erythropoietin by an established human renal carcinoma cell line: in vitro and in vivo studies," in *Advances in Experimental Medicine and Biology*, M. Tavassoli, E. D. Zanjani, J. L. Ascensao, N. G. Abraham, and A. S. Levine, Eds., pp. 319–328, Springer, Boston, MA, USA, 1988.

[26] T. Nohara, "Editorial comment to postoperative renal function after partial nephrectomy for renal cell carcinoma in patients with pre-existing chronic kidney disease: a comparison with radical nephrectomy," *International Journal of Urology*, vol. 18, no. 6, p. 477, 2011.

[27] B. H. Park, S. R. Bae, Y. S. Lee, S. H. Kang, and C. H. Han, "Tumor size is associated with compensatory hypertrophy in the contralateral kidney before and after radical nephrectomy in patients with renal cell carcinoma," *European Urology Supplements*, vol. 16, no. 3, pp. e1337–e1338, 2017.

[28] M. John, S. Hoernig, W. Doehner, D. Okonko, D. C. Witt, and S. D. Anker, "Anemia and inflammation in COPD," *Chest*, vol. 127, no. 3, pp. 825–829, 2005.

[29] A. G. El Gazzar, G. F. Al Mehy, T. M. Gouda, O. S. El-Shaer, and S. H. Mohammed, "Evaluation of erythropoietin hormone in chronic obstructive pulmonary disease patients during exacerbation and after remission," *Egyptian Journal of Chest Diseases and Tuberculosis*, vol. 66, no. 1, pp. 27–32, 2017.

[30] E. Sala, C. Balaguer, C. Villena et al., "Low erythropoietin plasma levels during exacerbations of COPD," *Respiration*, vol. 80, no. 3, pp. 190–197, 2010.

[31] K. La Ferla, C. Reimann, W. Jelkmann, and T. Hellwig-Bürgel, "Inhibition of erythropoietin gene expression signaling involves the transcription factors GATA-2 and NF-$\kappa$B," *The FASEB Journal*, vol. 16, no. 13, pp. 1811–1813, 2002.

[32] A. Vilaseca, N. Campillo, M. Torres et al., "Intermittent hypoxia increases kidney tumor vascularization in a murine model of sleep apnea," *PLoS One*, vol. 12, no. 6, p. e0179444, 2017.

[33] B. R. Konety, B. Shuman, M. Webster, D. L. Steed, and R. R. Bahnson, "Simultaneous radical nephrectomy and repair of abdominal aortic aneurysm," *Urology*, vol. 47, no. 6, pp. 813–818, 1996.

[34] G. F. Veraldi, S. Tasselli, G. De Manzoni, and C. Cordiano, "Surgical treatment of abdominal aortic aneurysm with concomitant renal cell carcinoma: a single-centre experience with review of the literature," *The Journal of Cardiovascular Surgery*, vol. 47, no. 6, pp. 643–649, 2006.

[35] S. Howe, R. Taylor, B. Halloran, S. Smith, T. Lynch, and B. Baxter, "Management of synchronous renal cell carcinoma and aortic disease," *The American Journal of Surgery*, vol. 170, no. 2, pp. 231–234, 1995.

[36] A. D. Silverstein, A. Z. Weizer, and E. E. Anderson, "Ruptured abdominal aortic aneurysm complicated by horseshoe kidney and renal cell carcinoma," *Urology*, vol. 60, no. 6, p. 1108, 2002.

[37] P. G. John and M. Ross, "Staged minimally invasive treatment of inflammatory abdominal aortic aneurysm and renal cell carcinoma," *The Canadian Journal of Urology*, vol. 16, no. 2, pp. 4596–4598, 2009.

# 9

# Superselective Embolization with Microcoil and Gelfoam for High-Flow Priapism Secondary to Bilateral Cavernous Fistulae: A Case Study

**Sarah Prattley, Timothy Bryant, and Rowland Rees**

*University Hospital Southampton, Tremona Road, Southampton, Hampshire SO166YD, UK*

Correspondence should be addressed to Sarah Prattley; sarah.prattley@nhs.net

Academic Editor: Khaled Madbouly

*Background.* High-flow priapism is rare, and bilateral arteriocavernous fistulae formation following trauma is rarer still. Management of high-flow priapism is conservative either through observation, use of ice packs, mechanical decompression, or intracavernosal injection of $\alpha$-adrenergic agonists, giving temporary results in selected cases. Alternatively, superselective arteriography with embolization is widely accepted. However, intervention needs to be mindful of the potential impact on long-term potency. We report the first case of bilateral arteriocavernous fistulae managed with both Gelfoam and microcoil embolization. *Case Study.* We present the case of a 35-year-old gentleman who attended the emergency department nine days following a fall from a moped, where he sustained bruising to his perineum, with persistent nonpainful erection. CT angiogram demonstrated bilateral arteriovenous fistulas. Management with superselective catheterisation and embolization with Gelfoam and microcoil was successful with resolution of symptoms. Long-term follow-up has shown return to normal erectile function twelve months following the injury. *Outcomes.* Concern regarding the effect to long-term erectile function has previously led to delayed bilateral embolization. Selection of embolization material can be tailored to the anatomical features of the fistula to help preserve function.

## 1. Introduction

High-flow priapism is rare, and bilateral arteriovenous fistulae formation following trauma is rarer still [1]. Intervention needs to be mindful of the potential impact on long-term potency [2]. We present the case of a 35-year-old gentleman who sustained bilateral arteriovenous fistulae secondary to a moped injury. Following superselective catheterisation and embolization with Gelfoam and microcoil his symptoms resolved. Long-term follow-up has shown return to normal erectile function twelve months following the injury.

## 2. Case Study

A 35-year-old gentleman presented nine days following a fall from a moped, where he sustained bruising to his perineum, but no other significant injuries. Since the incident he had developed a persistent priapism that was nonpainful, with just mild discomfort on walking. He had no lower urinary tract symptoms.

On examination there was a grade IV erection with a rigid base and shaft with slight dorsal curvature of 10 degrees, which was nontender. There was a superficial haematoma present to the scrotum and base of penis. A corporal blood gas was taken which showed pH 7.415, pCO2 5.55, and pO2 11.0, consistent with high-flow priapism.

The ultrasound Doppler did not demonstrate any evidence of fistula and had contradictory Doppler traces; therefore a CT angiogram was performed both to further evaluate the pathology and to provide anatomical arterial information. The CT demonstrated evidence of arterial pooling within the bulbar segments of the corpora cavernosa bilaterally, in-keeping with a high flow, nonischaemic priapism (Figure 1). A discussion was held with the patient regarding the options of embolization of both internal pudendal arteries versus conservative management, along with the risks of each. The patient opted for embolization.

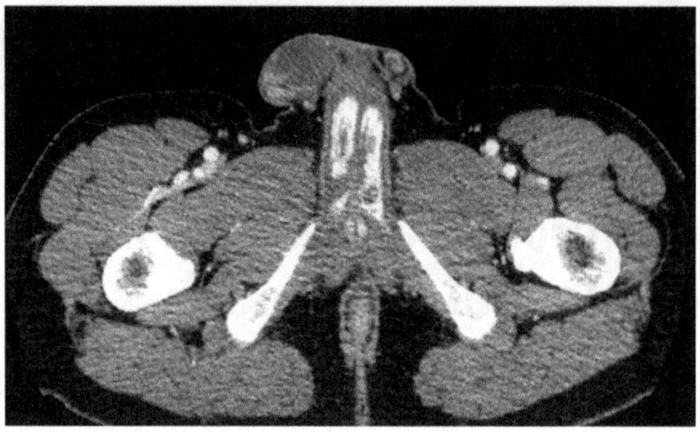

Figure 1: CT depicting bilateral arteriocavernous fistulae with pooling of contrast medium in the corpora.

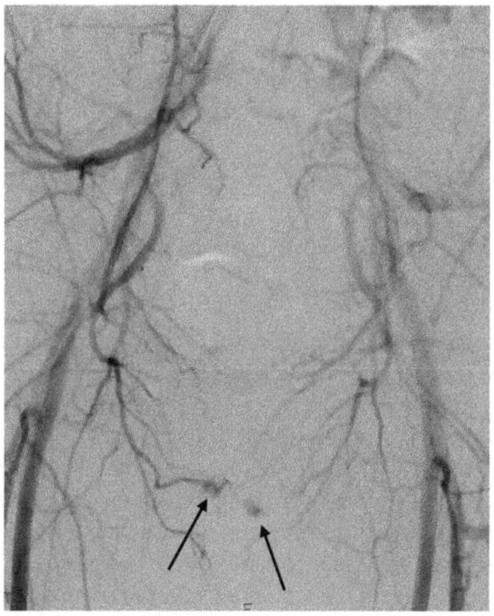

Figure 2: Angiography depicting extravasation of contrast at the sites of arteriocavernous fistulae.

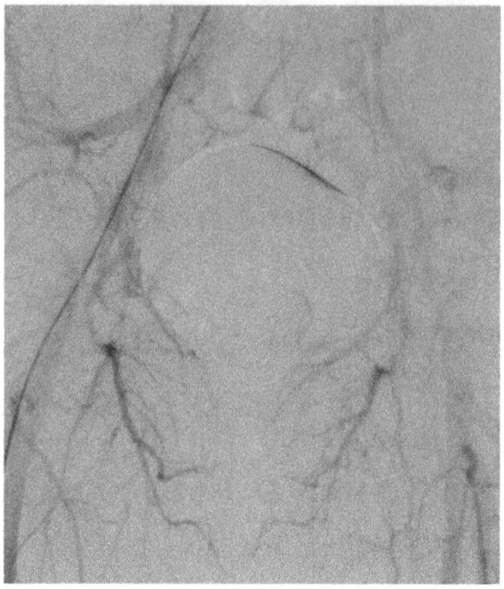

Figure 3: After procedure, no extravasation of contrast following successful embolization.

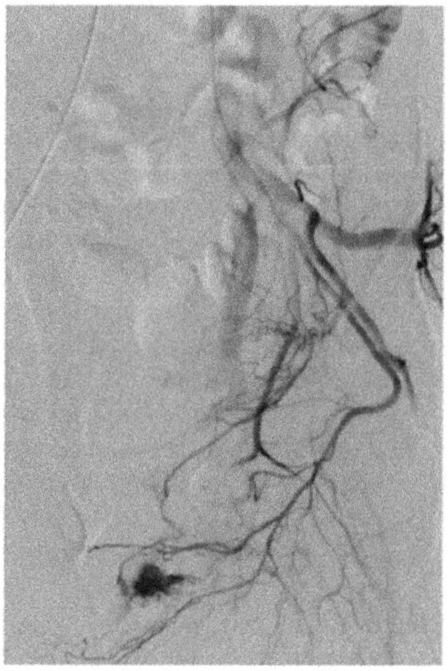

Figure 4: Left arteriocavernous fistula supplied by both the left internal pudendal artery and an accessory pudendal branch of the anterior prostatic artery from the obturator artery.

The right common femoral artery was cannulated under ultrasound guidance, and aortography was performed which confirmed bilateral cavernosal fistulae. The internal pudendal arteries were bilaterally catheterised using a 4-French C2 cobra catheter. The left fistula received supply from the branches of the left internal pudendal artery and an accessory pudendal branch of the anterior prostatic artery which came off the obturator (Figures 2 and 4). Both vessels were superselectively catheterised using a 2.4fr Direxion microcatheter and 0.016 Fathom guidewire. Due to the polyarterial supply to the fistula embolization with absorbable gelatine sponge (Spongostan, Ethicon, Johnson & Johnson Medical N.V, Belgium) was selected. Absorbable gelatine sponge (Gelfoam) is temporary embolic which resorbs within four to six weeks. The sponge sheet is cut into 1-2mm pledgets which are mixed with contrast and passed through a 3-way tap to create a slurry prior to injection. This resulted in satisfactory occlusion of the fistula and persistent good antegrade flow within the nontarget vessels (Figures 3 and 5). On the right a single fistula from a distal branch of the right internal pudendal was present (Figures 2 and 6) and superselectively catheterised beyond the dorsal penile branch and embolized just proximal to the fistula using microcoils (2mm Soft platinum Type-A, Cookmedical, Bloomington, USA) (Figure 7). Postembolization angiography showed satisfactory results with no further filling of the cavernosal fistulas (Figures 3 and 7).

This patient has been sequentially reviewed in our Urology Outpatient Clinic to assess his ongoing recovery. Self-reported erectile function has slowly improved over the course of twelve months, without the need to use PDE-5 inhibitors. At one year his erections have returned to baseline.

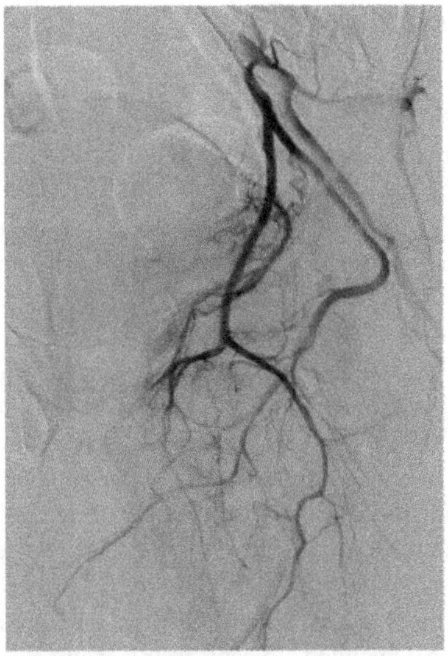

FIGURE 5: Cessation of fistula following Gelfoam embolization.

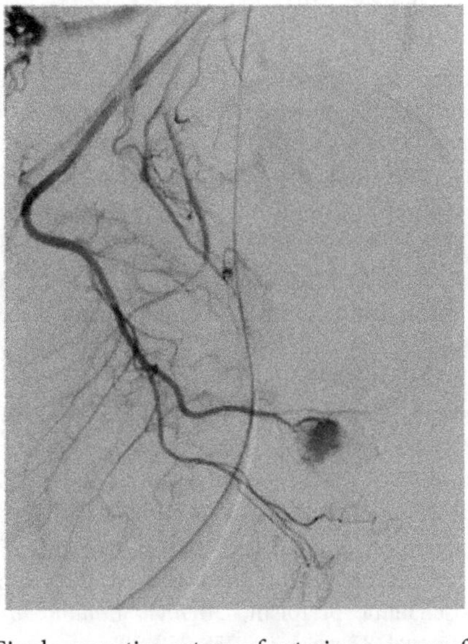

FIGURE 6: Single causative artery of arteriocavernous fistula being the distal branch of the right internal pudendal artery.

## 3. Discussion

First described by Burt *et al.* in 1960 following traumatic coitus, high-flow priapism is typically caused by trauma resulting in damage to the cavernosal artery, or one of its branches [3]. This leads to arteriovenous fistula formation and unregulated pooling of blood within the sinusoidal space propagating a nonischaemic erection due to the continuous supply of oxygenated blood. The corpora are typically tumescent but not rigid and lack the symptom of pain caused by ischaemia and can continue for a prolonged period of time [4].

Typically, ultrasound Doppler scan demonstrated "low resistance, high-velocity" arterial waveform, with the sensitivity being nearly 100% [5]. This, however, was not the case

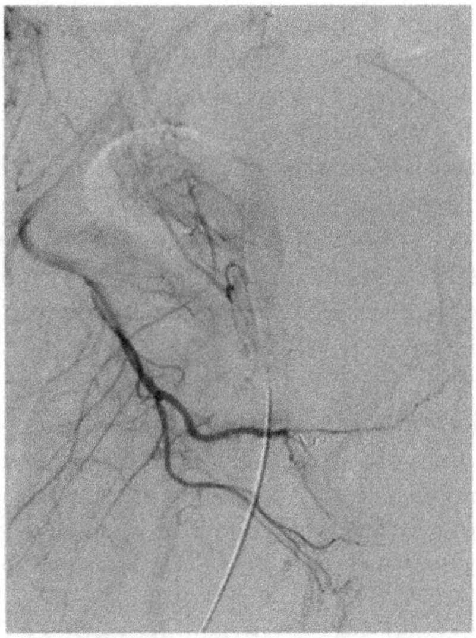

FIGURE 7: Microcoil embolization of the distal branch of the right internal pudendal artery.

with our patient and the colour Doppler result was not in-keeping with his clinical presentation; therefore progression to CT angiogram was necessary. The reason for this is not fully understood, but the proximal nature of the fistula may have degraded evaluation of the cavernosal arteries.

While arteriography is not used for diagnostic purposes due to its invasive nature, it is first assessed during superselective embolization for identification of the causative arteries. Penile arteriography will demonstrate outflow of the contrast medium into the corpora cavernosa from the arterial-sinusoidal fistula and will demonstrate a pooling effect (Figures 2, 4, and 6) [6]. Our patient had bilateral arteriocavernous fistulae; therefore it is essential that both sides were imaged accordingly.

Bilateral arteriocavernous fistulae formation is rare, with few cases being reported in current literature. Management of high-flow priapism is conservative either through observation, use of ice packs, mechanical decompression, or intracavernosal injection of $\alpha$-adrenergic agonists giving temporary results in selected cases [7]. Alternatively, superselective arteriography with embolization is widely accepted [7].

There is potential concern for erectile dysfunction in the treatment of bilateral arteriocavernous fistulae particularly with the use of microcoils [2]. In order to attempt to avoid bilateral embolization, a previously reported case from Davies *et al.* found adequate detumescence with unilateral embolization despite bilateral shunting [8]. Further reported attempts at unilateral embolization have not been as successful; the studies of both Lee et al. and Gujral et al. found that unilateral embolization resulted in return of symptoms shortly following the procedure [1, 9]. Lazinger *et al.* waited 20 days between autologous blood clot embolizations of each side to see if resolution occurred; however further embolization was required [10].

Bilateral embolization has been reported with the use of both Gelfoam and microcoil with excellent results, despite the potential for erectile dysfunction. Materials such as blood autologous clots and Gelfoam are typically preferred due to the recanalization of arterial supply following temporary interruption [11]. Accurate placement can be challenging as the material is nonopaque; however, it can be mixed with contrast to aid this. The use of microcoil for bilateral embolization is more of a concern due to the potential risk of erectile dysfunction [2]; however, to date it has also yielded good results with patients returning to normal erectile function at day two and six weeks after procedure [1, 9].

The selection of embolization material for our patient was based upon the arterial supply to his fistulae. The right side was supplied by a singular cavernosal branch off the internal pudendal artery; therefore a microcoil was used. The left side, however, was supplied by at least two arteries: the distal branches of the internal pudendal and an accessory internal pudendal branch of the anterior prostatic branch which came off the obturator artery. Therefore, to allow restoration of blood flow in the long-term and to reduce the risk of erectile dysfunction Gelfoam was selected. To our knowledge this is the first reported case to use multiple materials for embolization for this presentation.

Function following bilateral embolization for all patients appears to be excellent, with restoration of normal function in all cases within a year without the need for adjuncts [1, 8–10]. Timely nature of intervention may be essential for patients with high-flow priapism in order to reduce the risk of erectile dysfunction [11]. There is currently no recommended time interval to allow conservative measures to work and for spontaneous resolution of the fistula. In a case series by Zacharakis *et al.* six patients were reviewed who underwent conservative management for 2–12 weeks following presentation, average 4.5 weeks, which eventually led to embolization as a definitive form of management. Erectile dysfunction was noted in all six patients with a reduction in IIEF-5 score, with them requiring either PDE-5 inhibitors, intracavernosal injections, or a penile prosthesis [11]. Therefore, it may be prudent that definitive intervention with superselective embolization takes place without delay to avoid potential risk of erectile dysfunction, or that the patient is aware of this risk.

## 4. Conclusion

Bilateral arteriocavernous fistula for high-flow priapism is rare; however superselective embolization with either autologous clot, Gelfoam, or microcoil appears to yield good restorative outcomes with normal levels of potency at twelve months. Potential risk of erectile dysfunction needs to be borne in mind, particularly if multiple feeding arteries are present, with selection of absorbable material being recommended in this instance. Timely intervention needs to be considered to avoid the potential risk of erectile dysfunction in the long term from conservative measures.

## References

[1] Y. Lee, J. Shen, M. Shih, C. Chen, Y. Chou, and C. Huang, "Bilateral superselective arterial microcoil embolization in post-traumatic high-flow priapism: a case report," *Kaohsiung Journal of Medical Sciences*, vol. 19, no. 2, pp. 79–82, 2003.

[2] R. K. Kerlan Jr., R. L. Gordon, J. M. Laberge, and E. J. Ring, "Superselective microcoil embolization in the management of high-flow priapism," *Journal of Vascular and Interventional Radiology*, vol. 9, no. 1, pp. 85–89, 1998.

[3] F. B. Burt, H. K. Schirmer, and W. W. Scott, "A new concept in the management of priapism," *The Journal of Urology*, vol. 83, no. 1, pp. 60-61, 1960.

[4] G. A. Broderick, A. Kadioglu, T. J. Bivalacqua, H. Ghanem, A. Nehra, and R. Shamloul, "Priapism: pathogenesis, epidemiology, and management," *The Journal of Sexual Medicine*, vol. 7, no. 1, part 2, pp. 476–500, 2010.

[5] L. S. Hakim, H. Kulaksizoglu, R. Mulligan, A. Greenfield, and I. Goldstein, "Evolving concepts in the diagnosis and treatment of arterial high flow priapism," *The Journal of Urology*, vol. 155, pp. 541–548, 1996.

[6] K. Shigehara and M. Namiki, "Clinical management of priapism: a review," *The World Journal of Men's Health*, vol. 34, no. 1, pp. 1–8, 2016.

[7] D. K. Montague, J. Jarow, G. A. Broderick et al., "American urological association guideline on the management of priapism," *The Journal of Urology*, vol. 170, no. 4, pp. 1318–1324, 2003.

[8] N. Davies, F. Nuwayhid, and J. J. Froelich, "Idiopathic high-flow priapism due to bilateral internal pudendal artery shunting," *ANZ Journal of Surgery*, vol. 86, no. 12, pp. 1059–1061, 2016.

[9] S. Gujral, R. P. MacDonagh, and P. M. Cavanagh, "Bilateral superselective arterial microcoil embolisation in delayed post-traumatic high flow priapism," *Postgraduate Medical Journal*, vol. 77, no. 905, pp. 193-194, 2001.

[10] M. Lazinger, C. F. Beckmann, A. Cossi, and R. A. Roth, "Selective embolization of bilateral arterial cavernous fistulas for posttraumatic penile arterial priapism," *CardioVascular and Interventional Radiology*, vol. 19, no. 4, pp. 281–284, 1996.

[11] E. Zacharakis, D. J. Ralph, M. Walkden, and A. Muneer, "Distal corpus cavernosum fibrosis and erectile dysfunction secondary to non-ischaemic priapism," *Archivio Italiano di Urologia e Andrologia*, vol. 87, no. 3, pp. 258-259, 2015.

# 10

# Ureteral Guidewire Looping and Entrapment above an Impacted Ureter Stone

**Aikaterini Tsionga, Anastasios Anastasiadis, Wilbert Fana Mutomba, Dimitrios Memmos, Ioannis Vakalopoulos, and Georgios Dimitriadis**

*1st Department of Urology, Aristotle University of Thessaloniki, Ethnikis Aminis 41, 54635 Thessaloniki, Greece*

Correspondence should be addressed to Aikaterini Tsionga; kate.tsionga@hotmail.com

Academic Editor: Giorgio Carmignani

We present a rare case of a hydrophilic guidewire looping and entrapment in the ureter of a patient with an impacted stone in the proximal ureter during a simple double-J stent insertion. Looping of guidewire is a rare complication in urology and only few cases have been described. In that case, release and removal of the entrapped guidewire was possible only after one step fragmentation of the stone with laser lithotripsy.

## 1. Introduction

Guidewires play a significant role in many medical specialties [1]. They were initially developed for vascular procedures [2], but are also nowadays an essential tool in endourology. Although they are used by urologists to perform various advanced procedures, such as to insert a ureteral stent, to dilate the ureter or gain percutaneous access to the kidney, they are frequently associated with potential complications. Bleeding, kinking, false passages, and perforation are some of the usual complications [3]. Looping, usually combined with knotting, is a situation more commonly described during intravascular application of guidewires [1, 4]. Nevertheless, looping above the stone and entrapment of a guidewire inside the ureter is an extremely rare complication. There is only one case in the literature, where the authors present looping of a guidewire below the stone during rigid ureteroscopy and laser lithotripsy [5].

## 2. Case Presentation

A 57-year-old man was referred to our department by a district hospital, after a previous unsuccessful effort of a double-J ureteral stent placement without real-time fluoroscopy. The patient arrived at the emergency department with both parts of a guidewire (Terumo RadiofocusR Guidewire, 180 cm) protruding out of his urethral meatus (Figure 1). The intravenous urography (IVU), which had been performed at the district hospital after the failed stent insertion, revealed a right proximal ureteral obstructing stone with approximate maximal diameter 9 mm (9 × 4 × 6 mm) and the guidewire looping above it (Figure 2). IVU was performed instead of CT urography due to unavailability of CT urography at the referring center. The admission laboratory tests revealed no leukocytosis (WBC $10900 \times 10^3/\mu L$) and normal serum creatinine values (Cre 0.85 mg/dL). Rest of laboratory exams were normal. Also patient was in a good general clinical status.

Our first step was to pull gently one end of the guidewire under fluoroscopic guidance and local anesthesia, but our effort was unsuccessful. Next, we inserted another hybrid guidewire (Sensor™ Straight Tip, Boston Scientific), which could not bypass the stone and was looping under it. The retrograde urography showed full stop of the contrast at the level of the stone and no extravasation was revealed. Since the patient had no signs of infection, we decided to continue our handling under general anesthesia, so we could inspect the ureter with the semirigid ureteroscope (Karl Storz, 27002L, 43 cm length, 9.5 Fr). The ureteroscope was advanced easily up to the stone. The guidewire had initially perforated the mucosa of the ureter under the impacted stone, was looping intraluminally above the stone, returned submucosally and finally passed intraluminally to get out of the ureter orifice

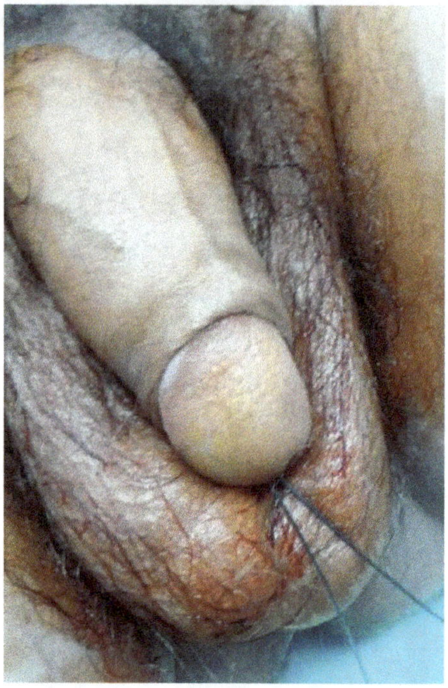

FIGURE 1: Both parts of the guidewire protruding out of the urethral meatus.

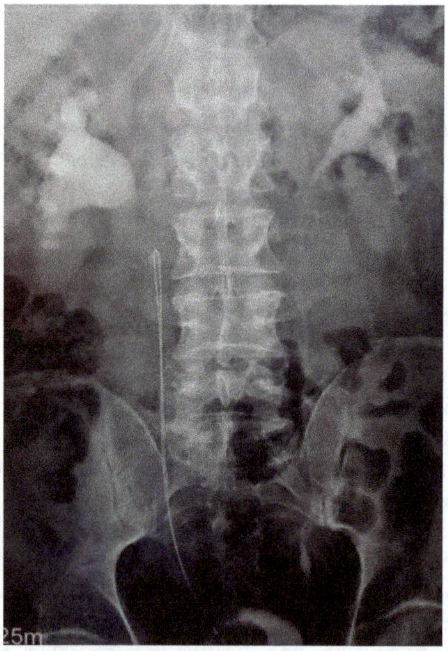

FIGURE 2: IVU reveals a right proximal ureteral obstructing stone and the guidewire looping above it.

and out of the meatus. Subsequently, we performed an active stone removal via laser lithotripsy (Dornier. Medilas H Solvo, laser fiber 600 $\mu$m). The entrapped guidewire was released after fragmentation of the stone and was easily removed from the ureter. Finally, a 7F-28 cm open-end double-J stent was placed over the second guidewire fluoroscopically. The patient was discharged the next day, with no complications after the ureteroscopy and the entrapped guidewire removal. The double-J was removed after two weeks under local anesthesia without any adverse events.

## 3. Discussion

As was mentioned before, guidewires are a frequently used tool that allows urologists to perform a great variety of endoscopic procedures, many times challenging and difficult ones. But, as with any tool in medicine, training is necessary to apply guidewires with safety and should be used by someone experienced [1]. There are basic principles and tips when using endourology tools, which could prevent undesirable complications.

In our case, the first attempt of double-J placement at the district hospital had been performed without fluoroscopic guidance. If the motion of the guidewire was monitored by fluoroscopy, looping direction might have been avoided. In addition, the length of the guidewire (180 cm, use in vascular surgery procedures) made it easier to form a loop inside the ureter, to come out of the ureteral orifice and out of the urethral meatus. Furthermore, if excessive force is applied when inserting the guidewire, the tip may perforate the wall and progress submucosally or advance outside the ureter. Especially, if the guidewire is forced blindly without fluoroscopy, it is difficult for the operator to realize in time the false route. Gentle maneuvers under fluoroscopy guidance and repositioning of the guidewire when operator feels resistance are important for a safe stent placement [1].

Also, when the urologist deals with impacted stones, needs to be aware that the ureteral wall at the level of the obstruction is oedematous and the guidewire may traumatize and perforate the ureteral wall even with the appliance of little force by the surgeon.

Guidewires can be found in various sizes, materials, tip design, and rigidity and each one has been developed for specific clinical use. They are used for achieving safe access to any part of the urinary system and as a guide over which stents and catheters can be passed. Guidewires with an atraumatic, flexible, and hydrophilic tip are appropriate for passing over obstructions in the urinary tract, while a wire with stiff shaft is required to place a stent over it [6]. Hybrid wires (nitilol guidewire with hydrophilic tip) seem to be the most preferable choice for safe access [7]. Different types of guidewires should be available at urology departments and the operators should be familiarized with them, as the selection of the appropriate guidewire is crucial for the success of the procedure used for.

Finally, it is very important to mention the necessity of nephrostomy tube insertion in case of urinary tract infection or elevated serum creatinine levels, before any endourological procedures. In our case, our therapeutic plan was at first to inspect the ureter with the semirigid ureteroscope. The lower part of the ureter was sufficiently large and the scope passed easily. We need to mention that we were without a normal placed guidewire, due to complete obstruction at the level of the stone. Our exit strategy, in case of unsuccessful ureterscopy, would be at the same session, the placement of a nephrostomy tube, a procedure that in our hospital is carried out by urologists. We made the same case presentation as an eposter in Berlin during 9th International Meeting "Challenges in Endourology" [8].

## 4. Conclusion

Many complications may occur during stent insertion with the aid of a guidewire. Surgeon's experience, adherence to the basic principles of endourology such as continuous imaging and appliance of little force, suspicion of impacted stone and availability of different types of guidewires are important factors to avoid various uncomfortable and difficult situations during endoscopic procedures.

## References

[1] M. Kipling, A. Mohammed, and R. N. Medding, "Guidewires inclinical practice: applications and troubleshooting," *Expert Review of Medical Devices*, vol. 6, no. 2, pp. 187–195, 2009.

[2] P. Fritzsche, J. D. Moorhead, P. D. Axford, and R. R. Torrey, "Urologic applications of angiographic guide wire and catheter techniques," *Journal of Urology*, vol. 125, no. 6, pp. 774–780, 1981.

[3] P. Geavlete, "Ureteroscopy complications," in *Smith's Textbook of Endourology*, A. Smith, G. Badlani, G. Preminger, and L. Kavoussi, Eds., pp. 506–518, Wiley-Blackwell, UK, 2012.

[4] H. E. Wang and T. A. Sweeney, "Subclavian central venous catheterization complicated by guidewire looping and entrapment," *The Journal of Emergency Medicine*, vol. 17, no. 4, pp. 721–724, 1999.

[5] I. Efthimiou, Z. Chousianitis, and K. Skrepetis, "Troubleshooting for ureteroscopy complicated by unexpected guidewire looping and entrapment," *Journal of Endourology Case Reports*, vol. 3, no. 1, pp. 84–86, 2017.

[6] M. Clayman, C. A. Uribe, L. Eichel, Z. Gordon, E. M. Mcdougall, and R. V. Clayman, "Comparison of guide wires in urology: which, when and why?" *Journal of Urology*, vol. 171, no. 6 Part 1, pp. 2146–2150, 2004.

[7] G. Liguori, F. Antoniolli, C. Trombetta et al., "Comparative experimental evaluation of guidewire use in urology," *Urology*, vol. 72, no. 2, pp. 286–289, 2008.

[8] A. Tsionga, A. Anastasiadis, W. F. Mutomba, D. Memmos, I. Vakalopoulos, and G. Dimitriadis, "Guidewire looping and entrapment above an impacted ureter stone: a case report," https://epostersonline.com/cie2019/node/176.

# 11

# A Case of Incomplete Removal of Horseshoe Kidney by Laparoscopic Nephrectomy in an Adult Leading to Urinary Leak: An Eye Opener

**S. Venkat Ramanan, P. Velmurugan, A. R. Bhaskar Prakash, Anuj Arora, and LeelaKrishna Karri**

*Department of Urology, Sri Ramachandra Medical College and Research Institute, Chennai, India*

Correspondence should be addressed to S. Venkat Ramanan; vramanan2001@yahoo.com

Academic Editor: Apul Goel

Horseshoe kidney is a common congenital fusion anomaly of the kidneys. It poses a challenge to surgeon because of its very variable anatomy in terms of location and lie, fusion, pelvicalyceal system, and the renal vessels. Here we describe a case of laparoscopic nephrectomy in a horseshoe kidney complicated by incomplete removal because of not realizing the lower and medial extent of pelvicalyceal system across midline to the contralateral side leading to persistent urine leak. The relevant anatomy and the necessary precautions to prevent such complication have been discussed.

## 1. Case Report

A 25-year-old man, driver by profession, presented with recurrent episodes of dull aching right flank pain of 6-year duration. The pain was affecting his work. The patient was thin built with a body-mass-index of 20 Kg/m$^2$. The preoperative CT scan revealed a horseshoe kidney (HSK) with the right side involved by ureteropelvic-junction obstruction (UPJO) causing gross hydronephrosis and parenchymal thinning (Figures 1 and 2). The relative renal function was 11% on DTPA renogram. The left renal moiety was functioning well with a GFR of 71.9 ml/min. The S. Creatinine was 0.9 mg%. The patient also had a history of epilepsy but there was no identifiable congenital anomaly other than the HSK. The options of right pyeloplasty and right nephrectomy with their pros and cons were discussed with the patient. The patient opted for nephrectomy. A transperitoneal laparoscopic right nephrectomy was done using five ports in the right lateral position. A preliminary retrograde pyelography (RGP) or right ureteric catheterization was not done. The right colon and duodenum were reflected medially to expose the kidney. As expected the right kidney was lying relatively lower and medially than what a normal kidney would be. Other than the main renal artery, the upper and the lower poles were supplied by accessory polar artery each. The upper polar artery itself had a very early branching and the lower polar artery was crossing the UPJ and causing obstruction. There were two right renal veins lying between the main renal artery and the lower polar artery. The right ureter was divided about 4 cm below the ureteropelvic junction. All the arteries and the veins were clipped with hem-o-lok clips and divided. The kidney was dissected within the Gerota's fascia from the upper pole downwards. The isthmus was mobilized to the extent possible and was divided just to left of inferior vena cava. Body side of the cut edge showed some brisk bleeding. The cut edge was sutured with 2'0 V-Loc sutures over a surgical bolster and hemostasis was secured. The specimen was removed using an endo-bag and a drain was placed. There was no intraoperative complication. The only abnormal event in the postoperative period was a persistent drain output of 100ml of urine every 24 hours. The drain fluid creatinine was 22mg%. The postoperative ultrasound examination of the abdomen did not reveal any significant intra-abdominal collection. Left retrograde pyelogram and

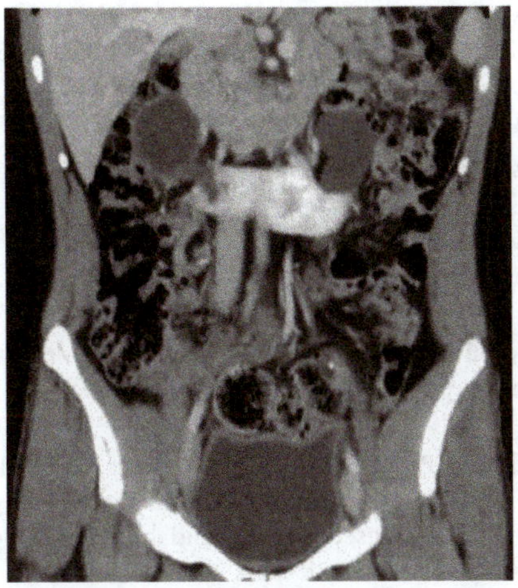

FIGURE 1: Initial preoperative CE-CT scan (coronal section) showing horseshoe kidney with right hydronephrosis.

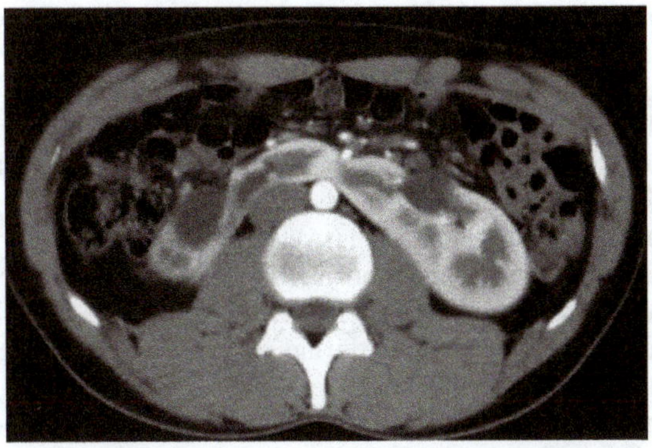

FIGURE 2: Initial preoperative CE-CT scan (axial section) showing horseshoe kidney with the fusion of the lower poles to the left of aorta.

right retrograde ureterogram done on the 14th postoperative day (POD) did not reveal any contrast leak either from the left side or from the right ureteric stump. Subsequently CT urogram was done which showed that a small residual stump of the right kidney fused to the lower pole of the left kidney was still viable and producing and leaking urine (Figure 3). This stump was supplied by a tiny arterial twig from the left renal artery. An exploratory laparotomy was done on the 16th POD through upper midline incision. The descending colon was reflected medially to expose the lower pole of the left kidney with the attached stump of the right kidney. The stump was densely adherent to the IVC and surrounding structures. For additional exposure and dissection, the mesentery of the transverse colon was opened lateral to the inferior mesenteric vein. The stump was freed from the IVC and delivered to the left side from underneath the inferior mesenteric artery (Figure 4). The stump was divided flush with the lower pole of the left kidney and the cut edge was sutured with 2'0 Vicryl over surgical bolster. The postoperative recovery was uneventful.

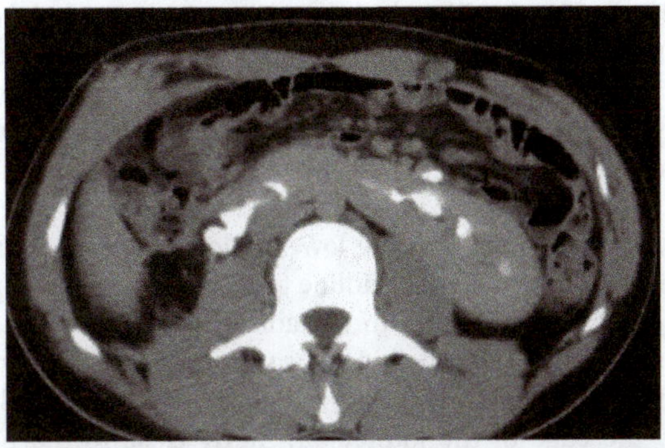

FIGURE 3: CE-CT following laparoscopic right nephrectomy showing leakage of contrast from the residual stump of the right lower pole.

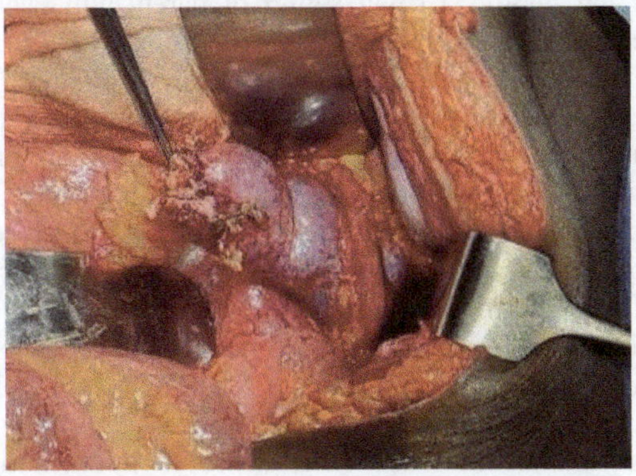

FIGURE 4: Intraoperative picture of exploratory laparotomy showing small residual stump of lower pole of right kidney fused to the lower pole of left kidney. Left ureter is seen running over the lower pole of left kidney.

## 2. Discussion

Horseshoe kidney is the commonest fusion anomaly of the kidneys and accounts for more than 90% of it [1, 2]. The reported incidence based on autopsy and radiographic data is 1:350 to 1:666 with a 2:1 male predominance [3–7]. HSK differs from crossed fused renal ectopia in that, unlike the latter in which only one kidney moves abnormally across the midline to fuse with the contralateral kidney, in HSK, both of the kidneys migrate abnormally and fuse. In 95% of cases the kidneys are fused at the lower poles. The lower polar fusion occurs in midline in 40 to 42% of cases giving rise to U-Shaped HSK or Symmetric HSK (Figure 5). In the remaining 58% to 60% of cases the fusion is lateral to the midline with one kidney being more horizontal and extending across the midline to fuse with the lower pole of the more vertical contralateral kidney (asymmetric HSK or L-shaped HSK) [7, 8]. The isthmus is composed of functioning renal parenchyma

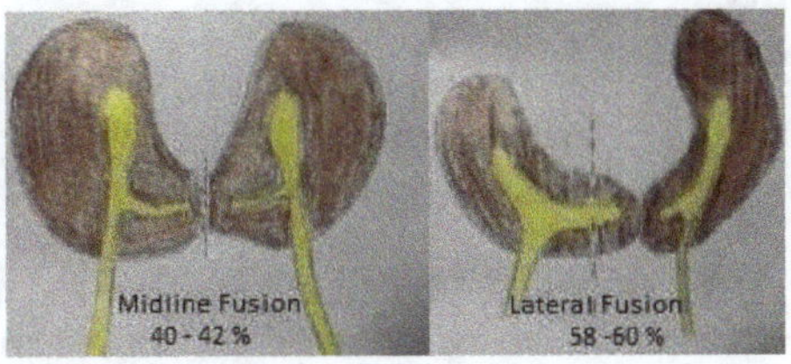


FIGURE 5: Midline lower polar fusion (40 to 42%) and lateral lower polar fusion (58% to 60%).

in majority of cases with only 4.4% to 15% of HSKs showing a fibrous isthmus [7, 9]. In 70% of the cases there are multiple renal vessels with variable origin and drainage patterns. The challenges in laparoscopic nephrectomy of a HSK pertain to dealing with multiple vessels as well as disconnecting the kidney at the isthmus. The issue of multiple vessels and variable vascular patterns is well recognized and it calls for a meticulous delineation of the vascular anatomy both preoperatively and intraoperatively and taking control of these vessels appropriately during surgery [10, 11]. However, the same kind of awareness regarding the anatomy of the isthmus during isthmectomy seems to be lacking. The reports of isthmectomy in the literature do not specify the type of isthmus that has been dealt with [12, 13]. As pointed out earlier, about 60% of HSKs with lower polar fusion have L-shaped kidney with fusion happening well beyond the midline on the contralateral side. Reaching the point of fusion well beyond the midline during laparoscopy may not be easy and it may result in incomplete removal. If only a small stump of a parenchymatous isthmus is left behind it may not be of any consequence. However, if that parenchymatous stump was also to contain a small portion collecting system within, then urinary leak is a potential possibility. In our case the HSK was L-shaped with the lower pole of the right kidney reaching well beyond the midline to fuse with the lower pole of the left kidney lateral to the aorta. The point of fusion was just a linear line. The kidney was grossly hydronephrotic with the dilated calices eroding the parenchyma and reaching up to the edge of the kidney and fairly close to the point of fusion. But this anatomy was somehow not appreciated in the first CT-Urogram prior to laparoscopic nephrectomy. Even though the isthmus was divided medial to the IVC, it still left behind a small stump of parenchyma with its contained collecting system. This led to a persistent urinary leak. This adverse outcome in our case could have been averted by clearly identifying the type of fusion and the anatomy of the isthmus in the preoperative imaging. In case of any uncertainty in the preoperative imaging, retrograde pyelography prior to nephrectomy would have clarified the relationship of pelvicalyceal system and the isthmus and how far medially the PCS was extending. This knowledge would have helped in avoiding cutting through the collecting system when dividing the isthmus. Moreover, if the point of division of the isthmus has to be beyond the lateral side of the contralateral great vessel, then laparoscopic approach may be extremely difficult and an open surgery may be a better option to prevent any incomplete removal.

## References

[1] S. Strauss, T. Dushnitsky, A. Peer, H. Manor, E. Libson, and P. D. Lebensart, "Sonographic features of horseshoe kidney: Review of 34 patients," *Journal of Ultrasound in Medicine*, vol. 19, no. 1, pp. 27–31, 2000.

[2] B.-K. Je, H. K. Kyung, and P. S. Horn, "Incidence and spectrum of renal complications and extrarenal diseases and syndromes in 380 children and young adults with horseshoe kidney," *American Journal of Roentgenology*, vol. 205, no. 6, pp. 1306–1314, 2015.

[3] A. Z. Weizer, A. D. Silverstein, B. K. Auge et al., "Determining the incidence of horseshoe kidney from radiographic data at a single institution," *The Journal of Urology*, vol. 170, no. 5, pp. 1722–1726, 2003.

[4] A. C. Allen, *The Kidney: Medical and Surgical Diseases*, Grune & Stratton, New York, NY, USA, 1951.

[5] P. H. Tan, G. S. Chiang, and A. H. Tay, "Pathology of urinary tract malformations in a paediatric autopsy series," *ANNALS Academy of Medicine Singapore*, vol. 23, pp. 838–843, 1994.

[6] E. F. Nation, "Horseshoe kidney: a study of thirty-two autopsy and nine surgical cases," *The Journal of Urology*, vol. 53, no. 6, pp. 762–768, 1945.

[7] B. Glodny, J. Petersen, K. J. Hofmann et al., "Kidney fusion anomalies revisited: clinical and radiological analysis of 209 cases of crossed fused ectopia and horseshoe kidney," *BJU International*, vol. 103, no. 2, pp. 224–235, 2009.

[8] K. Taghavi, J. Kirkpatrick, and S. A. Mirjalili, "The horseshoe kidney: Surgical anatomy and embryology," *Journal of Pediatric Urology*, vol. 12, no. 5, pp. 275–280, 2016.

[9] O. B. Stroosma, M. R. Scheltinga, B. M. Stubenitsky, and G. Kootstra, "Horseshoe kidney transplantation: An overview," *Clinical Transplantation*, vol. 14, no. 6, pp. 515–519, 2000.

[10] O. Olsson and M. Wholey, "Vascular abnormalities in gross anomalies of kidneys," *Acta Radiologica*, vol. 2, no. 5, pp. 420–432, 1964.

[11] L. Fazio, H. Razvi, and J. L. Chin, "Malignancy in horseshoe kidneys: review and discussion of surgical implications," *The Canadian Journal of Urology*, vol. 10, pp. 1899–1904, 2003 (Chinese).

[12] P. Jarzemski and S. Listopadzki, "Laparoscopic horseshoe kidney isthmusectomy: Four case reports," *Wideochirurgia i Inne Techniki Maloinwazyjne*, vol. 9, no. 1, pp. 115–120, 2014.

[13] A. Khan, A. Myatt, V. Palit, C. S. Biyani, and D. Urol, "Laparoscopic heminephrectomy of a horseshoe kidney," *Journal of the Society of Laparoendoscopic Surgeons*, vol. 15, no. 3, pp. 415–420, 2011.

12

# Non Typhoidal Salmonella Pyonephrosis in an Asymptomatic Immunocompetent Patient

Seif Mokadem ,[1] Mohamed Ali Nouioui ,[1] Salma Kalai,[2] Tarek Taktak,[1] Houssem Mediouni,[1] Ramzi Khiari,[1] and Samir Ghozzi[1]

[1]*Department of Urology, Military Hospital of First Instruction of Tunis, Tunisia*
[2]*Department of Microbiology, Military Hospital of First Instruction of Tunis, Tunisia*

Correspondence should be addressed to Seif Mokadem; mokadem.seif@gmail.com

Academic Editor: Tun-Chieh Chen

A 50-year-old man with no past medical history presented with 5 months history of right flank discomfort. Physical examination was unremarkable. CT-scan showed a large right renal pelvic calculi and upper pole hydronephrosis. He underwent open surgical procedure and we peroperatively discovered upper pole pyonephrosis. Bacteriological samples of pus grew group D Salmonella. We prescribed third generation cephalosporin for 14 days. The patient made a steady recovery. Non typhoidal salmonella (NTS) urinary tract infection (UTI) is extremely rare and usually associated with immunosuppressive chronic disease or genito urinary tract abnormalities. Pyonephrosis due to NTS have been reported twice. We report the first case of asymptomatic NTS pyonephrosis.

## 1. Introduction

Non typhoidal salmonella (NTS) is an enteroinvasive bacterium. Non typhoidal salmonellosis may have different clinical presentations [1]. Gastroenteritis is the most common form [1]. Urinary tract infection (UTI) due to NTS is extremely rare [2]. It is usually associated with immunosuppression or abnormalities of the genitourinary tract [1, 2]. The infection can be hematogenous or due to direct urethral invasion.

We present an unusual case of an incidental peroperative discovery of pyonephrosis due to NTS in an asymptomatic immunocompetent 50-year-old man.

## 2. Case Presentation

A 50-year-old man with no past medical history, presented with 5 months history of recurrent right flank discomfort. He denied any hematuria, passage of calculi, fever, chills, vomiting, diarrhea, constipation, or abdominal pain. He was not on any medication.

On examination, he was afebrile. Abdominal examination was normal and he had very soft right flank tenderness. Urine culture was negative.

Radiologic imaging including ultrasound and CT-scan showed a large right renal pelvic calculi and stones in the mid and inferior calix. It also showed upper calix hydronephrosis and thinned surrounding renal cortex (Figure 1). We proposed percutaneous nephrolithotomy (PCNL) but the patient refused any percutaneous or laparoscopic surgery. He underwent open surgical procedure. The upper pole of the kidney was adherent and surrounded by fibrotic tissue. We performed pyelolithotomy. While extracting the calculi, the urine was purulent so bacteriological samples have been taken. Pelvic suture was made after we placed Double-J ureteric stent.

Pus culture grew group D salmonella greater than $10^4$ colony-forming units (cfu) per mL of urine. Blood culture and HIV analysis were negative. Guided by measured antimicrobial susceptibility, we prescribed third generation cephalosporin (cefotaxim 2 g*3/g IV) for 14 days. The patient made a steady recovery and 16 days after admission he was discharged home.

## 3. Discussion

Urinary tract infections due to NTS are uncommon. It was mentioned the first time in 1946 [3]. Its frequency oscillates between 0.015% and 0.118% [2, 4]. It is commonly seen in

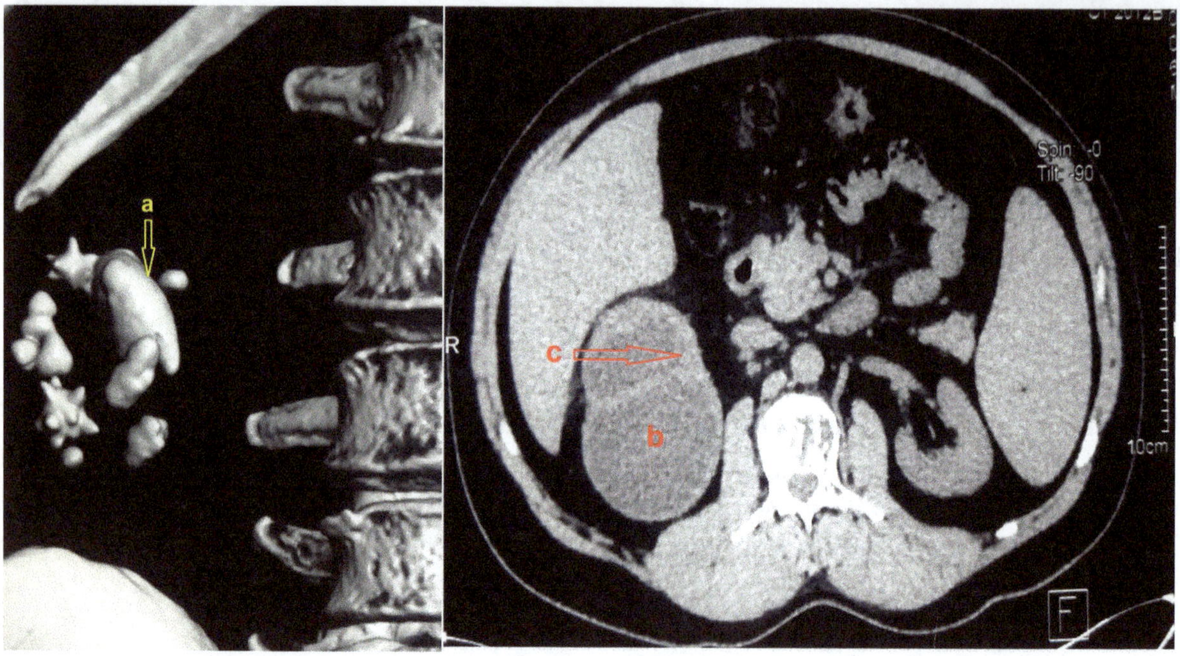


FIGURE 1: CT scan demonstrating large renal calculi and upper pole hydronephrosis: (a) large right renal pelvic calculi; (b) upper calix hydronephrosis; (c) thinned surrounding renal cortex.

TABLE 1: Characteristics of patients with pyonephrosis due to non typhoidal Salmonella.

| Case no (ref) | Age (Y)/ sex | Underlying disease(s) | Immuno suppressive therapy | Urologic predisposition | Salmonella serotype | Source of isolate(s) | Antecedent of diarrhea | Treatment | Outcome |
|---|---|---|---|---|---|---|---|---|---|
| 1 [10] | 47/M | None | None | Ureteral stone | Salmonella enterica | Urine and blood culture | No | Ceftriaxone gentamicin nephrectomy | Cured |
| 2 [11] | 7/M | None | None | Ureteropelvic junction stenosis | Salmonella infanitis | Urine culture | No | Fosfomycin norfloxacin | Cured |
| Our patient | 50/M | None | None | Renal stone | Group D salmonella | Urine culture | No | Pyelolitotomy cefotaxim | Cured |

infants and patients older than 60 years, not in healthy adults like our patient [5]. In our case, UTI was caused by group D salmonella but in a study including 799 UTI, the most frequent serotypes were C1 and E [6]. NTS can infect the urinary tract either hematogenously or directly via the urethra especially in women [4]. Several predisposing factors are incriminated in NTS-UTI such as immune deficiency, chronic illness, immunosuppressive therapy, and abnormalities of urinary tract [7, 8]. Our patient had no chronic disease or immunosuppressive therapy, but urolithiasis predisposed him to NTS-UTI. In his study, Paterson et al. [9] found that only 3 patients from the 23 included had structural abnormalities of urinary tract and none of them had immunosuppressive disease. However, Tena et al. [8] found that all the 19 patients of the study had chronic disease or urologic abnormalities. In the literature, NTS-UTI do not differ clinically from UTI caused by other bacteria [2, 4, 8]. Our case is the first reported asymptomatic NTS pyonephrosis. Indeed, in other reported cases of NTS pyonephrosis, the patients was febrile and one of them developed a systemic inflammatory response syndrome (Table 1) [10, 11].

## 4. Conclusion

NTS urinary tract infection is rare. When diagnosed, it should lead to investigations looking for immunosuppressive illness or urological abnormalities including urolithiasis. NTS pyonephrosis can be life threatening but asymptomatic forms can be seen.

## References

[1] J. L. Cohen, J. A. Bartlett, and R. Corey, "Extra-intestinal manifestations of Salmonella infections," *Medicine (Baltimore)*, vol. 66, no. 5, pp. 349–388, 1987.

[2] F. J. Allerberger, M. P. Dierich, A. Ebner et al., "Urinary tract infection caused by nontyphoidal *Salmonella*: report of 30 cases," *Urologia Internationalis*, vol. 48, no. 4, pp. 395–400, 1992.

[3] E. Seligmann, I. Saphra, and M. Wassermann, "*Salmonella* infections in the USA; a second series of 2,000 human infections recorded by the N.Y. salmonella center," *Journal of Immunology*, vol. 54, no. 1, pp. 69–87, 1946.

[4] J. M. Ramos, J. M. Augado, G.-C. Pilar, J. M. Alés, and F. Soriano, "Clinical spectrum of urinary tract infections due to nontyphoidal *Salmonella* species," *Clinical Infectious Diseases*, vol. 23, no. 2, pp. 388–390, 1996.

[5] R. B. S. Laing, F. W. Smith, and J. G. Douglas, "*Salmonella enteritidis* urinary infection associated with polycystic renal disease," *Journal of Infection*, vol. 27, no. 1, pp. 71–73, 1993.

[6] S. L. Abbott, B. A. Portoni, and J. M. Janda, "Urinary tract infections associated with nontyphoidal *Salmonella* serogroups," *Journal of Clinical Microbiology*, vol. 37, no. 12, pp. 4177–4178, 1999.

[7] A. Jehangir, D. Poudel, S. B. Fareedy et al., "Group D *Salmonella* urinary tract infection in an immunocompetent male," *Case Reports in Infectious Diseases*, vol. 2015, Article ID 608632, 2 pages, 2015.

[8] D. Tena, A. González-Praetorius, and J. Bisquert, "Urinary tract infection due to non-typhoidal *Salmonella*: report of 19 cases," *Journal of Infection*, vol. 54, no. 3, pp. 245–249, 2007.

[9] D. L. Paterson, M. W. Harrison, and J. M. B. Robson, "Clinical spectrum of urinary tract infections due to nontyphoidal *Salmonella* species," *Clinical Infectious Diseases*, vol. 25, no. 3, pp. 754–757, 1997.

[10] J. B. da Costa, J.-N. Cornu, D. Levgraverend et al., "Pyonephrosis caused by *Salmonella* typhi: a case report," *Urologia Internationalis*, vol. 96, no. 2, pp. 241–243, 2016.

[11] Y. Ogura, K. Kameda, N. Havashi, K. Arima, M. Yamagawa, and J. Kawamura, "A case of valve-like structure in ureter associated with pyonephrosis due to Salmonella infection," *Acta Urologica Japonica*, vol. 45, no. 4, pp. 261–264, 1999.

# 13

# Classic Testicular Seminoma in Men Aged 50 Years or Over: A Case Report and Review of the Literature

**Rawad Abou Zahr**,[1] **Khalil Chalhoub**,[1] **Imad Matta**,[1] **Sawsan Horani**,[2] **Zarouhie Bedoyan**,[3] **Georges El Hachem**,[4] **Imad Ghantous**,[1] and **Michel Jabbour**[1]

[1]*Department of Urology, University of Balamand, Saint George Hospital University Medical Center, Beirut 1100 2807, Lebanon*
[2]*University of Balamand, Faculty of Medicine and Medical Sciences, Beirut 1100 2807, Lebanon*
[3]*Department of Pathology, University of Balamand, Saint George Hospital University Medical Center, Beirut 1100 2807, Lebanon*
[4]*Department of Hematology-Oncology, University of Balamand, Saint George Hospital University Medical Center, Beirut 1100 2807, Lebanon*

Correspondence should be addressed to Michel Jabbour; drmjabbour@gmail.com

Academic Editor: David Duchene

Testicular cancer is the most frequent solid tumor detected in young adult men. Germ cell tumors (GCTs), particularly seminomas, are the most common type of testicular neoplasms seen in that age population. Most publications have reported decreasing incidence of GCTs in patients above forty years of age. Since the biologic activity of seminomas appears similar across ages, recommended management of senior adults involves a multimodal therapy of radical inguinal orchiectomy with radiation or cytotoxic treatment as needed. Attenuating chemotherapy dosages are critical to ensure better tolerability of associated adverse events. Here we report a case series of 2 men older than fifty years of age with metastatic testicular seminoma. We aim to emphasize a rare clinical entity encountered in the senior adult population.

## 1. Introduction

Testicular GCTs account for most testicular cancers in young adult men and have a peak incidence in the second and third decades of life [1, 2]. Of all reported testicular cancers in the United States, more than 95% are predominantly GCTs, half of which are seminomas [2, 3]. Globally, seminoma incidence rates were highest in European and Northern American countries and lowest in Asian and African countries [4]. The highest incidence rates were witnessed in Norway and Denmark (5.5/100,000 man-years), and the lowest rates were encountered in India and Uganda (<0.5/100,000 man-years) [4]. The World Health Organization's (WHO) 2016 updated classification of testicular GCTs now categorizes them based on histopathology into seminomas, non-seminomas, and spermatocytic tumors [5].

Despite their high incidence in young adults, testicular GCTs are rarely encountered in senior adults. Only less than 4% of patients with testicular GCTs are above sixty five years of age [6]. Recent epidemiologic studies highlight an increased incidence of seminomas across all age groups as well as an older age at diagnosis [7]. Mean age of diagnosis has shifted from 34 to 39 years for seminomas, as opposed to 26 to 31 years for non-seminomas [7]. In most clinicopathological studies seminomas, non-seminomas, and spermatocytic tumors account for 50–55%, 45–50% and 1% of testicular cancers, respectively [7, 8]. The biological phenotype and malignant potential remain the same across age groups suggesting that similar treatment regimens should be pursued [9].

Macroscopically, seminomas are well circumscribed, tan to pale yellow lesions with necrotic or hemorrhagic foci. The cells are arranged into nests and sheets with intercepting thin fibrovascular septa which have lymphocytes and sometimes syncytiotrophoblasts.

Cells have clear or eosinophilic cytoplasm with large nuclei and prominent nucleoli and they are immunoreactive to SALL4, OCT3/4, C-KIT, D2-40, and SOX17 [9]. Patients with seminomas can have elevated $\beta$-hCG and LDH but never AFP [8, 10]. Only about 30% of patients can have elevated $\beta$-hCG. LDH is a positive non-specific marker that reflect tumor burden [10].

Common metastatic sites of testicular seminomas involve the lungs and the liver. Rarely, it can also metastasize to the bones and the brain [11]. Even at advanced stages, testicular

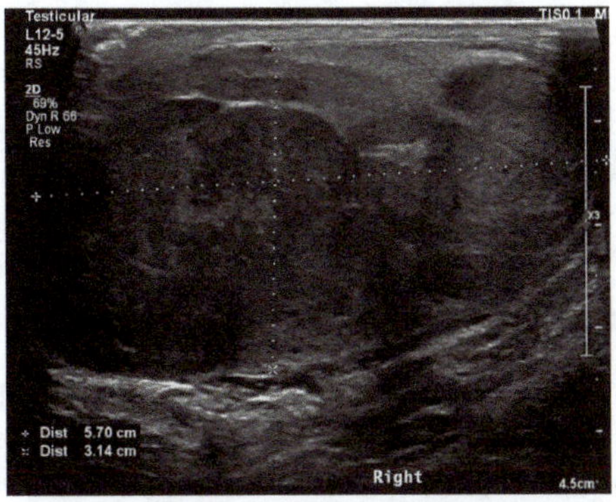


Figure 1: Ultrasound of right testicle.

seminomas can still have high cure rates. The most common stage of presentation, stage I seminoma, has a cure rate above 95% [12]. Considering all stages, the survival rate is 86% and 71% for the 5- and 10-year survival rate, respectively [9]. Important predictors of metastasis involve lymphovascular invasion by the primary tumor while predictors of relapse involve tumor size (>4 cm) and invasion of the rete testis. When both relapse predictors are absent, there is only a 6% risk of recurrence [12, 13].

## 2. Case 1

A 56-year-old male was presented to our facility for testicular pain of 3 weeks duration associated with progressive increase in the size and swelling of the right testicle. Physical examination revealed enlarged and rigid right testicle associated with tenderness.

Ultrasonography of the testicles revealed a hypoechoic heterogeneous well circumscribed lesion measuring more than 5.7 × 3.1 × 4.1 cm with nodularity and vascularity (Figure 1).

Metastatic work up included the Chest Abdomen Pelvis CT scan which revealed multiple enlarged retroperitoneal, para-aortic, and aorto caval lymphadenopathies. The largest lymph node was found in the left para aortic space with size 3 × 5 cm. Tumor markers were done upon admission showing negative AFP (2.31 ng/ml), slightly elevated BHCG (9.91 mIU/ml) and increased LDH levels (801 U/L). The patient underwent a right radical inguinal orchiectomy. The gross histology study demonstrated parenchyma of the testes occupied by a tan yellow, more or less well demarcated soft tumor mass measuring 5 × 2 × 2 cm with areas of yellow necrosis. Diagnosis concluded classic seminoma stage pT2, with lymphovascular invasion and negative spermatic cord margins. No evidence of invasion of the rete testis, tunica albuginea, tunica vaginalis, or epididymis. Immunostaining revealed positive expression of PLAP and SALL4 antibodies by tumor cells and negative anti-cytokeratin antibody.

Patient was diagnosed with stage IIB classical seminoma, he was started on cytotoxic chemotherapy consisting of 1 cycle of BEP protocol (Bleomycin, Etoposide, and Cisplatin) followed by 3 cycles of EP (Etoposide and Cisplatin) without Bleomycin because of pulmonary toxicity. A spirometry was performed since the patient was at high risk for pulmonary complications secondary to his smoking status and showed a 25% decrease in DLCO (Diffusing capacity of the Lungs for Carbon Monoxide), prompting bleomycin interruption [14]. He received 5 days of granulocytes colony stimulating factors (G-CSF) to prevent febrile neutropenia. The LDH normalized at the end of the first cycle. The Chest Abdomen Pelvis CT scan was repeated after the fourth cycle revealing an excellent partial response with persistence of 2 lymph nodes of 1.8 and 1.9 cm, with necrotic centers. The 4 cycles of chemotherapy were smooth without any renal, oto- or neuro-toxicity. He did not have any episode of febrile neutropenia. The DLCO re-increased by 15%, without reaching the pre-chemotherapy value. Since the remaining lymph nodes were less than 3 cm, close follow up with CT scan was

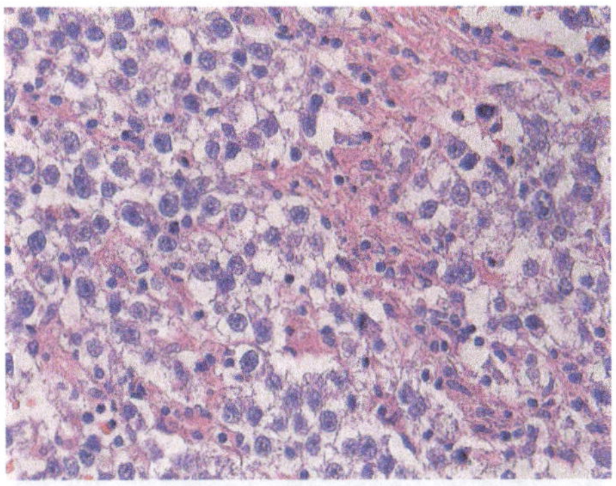

(a)

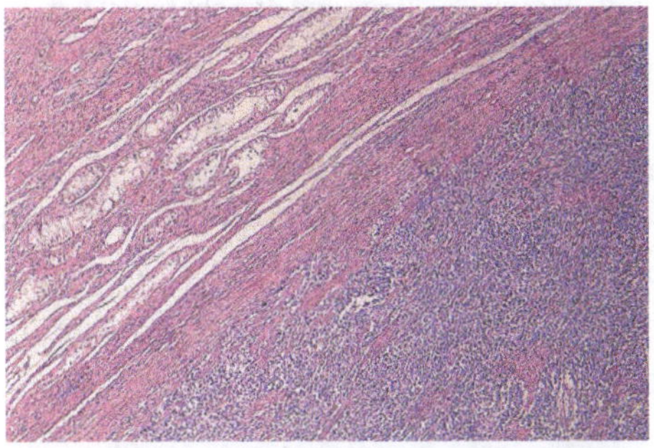

(b)

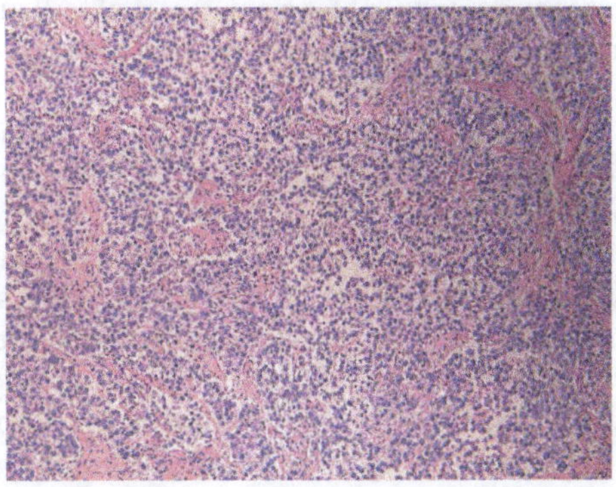

(c)

Figure 2: (a): High-power view shows round to polyhedral cells with distinct cell borders, and sparse lymphocytic infiltrate within fibrous septa, (b): Low-power view of the tumor (right) with background intratubular germ cell neoplasia (upper left), (c): Medium-power view of the tumor shows sheets of uniform clear cells divided into poorly demarcated lobules by delicate fibrous septa.

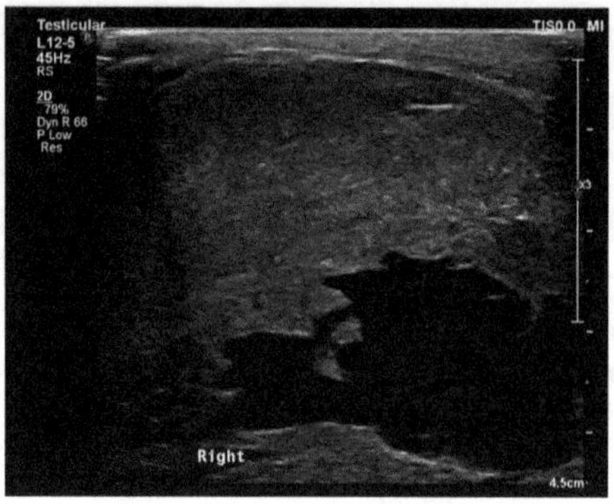


FIGURE 3: Ultrasound of right testicle.

scheduled on a bi-yearly basis for the first year and then yearly once for five years. To date the patient is being followed up 24 months after diagnosis and is doing well with no evidence of recurrence.

## 3. Case 2

A 65-year-old male patient, previously healthy, presented to our emergency department for a new onset of testicular pain following by swelling of his right testicle that started 4 weeks ago.

On physical examination, the patient had an apparent large and rigid right testicle with moderate tenderness upon palpation.

Ultrasonography of the testicles revealed a very large heterogenous vascularized mass in the right scrotum showing cystic components and containing fine echoes (Figure 3). The patient was admitted for further diagnosis and management. On the ward, tumor markers were done showing normal AFP and BHCG levels, 1.65 ng/ml and 3.63 mIU/ml respectively, and an elevated LDH level of 891 U/L.

The Chest Abdomen Pelvis CT scan was done as metastatic workup and showed few well circumscribed subpleural solid lung nodules measuring 1.4 cm in the apical segment of the right upper lobe, 2.5 × 2.8 cm in the anterior basal segment of right lower lobe and 3.3 × 1.6 cm in the posterior segment of the left lower lobe. Bulky necrotic retroperitoneal adenopathy was also noted in the portacaval region measuring up to 3.5 × 3 × 3 cm consistent with nodal metastases. After confirming the diagnosis, the patient underwent right radical orchiectomy. The final pathology came out as Classic Pure Seminoma, measuring 13 cm in largest dimension with extensive areas of necrosis and cystic degeneration. The Tumor focally invaded the tunica albuginea and reached the surface of the inked visceral layer of the tunica vaginalis. Invasion of the spermatic cord was also noted. Resection margin of the spermatic cord was free on neoplasia. Final diagnosis established a Classic Pure Seminoma stage pT3 N2 M1a.

The patient was classified to have good prognosis according to the International Germ Cell Cancer Collaborative Group (IGCCCG) risk classification and was started on 3 cycles of BEP protocol. His chemotherapy sessions were uneventful and smooth with no reported complications. A similar protocol of follow up with the Chest Abdomen Pelvis CT scan was scheduled on a bi-yearly basis for the first year and then once yearly for five years. To date, the patient is doing well 14 months post diagnosis and is currently being followed up as per the assigned protocol.

## 4. Discussion

Testicular GCTs is the number one cancer detected in young male adults, accounting for 21% of diagnosed invasive cancers in patients between 20 and 40 years of age. GCTs are rarely encountered in prepubertal males as well as senior adult men [15]. Most articles reviewed in the literature report showed declining incidence of testicular GCTs beyond the age of 40 [15, 16].

Histologically, studies showed that seminomas predominate in patients above fifty years old, while non-seminomas predominate in younger counterparts [16].

The clinical characteristics of seminomas in the elderly has had conflicting findings in the literature. The most common presenting symptom in older adults as well as young adults is a palpable, and painless scrotal mass that can be associated with discomfort [8]. Similarly, our patients were presented to our facility for a right testicular mass. According to Berney et al., seminomas in patients aged 50 and older tend to present at advanced stages and demonstrate aggressive behavior. Fifty cases were reviewed, and the results show that in senior adults with GCTs have a significantly larger macroscopic size and more frequent invasion of the rete testis and vascular invasion, as well as less frequent intratubular germ cell neoplasia [16].

One of the earliest publications on seminomas defines them as malignant GCTs that arise from the germinal epithelium of testicles and originate from precursor cells of the spermatogonium [17]. Rarely, however; about 5% of primary seminomas can also arise in extragonadal sites such as the pineal gland of the brain, the anterior mediastinum, and the retroperitoneum [18]. Primary GCTs in senior adults most commonly arise in the mediastinum followed by the retroperitoneum, and the CNS, while primary GCTs in young adult men are most commonly detected in the cranium [18].

A recent large-scale study by the Cancer Registration Committee of the Japanese Urological Association (2016) states that only 11% (123 out of 1119) of patients above 50 years old developed primary GCTs and 74.8% (91) of the GCTs in that age category were seminomas. 79.5% of the seminomas were stage I, 6.6% were stage II, and 13.9% were stage III according to the Union for International Cancer Control (UICC) classification. Furthermore, 84% of reported metastatic GCTs had a good prognosis as per the International Germ Cell Cancer Collaborative Group (IGCCC) vs. 16% and 0% had intermediate and poor prognosis, respectively. Survival, in months, included 72, 20 and 0 patients at 24, 48, and 60 months, respectively [19].

Wheater et al. studied 60 patients aged 60 and above. 44 patients were reported to have pure seminoma (73%) while the remaining 16 had non seminomatous and mixed tumors. Among the 44 patients with seminomas, 33 patients had stage I seminoma, 2 had stage II seminoma, and the rest had stage III seminoma. The median survival was 194 months for those with stage I seminoma and 70 months with metastatic disease [20].

In a case report written by Foell et al., an 86-year-old, the oldest patient in literature, with classic seminoma was compared with 4 patients under the age of 50. The authors state that the histologic features, biologic activity, and phenotype of the seminoma were similar and suggested following similar treatment algorithms [9]. The primary therapy for testicular seminoma is radical inguinal orchiectomy as it allows for accurate staging and histologic diagnosis of the tumor. Scrotal violations are avoided at all cost as they increased the risk of seeding of the scrotum and damaging regional lymphatic drainage [2].

Adjuvant therapy depends on staging but usually involves a multimodal approach. For stage I seminomas, active surveillance or carboplatin are recommended. Stage IIA and IIB seminomas are managed with dog-leg radiotherapy; the irradiation of the para-aortic lymph nodes with the ipsilateral iliac lymph nodes. Chemotherapy including 4 cycles of EP protocol (etoposide and cisplatin) or 3 cycles of BEP protocol (bleomycin, etoposide, and cisplatin), are used for stage IIA, IIB, IIC as an alternative to radiation as well as stage III seminomas [21]. For stage II seminomas, both radiotherapy and cisplatin-based chemotherapy are reported to be equally effective with the latter favored due to lower relapse rates. To note, carboplatin monotherapy has also been tried in stage II seminomas with reports of worse outcomes, however; when combined with radiotherapy it has been proven promising [21].

Testicular GCTs are highly responsive to chemotherapy and radiotherapy, thus; making a good outcome highly likely [16]. Both modalities, however, carry risks. Radiation runs the risk of secondary malignancies and cardiotoxicity, while the BEP protocol can cause cardiopulmonary toxicity, neurotoxicity, nephrotoxicity, and infertility as well as secondary cancer [3, 22]. Our patient was managed by a right radical inguinal orchiectomy and completed 1 cycle of the BEP protocol but was later switched to 3 cycles of EP as he developed a pulmonary reaction to Bleomycin at the start of his second cycle.

Most recent studies recommend following identical treatment algorithms, owing to the similar phenotype of seminomas in both age populations, but it is important to discuss factors hypothesized to lower treatment outcomes in senior adults. The age-related functional decline or associated comorbidities seen in this age bracket renders them less tolerable to the adverse effects and toxicities associated with chemotherapy. Prophylactic attenuation of chemotherapy dosage in senior adults is essential [23].

Those with contraindications to Bleomycin can alternatively receive 4 cycles of EP if they are in the good prognosis group and 4 cycles of VIP if they are in the intermediate or poor prognosis groups. The alternative EP and VIP regimens have been reported to have equivalent success rates, though the former regimen has been associated with lower rates of disease free survival [20, 22]. Wheater et al. modified the conventional BEP regimen by delivering a single empirically-reduced dose of 30,000 International Units of Bleomycin per cycle on the second day, without evidence of significant pulmonary toxicity [20]. To note, other trials have attempted to reduce Etoposide from the conventional dose of 500 $mg/m^2$ to 360 $mg/m^2$ with complete exclusion of Bleomycin but reported poorer outcomes [20].

For instance, advanced age and associated declining renal function in senior patients pose a 5% risk of Bleomycin pulmonary toxicity due to advanced age alone and a 20% risk when pooled with impaired renal function [19]. Thus, cautious selection of chemotherapeutic agents as well as dosages is necessary. According to Beyer et al., the BEP protocol is the mainstay of chemotherapy for senior patients with metastatic disease in good, intermediate, and poor prognosis groups [22].

Another concern is chemotherapy-induced nephrotoxicity particularly associated with cisplatin. The primary measures of mitigating cisplatin-related nephrotoxicity involve the combination of adequate hydration (≥3 L/day) and osmotic diuresis with mannitol during chemotherapy. Alternatively, patients with declining renal function could substitute cisplatin with carboplatin. Carboplatin dose setting based on renal function after target AUC has been established is also recommended [24].

The optimal salvage therapy for elderly patients with seminomas who relapse after surveillance, adjuvant carboplatin or adjuvant radiotherapy remains unknown. Several combinations of chemotherapy were used as a first-line salvage treatment, including conventional dose chemotherapy (CDCT) and high dose chemotherapy (HDCT). HDCT was reserved for patients with unfavorable prognostic factors and high risk of failure of salvage therapy. CDCT regimens included 4 cycles of VIP, TIP or VeIP, and HDCT which comprised of 2–3 sequential cycles of etoposide and carboplatin. In the second and third salvage therapy setting, other agents such as oxaliplatin, gemcitabine, and paclitaxel have been recommended as single agent or combination chemotherapy [21, 22].

If residual seminoma masses present post chemotherapy or radiotherapy, close monitoring with tumor serum markers and imaging is recommended, especially if residual masses are >3 cm. The Fluorodeoxyglucose (FDG)-PET scanning is a reliable imaging modality with high prognostic value for residual masses post treatment. Patients with positive FDG-PET scans for residual masses should get biopsied. Based on histology, further treatment options could include observation, chemotherapy, radiation or surgical resection [25].

Follow up protocols vary based on staging and consist of active surveillance, tumor markers, and imaging (the chest abdominopelvic CT, the brain CT and CXR) [12]. Testicular ultrasound is reserved for ambiguous exams [26]. For stage I seminoma, in the first 2 years post-surgery, tumor markers test and physical exam should be conducted every 4 months, and abdominopelvic CT and CXR every 6 months. In years 3–5, the physical exam and tumor markers test are to be done once per year and abdominopelvic CT on the third and fifth year. For metastatic seminoma, in the first 2 years, tumor markers test, physical exam, and CXR are to be done every 3 months, abdominopelvic CT every 6 months, and the brain and the chest CT every 12 months. For years 3–5, tumor markers, physical exam, and CXR should be done every 6 years, and the chest abdominopelvic CT and the brain CT every 12 months [12].

## 5. Conclusion

Testicular GCTs are neoplasms encountered frequently in young adults and are rarely seen in the senior adult population. Histologically, seminomas predominate in patients over fifty years old and have retained the phenotype, biologic activity, and malignant potential. Seminomas remain curable and have good prognosis in senior adults even at advanced stages. Treatment regimens similar to younger patients can be employed as long as chemotherapy dosages are empirically reduced, and precautions are taken to mitigate chemotherapy-related toxicities.

## References

[1] G. E. Hachem, S. Sideris, and T. Gil, "56 years-old, an old age for pure seminomatous germ cell tumor: Case report and review of the literature," *Cancer Reports and Reviews*, vol. 2, no. 1, pp. 1–4, 2017.

[2] N. Boujelbene, A. Cosinschi, N. Boujelbene et al., "Pure seminoma: a review and update," *Radiation Oncology*, vol. 6, no. 1, p. 90, 2011.

[3] A. A. Ghazarian, B. Trabert, S. S. Devesa, and K. A. McGlynn, "Recent trends in the incidence of testicular germ cell tumors in the United States," *Andrology*, vol. 3, no. 1, pp. 13–18, 2014.

[4] B. Trabert, J. Chen, S. S. Devesa, F. Bray, and K. A. Mcglynn, "International patterns and trends in testicular cancer incidence, overall and by histologic subtype, 1973-2007," *Andrology*, vol. 3, no. 1, pp. 4–12, 2014.

[5] S. R. Williamson, B. Delahunt, C. Magi-Galluzzi et al., "The World Health Organization 2016 classification of testicular germ cell tumours: a review and update from the International Society of Urological Pathology Testis Consultation Panel," *Histopathology*, vol. 70, no. 3, pp. 335–346, 2016.

[6] N. Ismaili, S. Naciri, S. Afqir et al., "A rare case of advanced testicular seminoma in a 78-year-old man managed successfully with carboplatin based chemotherapy: a case report," *Cases Journal*, vol. 1, no. 1, p. 357, 2008.

[7] C. G. Ruf, H. Isbarn, W. Wagner, M. Fisch, C. Matthies, and K. Dieckmann, "Changes in epidemiologic features of testicular germ cell cancer: age at diagnosis and relative frequency of seminoma are constantly and significantly increasing," *Urologic Oncology: Seminars and Original Investigations*, vol. 32, no. 1, pp. 33.e1–33.e6, 2014.

[8] J. Marko, D. J. Wolfman, A. L. Aubin, and I. A. Sesterhenn, "Testicular seminoma and its mimics: from the radiologic pathology archives," *RadioGraphics*, vol. 37, no. 4, pp. 1085–1098, 2017.

[9] K. Foell, M. Martens, and J. I. Izawa, "A rare case of classic testicular seminoma in an 86-year-old shows similar proliferation rate as in younger men," *Urology*, vol. 70, no. 5, pp. 1007.e7–1007.e9, 2007.

[10] C. G. Ruf, "Follow-up for testicular," in *Cancer Urologic Oncology*, A. Merseburger and M. Burger, Eds., pp. 1–11, Springer, Cham, 2019.

[11] S. Degirmencioglu and B. Degirmencioglu, "Isolated femoral muscle and bone metastases rarely encountered in testicular seminoma," *Case Reports in Oncological Medicine*, vol. 2013, Article ID 780493, 3 pages, 2013.

[12] P. Albers, W. Albrecht, F. Algaba et al., "Guidelines on testicular cancer: 2015 update," *European Urology*, vol. 68, no. 6, pp. 1054–1068, 2015.

[13] P. Warde, M. Gospodarowicz, D. Banerjee et al., "Prognostic factors for relapse in stage I testicular seminoma treated with surveillance," *Journal of Urology*, vol. 157, no. 5, pp. 1705–1710, 1997.

[14] J. Lauritsen, M. Kier, M. Bandak et al., "Pulmonary function in patients with germ cell cancer treated with bleomycin, etoposide, and cisplatin," *Journal Of Clinical Oncology*, vol. 34, no. 13, pp. 1492–1499, 2016.

[15] B. Hayes-Lattin and C. R. Nichols, "Testicular cancer: a prototypic tumor of young adults," *Seminars in Oncology*, vol. 36, no. 5, pp. 432–438, 2009.

[16] D. M. Berney, A. Y. Warren, M. Verma et al., "Malignant germ cell tumours in the elderly: a histopathological review of 50 cases in men aged 60 years or over," *Modern Pathology*, vol. 21, no. 1, pp. 54–59, 2007.

[17] J. Innes, W. F. Harvey, and E. K. Dawson, "Debatable tumors in human and animal pathology-iii," *Seminoma. Edinburgh Medical Journal*, vol. 45, no. 1, pp. 36–42, 1938.

[18] A. B. Shinagare, J. P. Jagannathan, N. H. Ramaiya, M. N. Hall, and A. D. Van den Abbeele, "Adult extragonadal germ cell tumors," *American Journal of Roentgenology*, vol. 195, no. 4, pp. W274–W280, 2010.

[19] T. Kawai and Y. Tanaka, "Clinical characteristics of testicular germ cell tumors in patients aged 50 years and older: a large-scale study from the cancer registration committee of the japanese urological association," *International Journal of Urology*, vol. 24, no. 2, pp. 124–128, 2016.

[20] M. J. Wheater, J. Manners, L. Nolan, P. D. Simmonds, M. C. Hayes, and G. M. Mead, "The clinical features and management of testicular germ cell tumours in patients aged 60 years and older," *BJU International*, vol. 108, no. 11, pp. 1794–1799, 2011.

[21] F. Honecker, J. Aparicio, D. Berney et al., "ESMO consensus conference on testicular germ cell cancer: diagnosis, treatment and follow-up," *Annals of Oncology*, vol. 29, no. 8, pp. 1658–1686, 2018.

[22] J. Beyer, P. Albers, R. Altena et al., "Maintaining success, reducing treatment burden, focusing on survivorship: highlights from the third European consensus conference on diagnosis and treatment of germ-cell cancer," *Annals of Oncology*, vol. 24, no. 4, pp. 878–888, 2013.

[23] J. Spermon, J. Witjes, and L. Kiemeney, "Difference in stage and morphology-adjusted survival between young and elderly patients with a testicular germ cell tumor," *Urology*, vol. 60, no. 5, pp. 889–893, 2002.

[24] S. Horie, M. Oya, M. Nangaku et al., "Guidelines for treatment of renal injury during cancer chemotherapy 2016," *Clinical and Experimental Nephrology*, vol. 22, no. 1, pp. 210–244, 2018.

[25] S. Krege, J. Beyer, R. Souchon et al., "European consensus conference on diagnosis and treatment of germ cell cancer: a report of the second meeting of the european germ cell cancer consensus group: part II," *European Urology*, vol. 53, no. 3, pp. 497–513, 2008.

[26] K. Sachdeva, "Testicular cancer follow-up," 2018, https://emedicine.medscape.com/article/279007-followup.

14

# Robot-Assisted Nephroureterectomy for Upper Tract Urothelial Carcinoma in a Patient with an Ileal Conduit

**Raymond A. Stemrich**,[1] **Neel Hasmukh Patel**,[2] **Jacob A. Baber**,[2] **and Mark J. Ferretti**[2]

[1]*Geisinger Health System, 100 N. Academy Avenue, Danville, PA 17822, USA*
[2]*Geisinger, Urology Associate, 1000 E. Mountain Boulevard, Wilkes-Barre, PA 18702, USA*

Correspondence should be addressed to Mark J. Ferretti; mferretti@geisinger.edu

Academic Editor: David Duchene

*Background.* Upper tract urothelial carcinoma remains an uncommon disease that is clinically difficult to identify early and surveil. Open nephroureterectomy is the gold standard for patients with high-grade disease, especially for patients in whom surveillance is complicated such as those with prior cystectomies/ileal conduits. This report presents a case of a patient with a history of radical cystectomy and ileal conduit construction who underwent a successful minimally invasive robotic surgery for treatment of upper tract urothelial carcinoma. *Case Presentation.* The patient is a 72-year-old Caucasian male with a history of recurrent superficial bladder tumors treated with cystoscopies with fulguration, Bacillus Calmette-Guerin, and a robot-assisted cystectomy with ileal conduit diversion presenting with recurrent urinary tract infections and hematuria secondary to a ureteral stricture. The patient was admitted previously for urosepsis during which time a percutaneous nephrostomy tube was inserted on the right side. Upon presentation, imaging revealed a lesion extending from the lower pole of the right kidney into the renal pelvis. The presence of a nephrostomy and urostomy allowed the surgical team to utilize a minimally invasive approach to remove the diseased kidney and ureter with visualization enhanced by indocyanine green. *Conclusion.* Minimally invasive robot-assisted approaches to treating upper tract urothelial carcinomas may offer an alternative to the open cases typically employed in cases of patients with prior ileal conduit. Furthermore, utilizing indocyanine green may expand the applicability of such approaches to uro-oncologic cases with greater complexity.

## 1. Introduction

Upper tract urothelial carcinoma (UTUC) remains an uncommon condition making up only 5% of urothelial carcinomas. Radical nephroureterectomy, whether an open, laparoscopic, or robotic approach, remains the standard treatment [1]. Although some aspects of these modalities demonstrate comparable perioperative, postoperative, and oncologic outcomes, further consideration is required before choosing an approach.

The laparoscopic and robotic approaches are minimally invasive with inherent advantages over open procedures, particularly in perioperative outcomes. Previous studies have found that minimally invasive nephroureterectomies require less intraoperative time and result in less mean blood loss. Postoperatively, they require shorter hospital stays, produce better cosmetic outcomes, and require less postoperative analgesics. Postoperative complications and oncologic outcomes were found to be comparable between the approaches [2, 3].

When comparing minimally invasive modalities, the robotic approach has been found to have longer operative times thought to be caused by the initial docking process [2, 4]. Furthermore, Veccia et al. found that the robotic approach had lower overall complications and shorter recovery times; however, these results were not statistically significant [4]. Other studies comparing oncologic outcomes

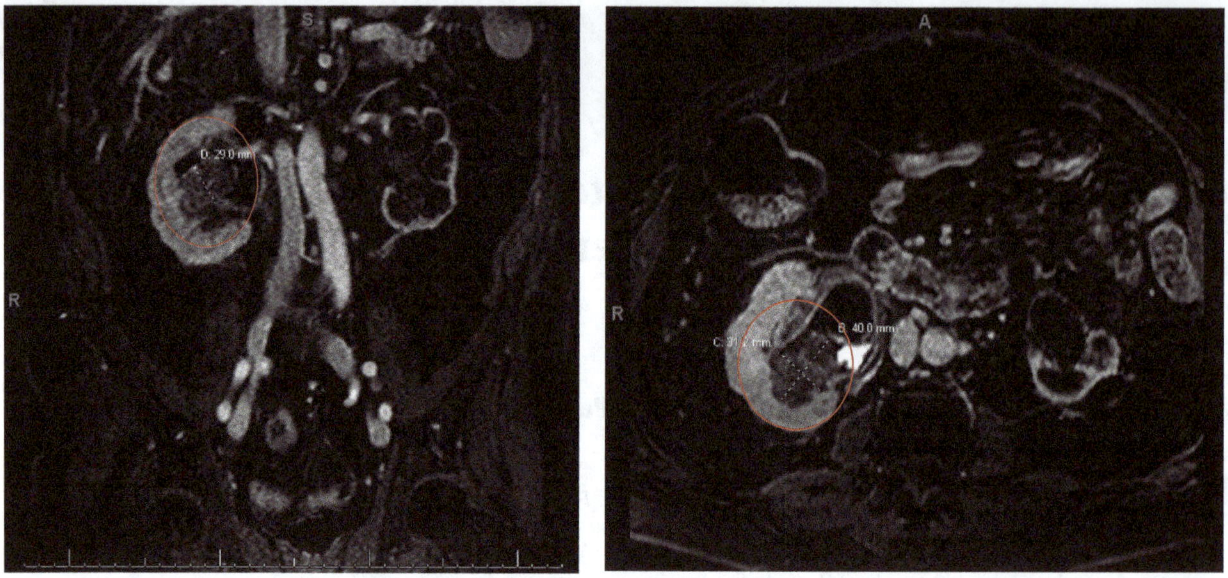

(a) (b)

FIGURE 1: (a) MR Urogram showing the coronal view of the lesion measuring 0.29 mm. (b) MR Urogram showing the axial view of the lesion measuring 31.2 mm × 40.0 mm.

(i.e., progression-free, cancer-specific, and overall survival) concluded that laparoscopic and robotic approaches were comparable [2, 4, 5]. The main advantages of the robotic approach include increased dexterity, improved accuracy, and enhanced visualization intraoperatively [2, 4]. Veccia et al. defined their "tetrafecta" outcome for robotic nephroureterectomies as concomitant occurrence of bladder cuff excision, lymph node dissection, no complications, and negative surgical margins as their measure of quality. They concluded that the improved versatility of robotic platforms overcomes the challenges with laparoscopic approaches achieving their "tetrafecta" [4].

This report presents the case of a patient who underwent a cystectomy with ileal conduit creation who subsequently developed UTUC. The surgical team elected to perform a robot-assisted nephroureterectomy with the use of indocyanine green (ICG) to improve visualization of the ureter and ileal conduit.

## 2. Case Presentation

A 72-year-old Caucasian male presented with intermittent hematuria and recurrent urinary tract infections secondary to a right ureteral stricture. The patient's significant past medical history included type 2 diabetes mellitus, dyslipidemia, coronary artery disease, stage 5 chronic kidney disease, and bladder cancer. He was initially diagnosed with superficial bladder carcinoma in 2000 and underwent multiple cystoscopies with fulguration of bladder tumors and intravesical Bacillus-Calmette-Guerin before a robot-assisted cystoprostatectomy was performed in 2010. An ileal loop diversion was performed with a Bricker ureteroileal anastomosis. Additionally, obturator and iliac lymph node dissections were performed, but no involvement was observed. Pathology at the time revealed extensive urothelial atypia consistent with high-grade carcinoma in situ. There was no evidence of an invasive process, but the right ureteral margin was positive for low-grade dysplasia. The final pathology report classified it as stage tis. After admission for urosepsis and placement

TABLE 1: Baseline renal function upon presentation to the clinic and renal function at the time of preoperative evaluation.

| | Presentation to clinic | Preoperative evaluation |
|---|---|---|
| BUN (mg/dL) | 72.0 | 36.0 |
| Creatinine (mg/dL) | 3.8 | 4.5 |
| Estimated GFR | 15.0 | 12.5 |

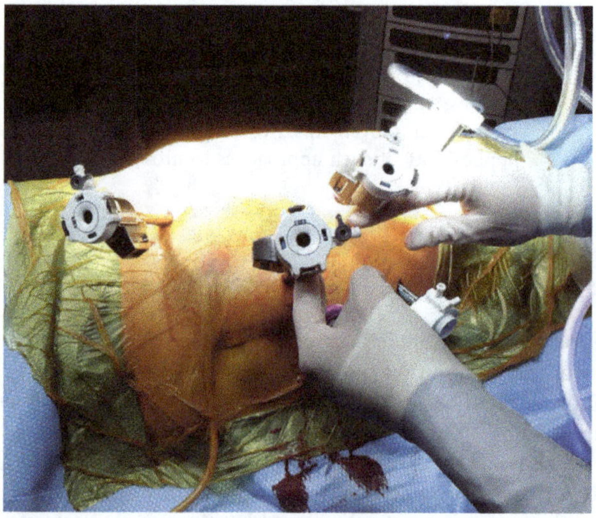

FIGURE 2: Placement of the ports.

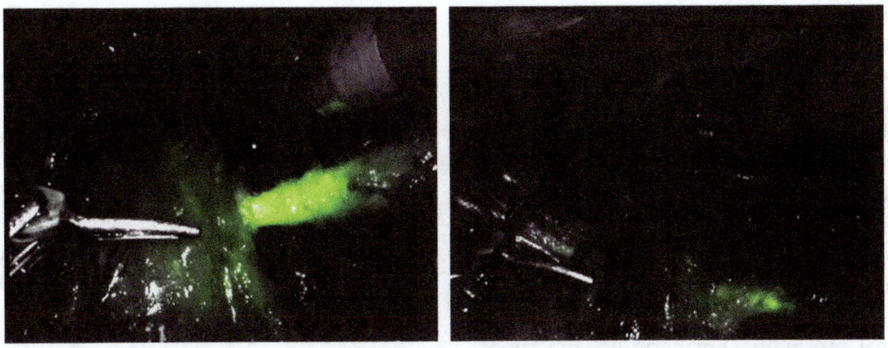

FIGURE 3: View of the ureter entering the ileal conduit after injection of indocyanine green (ICG).

of a right percutaneous nephrostomy (PCN), the patient presented to our clinic. MR Urogram demonstrated a right ureteroileal anastomosis stricture and a lobulated mass in the right kidney extending from the lower pole into the renal pelvis (Figure 1). Biopsy demonstrated high-grade urothelial carcinoma.

Preoperatively, a CT scan revealed that the patient's left kidney was severely atrophic and nonfunctioning. The planned removal of the right kidney would require the patient to undergo dialysis. Surgical options were discussed with the patient, including the possibility of a kidney-sparing procedure with aggressive endourologic resection and instillation of MitoGel. Ultimately, this was decided against due to the patient's worsening symptomatic azotemia. Upon presentation to the clinic, the patient's GFR was 14.2 and his creatinine was 3.8 mg/dL. Additionally, he was experiencing hypertension (systolic 152-178 mmHg, diastolic 72-84 mmHg) and hyperkalemia. On preoperative evaluation, his GFR declined to 8.5 and his creatinine was 4.5 mg/dL (renal function values in Table 1). In consultation with the patient's nephrologist, it was determined that dialysis was inevitable with his progressive renal impairment, so the patient elected to undergo a nephroureterectomy. A right-sided PCN and right lower quadrant urostomy allowed the surgical team to plan a robot-assisted nephroureterectomy utilizing indocyanine green (ICG) to improve visualization of the ureter and ileal conduit.

The patient was placed in a modified flank position and flexed at the hip. An 18F Foley catheter was inserted into the ileal conduit before the abdomen was insufflated and a Visiport, three robotic trocars, and two assistant trocars were inserted (Figure 2). After docking the da Vinci Xi® platform, a standard approach was employed until both poles of the kidney were visible at which time ICG was injected into the nephrostomy to improve visibility of the proximal ureter (Figure 3). At this point, the ureter was clipped, and the nephrectomy continued. Once the ureter was dissected to the level of the iliac vessels, ICG was injected through the urostomy to confirm the location of the ileal conduit and allow visualization of the anastomoses. A clip was placed on the distal ureter prior to entry into the conduit and excision of the conduit cuff around the ureter. The case was concluded in the usual fashion with the right kidney, ureter, and conduit cuff inserted into an EndoCatch bag and removed from the body cavity. Pathology revealed an invasive high-grade papillary urothelial carcinoma infiltrating the lamina propria with a final staging of pT1pNX.

Overall, operative time was four hours. Perioperative findings included moderate peritoneal adhesions and estimated blood loss of 50 mL with grossly negative margins. The patient tolerated the procedure well, but he developed an ileus postoperatively, which prolonged his hospital stay. He was discharged on postop day 10 and did well in follow up. In addition to monitoring the patient's chronic anemia secondary to chronic kidney disease, recurrence is surveilled with urine cytology obtained from the ileal conduit and the left kidney.

## 3. Discussion

Radical cystectomy serves as the standard treatment for muscle invasive bladder cancer, requiring urinary diversion such as an ileal conduit. This approach is generally curative for bladder cancers; however, patients may develop UTUC with an overall postcystectomy prevalence of 0.75-6.4% [6]. This prevalence after radical cystectomies may represent an underestimate given the pan-urothelial field defect theory and the high mortality associated with the initial bladder cancer diagnosis [6, 7]. Regardless, regular monitoring of the patient postoperatively is essential to identify recurrence early.

Surveillance itself poses challenges and remains a topic of ongoing discussion within the field. One study assessed the use of cytology and various imaging techniques (i.e., loopgraphy, urography, and computerized tomography) in the detection of UTUC. The rate of primary detection with urine cytology was only 8.9%; furthermore, the results of analysis may be difficult to interpret because the sample is often obtained from an ileal conduit or another urinary diversion. Despite these potential ambiguities, urine cytology is an inexpensive test to monitor recurrence and remains widely used by many providers. The primary detection rate for imaging modalities was 24.8%; however, roughly eight hundred radiologic assessments were performed to identify one case of UTUC. Additionally, many of these tests are conducted in tandem with other imaging techniques, making assessing the specificity and sensitivity of the individual methods challenging [6]. Regardless of detection method, UTUC is primarily treated with surgery unless deemed inoperable.

The gold standard treatment for high-grade UTUC, especially for patients with a history of cystectomy, is a radical open nephroureterectomy with excision of the bladder cuff; however, minimally invasive approaches are becoming more common and yielding improved outcomes. Despite acceptance of robot-assisted procedures in the treatment of prostate, kidney, and bladder cancers, its oncological results for UTUC remain unmeasured in the long term and thus the approach is not widely validated. In a retrospective study, De Groote et al. concluded that the minimally invasive robotic approach was safe with a low rate of major complications and low perioperative morbidity. Furthermore, the robot-assisted method produced oncologic outcomes similar to those of laparoscopic and open nephroureterectomies in the short term [1]. Several factors need to be considered in the planning stage of any robotic surgery. In the era of immunotherapy and the availability of novel agents such as Jelmyto, upper tract disease is increasingly able to be managed with renal preservation. In patients with salvageable kidneys, this may become the preferred route for both high-grade and low-grade disease when feasible. With dialysis already being planned for this patient, our decision was made to proceed with nephroureterectomy after discussion with patient.

In the case described above, the surgical plan took advantage of the ileal conduit urostomy and PCN to inject ICG to enhance visibility of key structures. ICG has a wide range of uses. Most notably in urology, it is employed to visualize lymph nodes during dissection, perfusion in transplants, and anatomy in ureteral procedures [8]. The operative plan for the patient in this case, included injecting ICG into the nephrostomy tube to highlight the ureter proximally, enabling clip placement near the renal pelvis. It was then injected into the urostomy, allowing visualization of the conduit and ureteroileal anastomoses. This step improved clip placement on the distal ureter and excision of the conduit cuff. Overall, utilization of ICG augments visibility during robot-assisted cases expanding both the approach's applicability and safety.

## 4. Conclusion

We reported a patient with upper tract urothelial carcinoma who underwent a robot-assisted nephroureterectomy utilizing ICG via a nephrostomy and urostomy to improve visualization of the ureter and ileal conduit anastomoses. This case report contributes to the growing body of evidence supporting the efficiency, safety, and flexibility of minimally invasive robotic approaches in complex urologic cases.

## References

[1] D. Groote, the YAU Robotic and Urothelial Group, K. Decaestecker et al., "Robot-assisted nephroureterectomy for upper tract urothelial carcinoma: results from three high-volume robotic surgery institutions," *Journal of Robotic Surgery*, vol. 14, no. 1, pp. 211–219, 2020.

[2] H. Lee, C. S. Ki, H. Sung et al., "Guidelines for the laboratory diagnosis of Middle East respiratory syndrome coronavirus in Korea," *Infection & Chemotherapy*, vol. 48, no. 1, pp. 61–69, 2016.

[3] G. Simone, R. Papalia, S. Guaglianone et al., "Laparoscopic versus open nephroureterectomy: perioperative and oncologic outcomes from a randomised prospective study," *European Urology*, vol. 56, no. 3, pp. 520–526, 2009.

[4] A. Veccia, U. Carbonara, H. Djaladat et al., "Robotic vs laparoscopic nephroureterectomy for upper tract urothelial carcinoma: a multicenter propensity-score matched pair "tetrafecta" analysis (ROBUUST Collaborative Group)," *Journal of Endourology*, 2022.

[5] A. A. Aboumohamed, L. S. Krane, and A. K. Hemal, "Oncologic outcomes following robot-assisted laparoscopic nephroureterectomy with bladder cuff excision for upper tract urothelial carcinoma," *The Journal of Urology*, vol. 194, no. 6, pp. 1561–1566, 2015.

[6] S. Picozzi, C. Ricci, M. Gaeta et al., "Upper urinary tract recurrence following radical cystectomy for bladder cancer: a meta-analysis on 13, 185 patients," *The Journal of Urology*, vol. 188, no. 6, pp. 2046–2054, 2012.

[7] F. G. Petros, "Epidemiology, clinical presentation, and evaluation of upper-tract urothelial carcinoma," *Translational Andrology and Urology*, vol. 9, no. 4, pp. 1794–1798, 2020.

[8] E. Kaplan-Marans, J. Fulla, N. Tomer, K. Bilal, and M. Palese, "Indocyanine green (ICG) in urologic surgery," *Urology*, vol. 132, pp. 10–17, 2019.

# 15

# Urethral Prolapse Case Report: Surgical and Social Considerations in Senegal

**Mohamed Jalloh**,[1] **Jennifer Heibig**,[2] **Oumar Gaye**,[1] **William Ghaul**,[2] **Gabrielle Yankelevich**,[2] **Medina Ndoye**,[1] **Mouhamadou Moustapha Mbodji**,[1] **Ayun Cassell**,[1] **Lamine Niang**,[1] **and Serigne Magueye Gueye**[1]

[1]*Service d'Urologie, Hopital General Idrissa Pouye, 134 Rue GY, 530 Dakar, Senegal*
[2]*Philadelphia College of Osteopathic Medicine (PCOM), 4170 City Ave, Philadelphia, PA 19131, USA*

Correspondence should be addressed to Mohamed Jalloh; jmohamed60@yahoo.fr

Academic Editor: Walid Farhat

We present three cases of urethral prolapse in prepubertal females in Senegal who presented with vulvar bleeding. Careful gynecologic and urologic physical exams were performed and revealed urethral origin and prolapse. Conservative versus surgical approaches were taken in different patients, but ultimately, each patient received a urethral meatoplasty. Surgical excision of these masses yielded a full recovery in the patients. A careful review of the literature was then undertaken and showed that surgical excision or ligation of the prolapse is preferable to more conservative treatment. The case series article discusses the rare occurrence of urethral prolapse, as well as the epidemiology and prognostic and therapeutic implications of urethral prolapse in prepubertal females. *Introduction.* Urethral prolapse is a rare condition occurring mostly in young black females. It can be worrying to the parents as it often causes vulvar bleeding. *Case Presentation.* We present three cases of urethral prolapse in prepubertal females who presented with vulvar bleeding. Physical exams were performed and revealed urethral origin and prolapse. Each patient underwent a urethral meatoplasty and subsequently experienced a full recovery after respective follow-up of 2 years, 1 year, and 1 year. *Conclusion.* Urethral prolapse is a rare condition which can be managed successfully by surgery. *Plain Language Summary.* This case report on pediatric urethral prolapse showcases the different presentations and modalities of treatment, as the literature does not show that a specific treatment is always undertaken. In some countries, there are strong social considerations and they demonstrate difficulty separating sexual abuse from genitourinary pathologies, which are important to address in the treatment of these conditions.

## 1. Introduction

Urethral prolapse is rare condition in which the proximal portions of the urethra tunnel into the distal portions. The most common presenting symptom of urethral prolapse is bleeding, which is frequently misdiagnosed as sexual abuse or vaginal trauma [1]. Due to the rarity of urethral prolapse, there are no specific algorithms for treatment. We report three cases of pediatric urethral prolapse that occurred at Hospital General Idrissa Pouye (HOGIP) in Dakar, Senegal. Moreover, this series reports on associated social and medicolegal facts.

## 2. Case Report

The first case is a 7-year-old female who was referred to gynecology for a second episode of vulvar bleeding. There was a suspicion for abuse noted by the gynecologist and referring physician. On examination, the patient had bleeding only at the urethral meatus, a circular bulging mass exceeding the limit of the meatus (Figure 1) and an intact hymen and vulva. She was diagnosed with urethral prolapse. After providing parental reassurance and education, the patient was managed surgically by excision and meatoplasty. She had no acute or chronic complications at 2-year follow-up.

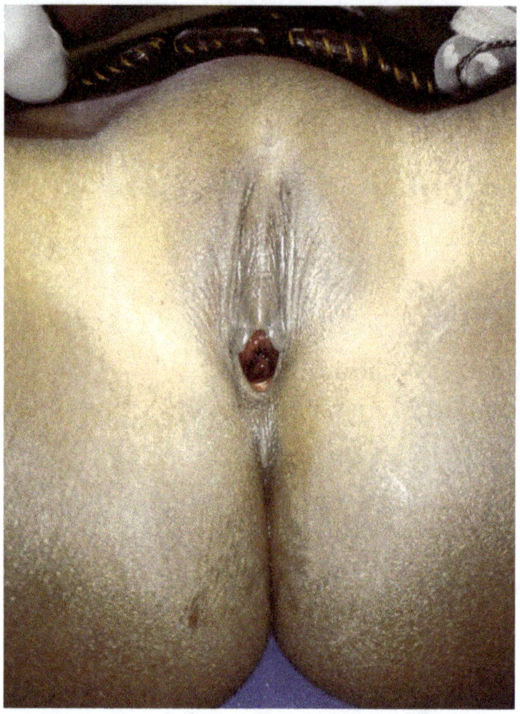

Figure 1: Blood at the meatus of a urethral prolapse in a 7-year-old girl.

The second case is a 4-year-old female referred to gynecology for vulvar bleeding, she was subsequently referred to urology. The patient had an intact hymen and a circular mass exceeding the limit of the meatus without bleeding leading to a diagnosis of urethral prolapse. This patient was managed conservatively with a 2-month course of estrogen ointment, which caused a reduction in bleeding but failed to completely resolve the bleeding and reduce the meatal mass. She was managed surgically with prolapse excision and meatoplasty. The patient resolved well postoperatively and had no acute or chronic complications at a 1-year follow-up.

The third case is a 7-year-old female who was referred to gynecology for vulvar bleeding. She was then referred to a urologist who noted bleeding from the urethra, a mass bulging at the urethra, and a normal hymen (Figure 2). She was diagnosed with urethral prolapse and was managed with excision and meatoplasty. The postoperative course assessed 1-year postoperatively was uneventful.

## 3. Discussion

This case series brings to light several important issues surrounding urethral prolapse, a condition which affects 1 : 3000 mostly prepubertal black females or postmenopausal Caucasian females [2]. Urethral prolapse is thought to be caused by weak attachments between longitudinal and circular oblique smooth muscle layers of the urethra, which can be precipitated by pathologies that increase intra-abdominal pressure or cause ligamentous and muscular laxity [2]. Patients with asthma, upper respiratory infections, trauma, surgery, and obesity have this increase in intra-abdominal pressure [3]. Estrogen deficiency may also play a role, as estrogen normally allows for stronger pelvic floor musculature, demonstrating why this occurs in prepubertal or postmenopausal populations [3].

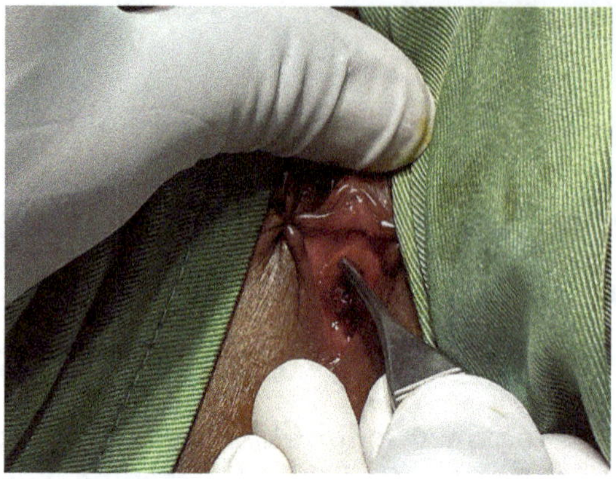

Figure 2: Urethral prolapse in a 7-year-old girl.

Important differential diagnoses, brought to light by multiple studies [1, 2, 4, 5], include ureterocele, penetrating injury, sexual abuse, foreign body, and urethral caruncle. As seen in this case series, every patient was referred to gynecology prior to urological involvement. Sexual abuse was a major concern for the physicians and parents but was absent despite the vulvar bleeding [6].

Urethral prolapse has two main treatment modalities: conservative and surgical. Conservative treatment consists mainly of local estrogen cream which targets at increasing muscle strength [2]. However, Valerie et al. [3] indicated that only 33% of patients were treated successfully with conservative management which is consistent with the findings of Jerkins et al. who found 67% of failure to medical treatment [8]. Surgical repair has two different modalities: excision or ligation, with some studies finding that excision has shorter postop hospital stays [7]. Surgical excision is performed by excising the redundant mucosa followed by anastomosis of the urethra to the vestibule [9, 10]. Surgical ligation is performed over a catheter and requires ligation of the prolapsed tissue. Surgical management has dramatically reduced recurrence rates compared to conservative management [11]. Supporting the current literature, all 3 patients in this series underwent surgical management with prior estrogen treatment in 1 case.

As seen in the first case, there was great parental concern regarding the possibility of sexual abuse. Taking that fact into consideration adds to the current body of knowledge in the literature. Therefore, patient education and reassurance are important.

## 4. Conclusion

Although rare, urethral prolapse is noticeable in the black pediatric population and has excellent outcomes when treated surgically. An interdisciplinary approach and a thorough differential are necessary in order to properly identify and treat urethral prolapse. Surgical management remains the gold standard.

## References

[1] C. Holbrook and D. Misra, "Surgical management of urethral prolapse in girls: 13 years' experience," *BJU International*, vol. 110, no. 1, pp. 132–134, 2012.

[2] S. Hillyer, U. Mooppan, H. Kim, and F. Gulmi, "Diagnosis and treatment of urethral prolapse in children: experience with 34 cases," *Urology*, vol. 73, no. 5, pp. 1008–1011, 2009.

[3] E. Valerie, B. F. Gilchrist, J. Frischer, R. Scriven, D. H. Klotz, and M. L. Ramenofsky, "Diagnosis and treatment of urethral prolapse in children," *Urology*, vol. 54, no. 6, pp. 1082–1084, 1999.

[4] P. Tomà, A. Magistrelli, and M. C. Lucchetti, "Urethral prolapse in a paediatric patient with urogenital bleeding: diagnosis by imaging," *International Urogynecology Journal*, vol. 28, no. 11, pp. 1755-1756, 2017.

[5] A. Aprile, C. Ranzato, M. R. Rizzotto, A. Arseni, L. Da Dalt, and P. Facchin, ""Vaginal" bleeding in prepubertal age: a rare scaring riddle, a case of the urethral prolapse and review of the literature," *Forensic Science International*, vol. 210, no. 1-3, pp. e16–e20, 2011.

[6] J. A. Adams, "Evolution of a classification scale: medical evaluation of suspected child sexual abuse," *Child Maltreatment*, vol. 6, no. 1, pp. 31–36, 2001.

[7] Y. Wei, S. Wu, T. Lin, D. He, X. Li, and G. Wei, "Diagnosis and treatment of urethral prolapse in children: 16 years' experience with 89 Chinese girls," *Arab Journal of Urology*, vol. 15, no. 3, pp. 248–253, 2017.

[8] G. R. Jerkins, K. Verheeck, and H. N. Noe, "Treatment of girls with urethral prolapse," *The Journal of Urology*, vol. 132, no. 4, pp. 732-733, 1984.

[9] A. Adesiyun and M. Samaila, "Childhood urethral mucosa prolapse: outcome of surgical treatment," *Nigerian Journal of Surgical Research*, vol. 8, no. 1-2, 2010.

[10] P. C. Devine and H. C. Kessel, "Surgical correction of urethral prolapse," *The Journal of Urology*, vol. 123, no. 6, pp. 856-857, 1980.

[11] Q. Ballouhey, P. Galinier, A. Gryn, A. Grimaudo, C. Pienkowski, and L. Fourcade, "Benefits of primary surgical resection for symptomatic urethral prolapse in children," *Journal of Pediatric Urology*, vol. 10, no. 1, pp. 94–97, 2014.

16

# The "Tri-Glide" Technique: A Case Report on a Novel Intraoperative Approach for Removal of Retained and Encrusted Ureteral Stents

**Alejandra Perez,[1] Adam Carl Nolte,[1] Giuseppe Maurici,[2] Alexander Charles Small,[3] Spencer Steve Liem,[1] Jorge Francisco Pereira,[1] Alan Scott Polackwich,[1] Rafael Yanes,[1] and Ojas Shah[4]**

[1]*Mount Sinai Medical Center, Department of Urology, 4302 Alton Road, MSOP Suite 540, Miami Beach, FL 33140, USA*
[2]*Olympus Medical Systems Corp., 4302 Alton Road, MSOP Suite 540, Miami Beach, FL 33140, USA*
[3]*Montefiore Medical Center, 1250 Waters Place, Bronx, NY 10461, USA*
[4]*Columbia University Irving Medical Center, Department of Urology, 161 Fort Washington Ave., New York, NY 10032, USA*

Correspondence should be addressed to Rafael Yanes; rafael.yanes@msmc.com

Academic Editor: David Duchene

*Background.* Retained ureteral stents can result in significant morbidity and can be surgically challenging to urologists. A multimodal approach is often necessary for removal, potentially including retrograde and antegrade procedures performed over multiple anesthetic sessions. We describe the novel "Tri-Glide" technique for treating retained stents, particularly those with stent shaft encrustation prohibiting safe removal. *Case Presentation.* Two patients with nephrolithiasis and retained, encrusted ureteral stents were managed with the "Tri-Glide" technique. Patient #1 was a 58-year-old man with a severely calcified ureteral stent, retained for 14 years. After undergoing simultaneous cystolitholapaxy and percutaneous nephrolithotomy to treat proximal and distal encrustations, the stent shaft remained trapped in the ureter due to heavy calcifications. Three hydrophilic guidewires were passed alongside the stent, allowing it to easily slide out of the ureter intact. Patient #2 was a 74-year-old man who after only 3-months of stent dwell time developed severe stent shaft encrustation preventing removal. After multiple maneuvers failed, the "Tri-Glide" technique was used to create a smooth track for stent to slide out intact with gentle traction. Both patients did well postoperatively with no complications. *Conclusion.* The "Tri-Glide" technique can aid in the management of complex encrusted stent extractions, especially when there is significant shaft encrustation.

## 1. Introduction

Since their first description in 1967, ureteral stents remain one of urologists' most commonly used tools for relief of renal and ureteral obstruction [1]. Regardless of the indication for stent placement, patient education, clear postoperative instructions, and proper record-keeping to coordinate removal are imperative to prevent prolonged stent retention. Long-term retained stents can lead to pain, encrustation, obstruction, urinary tract infections (UTI), and ultimately loss of kidney function. Encrustation is a multifactorial process involving biofilm formation, patient risk factors (e.g., stone history, UTI, and pregnancy), characteristics of individual stent materials, and most importantly duration of stent dwell time with some studies demonstrating exponential encrustation rate over time [1].

Retained and encrusted ureteral stents can lead to significant morbidity, sometimes requiring multiple complex procedures for removal [1]. In this report, we describe a novel intraoperative technique to aid in the removal of these stents. The "Tri-Glide" technique involves passage of three hydrophilic guidewires adjacent to a stent, creating a

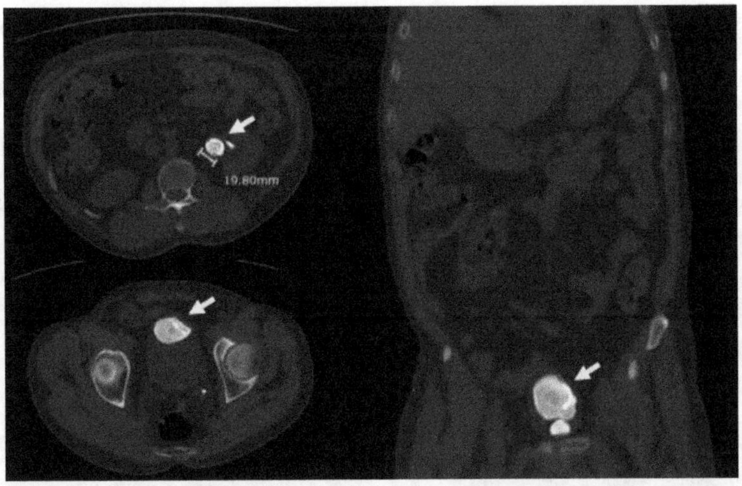


Figure 1: Patient 1 preoperative CT scan showing severe encrustation of the left ureteral stent at the proximal and distal coils (arrows).

hydrophilic track and allowing a stent to slide out with decreased friction. This approach is particularly useful for extraction of an encrusted stent body after other procedures such as cystolitholapaxy and/or percutaneous nephrolithotomy (PCNL) are used for large stone burdens at the proximal and/or distal coils of the stent. We demonstrate that in two patients, the "Tri-Glide" technique led to shortened operative times, fewer procedures, and decreased patient morbidity.

## 2. Cases

*2.1. Patient #1: Antegrade "Tri-Glide" Technique.* The first patient was a 58-year-old man found to have a retained left ureteral stent placed fourteen years prior for an episode of nephrolithiasis. On presentation, the patient had severe left-sided hydronephrosis and large proximal and distal encrustations encasing the stent (Figure 1). He first underwent nephrostomy tube placement, followed by cystolitholapaxy and left percutaneous nephrolithotomy (PCNL) in a Galdakao-modified Valdivia supine position to allow access to the bladder and kidney simultaneously. A 0.038″ Boston Scientific hybrid guidewire was initially placed as a safety wire. Once the proximal and distal ends of the stent were freed from the extensive encrustation, gentle traction was applied with a grasper through the nephroscope in an effort to remove the stent shaft through the PCNL tract. However, the stent was immobile and remained fixed in place. At this point, three 0.035″ Terumo hydrophilic guidewires were each advanced in an antegrade fashion adjacent to the stent until they were visualized in the bladder under fluoroscopy, and the hybrid guidewire was removed. On a second attempt to withdraw the encrusted stent, it slid out of the ureter easily and was removed intact. The shaft was noted to be severely encrusted. The ureter was cleared of residual stone fragments, and the procedure was concluded.

*2.2. Patient #2: Retrograde "Tri-Glide" Technique.* The second patient was a 74-year-old man with a long history of nephrolithiasis and recurrent UTIs requiring multiple surgical interventions, which led to development of a nonfunctional right kidney. Most recently, he had undergone left ureteroscopy with laser lithotripsy and stent placement for treatment of multiple renal calculi. Three months later, he presented for a second stage ureteroscopy and laser lithotripsy. During the procedure, a 0.038″ Boston Scientific hybrid guidewire was advanced to the kidney alongside the stent as a safety wire; however, the stent was unable to be completely extracted using gentle traction. The proximal coil was noted to be stuck in the midureter on fluoroscopy (Figure 2(a)). Semirigid ureteroscopy adjacent to the stent revealed the stent shaft to be severely encrusted. Ureteroscopy with laser lithotripsy was attempted to remove the encrustation, but the ureteroscope could not be safely advanced to the site of the proximal stent coil in the midureter. Therefore, the "Tri-Glide" technique was employed in a retrograde fashion—three 0.035″ Terumo hydrophilic guidewires were advanced alongside the stent until they were visualized in the kidney (Figure 2(b)). The hybrid guidewire was removed, and the encrusted stent was then removed easily and intact using gentle traction with a cystoscopic grasper.

## 3. Discussion

The removal of retained and encrusted ureteral stents can be surgically challenging, and various multimodal approaches can be employed to render patients stent and stone free. Combinations of percutaneous nephrolithotomy, shockwave lithotripsy, ureteroscopy with laser lithotripsy, cystolitholapaxy, and open surgical removal constitute endourologists' armamentarium for treating encrusted stents. The "Tri-Glide" technique is a successful new maneuver to add to this toolbox.

Despite the frequency of this problem, the available evidence for the optimal treatment of retained stents is primarily comprised of case reports and small series. Although no widely accepted guidelines exist, various authors have proposed algorithmic approaches for successful stent removal, which include degree of stent encrustation, stone size, and location. A classification system for forgotten, encrusted,

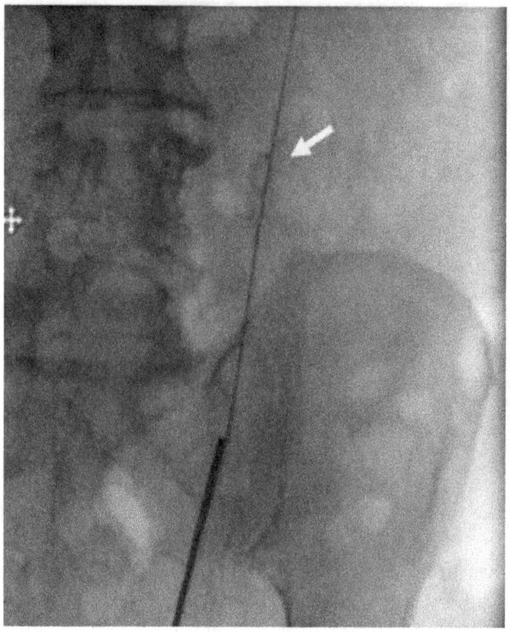

(a)

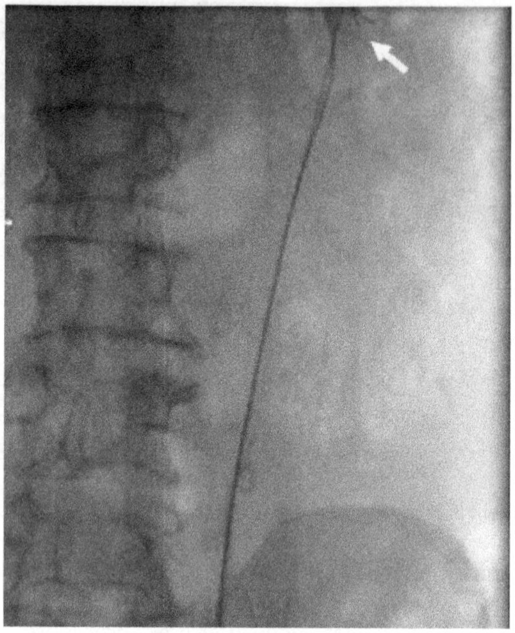

(b)

FIGURE 2: Intraoperative fluoroscopy images from patient #2. (a) The coiled stent in the midureter where it became lodged (arrow). The ureteroscope was unable to be advanced beyond the midureter. (b) 3 hydrophilic guidewires successfully passed to the kidney (arrow), at which point the stent was removed intact.

and calcified ("FECal") Double J stents was proposed by Acosta-Miranda et al. which describes the degree of stent encrustation (linear or bulky), stone size, and location in an algorithmic approach to guide treatment [2]. Murthy et al. also suggested an algorithm for forgotten, encrusted ureteral stents based on renal function, presence of infection, kidney salvageability, and finally, stone burden and site of encrustation as seen on imaging [3]. Generally, if there is lower coil calcification, cystolitholapaxy is indicated, while retrograde or antegrade ureteroscopy is performed for shaft encrustation [3]. If there is minimal upper coil encrustation, SWL is suggested, but if a large volume of proximal coil calcification exists, PCNL and antegrade ureteroscopy would likely be the next step [3]. Using the FECal stent classification, patient #1 would reflect a grade V level of encrustation with calcification found throughout the entirety of the stent. However, patient #2, who had primarily stent shaft encrustation with minimal distal or proximal coil calcifications, falls outside of the criteria for the FECal ureteral stent grading system and could potentially represent a rare, but important new category.

Retained stents often require multiple endourological procedures for removal with several series reporting averages of 2 to 4.2 procedures to render patients stent and stone free [3]. However, multiple single-step approaches have also been successful. These primarily describe the use of retrograde ureteroscopy with Holmium-YAG laser to treat stent calcifications along the way and in some instances fragment the stent itself in order to create more space in the ureter for the instruments. In a retrospective 2017 study, He et al. demonstrated that utilizing a smaller caliber ureteroscope 4.5/6.5 F can be effective in cases where the ureteral orifice or body cannot accommodate a larger, 8/9.8 F ureteroscope. In their series of 36 patients, ureteroscopy was found to be successful in removing encrusted stents in a single anesthetic session [4]. Use of a smaller ureteroscope can lead to reduction in the risk of mucosal injury, ureteral perforation, and ureteral avulsion as well as preclude the need for PCNL which has higher morbidity and complications [4].

Even with success of a ureteroscopic approach in multiple series, a percutaneous approach will be necessary in patients with large proximal coil stone burden and concomitant large renal stones. Indeed, the degree of proximal loop encrustation has been found to correlate with need for PCNL, multiple procedures, and risk of surgical complications [5]. Pais et al. published a multicenter retrospective study of 38 renal units that underwent PCNL for removal of encrusted ureteral stents with a mean dwell time of 28.2 months [5]. They concluded that PCNL alone was only sufficient in 21% of cases, and adjunctive procedures are often required at the time of PCNL or as a separate operation for stent removal [5].

The evolution in positioning for percutaneous nephrolithotomy has led to a shift towards prone and supine modifications that allow for simultaneous antegrade and retrograde access. In our series, a Galdakao-modified Valdivia supine position was utilized in patient 1 to allow two surgeons to work simultaneously to free the proximal and distal coils, thereby decreasing operative time. This can also be performed in a prone split-leg fashion to allow simultaneous access. In our patient, the 0.035″ Terumo hydrophilic guidewires were passed through the nephroscope in an antegrade fashion. However, the use of modified positioning would allow for the guidewires to be passed either retrograde or antegrade in the event of severe stent shaft encrustation, which is another advantage of the "Tri-Glide" technique.

Risks of retrograde ureteroscopy with laser lithotripsy include stent migration, ureteric injury, and perforation [3]. The use of the "Tri-Glide" technique can aid in the management of complex encrusted stent extractions, specifically when there is significant shaft encrustation or when the coils cannot be uncurled completely. It is a straightforward option in cases where a ureteroscope is unable to be advanced next to the stent secondary to severe encrustation or ureteral narrowing.

## 4. Conclusion

Encrustation and retention of ureteral stents can be a serious complication often requiring multiple procedures and a multimodal approach. During difficult extractions due to stent shaft calcification, we describe the novel "Tri-Glide" technique using three hydrophilic guidewires passed simultaneously adjacent to the stent to create a passage for an encrusted stent to be removed from the ureter in a single step.

## References

[1] S. Adanur and F. Ozkaya, "Challenges in treatment and diagnosis of forgotten/encrusted double-J ureteral stents: the largest single-center experience," *Renal Failure*, vol. 38, no. 6, pp. 920–926, 2016.

[2] A. Acosta-Miranda, J. Milner, and T. Turk, "The FECal double-J: a simplified approach in the management of encrusted and retained ureteral stents," *Journal of Endourology*, vol. 23, no. 3, pp. 409–415, 2009.

[3] K. V. Murthy, S. J. Reddy, and D. V. Prasad, "Endourological management of forgotten encrusted ureteral stents," *International Brazilian Journal of Urology*, vol. 36, no. 4, pp. 420–429, 2010.

[4] Z. He, H. Lei, C. Zhang, H. Wang, F. Tang, and G. Zeng, "Experience of retaining encrusted ureteral stents: URL by 4.5/6.5F ureteroscope can reduce the possibility of PCNL," *Urolithiasis*, vol. 46, no. 4, pp. 357–361, 2018.

[5] V. Pais, B. Chew, O. Shaw et al., "Percutaneous nephrolithotomy for removal of encrusted ureteral stents: a multicenter study," *Journal of Endourology*, vol. 28, no. 10, pp. 1188–1191, 2014.

# 17

# Plasmacytoid Urothelial Carcinoma of the Bladder that Manifests Disseminated Carcinomatosis of the Bone Marrow: A Case Report of Extremely Rapid Progression

**Nobuhiko Shimizu,[1] Yoshinobu Moritoki,[1,2] Nao Katsumi,[1] Takahiro Yanase,[3] Teruaki Sugino,[3] Kazuhiro Kanemoto,[1] Hidetoshi Akita,[1] and Takahiro Yasui[3]**

[1]*Department of Urology, Anjo Kosei Hospital, Anjo, Japan*
[2]*Department of Urology, Toyokawa City Hospital, Toyokawa, Japan*
[3]*Department of Nephro-Urology, Nagoya City University Graduate School of Medical Sciences, Nagoya, Japan*

Correspondence should be addressed to Yoshinobu Moritoki; moriji314@gmail.com

Academic Editor: Fumitaka Koga

Plasmacytoid urothelial carcinoma (PUC) of the bladder is a rare variant of invasive urothelial carcinoma (UC) with aggressive behavior. Despite its prognosis being poorer than that of conventional UC, a median overall survival of approximately 2 years is ensured when it is treated with radical cystectomy (RC), and few patients die within a few months of RC. In this paper, we report the case of a patient with PUC who developed widespread bone metastasis only 6 weeks after RC, which resulted in death within 2 months postoperatively.

## 1. Introduction

Plasmacytoid urothelial carcinoma (PUC) is a rare variant of invasive urothelial carcinoma (UC) and accounts for 1% to 3% of all invasive UCs [1]. Compared to conventional UC, PUC has a greater chance of higher-stage disease, metastasis at presentation, and poor prognosis [2]. Although clinical data on the prognosis of patients with PUC are limited, their median overall survival when treated with radical cystectomy (RC) and adjuvant cisplatin-based chemotherapy is 27.4 months (95% CI: 16.8-37.9 months) [3], and few patients die within a few months of RC. In this paper, we report a case of PUC that developed widespread bone metastasis 6 weeks after RC, which resulted in death within 2 months postoperatively.

## 2. Case Presentation

A 56-year-old man with hypertension and dyslipidemia was admitted to the hospital because of urinary bladder clot retention. The patient was asymptomatic until admission. He had smoked 54 pack-years. Magnetic resonance imaging (MRI) revealed a tumor and a hematoma in the bladder (Figures 1(a) and 1(b)). On account of continuous hemorrhage and anemia, transurethral electrocoagulation and resection of a nonpedunculated bladder tumor were performed. Hematoxylin and eosin (HE) staining of the bladder tumor showed discohesive malignant cells with eccentrically placed nuclei and abundant cytoplasm, resembling plasma cells. The resection specimen did not contain bladder muscle (Figure 2(a)). The tumor cells were immunoreactive for

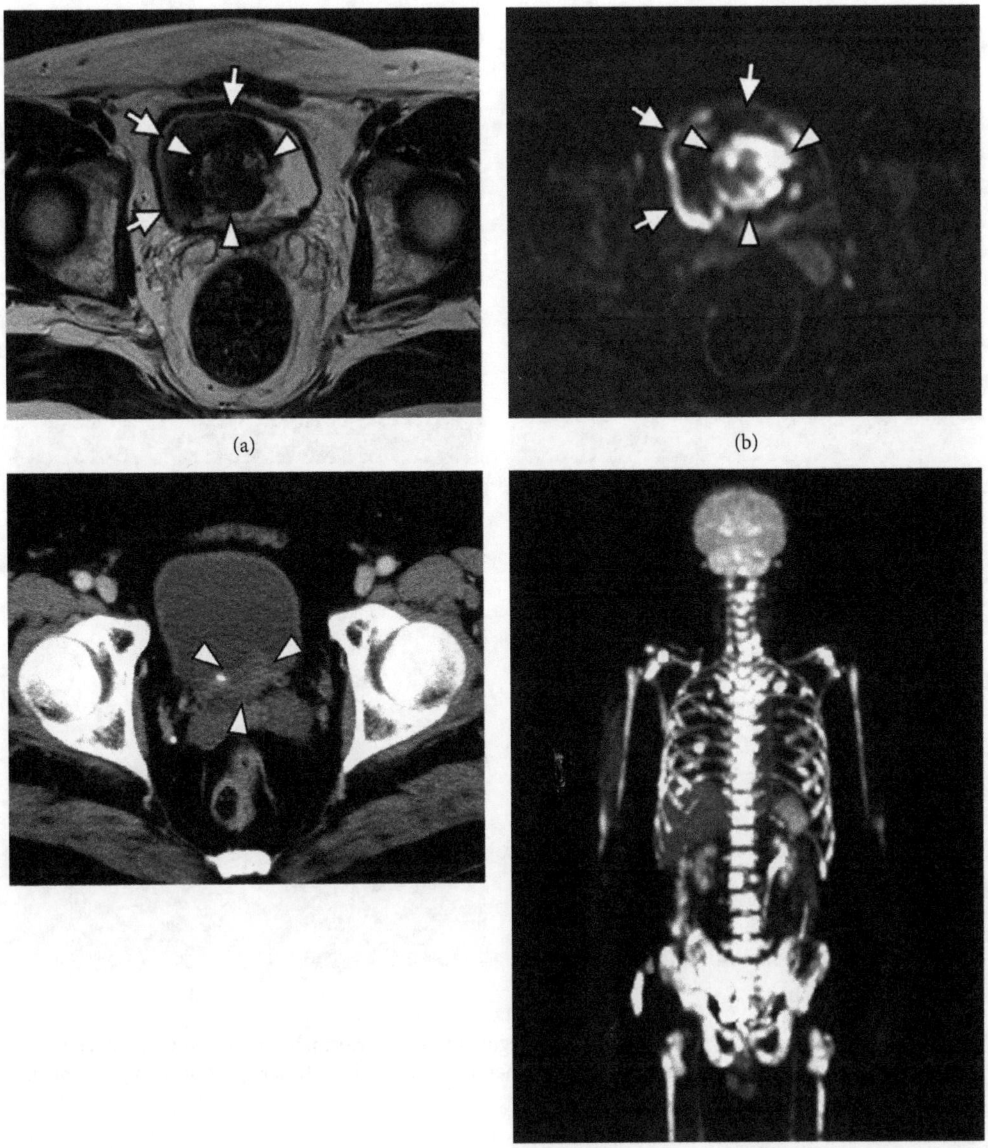

(a) (b) (c) (d)

FIGURE 1: (a) MRI T2-weighted image and (b) diffusion-weighted image showed a bladder tumor (white arrowheads) with hematoma (white arrows). (c) The CT image after NAC did not show rapid progression of the bladder tumor (white arrowheads). (d) The FDG-PET findings when the patient presented with low back pain after the RC.

pancytokeratin (Figure 2(b)), GATA3 (Figure 2(c)), and CD138 (Figure 2(d)), thereby leading to the diagnosis of invasive PUC, grade 3 (G3), pT1, or higher. Immunohistochemical staining for E-cadherin expression in PUC cells was negative, which suggested an aggressive phenotype of this bladder tumor (Figures 3(a) and 3(b)). Computed tomography (CT) did not show any metastasis in the lymph nodes or other organs, and MRI did not show any muscle invasion. Since upstaging of pT1 tumors diagnosed with transurethral resections is common, RC was performed, after three cycles of neoadjuvant chemotherapy (NAC) with gemcitabine and cisplatin. CT imaging obtained after NAC did not show rapid progression of the bladder tumor (Figure 1(c)). The pathological stage was pT3aN0 and RM0 with lymphovascular invasion. The postoperative course was uneventful, although the patient presented with low back pain on the 39$^{th}$ postoperative day. The hematologic examination on admission revealed a high white blood cell count (129,600 cells/$\mu$L), high serum alkaline phosphatase (1039 U/L), hypercalcemia (17.0 mg/dL), and low serum albumin level (3.3 g/dL). These findings are indicative of bone diseases such as primary myeloproliferative disease or bone metastasis. The $^{18}$F-fluorodeoxyglucose (FDG) positron emission tomography (PET) findings revealed significant FDG uptake in nearly all bones (Figure 1(d)). Histological findings of the bone marrow biopsy were negative for malignancy, which seemed to be a pseudonegative finding.

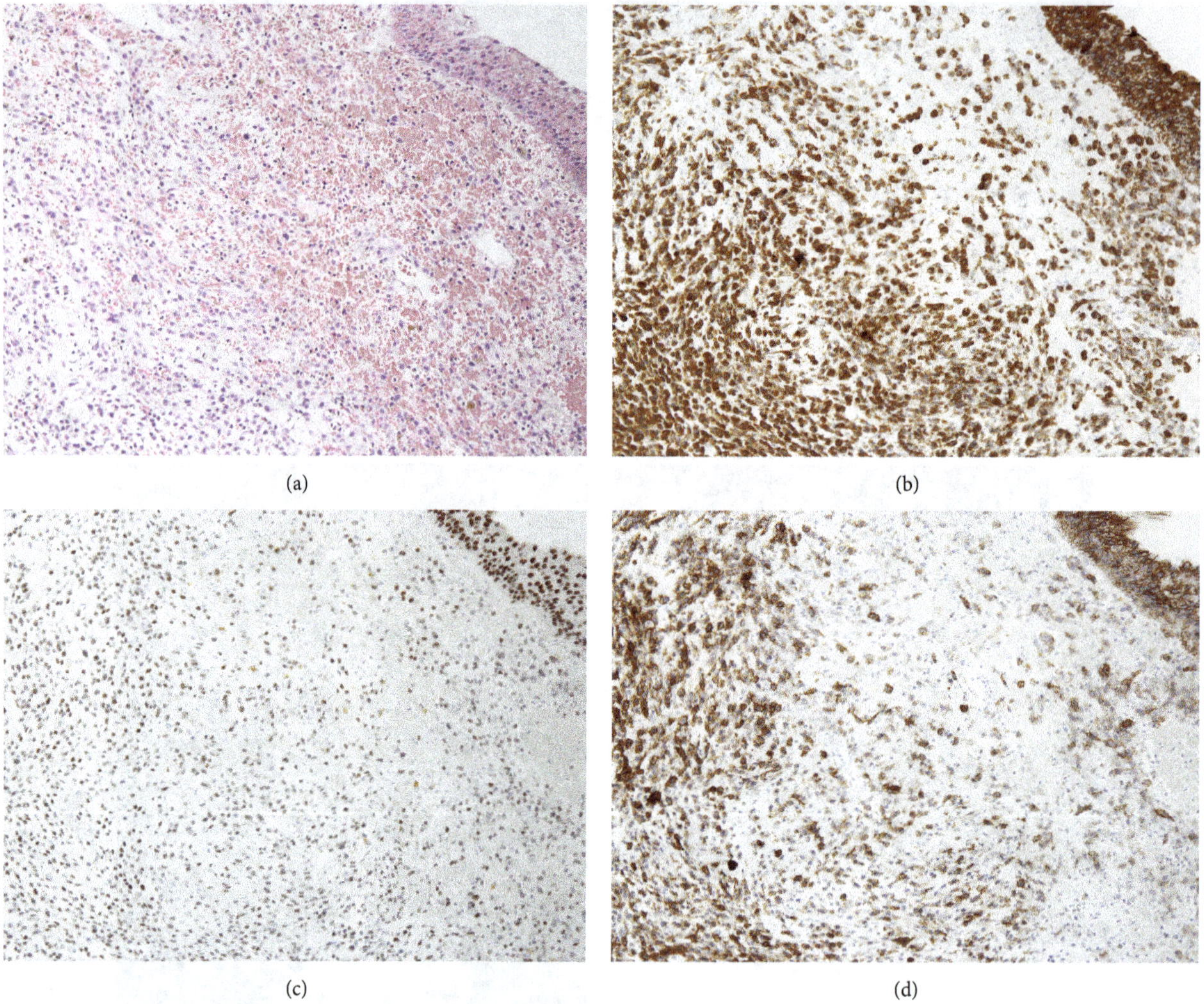

FIGURE 2: (a) HE staining of the tumor when transurethral electrocoagulation was performed. (b–d) Immunohistochemical staining findings of the tumor for pancytokeratin (b), GATA3 (c), and CD138 (d) when transurethral electrocoagulation was performed.

On the 53rd postoperative day, the patient passed away, which occurred just after a second bone marrow biopsy had been performed. Histological findings of the biopsy showed metastasis of the PUC (Figures 3(c) and 3(d)). The autopsy revealed metastasis of the bone marrow concomitant with small metastasis to the lung, chest wall, and spleen, which were not detected on the FDG-PET image.

## 3. Discussion

PUC is clinically aggressive and has a worse median overall survival (27.4 months) than does conventional UC (62.6 months; $P = 0.13$) when treated with RC and adjuvant cisplatin-based chemotherapy [3]. Its prognosis is worse, although it allows for 2 years of life expectancy after RC. However, in this case, the patient died 2 months after the surgery because of the extremely rapid progression of the disease.

A previous study reported that PUC has a poor response to NAC [4], whereas a systematic review reported that NAC was beneficial for PUC [5]. Therefore, the treatment strategies for PUC remain controversial. After we discussed whether to choose NAC or upfront RC, we decided on NAC for this patient in the hope that NAC could downstage the disease.

This patient was also diagnosed as having disseminated carcinomatosis of the bone marrow (CBM), which is characterized by widespread bone metastasis from solid tumors with coexistent hematologic disorders [6]. CBM is most frequently seen as a complication of gastric cancer, and only one case has been reported with urothelial carcinoma [7]. Despite the multidisciplinary treatment, the prognosis of CBM is quite poor (less than 1 year of life expectancy). In this patient, the prognosis was only within 2 months.

Investigators have noted that loss of E-cadherin expression may be associated with a plasmacytoid differentiation pattern in bladder UC, thereby explaining the aggressive

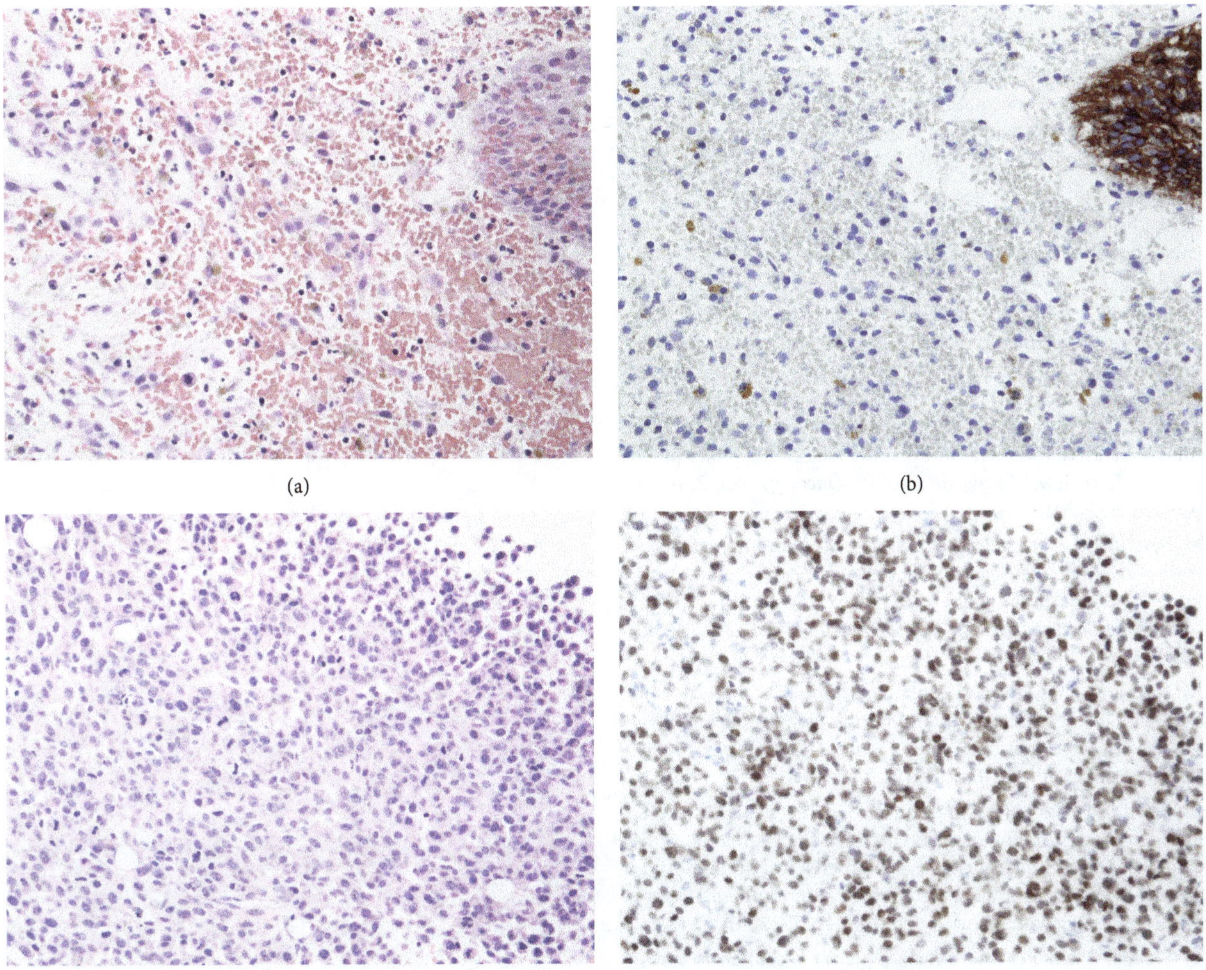

(a) (b) (c) (d)

FIGURE 3: (a) HE staining and (b) immunohistochemical staining for E-cadherin expression of the tumor when transurethral electrocoagulation was performed. (c) HE staining and (d) immunohistochemical staining for GATA3 from the second bone marrow biopsy.

behavior of PUC [1]. E-cadherin loss is associated with loss of cell differentiation and increased cell invasion, which leads to more aggressive pathology and poor prognosis in cases of bladder UC [8]. The effect of E-cadherin loss on the prognosis of PUC has not been established, although the complete loss of membranous E-cadherin expression was observed in as many as 76.2% of PUC cases [9]. In this patient, the tumor showed complete loss of membranous E-cadherin expression (Figure 3(b)), which may explain the poor prognosis in this patient.

According to previous studies [10, 11], an advanced pathological stage on RC after NAC and lymphovascular invasion is associated with a poor prognosis. Loss of E-cadherin, disseminated CBM, an advanced pathological stage after NAC, and lymphovascular invasion may have contributed to the extremely low life expectancy. A fact that must be noted is that some cases of PUC progress rapidly, even when the presurgical stage is non-muscle-invasive UC.

## Authors' Contributions

N.S., N.K., and Y.M. were responsible for drafting of the manuscript. N.S., T.Y., and Y.M. were responsible for conceptualization. T.S., K.K., and H.A. were responsible for the revision of the manuscript. Y.M. and T.Y. were responsible for the supervision. All authors have read and approved the final manuscript.

## References

[1] D. K. Kim, J. W. Kim, J. Y. Ro et al., "Plasmacytoid variant urothelial carcinoma of the bladder: a systematic review and meta-analysis of clinicopathological features and survival outcomes," *The Journal of Urology*, vol. 204, no. 2, pp. 215–223, 2020.

[2] S. Sood and G. P. Paner, "Plasmacytoid urothelial carcinoma: an unusual variant that warrants aggressive management and critical distinction on transurethral resections", *Archives of*

*Pathology & Laboratory Medicine*, vol. 143, no. 12, pp. 1562–1567, 2019.

[3] B. Keck, S. Wach, R. Stoehr et al., "Plasmacytoid variant of bladder cancer defines patients with poor prognosis if treated with cystectomy and adjuvant cisplatin-based chemotherapy," *BMC Cancer*, vol. 13, no. 1, p. 71, 2013.

[4] K. R. M. Leite, L. L. Borges, L. R. Filho et al., "Histological variants of urothelial carcinoma predict no response to neoadjuvant chemotherapy," *Clinical Genitourinary Cancer*, vol. 20, no. 1, pp. e1–e6, 2022.

[5] E. Veskimäe, E. L. Espinos, H. M. Bruins et al., "What is the prognostic and clinical importance of urothelial and nonurothelial histological variants of bladder cancer in predicting oncological outcomes in patients with muscle-invasive and metastatic bladder cancer? A European Association of Urology muscle invasive and metastatic bladder cancer guidelines panel systematic review," *European Urology Oncology*, vol. 2, no. 6, pp. 625–642, 2019.

[6] H. Iguchi, "Recent aspects for disseminated carcinomatosis of the bone marrow associated with gastric cancer: what has been done for the past, and what will be needed in future?," *World Journal of Gastroenterology*, vol. 21, no. 43, pp. 12249–12260, 2015.

[7] M. Kohno, K. Miyama, A. Gohbara, T. Onuki, S. Sugiura, and I. Ikeda, "Disseminated carcinomatosis of the bone marrow with urothelial carcinoma," *The Japanese Journal of Urology*, vol. 106, no. 2, pp. 114–117, 2015.

[8] F. Erdemir, F. Ozcan, I. Kilicaslan, B. S. Parlaktas, N. Uluocak, and O. Gokce, "The relationship between the expression of E-cadherin and tumor recurrence and progression in high-grade stage T1 bladder urothelial carcinoma," *International Urology and Nephrology*, vol. 39, no. 4, pp. 1031–1037, 2007.

[9] B. Keck, S. Wach, F. Kunath et al., "Nuclear E-cadherin expression is associated with the loss of membranous E-cadherin, plasmacytoid differentiation and reduced overall survival in urothelial carcinoma of the bladder," *Annals of Surgical Oncology*, vol. 20, no. 7, pp. 2440–2445, 2013.

[10] M. C. Mir, M. Marchioni, H. Zargar et al., "Nomogram predicting bladder cancer-specific mortality after neoadjuvant chemotherapy and radical cystectomy for muscle-invasive bladder cancer: results of an international consortium," *European Urology Focus*, vol. 7, no. 6, pp. 1347–1354, 2021.

[11] R. Mathieu, I. Lucca, M. Rouprêt, A. Briganti, and S. F. Shariat, "The prognostic role of lymphovascular invasion in urothelial carcinoma of the bladder," *Nature Reviews Urology*, vol. 13, no. 8, pp. 471–479, 2016.

# 18

# Melanosis of the Bladder: Possible Pathogenetic Mechanisms

**Justin E. Dupey**[1] **Sarah J. Wood**[2] **and Richard Y. Ball**[1]

[1]*Norfolk and Waveney Cellular Pathology Service, Norfolk and Norwich University Hospitals NHS Foundation Trust, Colney Lane, Norwich, Norfolk NR4 7UY, UK*
[2]*Department of Urology, Norfolk and Norwich University Hospitals NHS Foundation Trust, Colney Lane, Norwich, Norfolk NR4 7UY, UK*

Correspondence should be addressed to Richard Y. Ball; richard.ball@nnuh.nhs.uk

Academic Editor: Tun-Chieh Chen

Melanin accumulation within the bladder urothelium and/or macrophages in the lamina propria (melanosis of the bladder) is a very rare phenomenon of unknown pathogenesis. Its rarity argues for a complex, likely multifactorial, causation. We describe bladder melanosis developing after Botox therapy in an elderly woman with a history of overactive bladder, treated grade 2 uterovaginal prolapse, and episodes of urinary tract infection and speculate that one factor (probably of many) in its pathogenesis may be a derangement of local neurourothelial interactions.

## 1. Introduction

Melanosis of the bladder is the presence of melanin within the bladder urothelium and/or macrophages in the lamina propria. It was first recorded in humans in 1986 [1], since when about two dozen additional cases have been reported [2–21]. It affects middle-aged and older men and women (age range 43–86 years; median age = 65 years, including our case), with a slight male preponderance (M : F = 1.5). It is usually discovered when patients undergo cystoscopy to investigate various non-specific urinary tract symptoms. The pathogenesis is obscure.

In this report, we describe a case developing after botulinum toxin (Botox) therapy for an overactive bladder and discuss possible pathogenetic mechanisms.

## 2. Case Presentation

In September 2014, a 69-year-old woman presented to a gynaecologist with a history of urgency, urge incontinence, nocturia ×3–4, and occasional voiding difficulty. She had grade 2 uterovaginal prolapse on straining. A cystocoele, extending almost to the level of the hymen, was present. Subsequent urodynamic studies showed detrusor overactivity with minimal stress incontinence. She was advised to start anticholinergics for bladder overactivity and was counselled for surgery for the uterine prolapse. In October 2015, she underwent vaginal hysterectomy. Six months later, she complained of urgency, urge incontinence, and urine leakage on bending and standing. Gynaecological examination showed a well-supported wall and minimal cystocoele. Her symptoms continued, despite changing to mirabegron, and Botox therapy was discussed. She was taught how to undertake intermittent self-catheterisation (ISC) prior to Botox therapy. A urinary tract infection (UTI) was noted at first presentation for Botox injections, and the procedure was deferred.

In April 2017, cystoscopy under general anaesthesia (GA) revealed a normal urothelium; 100 units of Botox were injected into 10 sites in the bladder, sparing the trigone. At review two months later, her symptoms were no better. She had not attempted ISC postoperatively, and a residual urine volume at that time was 300 mL. She was again encouraged to perform SC twice daily to drain the residual urine.

Six months post-Botox, she continued to be symptomatic. She had not performed ISC (residual urine volume still

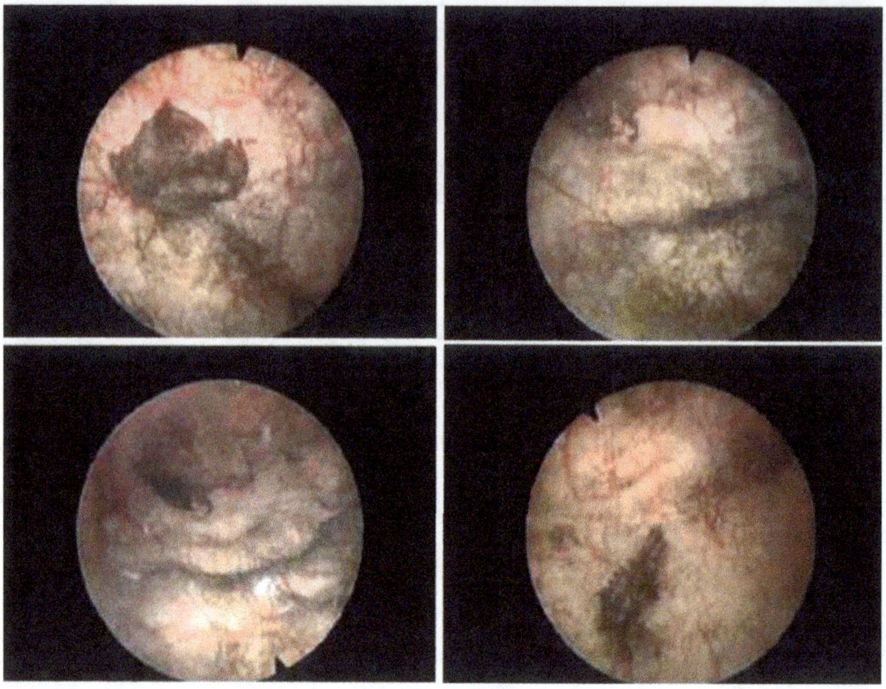

Figure 1: Cystoscopic images showing patches of melanosis of the bladder.

300 mL) and had problems with recurrent UTIs. Her infections were treated, and modifications in medication were tried to control her bladder overactivity.

In September 2018, she was referred to the Urology Department because of persistent nonvisible haematuria. She stated that her urinary symptoms, particularly urgency and urge incontinence associated with hesitancy on voiding, had not been controlled. Repeated MSUs had been positive despite being asymptomatic for infection. Ultrasound scan showed normal upper tracts and a postvoid residual urine volume of 260 mL. Flexible cystoscopy and subsequent GA cystoscopy revealed a normal urethra and a large-capacity bladder with dark-staining patches throughout (Figure 1), but sparing the trigone; there was no evidence of tumour. Four cold cup biopsies were obtained and cystodiathermy was undertaken.

She continued to have UTIs. Follow-up flexible cystoscopy 10 months after GA cystoscopy showed ongoing areas of pigmentation (which were possibly less severe than previously). She was started on low-dose antibiotics and was again advised to perform ISC.

In January 2020, because of ongoing infections, she was prescribed intravesical iAluRil weekly instillation for 4 weeks and further monthly single doses for the following 5 months, totalling 9 doses. She would sporadically perform ISC last thing at night only. This regime was interrupted because of the COVID-19 lockdown, and she had further problems with infections and incontinence.

In September 2020, cystoscopy showed patches of pigmentation dotted throughout the bladder, but they did not seem as marked as previously. She was again advised to increase ISC to twice daily (150 mL drained bd) and to recommence iAluRil instillations.

## 3. Histopathology Findings

The biopsies showed widespread dark brown cytoplasmic pigment in the urothelium, present at many levels but most abundant in the outer layers, especially the umbrella cells (Figure 2). It consisted of small to medium-sized granules with occasional course lumps and was positive with the Masson Fontana method (Figure 2). That reaction was abolished by prior treatment of the section with a bleach, confirming melanin and establishing the diagnosis of melanosis. The pigment was not ceroid/lipofuscin (negative with the Ziehl-Neelsen (ZN), modified ZN, oil-red-O and PAS.D methods) or haemosiderin (negative with Perls' method).

Immunohistochemical staining showed that the urothelium, including that containing pigment, was GATA-3-positive. Many (but not all) of the pigmented urothelial cells stained moderately strongly for S100 protein (Figure 2) and weakly for CD68. No definite melanocytes were recognised within the urothelium. There was no evidence of dysplasia or malignancy.

The superficial lamina propria showed focal mild nonspecific chronic inflammation. Granules of melanin were present in a few macrophages (CD68+).

## 4. Discussion

Bladder melanosis has been reported in patients with a variety of symptoms and findings, including: urinary obstruction, urgency, and incontinence; lower urinary tract symptoms; flank or loin pain; haematuria; and UTIs. It may be a transient phenomenon: one report [19] indicates that melanosis may completely resolve spontaneously within a year. It has also resolved after BCG therapy for urothelial

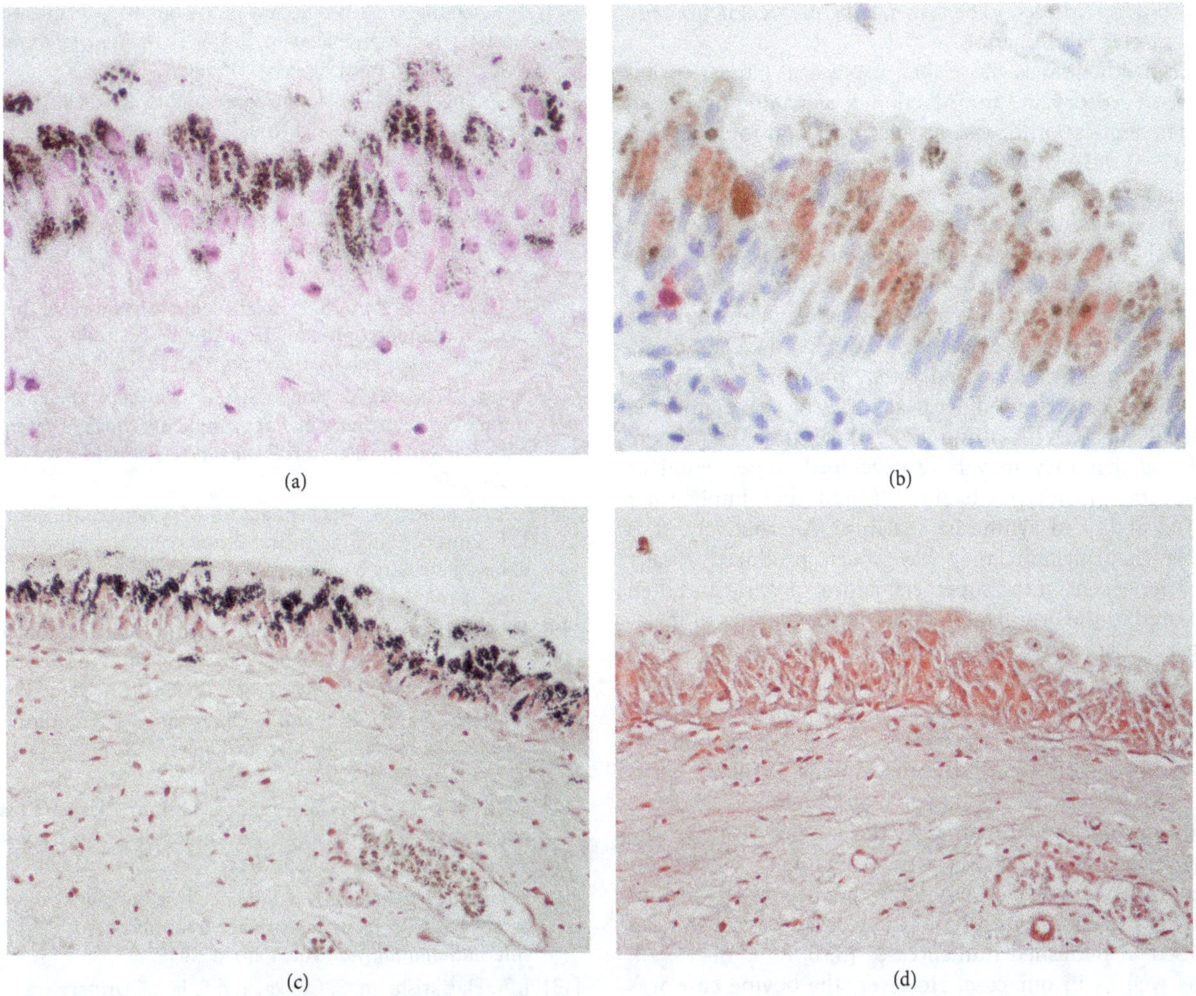

FIGURE 2: Histopathological preparations of bladder mucosa showing melanosis. (a) H&E-stained section showing melanin in the urothelium. (b) Many of the pigmented urothelial cells are immunoreactive for S100 protein (red stain). (c) The melanin is shown (black) in a Masson Fontana preparation. (d) The Masson Fontana reaction is abolished by prior treatment of the section with a bleach.

carcinoma [8]. Our patient, an elderly woman with an overactive bladder, treated grade 2 uterovaginal prolapse and subsequent episodes of UTI, resembled in many respects the typical patient with bladder melanosis. Her melanosis developed after a prolonged sequence of lower urinary tract symptoms associated with detrusor overactivity (followed by Botox therapy) and recurrent UTIs. Cystoscopy at the administration of Botox showed normal urothelium. While it may be tempting to believe that there was a causal link between the Botox therapy and the development of bladder melanosis, that association may be coincidental. The melanosis could perhaps have been caused by her UTIs. Such an association has been reported previously [8, 12].

Melanocytes are not a normal component of bladder urothelium. When discussing the origin of bladder melanosis, two main mechanisms, first mentioned by Rossen and Petersen [2], have been put forward to explain the assumed acquisition of melanocytes by the urothelium: migration of neural crest cells or their differentiation from local stem cells. However, very few reports indicate the presence of melanocytes in the urothelium, raising doubt about the validity of these proposals. However, it is possible that the acquisition of melanocytes by the urothelium is transient. A third possible process, melanuria, was mentioned by Pandian and colleagues [15], who noted that the melanin appeared to be within lysosomes, rather than melanosomes. If that were the case, melanosis of the bladder might be commoner in dark-skinned races than in white Caucasians. The race of the subjects is described in a minority of the case reports; where noted, Caucasians represent 80% and Afro-Caribbeans 20% of the subjects. While it cannot be excluded, melanuria seems an unlikely explanation.

If bladder melanosis is not the result of migration of neural crest cells, transdifferentiation of urothelial stem cells, or melanuria, how does it occur? Two other potential mechanisms might be considered: an abnormal reaction of the mucosal nerve plexus and the plasticity of urothelium. Our patient's melanosis developed after Botox therapy, which draws attention to the possible significance of the innervation of the bladder in the pathogenesis of melanosis. Some of the reported patients also had symptoms suggesting overactivity of the bladder or of outflow obstruction, conditions that would be expected to be associated with local neural and neuromuscular dysfunction.

The urothelium is more than a physical barrier: it has specialised sensory and transduction or signalling properties [22]. The expression of various receptors and ion channels implies that the urothelium can respond to a variety of stimuli. Nerve fibres are in close proximity to the urothelium. There may, therefore, be reciprocal communication between urothelial cells and nearby nerves and other cells types, such as smooth muscle cells and interstitial cells of Cajal [22].

Urothelium, both in its native state and when neoplastic, is recognised to have the potential to differentiate along various lines, often in a focal and patchy manner. The urothelium in our case showed focal staining of the pigmented urothelial cells (GATA-3-immunoreactive) for S100 protein, suggesting that they may have developed some neural or melanocytic phenotypic features. Might that imply their acquired ability to synthesise melanin? Alternatively, it is possible that melanin may have been produced focally within nerve cells in the superficial lamina propria and then transferred to the urothelium, rather in the manner of melanocytes and keratinocytes in the skin.

A unique case of melanosis of the bladder has been reported in a 7-year-old cow [23]. Melanin was present within the lamina propria in melanocytes and melanophages but was not seen in the urothelium. Bovine papilloma virus type 2 (BPV-2) DNA was detected, and there was evidence of mild chronic inflammation in the lamina propria. The authors suggested that the mild interstitial cystitis was related to BPV-2 infection but not to the melanosis. Melanophages in the lamina propria of the bladder have also been described in published human cases [3, 6, 8, 9, 14–16, 20, 21], as well as in our case. However, the bovine case was pathologically different from those so far reported in humans and the pathogenetic mechanisms may be different.

## 5. Conclusion

Melanosis of the bladder appears to be a rare acquired, sometimes transient, state. Its pathogenesis remains obscure. Given its rarity, the cause is likely to be complex and multifactorial; it may well be an idiosyncratic reaction. Published cases suggest the possibility that derangement of neural processes in the bladder wall and their interaction with the urothelium may be important. In our patient, an overactive bladder with episodes of UTI may have been significant underlying factors in pathogenesis, possibly exacerbated by the effects of Botox therapy.

## References


[1] J. Alroy, A. A. Ucci, J. A. Heaney, H. D. Mitcheson, V. E. Gavris, and W. Woods, "Multifocal pigmentation of prostatic and bladder urothelium," *Journal of Urology*, vol. 136, 1 Part 1, pp. 96-97, 1986.

[2] K. Rossen and M. M. Petersen, "Simple melanosis of the bladder," *Journal of Urology*, vol. 161, no. 5, p. 1564, 1999.

[3] F. K. Chong, G. Z. Wolfe, and W. J. Coukos, "Melanosis vesica urinaria: is it a premalignant lesion?," *The Journal of urology*, vol. 161, no. 6, pp. 1904-1905, 1999.

[4] P. F. Engelhardt, G. Hohlbrugger, and C. R. Riedl, "Melanose der Harnblase–Fallbericht mit Langzeitverlauf über 10 Jahre und Literaturübersicht," *Aktuelle Urologie*, vol. 37, no. 3, pp. 222–224, 2006.

[5] R. E. Wieringa, H. J. Blaauwgeers, and G. van Andel, "Pseudomelanosis of the bladder," *Acta Cytologica*, vol. 50, no. 4, pp. 473–475, 2006.

[6] F. Di Fiore, D. Pone, S. Domizio et al., "Melanosis of the bladder: a rare endoscopic and histopathological finding," *Urologia internationalis*, vol. 78, no. 2, pp. 185–187, 2007.

[7] B. Jin, S. Y. Zaidi, M. Hollowell, C. Hollowell, and H. Saleh, "A unique case of urinary bladder simple melanosis: a case report and review of the literature," *Diagnostic Pathology*, vol. 4, no. 1, p. 24, 2009.

[8] S. L. Sanborn, G. MacLennan, M. M. Cooney, M. Zhou, and L. E. Ponsky, "High-grade transitional cell carcinoma and melanosis of urinary bladder: case report and review of the literature," *Urology*, vol. 73, no. 4, 2009.

[9] G. A. Talmon, A. U. Khan, R. K. Koerber, and S. L. Johansson, "Simple melanosis of the bladder: a rare entity," *International Journal of Surgical Pathology*, vol. 18, no. 6, pp. 547–549, 2010.

[10] R. Sen Gupta, E. Seidl, and F. Oberpenning, "An unusual and rare case of urinary bladder melanosis," *Journal of Endourology*, vol. 24, no. 4, pp. 525-526, 2010.

[11] C. B. Willys, D. C. Winkle, and K. M. Kerr, "Urinary bladder melanosis: case report of a rare mucosal lesion," *Pathology*, vol. 43, no. 2, pp. 164–166, 2011.

[12] S. Lightowlers and A. Sengupta, "A case of bladder melanosis associated with recurrent urinary tract infections," *UroToday International Journal*, vol. 4, no. 6, 2011.

[13] J. A. Harikrishnan, S. Chilka, and S. Jain, "Urinary tract transitional cell carcinoma and melanosis of the bladder: a case report and review of the literature," *Annals of the Royal College of Surgeons of England*, vol. 94, no. 4, pp. e152–e154, 2012.

[14] P. Patel, G. Gotto, A. Kavanagh, S. Al Bashir, T. A. Bismar, and K. Trpkov, "Urinary bladder melanosis associated with urothelial dysplasia and invasive urothelial carcinoma: a report of two cases," *Analytical and Quantitative Cytopathology and Histopathology*, vol. 35, no. 5, pp. 294–300, 2013.

[15] S. S. Pandian, G. H. Rix, N. Jayasooriya, P. Conn, and D. Cano, "Melanosis of the urinary bladder – a case report and review of the literature," *Urology & Nephrology Open Access Journal*, vol. 3, no. 5, p. 00093, 2016.

[16] R. Godinho, E. Tavares, R. Oliveira, and P. Conceição, "Bladder melanosis: a rare case report," *Journal of Case Reports and Images in Urology*, vol. 1, no. 8, article 112016, 2016.

[17] S. E. Yau, E. J. Singer, Y. Sun, and M. H. Johnson, "Bladder melanosis with concurrent urothelial carcinoma," *Urology Case Reports*, vol. 15, pp. 30–32, 2017.

[18] S. L. Valente, J. M. Bieniek, and S. S. Kesler, "Urothelial melanosis of the bladder," *The Canadian Journal of Urology*, vol. 24, no. 5, pp. 9035–9037, 2017.

[19] Z. Mera, S. Patel, O. Qassid, and R. England, "Unusual case of simple urinary bladder melanosis with complete resolution," *BMJ Case Reports*, vol. 2018, 2018.

[20] D. M. Lopategui, R. C. Griffith, and J. Santos Cortes, "Melanosis of the bladder: a rare diagnosis," *Urology Case Reports*, vol. 33, article 101283, 2020.

[21] N. Barriobero, V. M. Nieto, H. A. Perez, and A. V. Diaz, "Melanosis of the bladder: a case report and review of the literature," *Medical Case Reports*, vol. 7, no. 1, p. 3, 2021.

[22] L. Merrill, E. J. Gonzalez, B. M. Girard, and M. A. Vizzard, "Receptors, channels, and signalling in the urothelial sensory system in the bladder," *Nature Reviews Urology*, vol. 13, no. 4, pp. 193–204, 2016.

[23] V. Russo, G. Borzacchiello, R. Brun et al., "Melanosis of the urinary bladder in a cow," *Veterinary Pathology*, vol. 45, no. 1, pp. 46–50, 2008.

# 19

# Complete Duplex of the Left Ureter with Lower Moiety Hydronephrosis Secondary to Ureteral Stone in Adult

**Masresha S. Dino, Alemayehu Tegegn Tefera, Kaleab Hebtemichael Gebreselassie, Sena Sefera Akkasa, and Ferid Ousman Mummed**

*St. Paul's Hospital Millennium Medical College, Department of Surgery, Urology Unit, Addis Ababa, Ethiopia*

Correspondence should be addressed to Masresha S. Dino; masreshasolomon412@gmail.com

Academic Editor: Tun-Chieh Chen

Ureteral duplication is a common embryologic abnormality of the kidney with an incidence rate of 0.8% in adults. However, complete duplex ureters opening independently into the urinary bladder are rarely present. We report a 35-year-old female who presented with left flank pain in the last three years. Abdominal CT scan showed left complete duplicated system with lower moiety hydroureteronephrosis and obstructed midureteral stone. The patient underwent left retroperitoneal exploration with complete excision of the hydronephrotic sac. The postoperative course was uneventful without complications. In conclusion, a complete duplex kidney with lower moiety hydronephrosis caused by mid ureteric stone is rare. The renal duplication system should be diagnosed and followed with image guidance periodically as the late diagnosis may have poor outcomes with loss of the kidney or part of it.

## 1. Introduction

Ureteral duplications are a common congenital anomaly of the kidney and the urinary tract system [1, 2]. It has an incidence rate of 0.8% in the healthy adult population, 0.3%–2.5% incidence in an autopsy, and 2–4% in patients investigated for urinary tract symptoms [3]. Complete duplication occurs in 40% of cases, whereas partial duplication occurs in 60% of the duplication [3].

Generally, duplex renal systems are asymptomatic and diagnosed incidentally; however, several conditions requiring treatment have been observed in association with duplex systems: obstruction, reflux disease, and urinary stones are not peculiar but may be commoner in duplex systems [4].

Concerning obstruction, the upper moiety may be at a greater risk caused by ureterocele and lower moiety is at risk of reflux nephropathy [5, 6]. To the best of our knowledge, only a few cases have been reported of a patient with unilateral complete ureteral duplication and ureteral stone [7]. We present a case of a hydronephrotic lower moiety of the left complete duplex system rather than the usual presentation of reflux hydronephrosis, caused by left midureteric stone in an adult female with a unilateral left duplex renal system which was asymptomatic for more than thirty years.

## 2. Case Report

*2.1. Patient Information.* A 35-year-old female patient presented with left flank pain in the last three years. The pain was a dull aching type that did not prevent her from accomplishing her daily work and not radiating without aggravating or relieving factors. The patient was visited by a primary health care personnel and diagnosed with renal stone without improvement with medical therapy. The patient had hypertension and was controlled with oral medication ten days ago.

*2.2. Clinical Findings.* On physical examination, her vital signs were normal. In the abdominal examination, she only had mild left costovertebral angle tenderness.

*2.3. Diagnostic Assessment.* Blood tests revealed a total white blood cell count of $9 \times 10$ [3]/ml, hemoglobin of 14.3 g/dl,

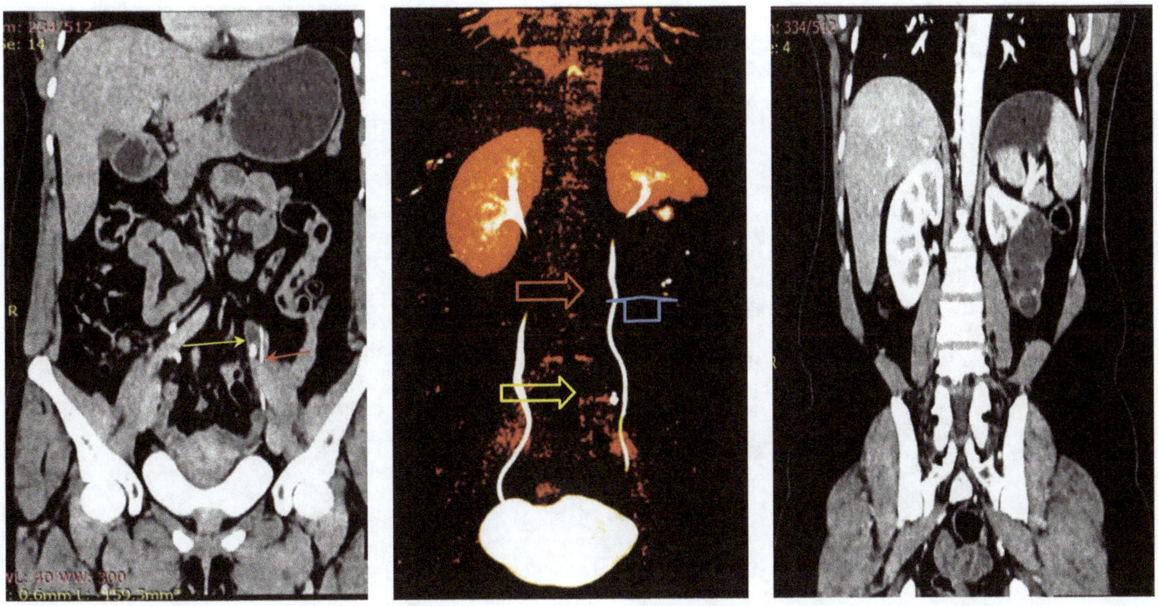

(a) (b) (c)

FIGURE 1: Abdominal CT scan showed the following: (a) coronal view shows both functioning (red arrow) and dilated ureter with proximal dilatation (yellow arrow); (b) 3D CT construction showing midureteric stone (yellow arrow), nonobstructed ureter with complete urinary drainage from upper segment (red arrow), and hydronephrotic segment (blue arrow); (c) contrast film showing lower pole nonfunctioning and hydronephrotic kidney.

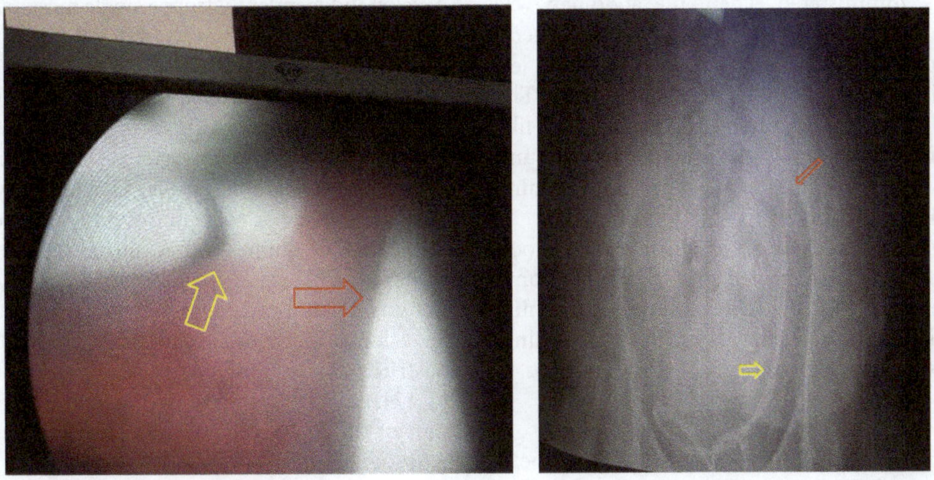

(a) (b)

FIGURE 2: (a) Preoperative cystoscopy showing the two left ureteric orifices where the medial is allowing JJ stent placement (yellow arrow) and the lateral one is intubated with a ureteric catheter (red arrow) (obstructed ureter). (b) KUB shows the two catheters where the lateral could not go beyond the mid sacrum because of ureteric stone (yellow arrow) and normally placed (red arrow) JJ stent.

blood urea nitrogen of 14 mg/dl, and creatinine of 0.52 mg/dl. Ultrasound of the kidney showed left multiple well-defined anechoic lesions with distal acoustic enhancement (fluid-filled structure) seen on the left kidney mid and lower pole. Computerized tomography (CT) scan of the urinary system (CT urography) showed normal excreting of the right kidney and ureter with no obstruction. The left kidney duplex pelvis with two complete ureters draining into the bladder where the lower kidney draining ureter was dilated to the level of the fourth lumbar vertebrae with obstructed stone measuring 7 mm in diameter (Figure 1).

Diagnostic cystoscopy showed a single right ureteric orifice and two left ureteric orifices where the nonobstructed ureteral orifice appears medial where JJ stent Fr 6 size was placed without difficulty. The obstructed ureteral orifice appears lateral and caudal where the ureteric catheter advanced till to the obstructed part (midureter) due to impacted stone with no association with ureterocele (Figure 2). A diagnosis of a complete duplex kidney with lower moiety hydronephrosis was made, and the patient was prepared for laparotomy. Ideally, laparoscopic surgery was preferred, but we did open surgery due to the low facility.

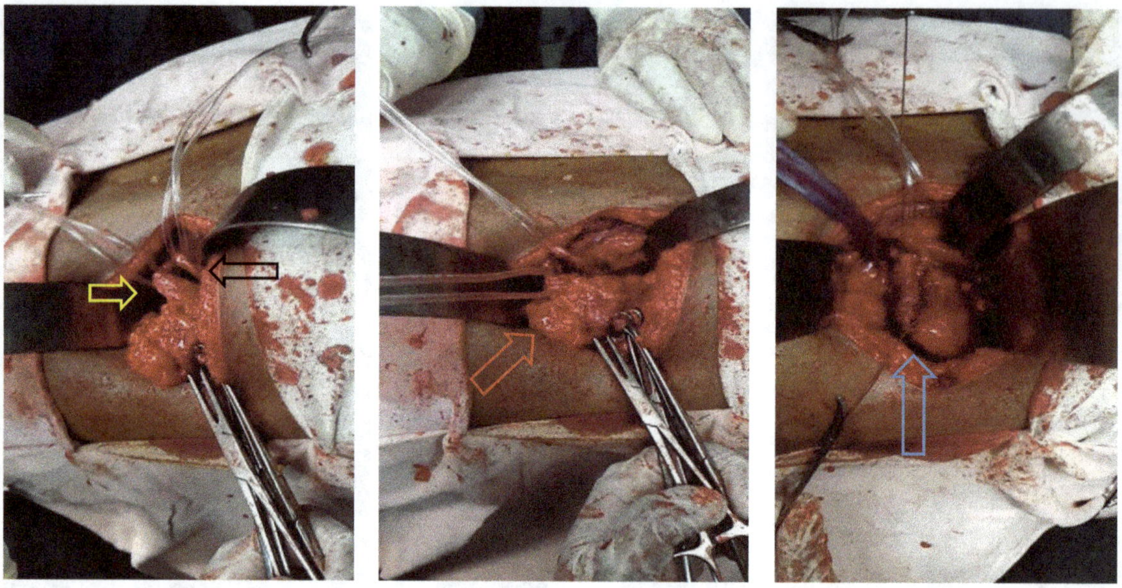

FIGURE 3: Intraoperative imaging. (a) Dilated proximal ureter draining lower moiety (yellow arrow), another ureter draining upper moiety (black arrow). (b) Hydronephrotic segment (red arrow). (c) Repair of the upper segment after lower pole resection (blue arrow).

*2.4. Therapeutic Interventions.* Preoperative antibiotic (ceftriaxone: 1 g) was administered. Then, the abdomen was entered through a left subcostal flank incision under general anesthesia. Retroperitoneal space was entered, and the left kidney was identified after Gerota's fascia was opened. The lower pole of the kidney was hydronephrotic and looked like a bag of fluid. The two ureters were identified and found with the upper pole insertion, and the other was draining the lower pole (Figure 3(a)).

The lower segment vasculature and upper moiety blood supply were identified, and the left partial nephrectomy was done (Figures 3(b) and 3(c). The lower pole draining ureter was ligated after stone removal. An intra-abdominal drain was left in situ, and the abdominal wall was closed in layers.

*2.5. Follow-Up and Outcome.* The patient had a smooth postoperative course following the surgery. The drainage tube was removed during a 36-hour postoperative period. The patient was discharged on her fifth postoperative day. On the 15th postoperative day, the patient was found to have a good condition without complications.

## 3. Discussion

The presence of two pelvicalyceal systems defines the duplex kidney system; the condition is a known congenital anomaly of the urinary tract [6, 8].

Most of them are incidental findings on routine imaging for other compliance; if it is symptomatic, it is caused by obstruction, reflux, or calculi alone or in combination with other associated anomalies, including ureterocele or ectopic ureter [4]. Females are more likely to have unilateral or bilateral duplex renal systems [9].

During embryonic development, two ureteral buds rarely develop independently from a single mesonephric duct, resulting in a duplex kidney with ureteral duplication [7, 10].

Even rarer is unilateral complete ureteral duplication with single renal parenchyma drained by two pyelocaliceal systems [4]. Urinary stone formation is possible comorbidity in patients with a duplex system. There have been few reports of patients with duplex systems and urinary stones who also have ureterocele or collecting system obstruction [7, 11].

Complete duplication is usually unilateral. Nevertheless, bilateral cases are also reported [4]. One of the complications associated with duplication is obstruction, which could be calculus (anywhere along the ureter) or noncalculus obstruction at a confluence of the ureter or bladder insertion [4, 12]. Our patient presented with ureteral calculus obstruction of the lower moiety draining ureter at the level of the mid ureter.

According to Meyer-Weigert-Rule, the upper pole is generally seen as ectopic and therefore dysplastic due to obstruction, whereas the lower pole is related to vesicoureteral reflux [13]. In our case, the patient had a left complete duplicated kidney with a lower draining ureter and left lower hydronephrotic segment, and a left mid ureteric stone caused a dilatation in the proximal part of the left kidney.

Amis et al. reviewed 11 cases of obstruction involving the lower pole moiety of kidneys. There were complete duplications in seven cases. The pathologic entities caused by ureteropelvic junction obstructions in 2 cases, bladder tumor in 2 cases, ectopic upper pole ureterocele compressing and obstructing the ureteral orifice to the lower pole in one case, and ureteral stones in two cases (located at the mid and ureterovesical junction) [5]. Similarly, our patient had a midureteric stone which caused prolonged obstruction unnoticed for an extended period.

The first modality used was ultrasound showing our patient's multicystic mid- and lower pole segments. Later, other imaging modalities used to confirm or rule out conditions must be held. These include voiding cystourethrography, which is used to rule out reflux. Intravenous urography IVP and CT urography to confirm the duplex system and other obstruction causes, and nuclear imaging to realize the split function and level of obstruction [4, 14]. In our case, CT urography was performed and showed a nonfunctional lower pole of the left kidney and dilated ureter.

Another option for clarifying the anatomy of duplication anomalies is preoperative cystoscopy combined with a retrograde ureteropyelogram prior to surgical correction [15].

Management depends on the cause of obstruction and the cortical loss in the renal moiety [4]. The majority of cases can be managed endoscopically and laparoscopically and through open surgery in resource-limited facilities [16]. The role of treatment is to relieve the obstruction cause or relieve the pain by removing part of the kidney (partial nephrectomy) [4]. In our patient, partial nephrectomy was performed. Several published reports mentioned a similar procedure [9, 17, 18].

Our patient might have benefited from a simple endoscopic procedure if the diagnosis had been made sooner. However, her delayed presentation to appropriate care due to her primary healthcare providers' low suspicion index resulted in this unfortunate complete renal moiety parenchymal loss; a similar result was reported by Anyimba et al. [4]

## 4. Conclusion

The previously asymptomatic duplex renal system may develop symptoms later in life. When identified without symptoms or evidence of renal function compromise, the integrity of the renal moieties may have to be closely monitored for the rest of its life. A thorough evaluation with a high index of suspicion is required in individuals presenting with flank pains to quickly identify missed duplex renal systems and duplex system associated disorders quickly and thus prevent the attendant renal moiety parenchymal loss.

## Ethical Approval

Ethical clearance was obtained from the Institutional Research and Ethics Review Committee (IRB) of SPHMMC for publication of the case report.

## Consent

Informed and written consent was taken from the patient to publish the case report.

## Authors' Contributions

MSD was involved in patient care, conceiving the study, and drafting the manuscript. ATT, KHM, SSA, and FOM were involved in inpatient care and critically revised the manuscript. MSD is the critical reviser of the manuscript and overall supervisor of the manuscript. All authors have read and approved the manuscript.

## Acknowledgments

We thank our patient for her consent in allowing us to share her experience. We also thank St. Paul's Hospital Millennium Medical College, Department of Surgery, Urology Unit, Addis Ababa, Ethiopia.

## References

[1] D. Sarma, S. K. Pratihar, T. P. Rajeev, S. K. Barua, P. K. Bagchi, and M. Phukan, "Duplex kidney anomalies and associated pathology: a single centre retrospective review," *International Surgery Journal*, vol. 7, no. 1, p. 76, 2019.

[2] J. O. Lynch, A. Cox, B. Rawal, S. Shelmerdine, N. Vasdev, and A. Patel, "Bilateral obstruction of bilaterally duplicated collecting systems requiring upper and lower moiety drainage," *The Annals of The Royal College of Surgeons of England*, vol. 98, no. 4, pp. e55–e58, 2016.

[3] J. T. Privett, W. D. Jeans, and J. Roylance, "The incidence and importance of renal duplication," *Clinical radiology*, vol. 27, no. 4, pp. 521–530, 1976.

[4] S. K. Anyimba, I. I. Nnabugwu, and C. A. Nnabugwu, "Obstructed right upper moiety in a bilateral partial duplex renal system in an adult," *Annals of African Surgery*, vol. 18, no. 2, pp. 119–122, 2021.

[5] E. S. Amis Jr., J. J. Cronan, and R. C. Pfister, "Lower moiety hydronephrosis in duplicated kidneys," *Urology*, vol. 26, no. 1, pp. 82–88, 1985.

[6] R. Aeron, A. K. Sokhal, M. Kumar, and S. Sankhwar, "Giant hydronephrosis in a case of ureterocele with a duplex system: an entity yet not reported," *BML Case Reports*, vol. 2017, 2017.

[7] A. Karakose, O. Aydogdu, and Y. Z. Atesci, "Unilateral complete ureteral duplication with distal ureteral stone: a rare entity," *Canadian Urological Association Journal*, vol. 7, no. 7-8, pp. 511-512, 2013.

[8] C. Başdaş, S. Çelebi, S. Özaydın et al., "Unusual presentation of duplex kidneys: ureteropelvic junction obstruction," *Advances in Urology*, vol. 2016, Article ID 7960794, 2016.

[9] R. G. Theophanous, A. T. Limkakeng, and J. S. Broder, "Duplicated or ectopic renal collecting system in two adult emergency department patients," *The Journal of Emergency Medicine*, vol. 58, no. 2, pp. e59–e61, 2020.

[10] R. T. Prakash, J. Venkatiah, A. K. Bhardwaj, D. K. Singh, and G. Singh, "Double ureter and duplex system: a cadaver and radiological study," *Urology Journal*, vol. 8, no. 2, pp. 145–148, 2011.

[11] A. Ghobashy, M. El-Shazly, A. Lari et al., "A case of complete renal duplex with h-shaped ureter," *Case Reports in Urology*, vol. 2012, Article ID 643207, 2 pages, 2012.

[12] W. Liu, L. Zhang, R. Ma, and R. Wu, "The morphology and treatment of coexisting ureteropelvic junction obstruction in lower moiety of duplex kidney," *International Journal of Surgery*, vol. 34, pp. 23–27, 2016.

[13] C. Darr, U. Krafft, A. Panic, S. Tschirdewahn, B. A. Hadaschik, and C. Rehme, "Renal duplication with ureter duplex not following Meyer-Weigert-rule with development of a megaureter of the lower ureteral segment due to distal stenosis - a case report," *Urology Case Reports*, vol. 28, article 101038, 2020.

[14] M. Haliloglu, E. Akpinar, and O. Akhan, "Lower-pole ureteropelvic junction obstruction with abnormal rotation in duplicated system," *European Journal of Radiology*, vol. 41, no. 1, pp. 78-79, 2002.

[15] D. Bruno, F. C. Delvecchio, and G. M. Preminger, "Successful management of lower-pole moiety ureteropelvic junction obstruction in a partially duplicated collecting system using minimally invasive retrograde endoscopic techniques," *Journal of Endourology*, vol. 14, no. 9, pp. 727–730, 2000.

[16] S. H. HosseiniSharifi, B. Nabavizadeh, S. Mozafarpour, and A. M. Kajbafzadeh, "Laparoscopic selective clipping of upper moiety vasculature and ureter without partial nephrectomy: a novel technique for pediatric urinary incontinence due to ectopic ureter associated with poor functioning upper renal moiety," *Journal of Pediatric Urology*, vol. 13, no. 2, pp. 217-218, 2017.

[17] C. Esposito, M. Escolino, G. Autorino et al., "Laparoscopic partial nephrectomy for duplex kidneys in infants and children: how we do it," *Journal of Laparoendoscopic & Advanced Surgical Techniques*, vol. 31, no. 10, pp. 1219–1223, 2021.

[18] C. T. Chen and S. F. Wang, "A case of left duplex kidney with hydronephrosis mimicking a left renal cyst in a 29-year-old woman," *The American Journal of Case Reports*, vol. 21, article e927430, 2020.

# 20

# The Management of Primary Hyperaldosteronism in a Poor Technology Environment

**Jean Sossa**,[1] **Dedjinnin Josue Georges Avakoudjo**,[2] **Dodji Magloire Ines Yevi**,[2] **Lionelle Fanou**,[1] **Gilles Natchagande**,[2] **Michel Michael Agounkpe**,[2] **Fred Hodonou**,[2] **Yao Felicien Hounto**,[1] **and Felix Atadokpede**[1]

[1]*Service d'Urologie, Hopital d'Instruction des Armees Centre Hospitalier Universitaire (HIA-CHU), Cotonou, Benin*
[2]*Clinique Universitaire d'Urologie-Andrologie, Centre National Hospitalier et Universitaire Hubert Koutoucou Maga (CNHU-HKM), Cotonou, Benin*

Correspondence should be addressed to Jean Sossa; feminawa@yahoo.com

Academic Editor: Claudio Simeone

We report a case of Conn's adenoma in a 35-year-old female successfully managed in a poor hospital technology environment.

## 1. Introduction

The primary hyperaldosteronism is the most frequent cause of secondary hypertension [1–4]. Diagnosis and management of the condition are often delicate. We report one case of a right aldosterone-producing adrenal adenoma or Conn's adenoma.

## 2. Case Presentation

The patient was a nulliparous 35-year-old female with a 3-year long history of recurrent dizziness and convulsions. She described a monthly frequency of up to 3 bouts of convulsions. Nine months before she consulted in our institution, a hypokalemia was discovered and treated with oral supplementation of potassium, one 600-milligram tablet daily. As the bouts of convulsions went more and more frequent, potassium tablet intake was progressively increased up to 6 tablets daily. Still, the bouts of convulsions which were said to have drastically decreased did not disappear. But the woman could not afford an evacuation abroad as her previous care provider advised her to do. Rather she resorted to our institution. On exam, a 172/110 millimeters of mercury high blood pressure was discovered. The cardiologist confirmed the hypertension and started treating it with amlodipine 10 mg daily. Potassium level was low, 2.10 milliequivalents per liter. Adrenal hormones' workup on a venous blood sampled at 09:15 am after the patient rested supine on a couch for more than 1 hour showed an elevated aldosterone level of $2.496 \times 10^{-9}$ mole per liter, i.e., 4.5 times the laboratory's $5.55 \times 10^{-10}$ moles per liter threshold. Were normal the levels of renin ($1.03 \times 10^{-2}$ International Unit per liter), cortisol ($1.85 \times 10^{-7}$ mole per liter), metanephrine ($2.7 \times 10^{-10}$ moles per liter), and normetanephrine ($9.4 \times 10^{-10}$ moles per liter). The elevated aldosterone to renin ratio (242, i.e., 3.78 times the laboratory's threshold 64) was indicative of a primary hyperaldosteronism. An abdominal computed tomography revealed a 24 mm diameter right adrenal mass in the woman (Figure 1). The nodule was hypodense, homogeneous, regularly limited, and exhibited a 65% washout rate. The diagnosis of an aldosterone-producing adenoma was quite evident. An electrocardiogram was performed which showed a left auricular hypertrophy and an overloaded left ventricle. Plasma levels of creatinine, glucose, and hemoglobin were normal, respectively, 7 milligrams per liter, 1.09 grams per liter, and 10 grams per deciliter. We performed a right adrenalectomy through a right subcostal incision under general anesthesia (Figure 2). We mobilized leftward the right hepatic flexure of the colon and entered into the renal fascia. Downward reclination of

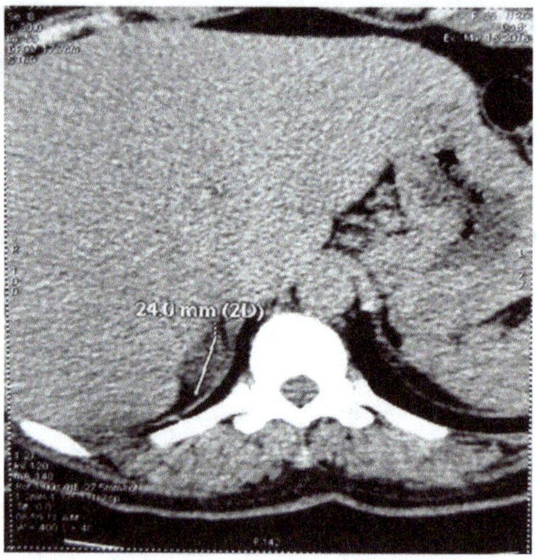


FIGURE 1: Right adrenal mass in the women.

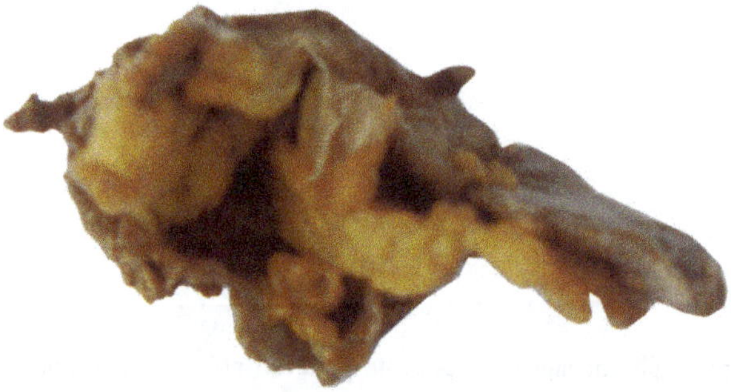

FIGURE 2: The right adrenal mass after adrenalectomy.

the kidney enabled us to dissect and remove the nodular right adrenal gland without any bleeding incident nor any injury to adjacent organs. The anesthesiologist corrected the potassium level which became 4.9 milliequivalents per liter on the eve of the surgery. The patient resumed walking on the second postoperative day. Amlodipine was discontinued on the third postoperative day. Potassium level was monitored daily. The patient was discharged from hospital on the seventh postoperative day with potassium intake completely stopped. Stitches were removed on the tenth postoperative day. One month after the operation, there was no complaint, the potassium level was 4.4 milliequivalents per liter, and the blood pressure was 130/90 millimeters of mercury. At the end of the sixteenth postoperative months, the patient was still good with a normal blood pressure = 127/96 millimeters of mercury. Four years after surgery, the potassium level was 4.5 milliequivalents per liter with no complaint.

## 3. Discussion

A deep hypokalemia alongside a hypertension and bouts of convulsions allowed the diagnosis of Conn's adenoma in our patient. As it abnormally produces aldosterone in excess, a Conn's adenoma triggers a sodium retention, a potassium depletion, and a reduction of renin production, leading to hypokalemia and hypertension. Nevertheless an aldosterone-producing adrenal adenoma may be hypokalemic or less commonly normal potassium leveled [5]. Also, other metabolic disorders such as a hypocalcemia may be associated with hyperaldosteronism [6]. The computed tomographic detection of a right adrenal mass in the woman has been crucial to the diagnosis and to the surgical treatment decision-making. In fact, primary hyperaldosteronism can come from other adrenal disorders such as a bilateral aldosterone-producing adrenal adenoma, a unilateral or bilateral adrenal hyperplasia, a unilateral aldosterone-producing adenoma associated with a contralateral adrenal hyperplasia, or even an aldosterone-producing adrenocortical carcinoma [7–10]. Pathological examination of the specimen has confirmed the presence of a Conn's adenoma, thereby excluding any primary hyperaldosteronism associated with a Cushing adenoma or a unilateral estrogen-producing adrenal adenoma [11–13].

We have performed an open right adrenalectomy in our patient. Surgery is the standard treatment for a unilateral aldosterone-producing adenoma. An adrenalectomy is best performed under laparoscopy or retroperitoneal endoscopy. The hospital sojourn is shorter after those mini-invasive procedures: the mean inward stay ranges from 1.1 to 2.6 days. [14, 15]. Obviously the little scars at the laparoscopic ports' sites are much more aesthetic than the one left by an open surgical incision. Anyway, the removal of the adenoma is the one that will suppress the hyperaldosteronism and its impacts, not the type of surgery. However, the clinician must inform the patient that the adrenalectomy does not always correct the hyperaldosteronism-driven hypertension: the older the patient is at surgery or the longer his hypertension has lasted before surgery, the less likely the total resolution of the hypertension [16–21]. Adrenal sparing surgery is feasible for bilateral aldosterone-producing adenoma [7].

The detection of aldosterone-producing adrenal adenoma amenable to surgery is not easy. Once primary hyperaldosteronism is diagnosed, selective adrenal vein sampling is the gold standard method to determine which one of the left and right adrenal glands is responsible for the disorder [7, 22–27]. Some researchers are assessing diagnostic tools less invasive than adrenal vein sampling such as the 18 oxo-cortisol plasma level [28]. Adrenal vein sampling is costly and requires special skill and equipment that are not yet available in Benin. Nevertheless, in patients less than 35 years old with evident hypokalemia and unilateral adrenal adenoma greater than 10 mm diameter, adrenal vein sampling is not mandatory [29, 30]: the clinician can rely on the aldosterone to renin ratio coupled with imaging. Best imaging for adrenals are computed tomography (sensitivity = 84.3%) and magnetic resonance imaging (sensitivity = 97%, specificity = 90%) [29]. Sometimes imaging can be normal, and reimaging months later may detect an adrenal adenoma [31].

## 4. Conclusion

In limited means' working conditions, a careful combination of aldosterone to renin ratio and imaging can help to successfully manage a primary hyperaldosteronism.

## References

[1] P. Milliez, X. Girerd, P. F. Plouin, J. Blacher, M. E. Safar, and J. J. Mourad, "Evidence for an increased rate of cardiovascular events in patients with primary aldosteronism," *Journal of the American College of Cardiology*, vol. 45, no. 8, pp. 1243–1248, 2005.

[2] S. Savard, L. Amar, P. F. Plouin, and O. Steichen, "Cardiovascular complications associated with primary Aldosteronism," *Hypertension*, vol. 62, no. 2, pp. 331–336, 2013.

[3] C. Schirpenbach, F. Segmiller, S. Diederich et al., "The diagnosis and treatment of primary hyperaldosteronism in Germany," *Deutsches Ärzteblatt International*, vol. 106, no. 18, pp. 305–311, 2009.

[4] G. P. Rossi, G. Bernini, C. Caliumi et al., "A prospective study of the prevalence of primary aldosteronism in 1,125 hypertensive patients," *Journal of the American College of Cardiology*, vol. 48, no. 11, pp. 2293–2300, 2006.

[5] P. Mulatero, M. Stowasser, K. Loh et al., "Increased diagnosis of primary aldosteronism including surgically correctable forms in centers from five continents," *The Journal of Clinical Endocrinology and Metabolism*, vol. 89, no. 3, pp. 1045–1050, 2004.

[6] S. G. Pai, K. N. Shivashankara, V. Pandit, and S. Sheshadri, "Symptomatic hypocalcemia in primary hyperaldosteronism: a case report," *Journal of Korean Medical Science*, vol. 24, no. 6, pp. 1220–1223, 2009.

[7] R. Morimoto, N. Satani, Y. Iwakura et al., "A case of bilateral aldosterone-producing adenomas differentiated by segmental adrenal venous sampling for bilateral adrenal sparing surgery," *Journal of Human Hypertension*, vol. 30, no. 6, pp. 379–385, 2016.

[8] I. Chatton Chambaz and A. Pechère-Bertschi, "Hyperaldosteronisme primaire," *Revue Médicale Suisse*, vol. 7, pp. 1736–1742, 2011.

[9] P. Mulatero, S. Monticone, C. Bertello et al., "Evaluation of primary aldosteronism," *Current Opinion in Endocrinology, Diabetes, and Obesity*, vol. 17, no. 3, pp. 188–193, 2010.

[10] L. Amar, P. F. Plouin, and O. Steichen, "Aldosterone-producing adenoma and other surgically correctable forms of primary aldosteronism," *Orphanet Journal of Rare Diseases*, vol. 5, p. 9, 2010.

[11] S. Vakkalanka, A. Zhao, and M. Samannodi, "Primary hyperaldosteronism: a case of unilateral adrenal hyperplasia with contralateral incidentaloma," *BML Case Reports*, vol. 2016, 2016.

[12] Y. Tezuka, Y. Yamazaki, Y. Ono et al., "Unique sex steroid profiles in estrogen-producing adrenocortical adenoma associated with bilateral hyperaldosteronism," *Journal of the Endocrine Society*, vol. 4, no. 2, pp. 1–8, 2020.

[13] K. Ren, J. Wei, Q. Liu et al., "Hypercortisolism and primary aldosteronism caused by bilateral adrenocortical adenomas: a case report," *BMC Endocrine Disorders*, vol. 19, no. 1, p. 63, 2019.

[14] B. K. P. Goh, Y. H. Tan, S. K. H. Yip, P. H. K. Eng, and C. W. S. Cheng, "Outcome of patients undergoing laparoscopic adrenalectomy for primary hyperaldosteronism," *Journal of the Society of Laparoendoscopic Surgeons*, vol. 8, no. 4, pp. 320–325, 2004.

[15] C. E. Costa Almeida, T. Caroço, M. A. Silva et al., "An update of posterior retroperitoneoscopic adrenalectomy - case series," *International Journal of Surgery Case Reports*, vol. 71, pp. 120–125, 2020.

[16] C. Y. Lo, P. C. Tam, A. W. C. Kung, K. S. L. Lam, and J. Wong, "Primary aldosteronism: results of surgical treatment," *Annals of Surgery*, vol. 224, no. 2, pp. 125–130, 1996.

[17] R. J. Weigel, S. A. Wells, J. C. Gunnells, and G. S. Leight, "Surgical treatment of primary hyperaldosteronism," *Annals of Surgery*, vol. 219, no. 4, pp. 347–352, 1994.

[18] T. Obara, Y. Ito, T. Okamoto et al., "Risk factors associated with postoperative persistent hypertension in patients with primary aldosteronism," *Surgery*, vol. 112, no. 6, pp. 987–993, 1992.

[19] C. A. G. Proye, E. A. R. Mulliez, B. M. L. Carnaille et al., "Essential hypertension: first reason for persistent hypertension after unilateral adrenalectomy for primary aldosteronism?," *Surgery*, vol. 124, no. 6, pp. 1128–1133, 1998.

[20] O. Celen, M. J. O'Brien, J. C. Melby, and R. M. Beazley, "Factors influencing outcome of surgery for primary aldosteronism," *Archives of Surgery*, vol. 131, no. 6, pp. 646–650, 1996.

[21] G. P. Rossi, M. Bolognesi, D. Rizzoni et al., "Vascular remodeling and duration of hypertension predict outcome of adrenalectomy in primary aldosteronism patients," *Hypertension*, vol. 51, no. 5, pp. 1366–1371, 2008.

[22] K. Okamura, T. Okuda, Y. Fukuda et al., "A case of primary aldosteronism due to a primary adrenal adenoma diagnosed by segmental adrenal venous sampling (S-AVS) using a modified catheter system and lateral cine angiography," *American Journal of Case Reports*, vol. 20, pp. 139–145, 2019.

[23] H. A. Sigurjonsdottir, M. Gronowitz, O. Andersson et al., "Unilateral adrenal hyperplasia is a usual cause of primary hyperaldosteronism. Results from a Swedish screening study," *BMC Endocrine Disorders*, vol. 12, no. 1, 2012.

[24] G. P. Rossi, R. J. Auchus, M. Brown et al., "An expert consensus statement on use of adrenal vein sampling for the subtyping of primary aldosteronism," *Hypertension*, vol. 63, no. 1, pp. 151–160, 2014.

[25] S. Monticone, F. Satoh, G. Giacchetti et al., "Effect of adrenocorticotropic hormone stimulation during adrenal vein sampling in primary aldosteronism," *Hypertension*, vol. 59, no. 4, pp. 840–846, 2012.

[26] A. Ganguly, J. Bergstein, C. E. Grim, M. O. Yum, and M. H. Weinberger, "Childhood primary aldosteronism due to an adrenal adenoma: preoperative localization by adrenal vein catheterization," *Pediatrics*, vol. 65, no. 3, pp. 605–609, 1980.

[27] P. C. Kahn, M. D. Kelleher, R. H. Egdahl, and J. C. Melby, "Adrenal arteriography and venography in primary aldosteronism," *Radiology*, vol. 101, no. 1, pp. 71–78, 1971.

[28] F. Satoh, R. Morimoto, Y. Ono et al., "Measurement of peripheral plasma 18-oxocortisol can discriminate unilateral adenoma from bilateral diseases in patients with primary aldosteronism," *Hypertension*, vol. 65, no. 5, pp. 1096–1102, 2015.

[29] O. Shidlovskyi Viktor, V. Shidlovskyi Oleander, M. Sheremet et al., "Laboratory diagnostics of primary hyperaldosteronism and its peculiarities (literature review)," *Journal of Medicine and Life*, vol. 12, no. 3, pp. 215–220, 2019.

[30] M. A. Reardon, J. F. Angle, N. Abi-Jaoudeh et al., "Intraprocedural cortisol levels in the evaluation of proper catheter placement in adrenal venous sampling," *Journal of Vascular and Interventional Radiology*, vol. 22, no. 11, pp. 1575–1580, 2011.

[31] B. T. Layden, A. J. Hahr, and D. M. Elaraj, "Primary hyperaldosteronism: challenges in subtype classification," *BMC Research Notes*, vol. 5, no. 1, 2012.

21

# Complaint of Testicular Discomfort in Patient with Esophageal Adenocarcinoma

**Kevin Krughoff**,[1] **Alan Schned**,[2] **Bing Ren**,[1] **and Vernon M. Pais Jr.**[1]

[1]*Department of Surgery/Section of Urology, Dartmouth-Hitchcock Medical Center, Lebanon, NH, USA*
[2]*VA Medical Center, White River Junction, VT, USA*

Correspondence should be addressed to Kevin Krughoff; krughoff@gmail.com

Academic Editor: Apul Goel

We report a case of esophageal cancer with solitary metastasis to the testicle in a 71-year-old man. The tumor was picked up on physical exam following new onset complaints of pain and swelling. While most testicular masses in older men are due to lymphoma, this case highlights the need to consider metastatic disease as a source of new symptoms in patients with a recent cancer diagnosis.

## 1. Introduction

The evaluation of scrotal discomfort requires consideration of a wide variety of etiologies, and the corner stone of assessment remains the physical exam. New testicular masses in men over the age of 60 are often due to lymphoma, but in a patient with a recent cancer diagnosis and new onset of pain, the consideration for metastatic disease should remain on the differential.

## 2. Case Presentation

A 71-year-old male presented with left testicle discomfort and swelling after failing to improve on a course of antibiotics. Physical exam demonstrated a small nodule of the left testicle. An ultrasound was requested, showing a heterogeneous left testicle with small rounded hypoechoic areas, increased blood flow, and small echogenic foci along the rete testis with moderate left hydrocele (Figure 1). A left inguinal orchiectomy was performed for suspicion of testicular cancer. The orchiectomy specimen showed an enlarged testicle nearly replaced by a firm, solid, pale tan neoplasm with scattered punctate foci of hemorrhage and necrosis, 6.5 cm in maximum diameter. The tumor focally extended beyond the tunica albuginea at the hilum. A separate, well-demarcated, nearly round tumor nodule was present in the head of the epididymis (Figure 2). Tumor markers AFP (2.5), beta HCG (<1.2), and CEA (1.4) were not elevated.

Immunohistochemical work-up was negative for multiple germ cell markers, including CD30, OCT3/4, PLAP, c-kit, and glypican and was positive for multiple epithelial markers, including cytokeratin AE1/3, cytokeratins 7 and 20 (focal), and epithelial membrane antigen. There was strong positivity for both monoclonal and polyclonal CEA and focal positivity for CDX-2. Markers for other potential primary tumor sites, including TTF-1 (lung), NKX 3.1 (prostate), PAX8 (renal), calretinin

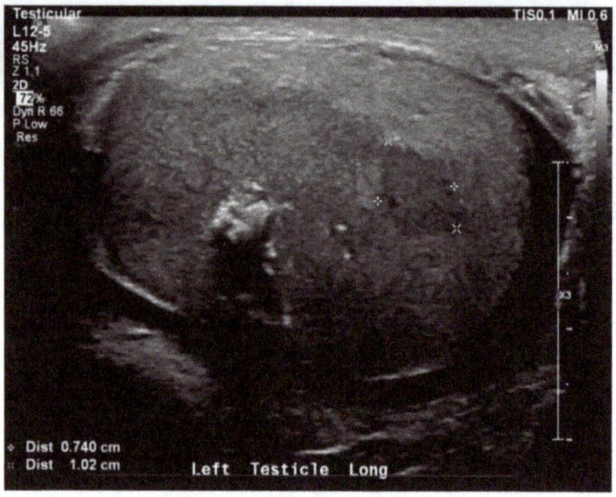


FIGURE 1: Scrotal ultrasound.

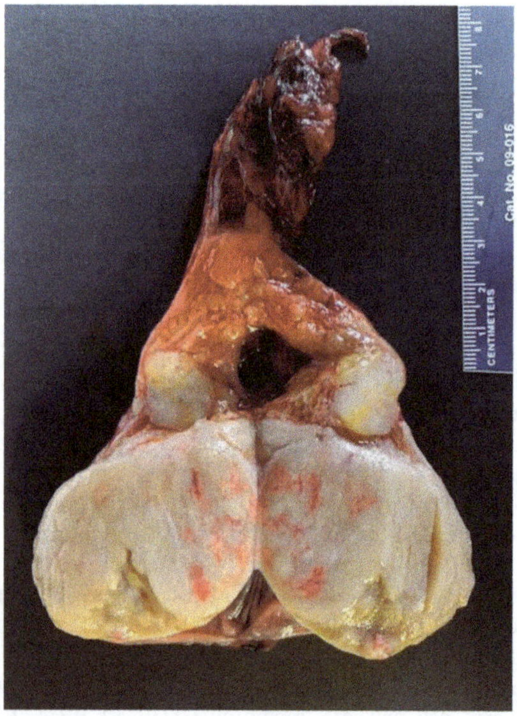


FIGURE 2: Gross specimen testicular tumor.

(mesothelial), and inhibin (adrenal plus testicular sex cord stromal tumors), were all negative. Histologically, the tumor in the testis was markedly similar to that in the esophagus, with both showing a majority solid growth pattern and focal glandular differentiation (Figure 3). Notably, both neoplasms showed positive staining patterns for CDX-2 and CEA, markers for a number of adenocarcinomas of gastrointestinal origin. Final pathology was consistent with metastatic esophageal cancer.

Ten months prior to orchiectomy, the patient had a salvage Ivor Lewis esophagectomy for esophageal adenocarcinoma, initially treated with neoadjuvant chemoradiation. Final pathology showed poorly differentiated adenocarcinoma of the esophageal gastric junction (ypT3N0) with negative margins and 0 of 22 examined lymph nodes. PET CT scans were obtained at initial diagnosis (21 months prior to orchiectomy) and preceding esophagectomy, both showing no distant metastases. A CT 6 months following esophagectomy was also unremarkable for metastatic disease. Finally, a third PET CT scan performed after orchiectomy suggested left periaortic region nodal metastasis but, again, no additional visceral metastases. Due to epididymal tumor involvement, he was then treated systemically with FOLFOX.

## 3. Discussion

Metastasis to the testicle from any cancer type is rare, with one autopsy study showing an incidence of 2.5% [1]. Metastatic testicular tumors are generally reported in older patients with a peak incidence in the fifth decade, with most originating from the prostate, lung, or colon [2–4]. Less commonly reported sites are the kidney (2), intestine (2), adrenal gland (1), malignant melanoma (1), and retinoblastoma (1) [2, 3]. In some cases, the testicular tumor discovery precedes that of the primary tumor, thus emphasizing a thorough immunohistochemical workup [5].

The lower esophagus is the most common site of esophageal cancer and the most common origin for unexpected metastases. Systemic organ metastases for esophageal cancer are as frequent as intrathoracic recurrences, with the most common sites being the regional lymph nodes, liver, lung, and bone [6]. Metastasis to the testicle with involvement of the epididymis, spermatic cord, and adjacent testicular tissues was reported once in the context of esophageal cancer with prior lymph node and cutaneous metastasis [7]. In the present report, the testicle constituted the only metastatic site despite negative surgical node status and repeated staging studies with no evidence of metastatic disease. The survival time for esophageal cancer patients decreases appreciably when recurrences are found at other locations, and the lymph nodes are uninvolved [8]. The patient went on to receive further chemotherapy following testicular diagnosis.

The esophageal origin of the testicular tumor in this case was based on morphologic similarities to the esophageal cancer, a similar immunohistochemical staining pattern, and an absence of other putative primary sites. The route of spread from a visceral cancer to the testicle in cases such as this is speculative, with previous reports suggesting lymphatic spread from the prostate, venous spread from the kidneys, or direct extension from retroperitoneal tumors [9]. The complex anatomical pathway of the esophageal lymphatic network has been found to show lymphatic nodal skip spread, both retrograde and bidirectional [2–4], which may lend support to

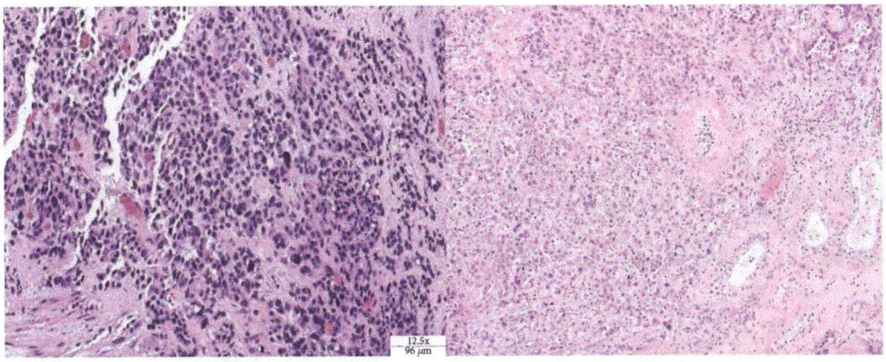


FIGURE 3: Esophageal tissue (left): sheets of neoplastic cells with high nucleus/cytoplasm ratio and nuclear hyperchromasia and pleomorphism. Immunohistochemical staining was positive for monoclonal CEA and negative for p63, synaptophysin, and chromogranin, supporting a diagnosis of poorly differentiated adenocarcinoma (H&E; ×12.5). Testicular tissue (right): poorly differentiated and loosely cohesive carcinoma with predominantly solid and some focal glandular architecture demonstrating considerable pleomorphism. Adjacent seminiferous tubule (H&E; ×10).

lymphatic spread to the testicle in this case. Despite an uncommon etiology for scrotal pain, testicular metastasis should be considered on the differential when evaluating new onset scrotal discomfort in a patient with a prior cancer diagnosis.

## References

[1] A. Tiltman, "Metastatic tumours in the testis," *Histopathology*, vol. 3, no. 1, pp. 31–37, 1979.

[2] K. Hanash, "Metastatic tumors to the testicles," *Progress in Clinical and Biological Research*, vol. 203, pp. 61–67, 1985.

[3] H. Haupt, R. Mann, D. Trump, and M. D. Abeloff, "Metastatic carcinoma involving the testis. Clinical and pathologic distinction from primary testicular neoplasms," *Cancer*, vol. 54, no. 4, pp. 709–714, 1984.

[4] N. Dutt, A. Bates, and S. Baithun, "Secondary neoplasms of the male genital tract with different patterns of involvement in adults and children," *Histopathology*, vol. 37, no. 4, pp. 323–331, 2000.

[5] R. B. Meacham, J. A. Mata, R. Espada, T. M. Wheeler, C. W. Schum, and P. T. Scardino, "Testicular metastasis as the first manifestation of colon carcinoma," *Journal of Urology*, vol. 140, no. 3, pp. 621-622, 1988.

[6] R. Ishihara, T. Oyama, S. Abe et al., "Risk of metastasis in adenocarcinoma of the esophagus: a multicenter retrospective study in a Japanese population," *Journal of Gastroenterology*, vol. 52, no. 7, pp. 800–808, 2017.

[7] S. Gillen, M. Feith, R. Gertler et al., "Testicular metastasis from adenocarcinoma of the esophagus," *The Annals of Thoracic Surgery*, vol. 87, no. 3, pp. 957–959, 2009.

[8] S. Law, M. Fok, and J. Wong, "Pattern of recurrence after oesophageal resection for cancer: clinical implications," *British Journal of Surgery*, vol. 83, no. 1, pp. 107–111, 1996.

[9] G. R. Bodon and J. A. Dressler, "Metastatic carcinoma of right testicle from primary carcinoma of the appendix," *Journal of Urology*, vol. 97, no. 5, pp. 885–887, 1967.

# 22

# First Report of Two Cases of Acute Gastric Ischemia after Robot-Assisted Radical Cystectomy

**Nikolaos Grivas,[1] Alexander D. Horsch,[2] Esther Wit,[1] Annemarie Bruining,[2] Johanna van Sandick,[3] and Henk G. van der Poel[1]**

[1]*Department of Urology, The Netherlands Cancer Institute-Antoni van Leeuwenhoek Hospital, Amsterdam, Netherlands*
[2]*Department of Radiology, The Netherlands Cancer Institute-Antoni van Leeuwenhoek Hospital, Amsterdam, Netherlands*
[3]*Department of Surgery, The Netherlands Cancer Institute-Antoni van Leeuwenhoek Hospital, Amsterdam, Netherlands*

Correspondence should be addressed to Nikolaos Grivas; nikolaosgrivas@hotmail.com

Academic Editor: Sigurdur Gudjonsson

Gastrointestinal ischemia is rare after small pelvis surgery. Minimal invasive robotic surgery requires adaptation of the surgical approach for cystectomy and derivation construction such as the use of pneumoperitoneum and Trendelenburg positioning of the patient. Two cases with gastric ischemic complications after robot-assisted radical cystectomy are described. The first case was a 68-year-old female who had prolonged gastroparalysis and blood in a replaced gastric tube at day 10 after robotic cystectomy and Bricker urinary derivation. Gastroscopy revealed ischemia of gastric and proximal duodenal mucosa while computed tomography showed multiple calcifications and thrombi in the coeliac trunk branches and splenic infarcts. The stenosis of the origin of the mesenteric superior artery was stented via an endovascular procedure, and the patient recovered with normal gastroscopy 1 month postoperatively. The second case was a 73-year-old male who developed abdominal pain and fever 5 days after robotic cystectomy and Bricker. On abdominal computed tomography imaging, subcutaneous emphysema, intra-abdominal air, and calcification at the origin of the coeliac trunk were found. At laparotomy 5 days after the cystectomy, a 3 cm hole in the fundus of the stomach was found which was removed with the major stomach curvature. Gastroscopy 5 days after hemigastrectomy revealed no remnant ischemia. The prolonged pneumoperitoneum during robotic cystectomy, the deep Trendelenburg position, and the preoperatively impaired vascular system can be the reasons of our first two cases of gastric ischemia. This rare complication should be kept in mind in patients with symptoms of gastric ischemia since it can result in gastric perforation.

## 1. Introduction

Radical cystectomy is the gold standard for the treatment of muscle-invasive bladder cancer and high-risk nonmuscle invasive disease. Despite the widespread application and the increasing surgical experience with robot-assisted radical cystectomy (RARC), Clavien – Dindo $\geq 2$ complications have been reported in 35-40% of the patients treated with RARC [1]. Ischemic complications can occur due to the increased intra-abdominal pressure associated with pneumoperitoneum applied during laparoscopic and robotic procedures, which can impair the splanchnic perfusion. Pneumoperitoneum itself and ischemia-reperfusion, after deflation of pneumoperitoneum, have been also found to decrease gastric pH and increase oxidative stress in patients undergoing robot-assisted radical prostatectomy with a prolonged duration of 4 hours [2]. Here, we present 2 cases with stomach ischemia after RARC both resulting in serious complications.

## 2. Case Presentation

*2.1. Case 1.* A 68-year-old female with a prior history of multiple sclerosis, peripheral vascular atherosclerosis with an arterial stent in the left external iliac artery developed a multifocal nonmuscle invasive high-grade bladder cancer. Due to

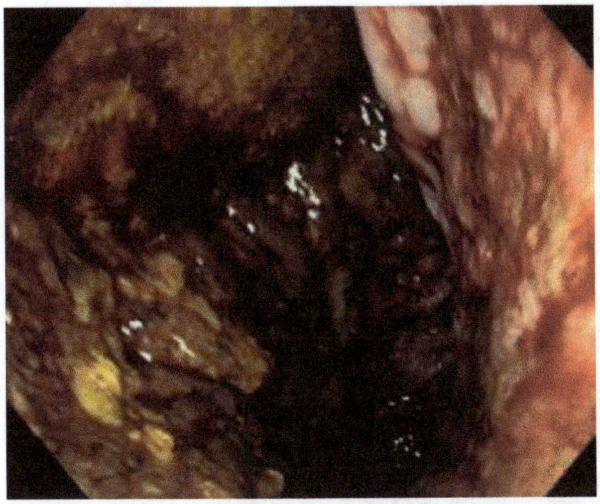

Figure 1: Gastroscopy 10 days postoperatively with gastric mucosal ischemia (case 1).

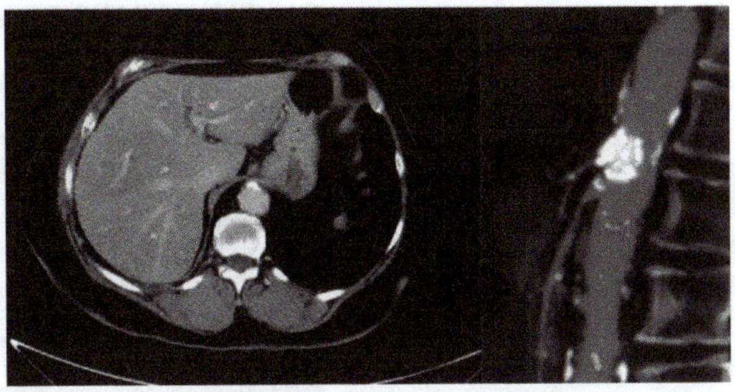

Figure 2: CT lateral view shows a severely calcified origin of the coeliac trunk and significant stenosis in the origin of the superior mesenteric artery. Axial image shows a thrombus inside the calcification (case 1).

a low compliance bladder, multifocal disease, and suspected/-potential muscle-invasive disease, it was decided to perform an anterior exenteration with the removal of bladder, urethra, uterus, and adnexes using a robot-assisted surgical approach. The procedure took 4 hours and included the construction of an intracorporeal Bricker urinary derivation. During the procedure, no bowel perfusion abnormalities were noted by the surgeons, but a remarkable short small-bowel mesentery was reported. Postoperative recovery was characterized by prolonged gastroparalysis and blood in a replaced gastric tube at day 10 postoperatively. Gastroscopy revealed ischemia of gastric and proximal duodenal mucosa (Figure 1). The Bricker stoma remained well perfused. Angio-computed tomography (CT) scan showed multiple calcifications and thrombi in the coeliac trunk branches and splenic infarcts (Figure 2). Stenosis of the origin of the mesenteric superior artery was stented (5 × 19 mm stent) via an endovascular procedure. One month after stent placement, there was a subsequent recovery with the improvement of clinical and gastroscopy findings. In the cystectomy specimen, a pTcisN0MxG3R0 urothelial carcinoma was found and the patient is recurrence-free three years after surgery.

*2.2. Case 2.* A 73-year-old male was seen with BCG-resistant carcinoma in situ of the bladder. The patient was known with hypercholesterolaemia, hypertension, and pulmonary embolism but no significant vascular disease. Five years after the primary diagnoses, RARC and pelvic node dissection with urine derivation according to Bricker was performed. Five days postoperatively, the patient developed abdominal pain, fever, and elevated serum CRP. On abdominal CT imaging, subcutaneous emphysema and intra-abdominal air were visible with perigastric and subphrenic fluid and renal ischemia on the left side, as well as calcification at the origin of the coeliac trunk (Figures 3 and 3(b)). At laparotomy 5 days after the RARC, a 3 cm hole in the fundus of the stomach was found with apparent ischemia of the major curvature of the stomach. The major curvature containing the hole in the stomach was removed using a surgical stapler, and the abdominal cavity was rinsed. Gastroscopy 5 days after hemigastrectomy revealed no remnant ischemia. The patient suffered pneumonia resulting in prolonged intensive care and showed a delayed recovery. The pathology of the cystectomy specimen revealed a pT1N0MxR0G3 urothelial carcinoma and a pT2N0MxR0GS3+4 prostate carcinoma. The gastrectomy specimen showed a perforation due to ischemia. The patient was discharged from the hospital 2 months after cystectomy but suddenly died in a nursing home 3 months after surgery. The autopsy revealed aorta sclerosis at the coeliac truncus but no signs of acute stomach ischemia.

## 3. Discussion

To the best of our knowledge, these are the first reported cases of gastric ischemia following RARC. In patients treated with robot-assisted radical prostatectomy, Luo et al. have shown that gastric pH is decreased by prolonged (4 hours) pneumoperitoneum [2]. It has been also found that low pH levels persist after termination of the pneumoperitoneum indicating that impaired splanchnic circulation continues even after deflation [2]. Moreover, the concentrations of malondialdehyde, which are the most reliable and producible markers of oxidative stress, were significantly elevated [2]. Ischemia-reperfusion can result in impaired myocardial and cerebral function, breakdown of the gastrointestinal barrier, and systemic and inflammatory response syndrome. Experimental models have also shown the clinical relevance of pneumoperitoneum-induced oxidative stress, with splanchnic ischemia while intestinal ischemia has been described after laparoscopic procedures [3, 4]. Since the severity of pneumoperitoneum-induced oxidative stress is time-dependent, splanchnic perfusion can be seriously impaired in a long operation as RARC (>4 h).

Patient-related risk factors can also impair splanchnic perfusion. Specific risk factors include advanced age, diabetes, hepatic and renal impairment, atherosclerosis, low cardiac output, cardiac arrhythmias, and medications (such as diuretics and beta-blockers) which can reduce intestinal perfusion [4]. In our study, both patients had cardiovascular disease symptoms and CT scans showed signs of vascular atherosclerosis, which could have predisposed to gastric

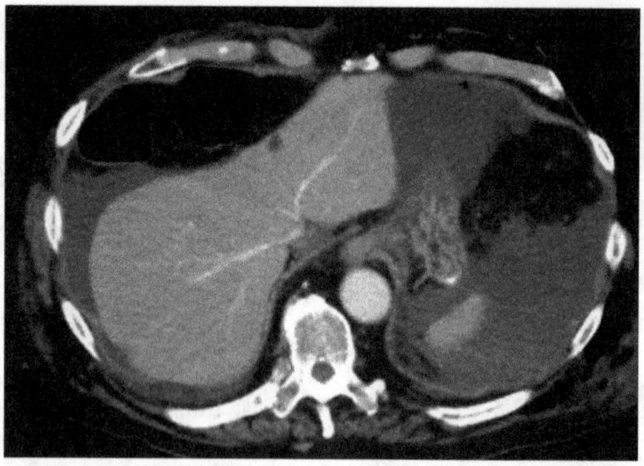

(a)

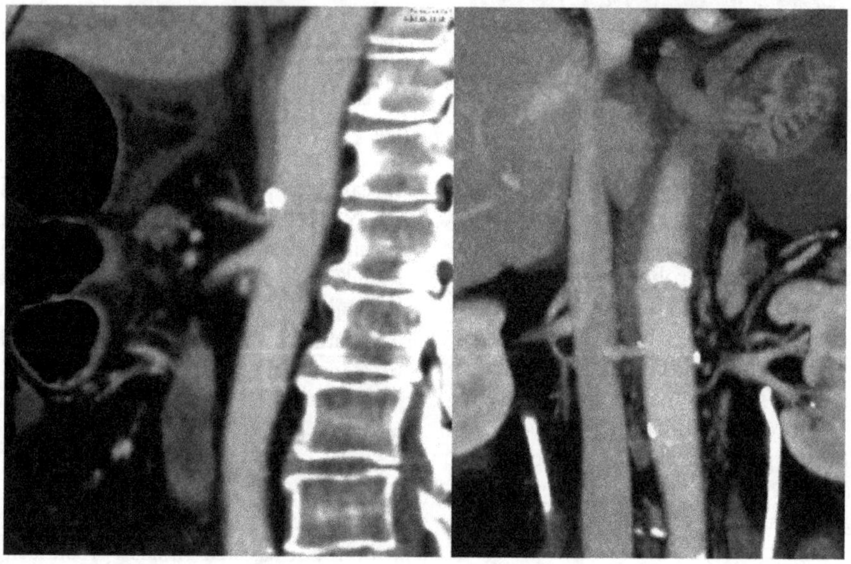

(b)

FIGURE 3: (a) CT with portovenous contrast shows intra-abdominal fluid around the stomach, spleen, and liver with free air suggestive of perforation (case 2). (b) CT lateral and axial views show a small-caliber coeliac trunk with calcification at the origin (case 2).

ischemia. Calcified atherosclerotic plaques at the level of the coeliac trunk level in the aorta were present in both patients prior to surgery.

Prolonged Trendelenburg position can be also associated with gastric ischemia since it has been reported to be the cause also of acute intestinal distress syndrome [5]. This syndrome can especially occur in patients with preexisting cardiac and respiratory diseases who are in a prolonged, high-pressure Trendelenburg position [5]. This situation can result in high central venous and pulmonary arterial pressures while the cardiac output is decreased. The combination of Trendelenburg position with high $CO_2$ pneumoperitoneum and a long surgical procedure can impair cardiac and vascular function, which could result in decreased gastric perfusion.

Measures to prevent this rare complication can be an increased intraoperative hydration, application of the lowest insufflation pressure possible, intermittent abdomen decompression, and use of novel smoke evacuation systems which combine stable intrabdominal pressure with constant suction via a mechanism of valve and insufflation. It has been associated with reduced need of $CO_2$ insufflation, absorption, and elimination. Immediate gastroscopy in patients with symptoms of gastric ischemia (abdominal pain, nausea, vomiting, gastrointestinal bleeding) will allow an early diagnosis and improved survival. Treatment should include vascular support, antibiotic therapy, and vigorous use of proton-pump inhibitors. Patients with signs of ischemic stomach perforation require abdominal exploration, endovascular reconstruction, and/or partial gastrectomy.

## 4. Conclusion

The prolonged pneumoperitoneum during RARC, the deep Trendelenburg position, and the preoperatively impaired vascular system can be the reasons of our first two cases of gastric ischemia. This rare complication should be kept in mind in patients with symptoms of gastric ischemia since it can result in gastric perforation.

## Abbreviations

RARC: Robot-assisted radical cystectomy
CT: Computed tomography.

## Consent

Written informed consent was obtained from the patients for publication of this case report and accompanying images.

## Authors' Contributions

All authors have read and approved the final version of the manuscript.

## References

[1] E. Mazzone, F. D'Hondt, S. Beato et al., "Robot-assisted radical cystectomy with intracorporeal urinary diversion decreases postoperative complications only in highly comorbid patients: findings that rely on a standardized methodology recommended by the European Association of Urology Guidelines," *World Journal of Urology*, 2020.

[2] C. F. Luo, Y. F. Tsai, C. H. Chang, C. T. Wu, and H. P. Yu, "Increased oxidative stress and gut ischemia caused by prolonged pneumoperitoneum in patients undergoing robot-assisted laparoscopic radical prostatectomy," *Acta Anaesthesiologica Taiwanica*, vol. 49, no. 2, pp. 46–49, 2011.

[3] W. Khoury, L. Schreiber, A. Szold, J. M. Klausner, and A. A. Wienbroum, "Renal oxidative stress following CO2 pneumoperitoneum-like conditions," *Surgical Endoscopy*, vol. 23, no. 4, pp. 776–782, 2009.

[4] H. M. Hasson, C. Galanopoulos, and A. Langerman, "Ischemic necrosis of small bowel following laparoscopic surgery," *Journal of the Society of Laparoendoscopic Surgeons*, vol. 8, no. 2, pp. 159–163, 2004.

[5] W. Al-Khyatt, J. D. Thomas, D. J. Humes, and D. N. Lobo, "Intestinal ischemia following laparoscopic surgery: a case series," *Journal of Medical Case Reports*, vol. 7, no. 1, 2013.

# 23

# Robotic Partial Cystectomy for Urachal Carcinoma: A Case Report and Review of the Literature

**Rawad Abou Zahr,[1] Valentin Colinet,[1] Aurore Mattlet,[1] Teddy Jabbour,[2] and Romain Diamand[1]**

[1]*Urology Department, Jules Bordet Institute, Université Libre de Bruxelles, Boulevard de Waterloo 121, 1000 Brussels, Belgium*
[2]*Urology Department, Saint George Hospital University Medical Center, University of Balamand, Beirut 1100 2807, Lebanon*

Correspondence should be addressed to Rawad Abou Zahr; rawad.abouzahr@gmail.com

Academic Editor: Fumitaka Koga

Urachal carcinoma is a very rare tumor, commonly found in the urachal remnant connecting the bladder dome to the umbilicus. Diagnosis is often challenging due to the location of the tumor and its late presentation. We hereby report the case of a 49-year-old female where the diagnosis of urachal carcinoma was made and a robotic partial cystectomy associated with en bloc resection of the umbilicus was performed. We aim to present the clinical aspects, presentation, and diagnosis of this rare entity along with a review of the literature.

## 1. Introduction

Embryologically, the urachus connects the allantois to the apex of the bladder; it later degenerates to become the median umbilical ligament. The urachus is located between the transverse fascia anteriorly, the peritoneum posteriorly, and the umbilical arteries laterally. Urachal remnants are found in almost one third of the population [1]. Urachal carcinoma was first reported by Begg in 1930; it is a rare but highly malignant epithelial cancer [2]. Histologically, urachal remnants resemble intestinal epithelium more closely than adjacent urothelium. As such, urachal tumors differ histologically and biologically from other bladder neoplasms, with adenocarcinoma being the most commonly encountered histological subtype [3].

Urachal tumors are rare and only represent less than 1% of bladder tumors and almost 0.01% of adult malignancies [4]. It is more common in men than in women with a ratio of 1.49 : 1, and it mostly presents after the age of 50 [2].

Hematuria especially macroscopic is the major clinical presentation of these tumors; it can be associated with pelvic pain, dysuria, and mucinuria [5]. None of these symptoms is specific to this particular entity of bladder tumor. Hence, the main diagnostic pathway remains the same as for usual bladder tumors which starts by cystoscopy to visualize and locate the tumor. Most lesions are located at the dome and anterior wall of the bladder. Urachal carcinoma can originate at any site between the umbilicus and the dome of the bladder, and thus, it may present with different clinical manifestations [6]. Urine cytology is only positive in 38% of cases which may be because of the extravesical location of the tumor [7]. Computed tomography (CT) and magnetic resonance imaging (MRI) may be used in the clinical evaluation of the tumor to determine the involvement of other organs and can serve to evaluate locoregional extension of the tumor [3, 8].

Biomarkers such as CEA, CA-125, and CA 19-9 may be elevated in 40–60% of patients; however, they are nonspecific and can be elevated in cancers of other origins [9].

## 2. Case Presentation

A 49-year-old female, nonsmoker, presented with persistent hematuria of one-month duration. She reported no pain or dysuria. Microscopic examination of the urine did not show evidence of infection. The patient has a BMI of 24 kg/m$^2$; she has a history of 2 normal vaginal deliveries and has no previous abdominal surgeries except for a tubal ligation 10 years ago. The patient has an office job and has no exposure to environmental or workplace toxins. She reported having regular menstrual cycles, was not following up regularly with her gynecologist, and has no family history of cancer.

Cystoscopic examination showed a mucinous lesion at the level of the bladder dome (Figure 1), followed by a Triphasic CT scan and MRI confirming the presence of a 6 cm mass at the level of the bladder dome. (Figure 2) A transurethral resection was then performed with the pathology report indicating a mucinous adenocarcinoma.

Due to the rarity of this tumor in the bladder, a complete gastroenterology evaluation to exclude a digestive primary tumor was performed. The gastroscopy and the colonoscopy were both normal.

An abdominal and pelvic MRI (Figure 2) completed the evaluation of this tumor to exclude a possible ovarian or appendicular origin. The appendix and annexes were normal, and the mass was localized in the bladder wall. The intensity of the signal and the contrast enhancement were in favor of a mucinous lesion. It corresponded to stage 2 urachal carcinoma according to the Mayo staging system. Tumor markers CA125 and CA19/9 were negative.

After a multidisciplinary team meeting, a robotic partial cystectomy with en bloc resection of the urachus and umbilicus was performed. Pelvic lymphadenectomy was excluded. The final evaluation of this tumor was made by laparoscopic exploration to exclude any potential peritoneal carcinomatosis.

The approach chosen for the intervention was minimally invasive, and hence, a robotic-assisted partial cystectomy with en bloc resection of the umbilicus was successfully performed (Figure 3). En bloc resection with the umbilicus, in addition to having a foley catheter in place during the procedure, limits tumor spread and spillage.

The operative piece measured $9 \times 5 \times 4.5$ cm, and the final histology confirmed a mucinous adenocarcinoma of the urachus (Figures 4 and 5). Margins were negative, and there was no sign of lymphovascular invasion; the pathological TNM staging was pT3bNx.

Immunohistochemistry tests were made on the operative piece; no microsatellite instability (MSI) was found. A pathologic mutation was detected in the TP53 gene.

Patient had an uneventful postoperative stay; she was discharged at day 5 postop, and a foley catheter left in place was removed at 10 days. No adjuvant therapy was given to our patient. Follow-up of her disease comprises of CT scan every 3 months for the first year. Her follow-up is negative for any recurrences to this date.

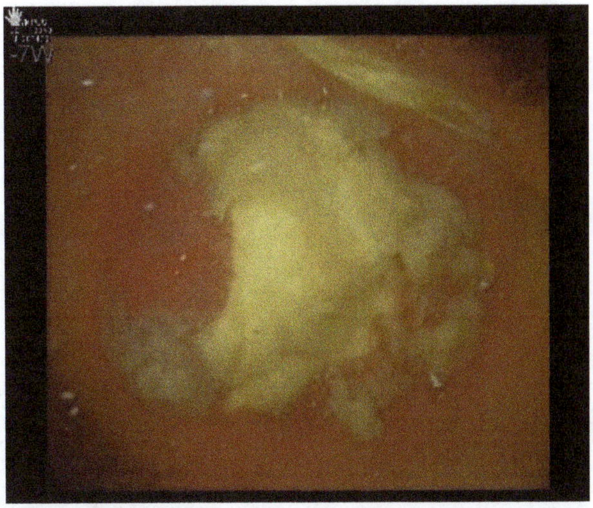

Figure 1: Cystoscopic examination showing a mucinous lesion at the bladder dome.

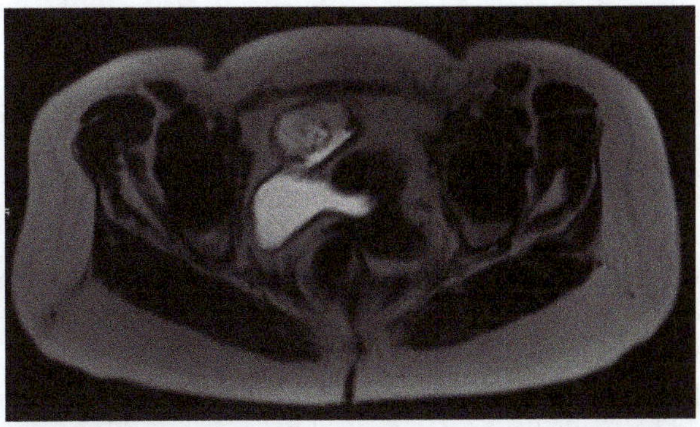

Figure 2: Magnetic resonance imaging showing a lesion at the expense of the bladder wall.

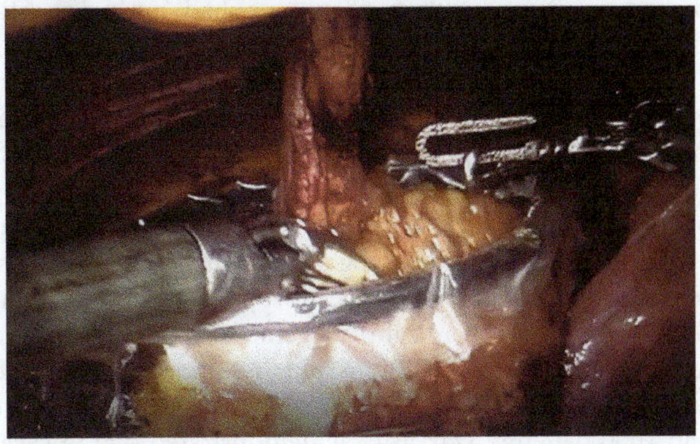

Figure 3: En bloc resection of bladder tumor with umbilicus.

## 3. Discussion

Urachal carcinoma is an uncommon tumor arising mostly from the urachal remnant. Due to its localization in the Retzius space, symptoms of urachal carcinoma do not appear in early stages of the disease [1]. Due to this, patients usually present with advanced or metastatic disease at presentation. The patient depicted in the case above presented with a sole complaint of gross hematuria of one-month duration and was found to have local disease with no extravesical extension.

There are two main staging systems to describe urachal carcinoma, the Mayo staging system and the Sheldon staging system. The former newer system was shown to be less complicated; however, both systems predicted cancer-specific mortality comparably [7]. Dhillon et al. showed that urachal

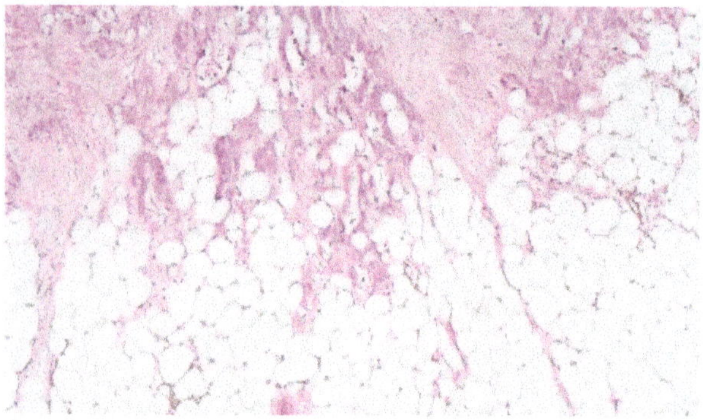

FIGURE 4: Focal conventional adenocarcinoma infiltrating perivesical fat.

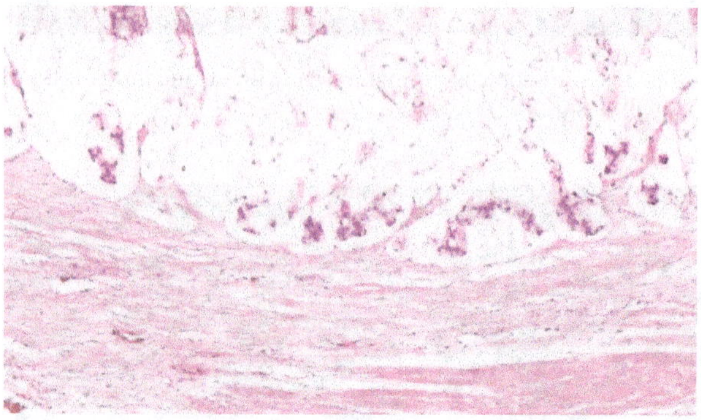

FIGURE 5: Predominant mucinous adenocarcinoma, with strands of glandular cells floating in abundant extracellular mucin.

adenocarcinoma is associated with a better prognosis than bladder urothelial carcinoma, with a cancer-specific survival of 45 months versus 27 months when compared at the same stage [1]. Tumor size and the presence of signet ring differentiation were controversially reported as prognostic factors, whereas mucinous tumor phenotype had no prognostic effect on survival [5].

Given that most urachal cancers are resectable, surgery remains the main treatment modality. Surgical treatment encompasses either partial cystectomy, radical cystoprostatectomy, or cystectomy [1]. It is worth to note that according to Gopalan et al., the incidence of local recurrence was higher in patients undergoing partial rather than radical treatment [10]. A defined surgical protocol is yet to be consolidated; however, surgical management should depend on tumor resectability, ability to obtain clear margins and patient factors. In a 2016 meta-analysis comprising more than 1000 patients, Szarvas et al. demonstrated that in cases where data on umbilectomy was available, 67% of these patients underwent umbilectomy in accordance with recommendations of most authors [5]. In fact, in their large retrospective review, Ashley et al. demonstrated that failure to perform umbilectomy was associated with increased cancer-specific mortality based on univariate analysis [7]. However, another review by Siefker-Radtke et al. concluded that umbilectomy in itself was not found to be a statistically significant factor in survival [3]. Different surgical approaches vary due to the lack of clear guideline recommendations. Hence, data regarding the benefit of umbilectomy has to be clearly highlighted to encourage clinicians to adopt this as an integral part of the surgical procedure.

The prognostic effect of lymph node dissection (LND) remains controversial at the time of surgery. However, its utility might be explained given the fact that patients with positive lymph nodes at the time of surgery carry a poorer survival outcome similar to those with distant metastasis [5]. This demonstrates a possible role for LND in accurate staging which might change treatment decisions depending on positivity. In the 2016 meta-analysis by Szarvas et al., only 17% of patients that underwent LND were found to be positive [11]. Such patients were allocated to LND given high-risk features and still yielded relatively low rates of positivity. Therefore, the benefit of LND in patients with urachal carcinoma still shows low levels of prognostic utility [5]. Future studies might be needed to demonstrate the utility of lymphadenectomy in patients with urachal cancer.

Given the fact that urachal cancer is relatively a clinically silent disease, >20% of patients present with metastatic disease at presentation. With urachal cancer histology being similar to that of colon cancer, 5FU combination chemotherapy regimens demonstrated most benefit in patients with recurrent or metastatic disease [5].

To demonstrate the oncological safety of the surgical technique, Knoedler et al. showed that when compared to patients who underwent radical cystectomy for all bladder cancers, patients that underwent partial cystectomy had no difference in metastasis-free or cancer specific survival. However, patients who opt to partial cystectomy remain at risk of local recurrence [12]. Given that the risk of "seeding" in adenocarcinoma remains significantly less than that of urothelial carcinoma of the bladder. In their retrospective study, Golombos et al. showed that adhering to traditional indications of ruling out CIS before partial cystectomy and having a tumor in a favorable location, this technique demonstrates both favorable recurrence and survival rates [11]. In our case, care was taken to remove the specimen en bloc with the umbilicus after suspending the whole specimen (Figure 3); resection was also done on an empty bladder with a foley catheter in place as to avoid urine spillage as much as possible.

## 4. Conclusion

Urachal carcinoma is a rare nonurothelial malignancy arising at the dome or anterior wall of the bladder. Given that the most common histology is adenocarcinoma, this highlights the importance of accurate diagnosis since a different staging and treatment path will be taken compared to urothelial cancer. Surgery remains the main modality of treatment either radical or partial with most surgeons advocating an umbilectomy en bloc. Lymph node dissection remains a controversial topic given the low prognostic yield available in the current literature. Robot-assisted partial cystectomy with en bloc umbilectomy seems to be an excellent treatment option for patients with evidence of localized disease with excellent oncological and cosmetic outcomes.

## Consent

Written consent was obtained from the patient for this case report.

## References

[1] K. S. Mylonas, P. O'Malley, I. A. Ziogas, L. el-Kabab, and D. Nasioudis, "Malignant urachal neoplasms: a population-based study and systematic review of literature," *Urologic Oncology: Seminars and Original Investigations*, vol. 35, no. 1, pp. 33.e11–33.e19, 2017.

[2] J. Zhang and J. Wu, "Options for diagnosis and treatment of urachal carcinoma," *Asia-Pacific Journal of Clinical Oncology*, vol. 9, no. 2, pp. 117–122, 2013.

[3] A. O. Siefker-Radtke, J. Gee, Y. U. Shen et al., "Multimodality management of urachal carcinoma: the M. D. Anderson Cancer Center experience," *The Journal of Urology*, vol. 169, no. 4, pp. 1295–1298, 2003.

[4] S. Krichen Makni, S. Ellouz, A. Khabir, J. Daoud, and T. Boudawara, "Primary signet ring cell carcinoma of urinary bladder. A case report," *Cancer/Radiothérapie*, vol. 9, no. 5, pp. 332–334, 2005.

[5] T. Szarvas, O. Módos, C. Niedworok et al., "Clinical, prognostic, and therapeutic aspects of urachal carcinoma–A comprehensive review with meta-analysis of 1,010 cases," *Urologic Oncology: Seminars and Original Investigations*, vol. 34, no. 9, pp. 388–398, 2016.

[6] J. R. Molina, J. F. Quevedo, A. F. Furth, R. L. Richardson, H. Zincke, and P. A. Burch, "Predictors of survival from urachal cancer," *Cancer*, vol. 110, no. 11, pp. 2434–2440, 2007.

[7] R. A. Ashley, T. J. Sebo, B. C. Leibovich et al., "Urachal carcinoma: clinicopathologic features and long-term outcomes of an aggressive malignancy," *Cancer*, vol. 107, no. 4, pp. 712–720, 2006.

[8] Z. Hamilou, S. North, C. Canil et al., "Management of urachal cancer: a review by the Canadian Urological Association and Genitourinary Medical Oncologists of Canada," *Canadian Urological Association Journal*, vol. 14, no. 2, pp. 57–64, 2019.

[9] A. Siefker-Radtke, "Urachal adenocarcinoma: a clinician's guide for treatment," *Seminars in Oncology*, vol. 39, no. 5, pp. 619–624, 2012.

[10] A. Gopalan, D. S. Sharp, S. W. Fine et al., "Urachal carcinoma: a clinicopathologic analysis of 24 cases with outcome correlation," *The American Journal of Surgical Pathology*, vol. 33, no. 5, pp. 659–668, 2009.

[11] D. M. Golombos, P. O'Malley, P. Lewicki, B. v. Stone, and D. S. Scherr, "Robot-assisted partial cystectomy: perioperative outcomes and early oncological efficacy," *BJU International*, vol. 119, no. 1, pp. 128–134, 2017.

[12] J. J. Knoedler, S. A. Boorjian, S. P. Kim et al., "Does partial cystectomy compromise oncologic outcomes for patients with bladder cancer compared to radical cystectomy? A matched case-control analysis," *Journal of Urology*, vol. 188, no. 4, pp. 1115–1119, 2012.

24

# Large Pelvic Hematoma after UroLift® Procedure for Treatment of BPH with Median Lobe

**Max J. Roehmholdt and Dennis F. Bentley**

*Cleveland Clinic Foundation – Akron General Medical Center, 1 Akron General Avenue, Akron, OH, USA 44307*

Correspondence should be addressed to Max J. Roehmholdt; roehmhm@ccf.org

Academic Editor: Claudio Simeone

The UroLift® procedure is a minimally invasive technique used to treat benign prostatic hyperplasia (BPH) in the office or hospital setting. As of 2021, over 200,000 of these procedures have been performed, with an excellent safety profile. We present a case report of a patient who underwent the UroLift® procedure and was found to have a 16.5 cm pelvic hematoma within 16 hours. This study was done as a retrospective chart review. In addition, a comprehensive review of the literature was performed, and all relevant government and company websites were reviewed for thorough evaluation. The patient had an uncomplicated inpatient UroLift® procedure for BPH using 5 implants and was discharged from the hospital without incident. The patient presented to the emergency department with abdominal pain 16 hours after the procedure, and a 16.5 cm pelvic hematoma was found on computerized tomography (CT) scan. Since 2015, there have been 27 cases of pelvic hematoma after UroLift® reported to the United States Food and Drug Administration (FDA), and only 2 cases published in the literature. Our patient required hospital admission for 3 days and 3 units of packed red blood cells, but no surgical exploration or intervention. The procedure was technically successful as it improved the patient's voiding and lower urinary tract symptoms (LUTS) as of 2-month follow-up. Potential etiologies include implant firing depth beyond the extent of the prostate, as well as treatment of the median lobe.

## 1. Introduction

The UroLift® prostatic urethral lift is a minimally invasive surgical technique to treat benign prostatic hyperplasia (BPH) in the office or hospital setting. The advance of pursuing this over the traditional approach of transurethral resection of the prostate is its favorable side effect profile and paucity of complications. As UroLift® is being utilized more frequently in the urologic community, more significant complications are being described. A rarely reported complication of a pelvic hematoma has been described in the literature in the past two years, and we describe another unique case of such, but this time in the setting of the treatment of the median lobe of the prostate, never before described.

## 2. Case Presentation

The patient is a 60-year-old male with a history of BPH with lower urinary tract symptoms (LUTS), managed with Flomax and Proscar once daily each, who wished to be off his BPH medications. He was otherwise healthy and did not take any other medications, including neither anticoagulants nor antiplatelet medications. He was interested in minimally invasive surgical management, including the UroLift® procedure. He then underwent office cystoscopy, which demonstrated a small but mobile median lobe of the prostate. Office transrectal ultrasound of the prostate was performed to determine prostate volume, which was 42 grams. All risks, benefits, and options were discussed, and the patient elected to proceed with the UroLift® procedure.

The patient had a preoperative urine culture, which was negative.

The patient underwent an ostensibly uncomplicated UroLift® procedure in the operating room, under general anesthesia. Intraoperatively, two implants were placed on the right (9 o'clock position between the verumontanum and 2 cm distal to the bladder neck), and three implants were placed on the left (3 o'clock position between the verumontanum and 2 cm distal to the bladder neck), with the third used to specifically address the small albeit mobile and median lobe and tack it to the left side. The implants were placed in the usual standard manner. Final cystoscopy demonstrated a patent anterior urethral channel and no significant bleeding at the implant sites. The patient was able to void spontaneously in the postanesthesia care unit and was discharged home the same day.

On postoperative day #1, 16 hours after the procedure, the patient presented to an emergency department (ED) with abdominal pain. He underwent a computerized tomography (CT) scan of his abdomen and pelvis, and a 14.5 cm by 15 cm by 16.5 cm pelvic extraperitoneal hemorrhage with extension into the left retroperitoneum was found (Figures 1 and 2).

Initial laboratory data at that time included leukocytosis of 26.5, hemoglobin of 13.6, creatinine of 0.89, lactic acid of <0.3, and international normalized ratio (INR) of 1.1. A 16 French Foley catheter was placed for initially pink urine, which turned yellow shortly thereafter in the ED. Blood and urine cultures were sent at that time.

In the ED, the patient was given 1 gram of intravenous (IV) ceftriaxone and 2 liters of IV normal saline fluid. Repeat laboratory values demonstrated leukocytosis of 19.7 and hemoglobin of 11. At that point, he was transferred to a tertiary care hospital for further care.

Upon admission to that hospital, repeat laboratory data showed leukocytosis increased to 25 and hemoglobin of 9.8. Urology assessed the patient and ordered a CT scan of the pelvis with cystogram, which was negative for extravasation, albeit was a poor cystogram, due to bladder filling limitations as the patient was experiencing severe bladder spasms (Figures 3 and 4).

On postoperative day (POD) #2 (hospital day (HD) #1), daily laboratory data showed leukocytosis improved to 14, hemoglobin of 7.2, and creatinine stable at 0.88. The patient was maintained on scheduled IV ceftriaxone and given 2 units of packed red blood cells. The patient's urine had remained yellow, so he was given a voiding trial and passed. Blood and urine cultures resulted with no growth.

On POD#3 (HD#2), laboratory data showed leukocytosis decreased to 10.9, hemoglobin of 8.2, and creatinine of 0.69.

On POD#4 (HD#3), laboratory data showed leukocytosis had resolved to 7.2, with hemoglobin slightly decreased to 7.5. The patient was on scheduled IV ceftriaxone, blood and urine cultures remained negative, and the decision was made to transfuse the patient 1 additional unit of packed red blood cells—3[rd] unit of his admission. Repeat hemoglobin was drawn after the transfusion, which was 9.2, and all of

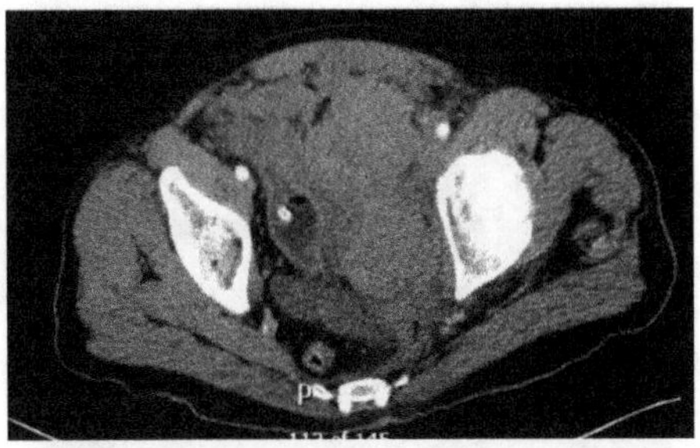

Figure 1: Initial CT abdomen and pelvis in ED (axial): 16 hours postop with large pelvic hematoma.

his vital signs were stable. The patient was discharged later that day in stable condition, voiding yellow urine.

Outpatient complete blood count on POD#11 demonstrated hemoglobin of 12, and follow-up visit in the office on POD#15 revealed some ecchymosis on the patient's left flank, penis, and scrotum, but the patient otherwise was voiding better and feeling well. Additional follow-up at 2 months postoperatively revealed that the patient's LUTS had resolved.

## 3. Discussion and Literature Review

UroLift® is a device manufactured by NeoTract for prostatic urethral lift, which delivers implants into the prostate to treat prostatic enlargement for the purpose of relieving lower urinary tract symptoms [1].

This was the first complication of its kind seen at our institution since the urologists began performing UroLift® in 2015.

After thorough discussion among the urologists at our institution and reflection on the case with UroLift® representatives, a few ideas were generated as to why such a significant pelvic hematoma may have formed.

One such idea is that the UroLift® device was compressed into the left side too deeply, and when deployed, one of the implants struck a vessel causing the hematoma. Another theory was that when the implant was placed to tack away the median lobe to the left, it may have advanced too proximally or posteriorly in the urethra and, again, struck a vessel, causing the hematoma. The UroLift® device deploys a needle 33 mm deep into the prostatic tissue, which has the potential to fire beyond the extent of the prostate, possibly leading to inadvertent vesicular vascular injuries. The depth can be adjusted based on the amount of compression given into the tissue by the device, prior to firing. The hematoma seen in this case (16.5 cm at its greatest dimension) was a significant size and presented with symptoms 16 hours postoperatively, so it is plausible that a small prostatic or vesicular arterial branch was struck by the implant, rather than a venous injury. Fortunately for the patient, the hematoma was retroperitoneal in nature and only required 3 units of packed red blood cells, without any further operative intervention. A possible solution to this theory could be for NeoTract to provide multiple options for the depth at which the UroLift® implant and needle fires, which could be based on preoperative transrectal ultrasound

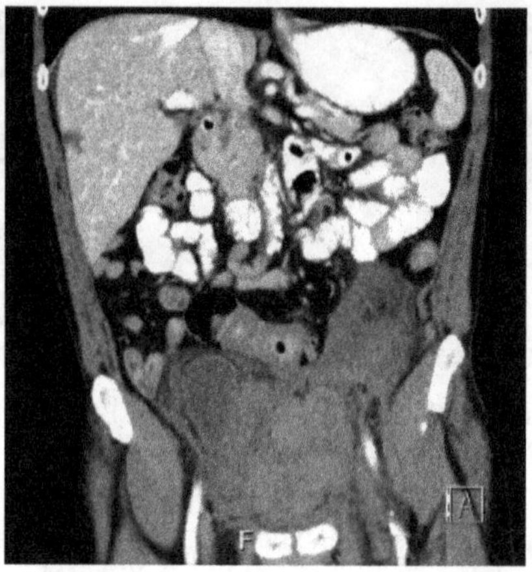

Figure 2: Initial CT abdomen and pelvis in ED (coronal): 16 hours postop with large pelvic hematoma.

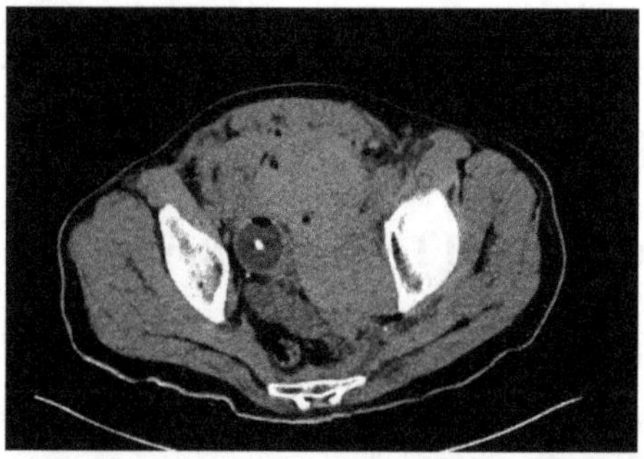

Figure 3: CT pelvis with cystogram at our hospital (axial): displaced bladder; poor cystogram without extravasation.

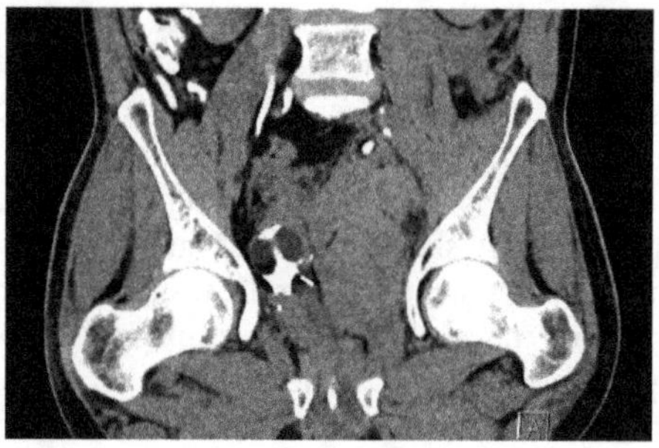

Figure 4: CT pelvis with cystogram at our hospital (coronal): displaced bladder; poor cystogram without extravasation.

measurements. Therefore, in patients with smaller prostate glands, a shallower depth implant could be used, which would theoretically provide the same clinical results for relief of lower urinary tract symptoms, without risking deeper vascular injuries.

Interestingly, this unique complication has only been described twice in the literature.

An article published in the Gold Journal of Urology in November 2019 described a case report of a patient undergoing UroLift® and having a postoperative pelvic hematoma [2]. The authors described it as the only known complication of its kind, in the literature [2]. The authors postulated that a short prostatic fossa, high bladder neck, and anterior deployment of the implants (at 2 and 10 o'clock positions) may have contributed to the hematoma in their patient [2].

This article generated some notable commentary on this complication.

One editorial, by Cai et al. from Weill Cornell (NY, NY), described a pelvic hematoma after UroLift® [3]. The patient required 3 units of packed red blood cells, vasopressors, and finally an exploratory laparotomy evacuating 1.5 liters of hematoma including fulguration and oversewing of a bleeding vessel on the left pubis [3]. Their input was that, "It seems that in rare cases, deploying an implant into the extraprostatic space without direct visualization of the final needle path can result in severe complications as described [3]."

Another editorial came from two groups: Tan et al. from the National University Hospital (Singapore) and Gange and Mueller from Summit Urology (Salt Lake City, UT) [4]. They sourced data from the United States Food and Drug Administration's (FDA) Manufacturer and User Facility Device Experience (MAUDE) [4]. Within this database, there was found to be 18 reports of pelvic hematoma since the UroLift® device was introduced [4]. Of these 18 patients, 14 required blood transfusions, 4 required prostatic artery embolization, and 3 required surgery: 1 of those was an open intervention (Cornell editorial), 2 died, and 1 required percutaneous nephrostomy tubes and hemodialysis [4]. Their input included describing how 175,000 patients were treated with UroLift®, which makes a 0.009% estimated pelvic hematoma occurrence [4]. They postulated that the number and percentage was likely lower than in reality, so they encouraged all urologists to report any complications to the MAUDE surveys [4].

A recent article from the University of Buffalo reported a case of pelvic hematoma after UroLift® causing a progression of the patient's chronic kidney disease, requiring 10 units of packed red blood cells and initiation of dialysis [5].

Currently, on the FDA's website for UroLift® MAUDE, since 2015, there have been a total of 27 reports of the adverse event of pelvic hematoma after UroLift® [6]. As of 2021, NeoTract/Teleflex reported that there have been over 200,000 patients treated with UroLift®, culminating in a reported 0.0135% incidence of hematoma.

We hypothesize that since these hematomas formed and were found after UroLift®, then there is a significant possibility that clinically insignificant hematomas also form but never cause enough of an issue to the patient to require hospital visits or imaging studies to discover them. In addition, contributing to this database requires urologists to submit their adverse events, which requires knowledge of where to submit them, as well as being time-consuming. Perhaps, hematoma after UroLift® is more common than is known.

Further studies could be performed to assess patients treated with UroLift®, who have median lobes of the prostate and then determine if there is a higher rate of pelvic hematoma.

According to the MedLift study, there is good data to support the use of UroLift® in patients even with a small median lobe, but there is a possibility that in addressing the median lobe, there is a higher chance of striking a vessel with the implant, causing a hematoma [7]. Therefore, we advise additional caution be taken when using the UroLift® device on a patient with a median lobe of the prostate.

We present a rare complication of a large pelvic hematoma after a minimally invasive BPH procedure, the UroLift®. Potential etiologies include implant firing depth beyond the extent of the prostate, as well as treatment of the median lobe. We encourage all urologists to report any complications of the UroLift®, to ensure there is an accurate representation of the risks of the procedure, and to bring more attention to this potential complication.

## Consent

Patient information was anonymized prior to submission of the case report.

## Disclosure

The authors certify that they have no affiliations with or involvement in any organization of entity with any financial interest or nonfinancial interest in the subject matter discussed in this manuscript.

## Acknowledgments

We thank Kimberly Stakleff, Ph.D, for her assistance in editing and supporting this manuscript.

## References

[1] L. P. Walsh, "State of the art: advanced techniques for prostatic urethral lift for the relief of prostate obstruction under local anesthesia," *The Canadian Journal of Urology*, vol. 24, no. 3, pp. 8859–8864, 2017.

[2] G. R. Pollock, A. Bergersen, F. M. Chaus, and M. Gretzer, "Pelvic hematoma following UroLift procedure for BPH," *Urology*, vol. 133, pp. e3–e4, 2019.

[3] P. Y. Cai, C. Gaffney, R. W. Vanden Berg, J. E. Shoag, and R. K. Lee, "Pelvic hematoma following Urolift Procedure for BPH," *Urology*, 2020.

[4] S. N. Gange and T. J. Mueller, "Re: Pelvic hematoma following UroLift procedure for BPH, [Urology 2020; 137: 208]," *Urology*, vol. 142, pp. 245-246, 2020.

[5] B. Ewing, N. Alavi-Dunn, H. Hamann, and T. Danforth, "Large pelvic hematoma following UroLift procedure causing renal failure requiring dialysis," *Urology Case Report*, vol. 34, article 101514, 2020.

[6] "Neotract Urolift-Maude-Manufacturer and User Facility Device Experience," 2021, http://www.accessdata.fda.gov/scripts/cdrh/cfdocs/cfmaude/results.cfm?start_search=1&productcode=PEW&productproblem=2993&patientproblem=&devicename=&modelNumber=&reportNumber=&manufacturer=&brandname=&eventtype=&reportdatefrom=01%2F1%2F2007&reportdateto=&pagenum=10.

[7] D. Rukstalis, D. Grier, S. P. Stroup et al., "Prostatic urethral lift (PUL) for obstructive median lobes: 12 month results of the MedLift study," *Prostate Cancer and Prostatic Diseases*, vol. 22, no. 3, pp. 411–419, 2019.

# Adult Granulosa Cell Tumor of the Testis: A Case Report with a Review of the Literature

**Klaus-Peter Dieckmann,[1] Julia Bertolini,[2] and Christian Wülfing[1]**

[1]*Asklepios Klinik Altona, Abteilung Urologie/Hodentumorzentrum, Hamburg, Germany*
[2]*MVZ Hanse Histologikum, Hamburg, Germany*

Correspondence should be addressed to Klaus-Peter Dieckmann; dieckmannkp@t-online.de

Academic Editor: Nicola Zampieri

Adult granulosa cell tumor (AGCT) of the testis represents a very rare testicular neoplasm that is poorly understood clinically. Here we report the case of a 22-year-old male who presented with unspecific scrotal symptoms. Scrotal sonography disclosed a 6 mm hypoechoic intratesticular lesion. Histological examination after orchiectomy revealed a homogeneous and well demarcated neoplasm with monomorphic cells with nuclear grooving and microfollicular formation of the so-called Call-Exner bodies. Immunohistology showed positive stainings of vimentin, calretinin, and inhibin with negative stainings of the typical germ cell tumor markers. Thus, the diagnosis of a benign AGCT was made. The patient is well one year after surgery. A total of 91 previous AGCT cases were identified in the literature. Median age of the cases reported to date is 44 years, median tumor size 3.2 cm. 54.3% of the AGCT cases were located on the left side. 12 cases (13.2%) were of malignant nature. Testis-sparing surgery would be the treatment of choice, but only two of all cases had received that procedure. The present report aims to increase the clinical knowledge of AGCT and specifically to increase the clinician's vigilance with respect to testis-sparing surgery in probably benign testicular masses.

## 1. Introduction

Histologically, about 90% of all testicular neoplasms comprise germ cell tumors (GCTs) while the remainder involves sex cord gonadal stromal tumors, malignant lymphomas, secondary tumors, and other very rare new growths [1, 2]. Among the gonadal stromal tumors, Leydig cell tumors and Sertoli cell tumors are the most common subtypes encompassing 1-2% and 0.5%, respectively, of all testis tumors [3]. The third subtype is the granulosa cell tumor which represents a truly rare neoplasm. Granulosa cell tumors arising in the testis are histologically identical with their ovarian counterparts. With respect to the pathogenesis of these unusual testicular neoplasms, Teilum postulated that cells of the male gonadal stroma retain their embryological ability to differentiate into both male or female specialized stromal cells, i.e., Leydig or Sertoli cells and granulosa or theca cells, respectively [4]. Thus, in the case of neoplastic growth of gonadal stromal cells the tumor cell types of both genders may evolve. Regarding granulosa cell tumors, two subtypes must be considered, the juvenile type occurring only in the first year of life and the adult type occurring later in life [5]. The clinical behavior of gonadal stromal tumors and particularly that of the adult granulosa cell tumor (AGCT) is poorly understood so far. The overall experience rests on a few small case series [6] and predominantly on single case reports [7]. The aim of the present report is to document another case of AGCT and to summarize the knowledge regarding this rare tumor.

## 2. Case Presentation

This 22-year-old man of European descent presented with unspecific scrotal discomfort lasting for two weeks. Clinical history is uneventful. The patient is unmarried and has no children so far. He is an untrained workingman by profession. Both testicles were of normal size and nonsuspicious upon palpation with only some tenderness on the

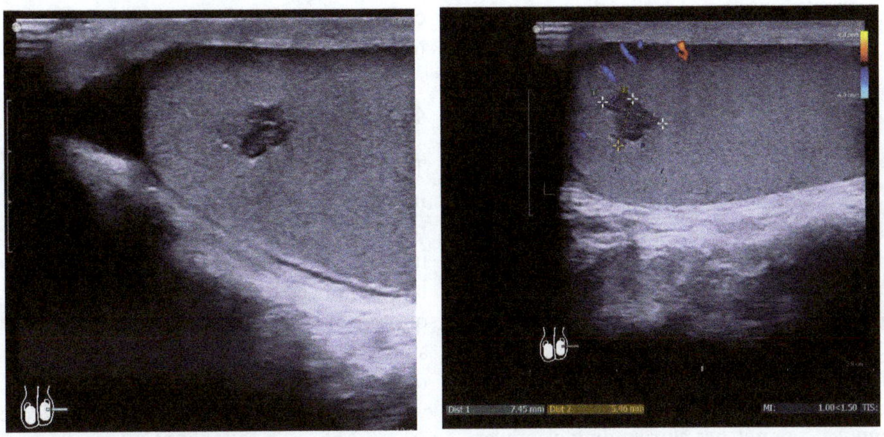

(a) (b)

FIGURE 1: (a) Sonographic appearance of the adult granulosa cell tumor in the 22-year-old patient. Note the lobulated but well circumscribed shape and homogeneous hypoechoic appearance. (b) The same patient, color-coded duplex sonography showing duplex signals within the hypoechoic lesion.

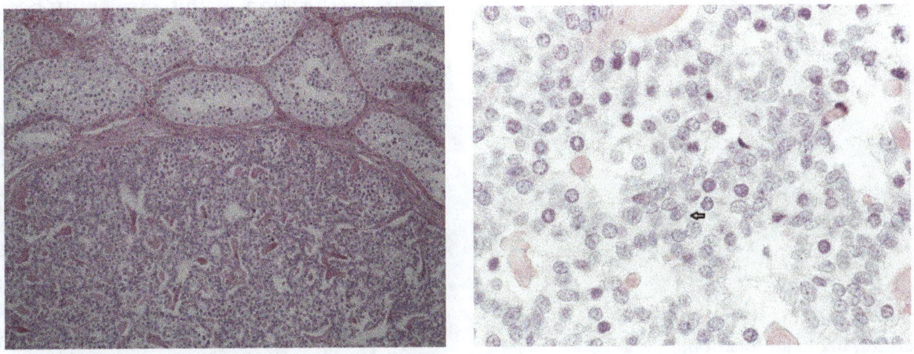

(a) (b)

FIGURE 2: (a) Histological section of the neoplasm, hematoxylin-eosin stain. Well demarcated rim of the testicular neoplasm, no clear encapsulation. Normal testicular parenchyma, upper part of image. 10x magnification. (b) Histological section of the neoplasm. The tumor cells have scant cytoplasm and elongated nuclei with numerous grooves (arrow). Hematoxylin-eosin stain, magnification x20.

left scrotal side. Scrotal sonography revealed a 1 cm sized lobulated hypoechoic lesion at the cranial pole of the left testis (Figure 1(a)) showing intense color duplex signals within the lesion (Figure 1(b)). Laboratory workup disclosed no abnormal results. Specifically, the germ cell tumor markers alpha fetoprotein, beta-human chorionic gonadotropin, and lactate dehydrogenase were within normal limits, as were the serum testosterone level (6.57 ng/ml; reference limits 2.4–8.7) and the gonadotropins LH (1.69 U/l) and FSH (2.78 U/l). Upon surgical exploration, a well circumscribed greyish-tan lesion of about 1 cm in size was identified at the cranial pole. Inguinal radical orchiectomy with placement of a silicone testicular implant and contralateral testicular biopsy were performed accordingly. The postoperative course was uneventful. Computed tomography of chest and abdomen did not reveal any metastases. No further treatment was applied. The patient is well and without recurrence of the disease one year after surgery.

Pathohistological analysis showed a well demarcated solid neoplasm of 8 mm in size (Figure 2(a)). Histologically, the lesion consisted of monomorphic cells resembling typical ovarian granulosa cells. Many of the cells had large nuclei with many of them having a grooved shape mirroring the appearance of coffee beans (Figure 2(b)). The growth pattern was solid in most parts of the neoplasm but in some areas microfollicular structures prevailed resembling Call-Exner bodies (Figure 3). Mitotic figures were very rare. No necrotic areas were detected. The tumor-surrounding testicular tissue showed normal spermatogenesis. Germ cell neoplasia in situ was detected neither in the ipsilateral parenchyma nor in the contralateral testicular tissue. Immunohistochemical workup revealed positive staining of inhibin, vimentin, and calretinin (Figure 4) and negative staining for Oct 4 and chromogranin A. Staining of progesterone receptor was negative, too. The MIB-1 labeling index revealed a growth fraction of < 1%. The histopathological findings were thus consistent with the

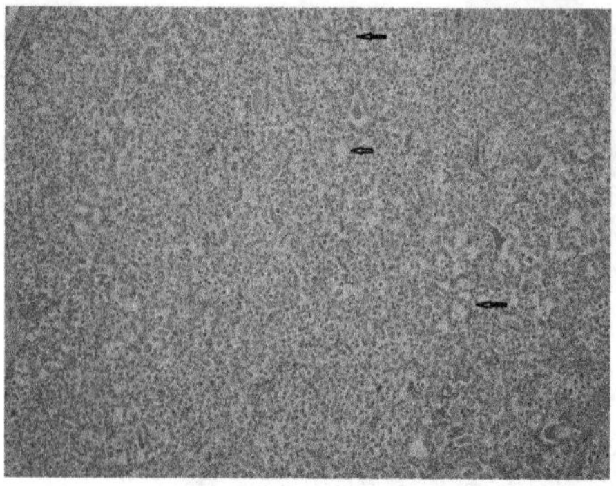

FIGURE 3: Histological section of the tumor. Adult granulosa cell tumor with microfollicular pattern. Call-Exner body: coffee bean-like tumor cells with groove core notches surrounding glandular cavities containing eosinophilic material and tumor cells detached from the dressing (arrows). Hematoxylin-eosin stain, 10x magnification.

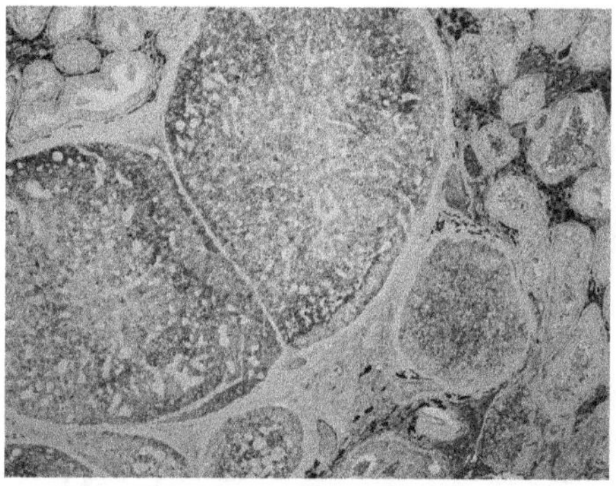

FIGURE 4: Immunohistological stain of calretinin. All neoplastic cells stain positive for calretinin, 10x magnification.

diagnosis of a benign adult type granulosa cell tumor of the testis.

## 3. Literature Survey

A total of 91 cases could be identified from the literature by using the PUBMED database and by hand-searching the reference lists of previous reports (Table 1). Not all of the case reports specified details regarding all of the clinical characteristics. Therefore, the various clinical features had to be analyzed with different sample sizes. With regard to age, 86 cases are eligible and the median age is 44 years (interquartile range (IQR) 26–55 years; range 12–87 years). With regard to tumor size, 80 cases are evaluable, with the median size amounting to 3.2 cm (IQR 1.5–5.0 cm; range 0.5–18.0 cm). Laterality is specified in 81 reports showing a slight preponderance of the left side with 44 cases (54.3 %; 95% confidence intervals (CIs) 42.9–65.4%) as opposed to 37 cases located on the right side (45.7%, 95% CI 34.6–57.1%). Malignancy was documented in 12 cases (13.2%) with 4 of these cases surviving more than 2 years. Endocrine symptoms were not systematically documented, but gynecomastia was reported in 8 cases. With regard to primary treatment, orchiectomy was the standard therapy. Only two cases had testis-sparing surgery.

## 4. Discussion

The first documentation of an AGCT is credited to Laskowski in 1952 [8]. By the year 2000, another 28 cases had been reported. In 2014, Schubert et al. summarized 43 cases of the literature [7]. In the same year, Cornejo et al. published the largest consecutive series of 32 patients [6]. Isolated cases not quoted by Schubert [36–39] and several cases documented since 2014 bring the total number to 91 cases reported to date (Table 1). Some more cases are briefly mentioned without providing details in several case series on gonadal stromal tumors [3, 55–57]. Thus, the total number of cases referred to in the medical literature is probably more than one hundred. And as a matter of fact, a large number of cases remained unreported. The number of documented cases has apparently increased since the year 2000. However, this statistical trend does probably not indicate a true increase of the incidence of AGCT but rather reflects a lower rate of misclassification of this rare entity because of increasing knowledge regarding testicular tumors [58]. One additional factor could be publication bias because the possibilities of publishing minor reports have much improved since the beginning of this century because of the ever increasing number of Internet-based scientific journals.

The age of the present patient is 22 years which is clearly lower than the median age of 44 years and even lower than the inter quartile range (26 -55 years) as observed in the literature survey. The lowest age ever observed in AGCT is 12 years [31] while the oldest subject is aged 87 years [6].

The tumor size of 8 mm found in our case is clearly smaller than the median size of 3.2 cm observed in the literature survey and it lies in the lowest quartile of reported findings. Obviously, granulosa cell tumors of the adult type may occur with a wide variety of sizes since seven cases with tumor sizes of less than 1 cm were reported (Table 1) and on the other side there were at least eight patients with giant tumors sized >10 cm. The median size of AGCT is very similar to the sizes of 3.2–3.5 cm and 2.8–3.5 cm found in nonseminomatous and seminomatous germ cell tumors, respectively [59, 60]. Probably, the presenting size of different histological types of testicular tumors does not relate to biological reasons but rather to sensual-cognitive structures of patients. Putatively, a diameter of around 3 cm represents the threshold where the majority of men will recognize a mass in the testicle. Most of the patients with AGCT presented with slowly growing painless testicular masses with several of whom reporting a duration of symptoms for many years [7, 22, 30]. On the other hand, eight cases were sized <1cm that were found incidentally upon autopsy [9] or with ultrasonography [25, 43]. Overall, a palpable mass is probably the typical presenting symptom of AGCT as it is with testicular germ cell tumors [6, 38, 45]. Endocrine-related symptoms were infrequently reported in previous cases, but eight patients of the survey were reported to present with gynecomastia. This symptom is not specific for AGCT because it is frequently observed in Leydig cell tumors

TABLE 1: Synopsis of cases with adult granulosa cell tumor of the testis reported in 1953–2018.

| *Author* (first) | *year* | *reference* (#) | *age* (years) | *tumor size* (cm) | *right side* | *malignant* | *presenting symptom* | *endocrine symptoms* | *F/U* |
|---|---|---|---|---|---|---|---|---|---|
| Laskowski | 1952 | [8] | 35 | 9,00 | R | | | gynecomastia | 8,5 yrs |
| Cohen | 1953 | [9] | 21 | <1 cm | L | | incidental | gynecomastia | ns |
| Massachusetts case * | 1955 | [7] | 53 | 10 cm | R | | | gynecomastia | ns |
| Melicow | 1955 | [10] | 52 | 13,00 | R | | | | ns |
| Mostofi | 1959 | [11] | 41 | 10,10 | L | malignant | | gynecomastia | DOD 5 m |
| Marshall | 1977 | [12] | 53 | 10,00 | ns | | mass, no pain | gynecomastia | 17 yrs |
| Talerman | 1985 | [13] | 44 | 3,50 | R | | mass, no pain | | 3 yrs |
| Gaylis | 1989 | [14] | 41 | 1.8 cm | R | | | | ns |
| Düe | 1990 | [15] | 83 | 18 cm | L | | mass, no pain | | DOC 1 m |
| Nistal | 1992 | [16] | 61 | 5,00 | R | | | | ns |
| Matoska | 1992 | [17] | 26 | 10,00 | L | malignant | painful mass | gynecomastia | 14 yrs NED |
| Sasano | 1992 | [18] | ns | ns | ns | | | | ns |
| Monobe | 1992 | [19] | 42 | ns | L | malignant | | | AWD |
| Jiminez-Quintero | 1993 | [20] | 57 | 2,50 | R | | | | 3y DOC |
| Jiminez-Quintero | 1993 | | 55 | 1,30 | L | | | | ns |
| Jiminez-Quintero | 1993 | | 60 | 7,00 | L | malignant | | | DOD 11 yrs |
| Jiminez-Quintero | 1993 | | 39 | 4,00 | L | | | | 3 yrs NED |
| Jiminez-Quintero | 1993 | | 29 | 7,50 | R | malignant | | | |
| Jiminez-Quintero | 1993 | | 76 | 0,70 | L | | | | NED 1 m |
| Renshaw | 1997 | [21] | ns | ns | ns | | | | ns |

Table 1: Continued.

| *Author* (first) | *year* | *reference* (#) | *age* (years) | *tumor size* (cm) | *right side* | *malignant* | *presenting symptom* | *endocrine symptoms* | *F/U* |
|---|---|---|---|---|---|---|---|---|---|
| Renshaw | 1997 | | ns | ns | ns | | | | ns |
| Renshaw | 1997 | | ns | ns | ns | | | | ns |
| Morgan | 1999 | [22] | 49 | 2,60 | L | | | | 2 yrs NED |
| Al-Bozom | 2000 | [23] | 48 | 5,00 | R | | | | 7 m NED |
| Wang | 2002 | [24] | 54 | ns | L | | hydrocele, asymptomatic | | ns |
| Guzzo | 2004 | [25] | 33 | 1,00 | L | | | | ns |
| Suppiah | 2005 | [26] | 51 | ns | L | malignant | | | 6 yrs AWD |
| Hisano | 2006 | [27] | 59 | 15,00 | L | | | | 4 yrs NED |
| Arzola | 2006 | [28] | 32 | 2,10 | L | | painless mass | | |
| Lopez | 2007 | [29] | 77 | 4,00 | L | | | | ns |
| Ditonno | 2007 | [30] | 45 | 6,50 | R | | painless mass | | 2 yrs NED |
| Gupta | 2008 | [31] | 12 | 8,00 | L | | | | 1 yr NED |
| Hammerich | 2008 | [32] | 55 | ns | ns | malignant | | | 3 yrs NED |
| Song | 2011 | [33] | 28 | 2,60 | L | | | | ns |
| Hanson | 2011 | [34] | 21 | 1,00 | L | | | | 2 yrs NED |
| Lima | 2012 | [35] | 77 | 2,50 | R | | | | ns |
| Lima | 2012 | | 22 | 1,00 | L | | | | ns |
| Lima | 2012 | | 40 | 2,10 | L | | | | |
| Schubert | 2014 | [7] | 78 | 1,3 | L | | painless mass | | 23 m NED |
| Cornejo | 2014 | [6] | 49 | 3,00 | R | | | | 137 m, DOOD |
| Cornejo | 2014 | | 22 | 3,30 | L | | | | 48 m |
| Cornejo | 2014 | | 50 | 0,90 | L | | | | 59 m |

Table 1: Continued.

| *Author* (first) | *year* | *reference* (#) | *age* (years) | *tumor size* (cm) | *right side* | *malignant* | *presenting symptom* | *endocrine symptoms* | *F/U* |
|---|---|---|---|---|---|---|---|---|---|
| Cornejo | 2014 | | ns | 3,00 | L | | | | lost |
| Cornejo | 2014 | | 27 | 1,80 | R | | | | 60 m |
| Cornejo | 2014 | | 87 | ns | ns | | | | 169 m |
| Cornejo | 2014 | | 47 | 4,50 | R | | | | lost |
| Cornejo | 2014 | | 51 | 2,10 | R | | | | 58 m |
| Cornejo | 2014 | | 47 | 0,50 | L | | | | lost |
| Cornejo | 2014 | | 55 | 2,10 | L | | | | 80 m |
| Cornejo | 2014 | | 25 | 2,00 | R | | | | lost |
| Cornejo | 2014 | | 45 | 1,40 | R | | | | lost |
| Cornejo | 2014 | | 74 | 3,50 | L | | | | 104 m |
| Cornejo | 2014 | | 27 | 1,40 | R | | | | 36 m |
| Cornejo | 2014 | | 32 | 4,20 | R | | | | lost |
| Cornejo | 2014 | | 18 | 3,20 | L | | | | lost |
| Cornejo | 2014 | | 60 | 6,00 | R | | | | lost |
| Cornejo | 2014 | | 23 | 1,40 | R | | | | 65 m |
| Cornejo | 2014 | | 20 | 4,50 | L | | | | 1 m |
| Cornejo | 2014 | | 52 | 4,30 | R | malignant | | | 24 m AWD |
| Cornejo | 2014 | | 14 | 0,80 | R | | | | lost |
| Cornejo | 2014 | | 21 | 3,00 | R | | | | 37 m |
| Cornejo | 2014 | | 17 | 1,50 | R | | | | lost |
| Cornejo | 2014 | | 64 | 2,40 | R | | | | 28 m |
| Cornejo | 2014 | | 14 | 3,50 | R | | | | 35 m |
| Cornejo | 2014 | | 28 | 2,60 | L | | | | lost |
| Cornejo | 2014 | | 51 | 3,00 | L | | | | lost |
| Cornejo | 2014 | | 63 | 1,00 | L | | | | 25 m |
| Cornejo | 2014 | | 25 | 5,50 | R | | | | 1 m |
| Cornejo | 2014 | | 44 | 1,20 | L | | | | 1 m |
| Cornejo | 2014 | | 50 | 4,70 | R | | | | 1 m |
| Köksal | 2003 | [36] | 40 | 3,50 | R | | 8-month mass | no | 20 m |

Table 1: Continued.

| *Author* (first) | *year* | *reference* (#) | *age* (years) | *tumor size* (cm) | *right side* | *malignant* | *presenting symptom* | *endocrine symptoms* | *F/U* |
|---|---|---|---|---|---|---|---|---|---|
| Mitra | 2008 | [37] | 25 | 0,50 | L | | scrotal pain 2 weeks | | ns |
| Kucukodaci | 2008 | [38] | 21 | 1,50 | L | | incidental | no | 1 yr |
| Harrison | 2009 | [39] | 65 | 5,00 | L | malignant | | | DOD |
| Miliaris | 2013 | [40] | 37 | 4,20 | L | | painless mass | no | 2 yrs |
| Norman | 2013 | [41] | 68 | ns | R | | | | 18 m |
| Rane | 2014 | [42] | 34 | 5,00 | R | | | | 6 m |
| Rane | 2014 | | 46 | 65,00 | L | | | | 2,5 yrs |
| Rane | 2014 | | 46 | 11,00 | R | malignant | | | 3 m |
| Tanner | 2014 | [43] | 22 | 0,60 | L | | | | ns |
| Tsitouridis | 2014 | [44] | 29 | 2,50 | R | | | | 1 yr |
| Giulianelli | 2015 | [45] | 80 | 6,00 | R | | mass, no pain | gynecomastia | 1 yr |
| Vallonthaiel | 2015 | [46] | 43 | 6,00 | L | | painless mass | | 1 yr |
| Gomez-Valcarcel | 2016 | [47] | 23 | ns | ns | | | | ns |
| Mohapatra | 2016 | [48] | 57 | 4,7 | L | malignant | incidental | gynecomastia | 32 m NED |
| Al-Alao | 2016 | [49] | 48 | 1,20 | L | | | | ns |
| Bani | 2016 | [50] | 20 | 2,00 | R | | | | 4 m NED |
| Elbachiri | 2017 | [51] | 40 | 5,50 | L | malignant | painless growing mass | | 2 yrs NED |
| Mezentsev | 2017 | [52] | 74 | 5,00 | R | | painless mass | | ns |
| Meilan | 2017 | [53] | 59 | 3,30 | ns | | | | ns |
| Nunes-Carneiro | 2017 | [54] | 31 | 4,50 | ns | | | | 10 yrs |

∗As cited by Schubert et al. 2014.
Ns: not stated.
NED: no evidence of disease; DOD: dead of disease; DOC: dead of complication; AWD: alive with disease; DOOD: dead of other disease.
yrs: years; m: months.
R: right side; L: left side; F/U: follow-up.

and sometimes also in beta-human chorionic gonadotropin secreting germ cell tumors [61]. Our patient presented with unspecific scrotal symptoms that were not related to the tiny testicular tumor that was only detected with ultrasonography. Sonographic features were frequently reported and typically involve hypoechoic well circumscribed masses with positive color-coded sonographic signals [37, 49]. But anechoic areas corresponding to cystic parts of the tumor have also been observed [7, 52].

Regarding laterality of AGCT, our patient presented with a left sided tumor which corresponds to the findings in the majority of cases of the survey where 54.3% (95% CI 42.9–65.4%) had left sided tumors as opposed to 45.7% (95% CI 34.6–57.1%) right sided tumors. However, in view of the overall small database and overlapping confidence intervals of the proportions there is probably no clear evidence for a predisposition of one side. The same is true with germ cell tumors where no clear preponderance of one particular side has been found [59].

The neoplasm detected in our patient was a clearly benign lesion. Among the 91 cases listed in the survey, 12 were malignant (13.2%). A 15% proportion of malignancy was likewise reported by Rove et al. [57] and two additional malignant cases were briefly mentioned by Featherstone et al. [56]. Reportedly, clinical features of malignancy involve tumor size > 5 cm and age > 50 years [34, 57]. Histologically, >3 mitoses per high-power field, invasion of rete testis, vascular invasion, and cellular atypia are considered as characteristics of malignancy [51, 58].

Histologically, AGCT consist of monomorphic cells identical with ovarian granulosa cells with a scanty cytoplasm. Many of the cells may show coffee bean-like nuclei with small grooves [6, 45]. The cells are mostly arranged in trabeculae and sheets and some may form microfollicular structures, the so-called Call-Exner bodies [62]. The histological diagnosis mainly rests on immunohistochemical findings with positive stainings of inhibin, vimentin, and calretinin and negative stainings for pancytokeratin and the typical germ cell tumor specific markers like placental alkaline phosphatase, D2-40, and Oct 3/4 [7, 18, 20, 21, 62].

With regard to treatment, testis-sparing surgery would be the treatment of choice, as only few cases are malignant. As age >50 years and tumor size are the most important characteristics of malignancy the cases qualifying for conservative surgery could in principle be easily identified, preoperatively.

Hence, only two of the cases of the survey received that appropriate therapy and also the present case was submitted to orchiectomy. Clearly, in everyday clinical practice it is difficult to sort out benign tumors from malignant ones by means of clinical assessment only. As malignant tumors of the testis are far more common than benign growths most of the urologic surgeons will proceed to radical orchiectomy. However, as shown in the present case and in many cases of the survey, benign tumors of the testis do actually occur, and small size is one of the leading characteristics of benign nature though not specific. The present case report is thought to increase the overall knowledge of testicular granulosa cell tumors, and it particularly aims to increase the vigilance of urologic surgeons to consider conservative surgery in cases with small testicular neoplasms. Practically, a conservative approach with intraoperative frozen section examination could help to save more testicles and avoid unnecessary orchiectomies.

## Consent

Written consent was obtained from the patient for publication of this report and accompanying images.

## References

[1] H. M. Rosevear, A. Mishail, Y. Sheynkin, and M. Wald, "Unusual scrotal pathology: an overview," *Nature Reviews Urology*, vol. 6, no. 9, pp. 491–500, 2009.

[2] S. R. Williamson, B. Delahunt, C. Magi-Galluzzi et al., "The World Health Organization 2016 classification of testicular germ cell tumours: a review and update from the International Society of Urological Pathology Testis Consultation Panel," *Histopathology*, vol. 70, no. 3, pp. 335–346, 2017.

[3] D. S. Conkey, G. C. W. Howard, K. M. Grigor, D. B. McLaren, and G. R. Kerr, "Testicular sex cord-stromal tumours: the Edinburgh experience 1988-2002, and a review of the literature," *Clinical Oncology*, vol. 17, no. 5, pp. 322–327, 2005.

[4] G. Teilum, *Special tumors of ovary and testis and related extragonadal lesions*, Munksgaard, Copenhagen, Denmark, 2nd edition, 1976.

[5] L. M. Roth, B. Lyu, and L. Cheng, "Perspectives on testicular sex cord-stromal tumors and those composed of both germ cells and sex cord-stromal derivatives with a comparison to corresponding ovarian neoplasms," *Human Pathology*, vol. 65, pp. 1–14, 2017.

[6] K. M. Cornejo and R. H. Young, "Adult granulosa cell tumors of the testis: A report of 32 cases," *The American Journal of Surgical Pathology*, vol. 38, no. 9, pp. 1242–1250, 2014.

[7] T. E. O. Schubert, R. Stoehr, A. Hartmann, S. Schöne, M. Löbelenz, and G. Mikuz, "Adult type granulosa cell tumor of the testis with a heterologous sarcomatous component: case report and review of the literature," *Diagnostic Pathology*, vol. 9, article 107, 2014.

[8] J. Laskowski, "Feminizing tumours of testis; general review with case report of granulosa cell tumour of testis," *Endokrynologia Polska*, vol. 3, pp. 337–343, 1952.

[9] J. Cohen and J. Diamond, "Leontiasis ossea, slipped epiphyses and granulosa cell tumor of the testis with renal disease," *Archives of Pathology & Laboratory Medicine*, vol. 56, pp. 488–500, 1953.

[10] M. M. Melicow, "Classification of tumors of testis: a clinical and pathological study based on 105 primary and 13 secondary cases in adults, and 3 primary and 4 secondary cases in children," *The Journal of Urology*, vol. 73, no. 3, pp. 547–574, 1955.

[11] F. K. Mostofi, E. A. Theiss, and D. J. B. Ashley, "Tumors of specialized gonadal stroma in human male patients. Androblastoma, sertoli cell tumor, granulosa-theca cell tumor of the testis, and gonadal stromal tumor," *Cancer*, vol. 12, no. 5, pp. 944–957, 1959.

[12] F. F. Marshall, W. S. Kerr Jr., B. Kliman, and R. E. Scully, "Sex cord stromal (gonadal stromal) tumors of the testis: a report of 5 cases," *The Journal of Urology*, vol. 117, no. 2, pp. 180–184, 1977.

[13] A. Talerman, "Pure granulosa cell tumour of the testis. report of a case and review of the literature," *Applied Pathology*, vol. 3, no. 3, pp. 117–122, 1985.

[14] F. D. Gaylis, C. August, A. Yeldandi, A. Nemcek, and J. Garnett, "Granulosa cell tumor of the adult testis: Ultrastructural and ultrasonographic characteristics," *The Journal of Urology*, vol. 141, no. 1, pp. 126-127, 1989.

[15] W. Düe, K.-P. Dieckmann, G. Niedobitek, G. Bornhoft, V. Loy, and H. Stein, "Testicular sex cord stromal tumour with granulosa cell differentiation: detection of steroid hormone receptors as a possible basis for tumour development and therapeutic management," *Journal of Clinical Pathology*, vol. 43, no. 9, pp. 732–737, 1990.

[16] M. Nistal, R. Lázaro, J. García, and R. Paniagua, "Testicular granulosa cell tumor of the adult type," *Archives of Pathology & Laboratory Medicine*, vol. 116, pp. 284–287, 1992.

[17] J. Matoška, D. Ondruš, and A. Talerman, "Malignant granulosa cell tumor of the testis associated with gynecomastia and long survival," *Cancer*, vol. 69, no. 7, pp. 1769–1772, 1992.

[18] H. Sasano, N. Nakashima, O. Matsuzaki et al., "Testicular sex cord-stromal lesions: Immunohistochemical analysis of cytokeratin, vimentin and steroidogenic enzymes," *Virchows Archiv A Pathological Anatomy and Histopathology*, vol. 421, no. 2, pp. 163–169, 1992.

[19] Y. Monobe and T. Manabe, "Malignant sex-cord stromal tumor of the testis: report of a case with special reference to its unusual intracytoplasmic substructures," *Japanese Journal of Clinical Oncology*, vol. 22, no. 6, pp. 414–420, 1992.

[20] L. P. Jimenez-Quintero, J. Y. Ro, A. Zavala-Pompa et al., "Granulosa cell tumor of the adult testis: a clinicopathologic study of seven cases and a review of the literature," *Human Pathology*, vol. 24, no. 10, pp. 1120–1126, 1993.

[21] A. A. Renshaw, M. Gordon, and C. L. Corless, "Immunohistochemistry of unclassified sex cord-stromal tumors of the testis with a predominance of spindle cells," *Modern Pathology*, vol. 10, no. 7, pp. 693–700, 1997.

[22] D. R. Morgan and K. G. Brame, "Granulosa cell tumour of the testis displaying immunoreactivity for inhibin," *BJU International*, vol. 83, no. 6, pp. 731-732, 1999.

[23] I. A. Al-Bozom, S. R. El-Faqih, S. H. Hassan, and A. E. El-Tiraifi, "Granulosa cell tumor of the adult type: a case report and review of the literature of a very rare testicular tumor," *Archives of Pathology & Laboratory Medicine*, vol. 124, pp. 1525–1528, 2000.

[24] B. Y. Wang, D. S. Rabinowitz, R. C. S. Granato, and P. D. Unger, "Gonadal tumor with granulosa cell tumor features in an adult testis," *Annals of Diagnostic Pathology*, vol. 6, no. 1, pp. 56–60, 2002.

[25] T. Guzzo, M. Gerstein, and J. H. Mydlo, "Granulosa cell tumor of the contralateral testis in a man with a history of cryptorchism," *Urologia Internationalis*, vol. 72, no. 1, pp. 85–87, 2004.

[26] A. Suppiah, M. M. Musa, D. R. Morgan, and A. D. North, "Adult granulosa cell tumour of the testis and bony metastasis: a report of the first case of granulosa cell tumour of the testicle metastasising to bone," *Urologia Internationalis*, vol. 75, no. 1, pp. 91–93, 2005.

[27] M. Hisano, F. M. Mascarenhas Souza, D. M. A. Costa Malheiros, A. C. Lima Pompeo, and A. M. Lucon, "Granulosa cell tumor of the adult testis. Report of a case and review of the literature," *Clinics*, vol. 61, no. 1, pp. 77-78, 2006.

[28] J. Arzola, R. L. Hutton, S. M. Baughman, and R. V. Mora, "Adult-type testicular granulosa cell tumor: Case report and review of the literature," *Urology*, vol. 68, no. 5, pp. 1121.e13–1121.e16, 2006.

[29] J. I. López, "Adult-type granulosa cell tumor of the testis. report of a case," *Tumori*, vol. 93, no. 2, pp. 223-224, 2007.

[30] P. Ditonno, G. Lucarelli, M. Battaglia et al., "Testicular granulosa cell tumor of adult type: a new case and a review of the literature," *Urologic Oncology: Seminars and Original Investigations*, vol. 25, no. 4, pp. 322–325, 2007.

[31] A. Gupta, S. Mathur, C. Reddy, and B. Arora, "Testicular granulosa cell tumor, adult type," *Indian Journal of Pathology and Microbiology*, vol. 51, no. 3, pp. 405-406, 2008.

[32] K. H. Hammerich, S. Hille, G. E. Ayala et al., "Malignant advanced granulosa cell tumor of the adult testis: case report and review of the literature," *Human Pathology*, vol. 39, no. 5, pp. 701–709, 2008.

[33] Z. Song, D. J. Vaughn, and Z. Bing, "Adult type granulosa cell tumor in adult testis: report of a case and review of the literature," *Rare Tumors*, vol. 3, no. 4, article e37, pp. 117–119, 2011.

[34] J. A. Hanson and A. B. Ambaye, "Adult testicular granulosa cell tumor: a review of the literature for clinicopathologic predictors of malignancy," *Archives of Pathology & Laboratory Medicine*, vol. 135, pp. 143–146, 2011.

[35] J. F. Lima, L. Jin, A. R. de Araujo et al., "Medeiros FOXL2 mutations in granulosa cell tumors occurring in males," *Archives of Pathology & Laboratory Medicine*, vol. 136, no. 7, pp. 825–828, 2012.

[36] I. T. Köksal, M. Usta, A. Ciftcioglu, T. Erdogru, E. Kukul, and M. Baykara, "Sex cord tumour of the adult testis," *International Urology and Nephrology*, vol. 35, no. 3, pp. 365–367, 2003.

[37] A. Mitra, V. Palit, R. Paes, and M. Ferro, "Sonographic features of an adult granulosa cell tumor of the testis," *Radiology Case Reports*, vol. 3, article 188, 2008.

[38] Z. Kucukodaci, M. Keles, T. Yapanoglu, B. F. Alp, Y. Aksoy, and I. Ozbey, "Adult type granulosa cell tumor of the testis: case report and review of the literature," *The Eurasian Journal of Medicine*, vol. 40, pp. 39–41, 2008.

[39] M. R. Harrison, W. Huang, G. Liu, and J. Gee, "Response to antiangiogenesis therapy in a patient with advanced adult-type testicular granulosa cell tumor," *Oncology (Williston Park)*, vol. 23, pp. 792–795, 2009.

[40] D. Miliaras, E. Anagnostou, and I. Moysides, "Adult type granulosa cell tumor: a very rare case of sex-cord tumor of the testis with review of the literature," *Case Reports in Pathology*, vol. 2013, Article ID 932086, 4 pages, 2013.

[41] R. W. Norman, A. Sheridan-Jonah, J. Merrimen, and R. Gupta, "Adult granulosa cell tumor of the testicle," *Canadian Journal of Urology*, vol. 20, no. 1, pp. 6640–6642, 2013.

[42] S. U. Rane, S. Menon, S. Desai, G. Bakshi, and A. Joshi, "Granulosa cell tumor of testis: clinicopathological correlation of a rare tumor," *Indian Journal of Pathology and Microbiology*, vol. 57, no. 4, pp. 564–573, 2014.

[43] S. B. Tanner, D. B. Morilla, and J. D. Schaber, "A case of adult granulosa cell tumor of the testis," *The American Journal of Case Reports*, vol. 15, article 471, 2014.

[44] I. Tsitouridis, C. Maskalidis, A. Sdrolia, S. Pervana, E. Pazarli, and E. P. Kariki, "Adult type granulosa cell tumor of the testis: radiological evaluation and review of the literature," *Turkish Journal of Urology*, vol. 40, no. 2, pp. 115–119, 2014.

[45] R. Giulianelli, G. Mirabile, G. Vincenti, F. Pellegrino, and G. Soda, "A very rare case of adult-type granulosa cell tumor," *Archivio Italiano di Urologia, Andrologia*, vol. 87, no. 1, pp. 98-99, 2015.

[46] A. G. Vallonthaiel, A. Kakkar, A. Singh, P. N. Dogra, and R. Ray, "Adult granulosa cell tumor of the testis masquerading as

hydrocele," *International Brazilian Journal of Urology*, vol. 41, no. 6, pp. 1226–1231, 2015.

[47] J. Gómez-Valcárcel, J. d. Barranco-García, and I. García-Muñoz, "Tumor de células de la granulosa de tipo adulto. Un caso raro de tumor testicular," *Presentación Y Discusión De Tres Casos Clínicos*, vol. 49, no. 1, pp. 62–65, 2016.

[48] A. Mohapatra, A. M. Potretzke, B. A. Knight, M. Han, and R. S. Figenshau, "Metastatic granulosa cell tumor of the testis: clinical presentation and management," *Case Reports in Urology*, vol. 2016, Article ID 9016728, 4 pages, 2016.

[49] O. Al-Alao, T. Gul, A. Al-Ani, I. A. Bozom, and K. Al-Jalham, "Adult-type granulosa cell tumour of the testis: report of a case and review of the literature," *Arab Journal of Urology*, vol. 14, no. 1, pp. 44–49, 2016.

[50] M. A. Bani, A. Zehani, I. Chelly, A. Fethi, S. Haouet, and N. Kchir, "Adult granulosa cell tumor of the testis: a case report," *La Tunisie Médicale*, vol. 94, no. 12, pp. 897-898, 2016.

[51] M. Elbachiri, A. Taleb, N. Derrabi et al., "Adult-type granulosa cell tumor of the testis: Report of a case and review of literature," *Pan African Medical Journal*, vol. 26, article 198, 2017.

[52] V. Mezentsev, H. Ali, J. McKenzie, and J. Virdi, "Adult type granulosa cell tumour of the testis: a case report," *Onkourologiya*, vol. 13, no. 1, pp. 134–138, 2017.

[53] E. Meilán, C. Esquinas, I. Romero, J. Duarte, and A. García-Tello, "Adult type granulosa cell testicular tumor. case report and bibliographic review," *Archivos Espanoles De Urologia*, vol. 70, pp. 617–620, 2017 (Spanish).

[54] D. Nunes-Carneiro, A. Marques-Pinto, V. Cavadas, and A. Fraga, "Adult testicular granulosa cell tumour: an extremely rare entity," *BMJ Case Reports*, 2018.

[55] A. A. Mosharafa, R. S. Foster, R. Bihrle et al., "Does retroperitoneal lymph node dissection have a curative role for patients with sex cord-stromal testicular tumors?" *Cancer*, vol. 98, no. 4, pp. 753–757, 2003.

[56] J. M. Featherstone, H. S. Fernando, J. M. Theaker, P. D. Simmonds, M. C. Hayes, and G. M. Mead, "Sex cord stromal testicular tumors: a clinical series-uniformly stage i disease," *The Journal of Urology*, vol. 181, no. 5, pp. 2090–2096, 2009.

[57] K. O. Rove, P. D. Maroni, C. R. Cost et al., "Pathologic risk factors for metastatic disease in postpubertal patients with clinical stage i testicular stromal tumors," *Urology*, vol. 97, pp. 138–144, 2016.

[58] F. Bremmer, C. L. Behnes, H.-J. Radzun, M. Bettstetter, and S. Schweyer, "Sex cord gonadal stromal tumors," *Pathologe*, vol. 35, pp. 245–251, 2014.

[59] K.-P. Dieckmann, H. Richter-Simonsen, M. Kulejewski et al., "Testicular germ-cell tumours: a descriptive analysis of clinical characteristics at first presentation," *Urologia Internationalis*, vol. 100, no. 4, pp. 409–419, 2018.

[60] C. Rothermund, C. Thurneysen, R. Cathomas et al., "Baseline characteristics and patterns of care in testicular cancer patients: First data from the Swiss Austrian German Testicular Cancer Cohort Study (SAG TCCS)," *Swiss Medical Weekly*, vol. 148, no. 29-30, article w14640, 2018.

[61] P. Zeuschner, C. Veith, J. Linxweiler, M. Stöckle, and J. Heinzelbecker, "Two years of gynecomastia caused by leydig cell tumor," *Case Reports in Urology*, vol. 2018, Article ID 7202560, 4 pages, 2018.

[62] F. Bremmer and S. Schweyer, "Leydig cell, Sertoli cell and adult granulosa cell tumors," *Pathologe*, vol. 37, no. 1, pp. 71–77, 2016.

# 26

# Intratesticular Angiolipoma: A Rare Case of Adipose Tissue Presence in the Testis

V. Kalyvas,[2] C. Gkekas,[1] D. Papadopoulos,[1] A. Malioris,[1] S. Milias,[3] M. Papathanasiou,[1] N. Kalinderis,[2] K. Moysidis,[2] and K. Hatzimouratidis[2]

[1] *Department of Urology, 424 General Military Hospital of Thessaloniki, Greece*
[2] *2nd Department of Urology, Aristotle University of Thessaloniki, Greece*
[3] *Department of Pathology, 424 General Military Hospital of Thessaloniki, Greece*

Correspondence should be addressed to D. Papadopoulos; papadopoud@gmail.com

Academic Editor: Khaled Madbouly

*Introduction.* Solid, fat-containing tumors of the testes are extremely rare with only a few cases having been reported so far, contrary to the more frequent occurrence of paratesticular lipomatosis. Testicular angiomyolipomas and gonadal involvement in Cowden's disease, although infrequently occurring, are known examples of fat-bearing testicular lesions. Hereby, we present an extremely rare case of intratesticular angiolipoma. Angiolipomas are benign tumors of the subcutaneous tissue commonly occurring in the trunk and the extremities. Histologically, they are characterized by ample vascularity and an excess of mature adipocytes. Definitive diagnosis is established by biopsy of the lesion. *Presentation of the Case.* A 35-year-old patient presented to our andrology outpatient clinic for fertility assessment. Physical examination of external genitalia revealed no significant pathology. Testicular ultrasound however depicted an isoechoic lesion on the upper pole of the right testis measuring $1.8\,\text{cm} \times 0.8\,\text{cm} \times 1\,\text{cm}$ and exhibiting intense arterial flow. After sonographic and MRI investigation, the patient was referred for semen analysis and cryopreservation. Subsequently, the patient underwent testicular biopsy (frozen section biopsy) and right partial orchiectomy. Final histology reported a noninfiltrating testicular angiolipoma. No recurrences have been observed in the follow-up period. *Discussion.* Angiolipomas, which mainly occur in the trunk and extremities, are classified as infiltrating and noninfiltrating. The diagnosis is based on both clinical and histologic criteria, and the main method of treatment for both types is by surgical excision. The infiltrating type exhibits higher recurrence rates. *Conclusion.* Angiolipomas commonly occur in the subcutaneous tissue and have been invariably treated by radical excision. Hereby, we report the first case of an intratesticular, noninfiltrating type angiolipoma which was treated by partial orchiectomy.

## 1. Introduction

Angiolipomas are benign tumors, commonly occurring in the subcutaneous tissue. They are either encapsulated or nonencapsulated fatty tumors and are distinguished from other lipomas by the excessive degree of vascular proliferation and abundance of mature adipocytes. They more often occur in the trunk and extremities, rarely in the maxillofacial area [1] and are usually diagnosed histologically [2]. We report the first case of an intratesticular angiolipoma.

## 2. Case Presentation

A 35-year-old patient presented to our andrology outpatient clinic for fertility assessment. Physical examination of the external genitalia was insignificant. There was neither history of testicular trauma nor any sexually transmitted disease in his medical record.

Testicular ultrasound revealed a solitary isoechoic, highly vascularized lesion of the upper pole of the right testis measuring $1.8\,\text{cm} \times 0.8\,\text{cm} \times 1\,\text{cm}$ distinctly separated from the

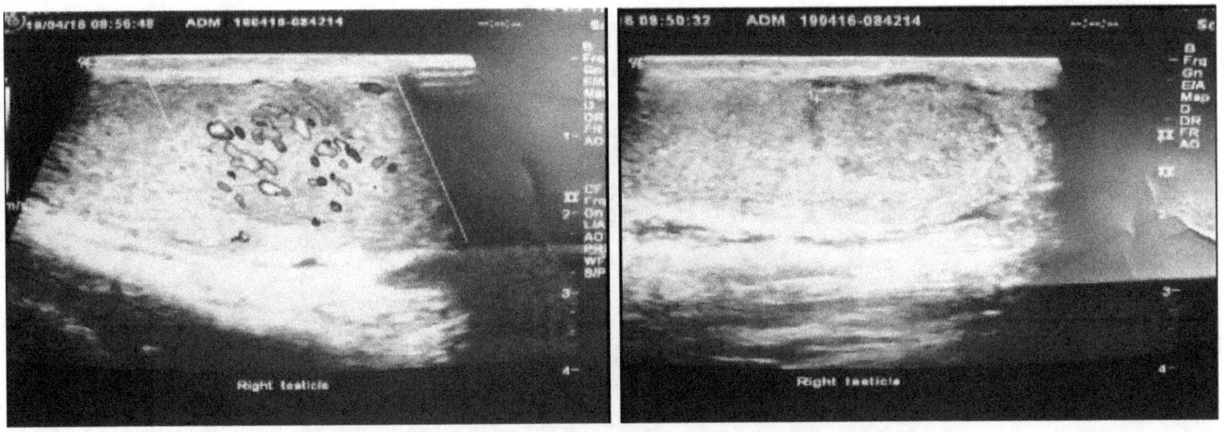


FIGURE 1: Scrotal ultrasound: right testicle.

TABLE 1: Hormonal testing.

| | |
|---|---|
| FSH | 2.17 mIU/ml |
| LH | 3.7 mIU/ml |
| Testosterone | 3.1 ng/ml |
| $\beta$-hCG | <1.2 mIU/ml |
| aFP | 3.7 ng/ml |

TABLE 2: Semen analysis.

| | |
|---|---|
| Ejaculate volume (ml) | 2.1 |
| pH | 7.3 |
| Total sperm number (10/ejaculate) | 29.4 |
| Sperm concentration (10/ml) | 14 |
| Total motility (PR+NP) | 39 |
| Progressive motility (PR, %) | 32 |
| Vitality (live spermatozoa, %) | 59 |
| Sperm morphology (normal forms, %) | 4 |

PR = progressive; NP = nonprogressive.

adjacent healthy parenchyma by a well-defined hypoechoic capsule (Figure 1). No additional testicular or epididymal pathology was identified on both sides.

Hormonal testing (FSH, LH, Testosterone, $\beta$-hCG, and aFP) and semen analysis fell within the normal range (Tables 1 and 2).

CT scan of the thorax, abdomen, and pelvis revealed no retroperitoneal lymphadenopathy or other abnormalities.

MRI of the scrotum demonstrated a well-defined encapsulated mass, located in the upper pole of the right testis measuring 1.9 cm × 0.9 cm × 1.2 cm.

After semen cryopreservation, the patient underwent surgical exploration. Intraoperative frozen section analysis reported a nonmalignant lesion, possibly an angiolipoma. A right partial orchiectomy was subsequently performed. The final histology reported a 1.9 cm × 0.9 cm × 1.2 cm lesion composed of adipocytes and small vessels with fibrous microthrombi, identified as noninfiltrating type angiolipoma. The tumor was circumscribed and partially encapsulated. Capillaries and mature adipocytes were observed. Few vascular channels contained microthrombi. Around the periphery of the tumor, the capillaries and the adipocytes entrapped the seminiferous tubules. This finding, which is also observed in testicular hemangiomas, perhaps predicts a more aggressive behavior of the tumor with higher possibility of recurrence in cases of partial orchiectomy (Figures 2–5).

Follow-up visits included physical examination, hormonal assessment, and scrotal ultrasound every three months for the first two years, every six months for the next two years, and subsequently on a yearly basis. The patient has currently been free of recurrence.

## 3. Discussion

Angiolipomas consist a variant of lipomas which was first described by Bowen in 1912 [1]. In 1960, Howard [3] classified angiolipomas as a new entity, because of their distinct clinical and pathological differences with lipomas. The presence of adipocyte cells in the testis has previously been described in angiomyolipomas (AML), which are mostly benign mesenchymal tumors composed of fat, smooth muscle cells, and tortuous, thick-walled blood vessels [4, 5]. Likewise, in testicular lipomatosis or Cowden's disease, nested fat cells have been identified in the testicular parenchyma [6]. Additionally, fat cells have been reported in Leydig cell tumors, coupled with atypical features, such as calcification, ossification, and spindle cell proliferation [7].

Based on cytogenetic analysis, the karyotype of angiolipomas differs from that of other benign lipomatous tumors [8] which suggests that the hamartomatous origin of angiolipomas may be different from the rest of the lipomas. They commonly develop in the trunk and extremities and rarely in the gastrointestinal tract [1]. They are usually encountered as multiple, small tumors (less than 2 cm in diameter each), which produce no symptoms [9]. There is no reference in the existing literature of testicular angiolipomas.

Angiolipomas can easily be distinguished from other lipomas from their excess of vascular elements [10]. There are various factors that are related to the etiology of

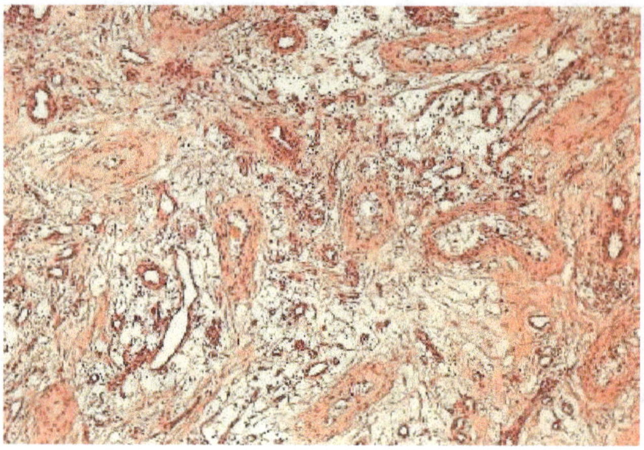

FIGURE 2: Testicular tumor composed of mature adipose tissue and small vessels: seminiferous tubules with thickened basement membrane and atrophic are also observed (H&E stain ×10).

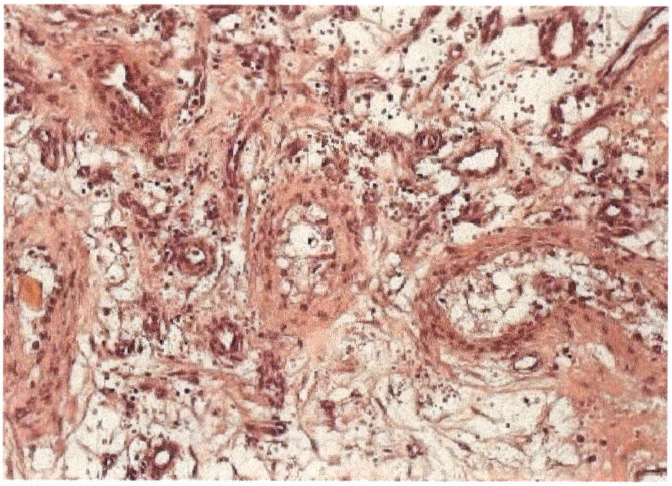

FIGURE 3: Same area under higher magnification (H&E stain ×20).

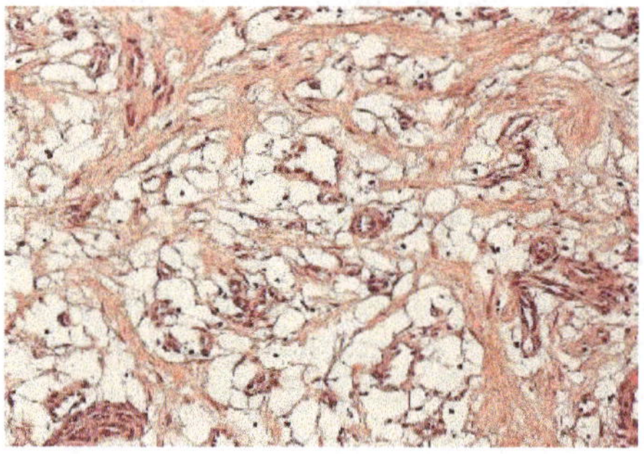

FIGURE 4: Area with numerous adipocytes and small vessels, some of them including erythrocytes in their lumen (H&E stain ×20).

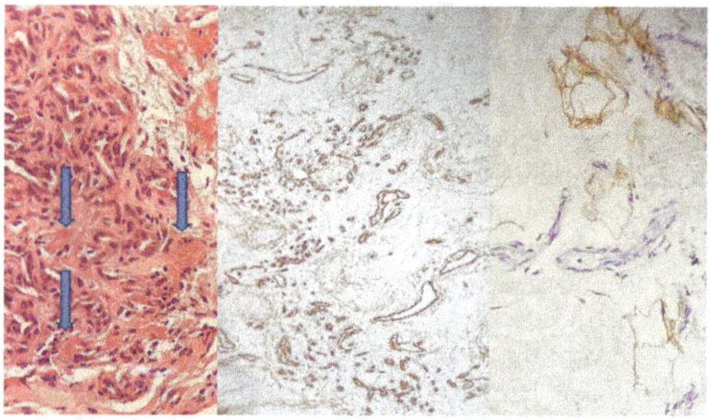

(a) (b) (c)

FIGURE 5: (a) Microthrombi in capillaries (blue arrows) (H&E stain ×20). (b) Endothelial cells of the vascular capillaries are positive (CD34 immunohistochemistry ×10). (c) Adipocytes are positive (S100 Protein Immunohistochemistry ×40).

angiolipomas such as a history of trauma, vascular transformation of a lipoma, and hormonal imbalances [3].

J. J. Lin and F. Lin classified angiolipomas into infiltrating and noninfiltrating types [8]. The noninfiltrating type which is the most common occurs in younger individuals and presents as a painless subcutaneous nodule [8, 10]. Histologically, it is encapsulated and consists a mixture of mature adipocytes interspersed between thin-walled vessels [11]. The infiltrating angiolipoma which rarely has a capsule occurs in older patients, invades into the adjacent

TABLE 3: Histologic guidelines for diagnosis of noninfiltrating angiolipoma [1].

| |
|---|
| Evidence of 50% mature adipocytes in the tumor |
| Interspersed angiomatous proliferation in the tumor |
| Well encapsulated |
| Fibrinous microthrombi |
| Absence of other mesenchymal elements |

structures, and is more common in the head and neck region [10]. The diagnosis is based on both clinical and histological criteria (Table 3).

The main treatment for both types is by complete excision. Noninfiltrating angiolipomas have no tendency to recur after surgical removal; therefore, a simple excision of the lesion will probably be curative. In the case of infiltrating angiolipomas, the recurrence rate is higher and a wide surgical excision is imperative [8, 12, 13].

## 4. Conclusion

Angiolipomas are benign tumors, commonly occurring in the subcutaneous tissue. This is the first recorded case of an intratesticular, noninfiltrating type angiolipoma which was treated by organ-sparing surgery. Two years after the procedure, there were no recurrences. The rarity of the specific entity and the lack of published experience impede the construction of an evidence-based treatment algorithm. Every case report adds to the growing body of evidence.

## References


[1] J. Arenaz Búa, R. Luáces, F. Lorenzo Franco et al., "Angiolipoma in head and neck: report of two cases and review of the literature," *International Journal of Oral and Maxillofacial Surgery*, vol. 39, no. 6, pp. 610–615, 2010.

[2] L. Wang, P. Chen, L. Zong, G. Y. Wang, and H. Wang, "Colon angiolipoma with intussusception: a case report and literature review," *World Journal of Surgical Oncology*, vol. 11, no. 1, p. 69, 2013.

[3] S. Pattipati, M. N. Kumar, and B. P. K. Ramadevi, "Palatal lipoma: a case report," *Journal of Clinical and Diagnostic Research*, vol. 7, no. 12, pp. 3105-3106, 2013.

[4] C. P. Nelson and M. G. Sanda, "Contemporary diagnosis and management of renal angiomyolipoma," *The Journal of Urology*, vol. 168, 4 Part 1, pp. 1315–1325, 2002.

[5] E. Cibas, G. Goss, M. Kulke, G. Demetri, and C. Fletcher, "Malignant epithelioid angiomyolipoma (`sarcoma ex angiomyolipoma') of the kidney: a case report and review of the literature," *The American Journal of Surgical Pathology*, vol. 25, no. 1, pp. 121–126, 2001.

[6] J. B. Woodhouse, B. Delahunt, S. F. English, H. H. Fraser, and M. M. Ferguson, "Testicular lipomatosis in Cowden's syndrome," *Modern Pathology*, vol. 18, no. 9, pp. 1151–1156, 2005.

[7] T. M. Ulbright, J. R. Srigley, D. K. Hatzianastassiou, and R. H. Young, "Leydig cell tumors of the testis with unusual features. Adipose differentiation, calcification with ossification, and spindle-shaped tumor cells," *The American Journal of Surgical Pathology*, vol. 26, no. 11, pp. 1424–1433, 2002.

[8] J. J. Lin and F. Lin, "Two entities in angiolipoma(*A study of 459 cases of lipoma with review of literature on infiltrating angiolipoma*)," *Cancer*, vol. 34, no. 3, pp. 720–727, 1974.

[9] G. B. Davis, P. J. W. Stoelinga, H. Tideman, and F. Bronkhorst, "Angiolipoma of the hard palate: a case report and review of the literature," *Journal of Maxillofacial Surgery*, vol. 4, no. 4, pp. 242–244, 1976.

[10] J. J. Flaggert III, L. V. Heldt, and W. M. Keaton, "Angiolipoma of the palate: Report of a case," *Oral Surgery, Oral Medicine, Oral Pathology*, vol. 61, no. 4, pp. 333–336, 1986.

[11] J. S. Reilly, D. R. Kelly, and S. A. Royal, "Angiolipoma of the parotid: case report and review," *The Laryngoscope*, vol. 98, no. 8, pp. 818–821, 1988.

[12] S. Dalambiras, I. Tilaveridis, S. Iordanidis, T. Zaraboukas, and A. Epivatianos, "Infiltrating angiolipoma of a the oral cavity: report of a case and literature review," *Journal of Oral and Maxillofacial Surgery*, vol. 68, no. 3, pp. 681–683, 2010.

[13] M. H. Ali and F. El Zuebi, "Angiolipoma of the cheek: report of a case," *Journal of Oral and Maxillofacial Surgery*, vol. 54, no. 2, pp. 213–215, 1996.

27

# Intranodal Lymphangiography during Surgical Repair of Pelvic Lymphorrhea after Radical Cystectomy

**Yasuyuki Onishi,[1] Yusaku Moribata,[1] Hironori Shimizu,[1] Kosuke Shimizu,[2] Takeshi Sano,[2] Takashi Kobayashi,[2] and Yuji Nakamoto[1]**

[1]*Department of Diagnostic Imaging and Nuclear Medicine, Kyoto University Graduate School of Medicine, Japan*
[2]*Department of Urology, Kyoto University Graduate School of Medicine, Japan*

Correspondence should be addressed to Yasuyuki Onishi; goforawalktoday@yahoo.co.jp

Academic Editor: Apul Goel

Lymphorrhea can develop after various types of surgeries. Surgical closure of the lymphatic leakage point is an effective treatment option. However, it is difficult to identify the leakage point sometimes. Here, we report a case of pelvic lymphorrhea after radical cystectomy for bladder cancer. Identification of the leakage point was difficult during laparoscopic surgical repair of lymphorrhea. Intranodal lymphangiography was performed via the inguinal lymph node by injection of lipiodol, followed by injection of indigo carmine. Laparoscopy revealed extravasation of lipiodol and indigo carmine from the pelvic wall. The leakage point was successfully cauterized using an electric scalpel. Lymphorrhea improved after the surgical repair. This case suggests that intranodal lymphangiography may be useful for detecting the site of lymphatic leakage during the surgical repair of lymphorrhea.

## 1. Introduction

Lymphorrhea can occur after various types of surgeries, including esophagectomy, pneumonectomy, gastrectomy, pancreaticoduodenectomy, kidney transplantation, hysterectomy, prostatectomy, and lymph node resection [1]. Dehydration, nutritional deficiency, and immunological dysfunction may develop due to lymphorrhea [2]. Conservative management, such as dietary therapy, total parenteral nutrition, pharmacotherapy, and abdominal paracentesis, is an effective initial treatment [3]. If conservative management fails, surgical closure of the site of lymphatic leakage is the ideal treatment [3, 4]. However, the leakage point is occasionally not identified during surgery [3]. Intraoperative lymphangiography is an effective method for identifying the leakage point. Herein, we describe a case of postoperative lymphorrhea that was treated with surgical repair. Intranodal lymphangiography was performed during the repair to identify the site of leakage.

## 2. Case Presentation

A 79-year-old man presented with high-grade muscle-invasive bladder cancer and underwent robot-assisted laparoscopic radical cystoprostatectomy with urethrectomy, extended pelvic lymph node dissection, and intracorporeal urinary diversion. One week after surgery, clear fluid started leaking from the external urethral orifice. The leakage output was 300 mL per day. CT revealed a medium amount of ascites. Biochemical examination of the ascitic fluid was suggestive of lymphorrhea. A low-fat diet was started, but the leakage output did not decrease. Two months after surgery, intranodal lymphangiography was performed to detect the site of leakage and reduce the amount of lymphatic leakage. Under local anesthesia, bilateral inguinal lymph nodes were punctured with a 23-gauge cathelin needle under ultrasound guidance (Figure 1). Lipiodol was injected slowly under fluoroscopy, showing a network of lymphatic vessels in the pelvis. Lymphatic leakage from the left pelvic wall into the

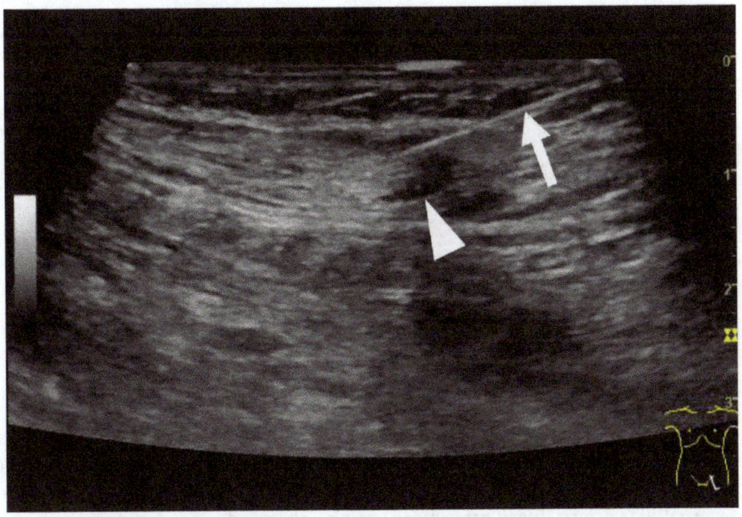

FIGURE 1: Ultrasonography performed during intranodal lymphangiography demonstrating a 23-gauge needle (arrow) being advanced into an inguinal lymph node (arrowhead).

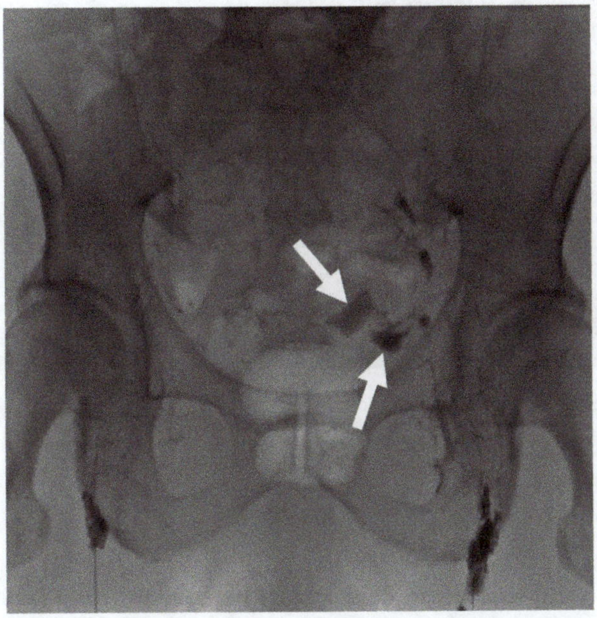

FIGURE 2: Pelvic X-ray performed during intranodal lymphangiography demonstrating leakage of lipiodol (arrows) from the left wall of the pelvis into the peritoneal cavity.

peritoneal cavity was detected (Figure 2). Although the therapeutic effect of lipiodol lymphangiography was expected, the amount of lymphatic leakage did not change after lymphangiography. Thus, laparoscopic surgical repair of lymphorrhea was performed two weeks later. During the repair, a dent was found on the left wall of the pelvis just above the external iliac artery, from which the serous fluid slowly leaked into the peritoneal cavity. Although the dent was suspected to be the lymphatic leakage point, the laparoscopic findings alone were not conclusive. We decided to perform intraoperative lymphangiography to confirm that the dent was the leakage point and to exclude other sites of leakage. A left inguinal lymph node was punctured under ultrasound guidance and lipiodol was slowly injected, showing leakage from the left wall of the pelvis. Then, indigo carmine diluted 10-fold with normal saline was slowly injected. In total, 1 mL of lipiodol and 1 mL of diluted indigo carmine were used. Three minutes after administering lipiodol injection, laparoscopy revealed extravasation of lipiodol and indigo carmine from the dent (Figures 3 and 4 and Supplementary Video). We also confirmed the absence of other leakage sites. The lymphatic leakage point on the left wall of the pelvis was close to the external iliac artery, and suturing the leakage point was a risk factor for vascular injury. Thus, the leakage point was cauterized using an electric scalpel. Additionally, a defect was observed at the pelvic floor region that was sutured at the completion of the previous surgery, and the lymph was considered to have leaked from the external urethral orifice through the defect. The defect was closed with 3-0 Vicryl sutures. No complications were observed. After surgical repair, lymphatic leakage from the external urethral orifice was no longer observed. Abdominal ultrasound revealed a decrease in ascites. One month later, the patient was discharged home.

## 3. Discussion

A small number of studies have reported the usefulness of intraoperative lymphangiography in detecting the leakage point in patients with postoperative lymphorrhea [5–8]. In previous studies, intertoe injection of iso-sulphan blue or indocyanine green, or subcutaneous injection of indocyanine green dye in the inguinal region was performed [5, 7, 8]. In contrast, we performed intranodal lymphangiography in the present case. The clinical outcome of this patient indicates the clinical usefulness of intranodal lymphangiography as it appropriately showed the lymphatic leakage point during surgery.

Intranodal lymphangiography is a relatively new technique, which requires puncture of the inguinal lymph nodes and injection of lipiodol, and it has previously been

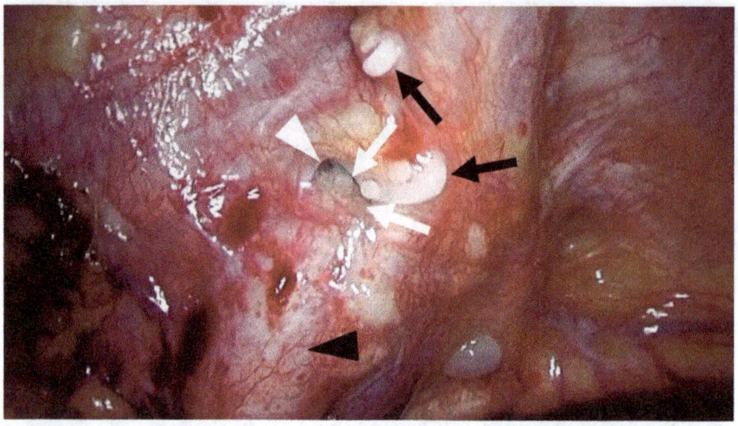

Figure 3: Laparoscopic image taken during surgical repair of lymphorrhea demonstrating droplets of lipiodol (white arrows) flowing out from a dent (white arrowhead) on the left wall of the pelvis; surgical clips (black arrows) that were placed during cystectomy to prevent lymphatic leakage and the left external iliac artery (black arrowhead) can be observed.

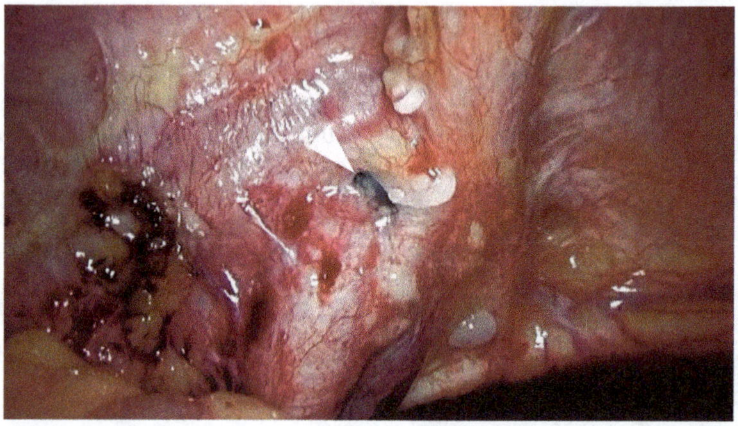

Figure 4: Laparoscopic image taken during surgical repair of lymphorrhea demonstrating indigo carmine (arrowhead) flowing out from a dent on the left wall of the pelvis.

performed under fluoroscopy guidance to detect lymphatic leakage points [9]. Additionally, this technique is reportedly therapeutically effective for lymphatic leakage [9]. Compared with the conventional pedal lymphangiography, which requires the isolation and cannulation of pedal lymphatic vessels and injection of lipiodol, intranodal lymphangiography is less time-consuming and easier to perform [10].

In patients with postoperative lymphorrhea, the leakage point may be difficult to localize during surgical repair, and unsuccessful surgical repair is not uncommon [11]. Additionally, there can be multiple leakage points, and successful ligation of one leakage point does not always lead to alleviation of the symptoms [6]. The lymphatic system can be clearly visualized on intranodal lymphangiography, and it is also easy to perform during surgical repair. It probably has a higher leakage point detection rate than other methods of lymphangiography.

In conclusion, we report a case in which intranodal lymphangiography made it possible to determine the lymphatic leakage point and to confirm the absence of other leakage points. This technique may be beneficial during surgical repair of lymphorrhea.

## References


[1] C. M. Sommer, C. C. Pieper, F. Offensperger et al., "Radiological management of postoperative lymphorrhea," *Langenbeck's Archives of Surgery*, vol. 406, no. 4, pp. 945–969, 2021.

[2] S. Lv, Q. Wang, W. Zhao et al., "A review of the postoperative lymphatic leakage," *Oncotarget*, vol. 8, no. 40, pp. 69062–69075, 2017.

[3] S. A. Al-Busa fi, P. Ghali, M. Deschenes, and P. Wong, "Chylous ascites: evaluation and management," *ISRN Hepatology*, vol. 2014, 240410 pages, 2014.

[4] A. Cardenas and S. Chopra, "Chylous ascites," *The American Journal of Gastroenterology*, vol. 97, no. 8, pp. 1896–1900, 2002.

[5] P. J. Rubis, J. Tisnado, J. I. Hirsch, and J. Capehart, "Intraoperative identification of chylous fistulas using iso-sulphan blue dye," *AJR. American Journal of Roentgenology*, vol. 139, no. 1, pp. 186-187, 1982.

[6] S. Kohnoe, I. Takahashi, H. Kawanaka, M. Mori, K. Okadome, and K. Sugimachi, "Combination of preoperative lymphangiography using lipiodol and intraoperative lymphangiography using Evans Blue facilitates the accurate identification of post-

operative chylous fistulas," *Surgery Today*, vol. 23, no. 10, pp. 929–931, 1993.

[7] K. Kamiya, N. Unno, and H. Konno, "Intraoperative indocyanine green fluorescence lymphography, a novel imaging technique to detect a chyle fistula after an esophagectomy: report of a case," *Surgery Today*, vol. 39, no. 5, pp. 421–424, 2009.

[8] R. Shirotsuki, H. Uchida, Y. Tanaka et al., "Novel thoracoscopic navigation surgery for neonatal chylothorax using indocyanine-green fluorescent lymphography," *Journal of Pediatric Surgery*, vol. 53, no. 6, pp. 1246–1249, 2018.

[9] E. W. Lee, J. H. Shin, H. K. Ko, J. Park, S. H. Kim, and K. B. Sung, "Lymphangiography to treat postoperative lymphatic leakage: a technical review," *Korean Journal of Radiology*, vol. 15, no. 6, pp. 724–732, 2014.

[10] G. J. Nadolski and M. Itkin, "Feasibility of ultrasound-guided intranodal lymphangiogram for thoracic duct embolization," *Journal of Vascular and Interventional Radiology*, vol. 23, no. 5, pp. 613–616, 2012.

[11] I. Leibovitch, Y. Mor, J. Golomb, and J. Ramon, "The diagnosis and management of postoperative chylous ascites," *The Journal of Urology*, vol. 167, pp. 449–457, 2002.

# 28

# Giant Cell Urothelial Carcinoma of Bladder

**Harshima Disvini Wijesinghe**[1] **and Ajith Malalasekera**[2]

[1]*Department of Pathology, Faculty of Medicine, University of Colombo, Sri Lanka*
[2]*Department of Anatomy, Faculty of Medicine, University of Colombo, Sri Lanka*

Correspondence should be addressed to Harshima Disvini Wijesinghe; harshima@path.cmb.ac.lk

Academic Editor: ChunHou Liao

Giant cell urothelial carcinoma is a rare variant of bladder cancer recognized by the current World Health Organization classification of urologic tumours. It is an aggressive tumour with a poor prognosis that usually presents at an advanced stage. It is characterized histologically by pleomorphic giant cells. We discuss a case of giant cell urothelial carcinoma presenting at an early stage in a previously well 62-year-old woman. Histology showed a tumour comprising pancytokeratin positive bizarre mononuclear and multi-nuclear giant cells admixed with areas of conventional urothelial carcinoma and carcinoma in situ. Three-month follow-up cystoscopy and magnetic resonance imaging showed no evidence of recurrence or pelvic lymphadenopathy.

## 1. Introduction

Giant cell urothelial carcinoma is a rare aggressive variant of urothelial carcinoma characterized by the presence of highly pleomorphic bizarre tumour giant cells. We report a case of giant cell urothelial carcinoma in a 62-year-old woman. The approach to diagnosis and differential diagnosis is discussed.

## 2. Case History

A 62-year-old woman presented with visible haematuria. Cystoscopy showed a 15 mm papillary growth with a broad base in the left wall of the bladder. She underwent transurethral resection of the bladder tumour. The entire tumour was processed and examined microscopically. Microscopic examination showed bladder tissue infiltrated by a high-grade (Grade 3) urothelial carcinoma with a component of giant cell urothelial carcinoma. The tumour was composed predominantly of cells arranged in diffuse sheets and solid nests. The constituent cells had enlarged, markedly pleomorphic, hyperchromatic nuclei, and frequent mitoses. Admixed bizarre mononuclear and multinuclear giant cells were seen (Figure 1(a)). The giant cells were positive for pancytokeratin (AE1/AE3) (Figure 1(b)). Areas of conventional urothelial carcinoma (Figure 1(c)) with overlying carcinoma in situ were present (Figure 1(d)). The tumour showed extensive invasion of the lamina propria and muscularis mucosa, but the invasion of muscularis propria was not seen. Lymphovascular invasion was present. Follow up cystoscopy at three months did not show any recurrence in the bladder. There was no residual tumour or pelvic lymphadenopathy on a magnetic resonance imaging scan done at four months.

## 3. Discussion

Giant cell urothelial carcinoma is a rare aggressive carcinoma [1]. A variant of UC with highly pleomorphic tumour giant cells has been described in several publications since it was first reported in 1997 [2]. There are two case series and a few case reports that describe the clinical and pathological features of giant cell urothelial carcinoma [3–5] (Tables 1 and 2), including an interesting case of polyomavirus- (BK-) associated pleomorphic giant cell carcinoma of the urinary bladder associated with areas of trophoblastic differentiation [5].

Giant cell urothelial carcinoma has also been called pleomorphic giant cell carcinoma and large-cell undifferentiated carcinoma. Like most urothelial carcinomas, giant cell

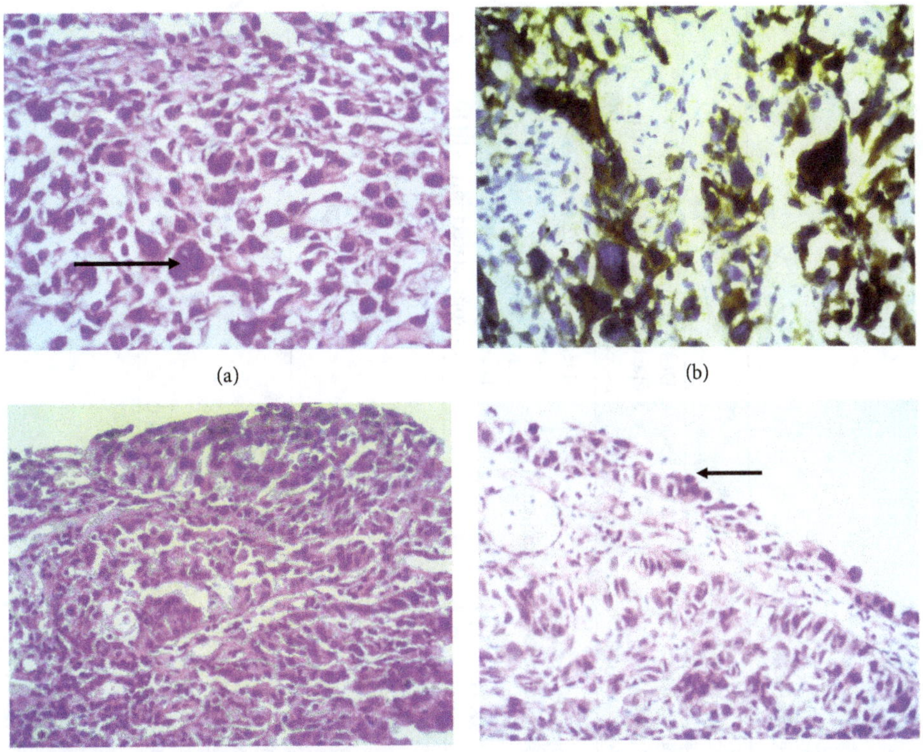

(a) (b) (c) (d)

Figure 1: Histological appearance of the tumour. Giant cell urothelial carcinoma comprising sheets of pleomorphic cells with admixed bizarre mononuclear and multinuclear giant cells ((a), haematoxylin and eosin ×400) which were positive for pancytokeratin ((b), AE1/AE3 ×400) admixed with areas of conventional urothelial carcinoma (c) and carcinoma in situ (d).

urothelial carcinoma occurs more commonly in older males (ages ranging from 53 to 92 years). It presents with haematuria, dysuria, or frequency [1.3.4]. It is characterized histologically by the presence of highly pleomorphic bizarre tumour giant cells similar to those seen in giant cell carcinoma of the lung. These tumours usually show muscularis propria invasion and extensive necrosis, although they were not identified in the present case. The current guidelines recommend that ideally all the bladder tumour tissue resected by transurethral resection is submitted, for pathological assessment. In large specimens where this is not feasible, it is recommended to submit the first 20 g (10 cassettes) of tissue plus one cassette for every additional 5 g [6]. This will facilitate accurate staging and histopathological subtyping of the tumour. This was a small tumour and it was sampled in its entirety.

The current World Health Organization (WHO) classification defines giant cell carcinoma as a rare form of infiltrating urothelial carcinoma resembling giant cell carcinoma of the lung in which the proliferating cells may appear undifferentiated [1]. Giant cell urothelial carcinoma shows expansile masses of the pleomorphic epithelioid tumour with bizarre anaplastic multinucleated and mononucleated tumour giant cells. Tumour cells have abundant cytoplasm and show frequent typical or atypical mitotic figures. Giant cell urothelial carcinoma has been reported in association with both conventional urothelial carcinoma and variants such as micropapillary, plasmacytoid, and lymphoepithelioma-like urothelial carcinoma [3–5]. It has also been reported with carcinomas with areas of trophoblastic differentiation [5]. The pleomorphic giant cell component, which accounted for 50% of the tumour in the present case, has been reported to range from 20% to 100% of the tumour [3].

Giant cell urothelial carcinoma must be distinguished from sarcomatoid carcinoma. The bladder and prostate cases with a significant spindle cell component [1] are called sarcomatoid carcinoma and are considered to be distinct from giant cell urothelial carcinoma which lacks a malignant spindle cell component. This is in contrast to organs such as the lung where according to the WHO classification of lung tumours, giant cell carcinoma is considered to be a subtype of sarcomatoid carcinoma [7].

Giant cell urothelial carcinoma must be differentiated from other primary bladder tumours that can contain giant cells, including osteoclast rich undifferentiated carcinoma and urothelial carcinoma with trophoblastic differentiation. The giant cells in giant cell urothelial carcinoma are morphologically different from the giant cells seen in these two entities [1, 8]. In contrast to giant cell urothelial carcinoma, osteoclast-rich undifferentiated carcinoma has a biphasic appearance. Giant cells resembling osteoclastic giant cells have numerous small bland nuclei and are present in a background of mononuclear cells [1, 8, 9]. These giant cells are positive for CD68 and LCA and negative for cytokeratins and epithelial membrane antigen.

Giant cell urothelial carcinoma must also be distinguished from metastasis from a giant cell carcinoma, melanoma, or

Table 1: Clinical features of reported cases of giant cell urothelial carcinoma.

| Case series/case report | Number of cases | M : F | Age (years) | Presentation | Type of specimen | Prognosis |
|---|---|---|---|---|---|---|
| Lopez et al. 2009 [3] | 8 | 3 : 1 | Mean age—67<br>Range (55-88) | Haematuria—8 (100%)<br>Frequency—2 (25%)<br>Dysuria—2 (25%) | Transurethral resection of bladder—3 (37.5%)<br>Cystoprostatectomy—3 (37.5%)<br>Cystectomy with hysterectomy—2 (25%) | Death within 17 months—5 (62.5%)<br>Metastasis at 11 and 19 months—2 (25%)<br>Disease free at 74 months—1 (12.5%) |
| Samaratunga et al. 2016 [4] | 13 (IHC and follow-up available in 10 cases) | 9 : 4 | Mean age—72<br>Range—53-92 | Haematuria—13 (100%)<br>Voiding dysfunction—7 (53.8%) | Cystoprostatectomy—2 (15.4%)<br>Transurethral resection specimens of bladder (TURBT) —11 (84.6%) | Death within 12 months—5 (50%)<br>Metastasis at 17 months—1 (10%)<br>Recurrent high grade tumour—3 (30%)<br>Disease free at 46 months following cystoprostatectomy—1 (10%) |
| Alexiev et al. 2013 [5] | 1 | Male | 77 | Renal transplant recipient—12 years post-transplant voided urine samples were positive for malignancy and decoy cells | Cystoprostatectomy | Distant metastasis at 4 months |
| Kimura et al. 2019 [11] | 1 | Male | 73 | Haematuria | Transurethral resection of bladder tumour followed by radical cystectomy and lymphadenectomy following two cycles of neoadjuvant chemotherapy with gemcitabine and cisplatin. | Disease free at 4 years |

TABLE 2: Pathological features of reported cases of giant cell urothelial carcinoma.

| Case series/case report | CIS/conventional urothelial CA/variants of UC | Proportion of giant cell UC | IHC | Stage at presentation |
|---|---|---|---|---|
| Lopez et al. 2009 [3] | Lymphoepithelioma like urothelial CA—1 (12.5%)<br>Micropapillary carcinoma—1 (12.5%) | 20-100%<br>100%—1 (12.5%) | CK8/18—8 (100%)<br>AE1/AE3—8 (100%)<br>EMA—8 (100%)<br>CK7—8 (100%) | pT3—6 (75%)<br>pT4—2 (25%)<br>Lymph node metastasis—6 (75%) |
| Samaratunga et al. 2016 [4] | CIS—5 (38.5%)<br>Conventional UC—8 (61.5%)<br>Micropapillary UC—3 (23.15)<br>Plasmacytoid UC—1 (7.7%)<br>None—3 (23.1%) | 40-100%<br>40%—3 (23.1%)<br>50%—3 (23.1%)<br>80%—3 (23.1%)<br>95%—1 (7.75)<br>100%—3 (23.1%) | CK8/18—10 (100%)<br>AE1/AE3—10 (100%)<br>CK7—9 (90%)<br>CK20—9 (90%)<br>P63—3 (30%)<br>Uroplakin—9 (90%)<br>GATA 3—9 (90%) | pT1—8 (61.5%)<br>pT2—3 (23.15%)<br>pT3—2 (15.4%) |
| Alexiev et al. 2013 [5] | Conventional high-grade urothelial carcinoma (20%)<br>Trophoblastic differentiation (10%). | 70% | Pleomorphic giant cells were positive for CK903, CK7 p63, p53, and p16.<br>HCG expression was present in scattered giant cells.<br>Tissue sections from the primary pleomorphic giant cell carcinoma and the omental metastasis were positive for SV40. | pT3bNxM1 (omental node metastasis were present) |
| Kimura et al. 2019 [11] | Conventional urothelial carcinoma | 70% | Not available | cT3bN2M0→ypT3aN0M0 |

sarcoma and direct extension from a pleomorphic giant cell carcinoma of the prostate. Coexisting carcinoma in situ and conventional urothelial carcinoma have been reported in the vast majority of cases [4] and were seen in this case. This helps to exclude a metastatic malignancy. It also raises the possibility that this is not a specific subtype of urothelial carcinoma but is instead a feature of extreme dedifferentiation. Small biopsies may not show areas of conventional urothelial carcinoma, carcinoma in situ, or variants of urothelial carcinoma making diagnosis difficult. In such cases, immunostaining, particularly with CK7, CK20, melanocytic markers, GATA3, and uroplakin III, needs to be performed.

The cells of the giant cell urothelial carcinoma component show positivity for CK 8/18 and AE1/AE3. Studies have also shown positivity for CK7, CK20, uroplakin III, and GATA3 in 90% of cases [4]. Some cases have shown positivity for p63 [4]. Uroplakin III has value as a marker for urothelial carcinoma. However, the use of this immunostain alone can be misleading, as carcinoma metastatic to the bladder can be positive. GATA3 is of greater utility [10]. When the differential diagnosis is giant cell urothelial carcinoma of the prostate, a panel including prostate-specific antigen, prostate-specific acid phosphatase, p63, and GATA3 would be diagnostic. Additionally, negativity for $\beta$HCG and CD68 helps to differentiate the giant cells from trophoblastic giant cells and osteoclast-type cells, respectively. Molecular characteristics of giant cell urothelial carcinoma are yet unknown [9].

This tumour has a very poor prognosis. Patients often have advanced stage cancer at presentation. Death within a short period, metastasis, or recurrent high-grade urothelial carcinoma has been reported in the majority. In the case series of 8 cases, reported by Lopez [3], all patients presented with ≥T3 disease. Six had lymph node metastases. Seven of the eight patients were either dead of disease or alive with metastases after fewer than two years' follow-up. In the case series reported by Samaratunga et al. [4], five of ten patients died within 12 months. One patient developed metastatic disease at 17 months following cystectomy, even though the initial staging on TURBT was pT1. Three other patients had recurrent high-grade urothelial carcinoma within three years. Only three of twenty-three patients reported in the literature were disease free for over three years. All three had pT3 disease and had undergone cystoprostatectomy, one following neoadjuvant chemotherapy [3, 4, 11].

This patient presented with T1 disease and was disease free at three-month follow-up. However, she had a stage T1, high-grade (Grade 3) tumour, and carcinoma in situ which places her in a high-risk category based on the European Association of Urology guidelines for the management of nonmuscle invasive bladder cancer. The probability of recurrence and progression at one year is 24% and 17%, respectively [12]. Based on the above guidelines, she would require follow-up with cystoscopy and cytology every three months for a period of two years, every six months thereafter until five years and then yearly. Annual upper tract imaging with computed tomography-intravenous urography (CT-IVU) or IVU is also recommended [12].

## References

[1] H. Moch, P. A. Humphrey, T. M. Ulbright, and V. Reuter, *WHO Classification of Tumours of the Urinary System and Male Genital Organs*, International Agency for Research on Cancer, Lyon, France, 2016.

[2] J. N. Eble and R. H. Young, "Carcinoma of the urinary bladder: a review of its diverse morphology," *Seminars in Diagnostic Pathology*, vol. 14, no. 2, pp. 98–108, 1997.

[3] A. Lopez-Beltran, A. Blanca, R. Montironi, L. Cheng, and J. C. Regueiro, "Pleomorphic giant cell carcinoma of the urinary bladder," *Human Pathology*, vol. 40, no. 10, pp. 1461–1466, 2009.

[4] H. Samaratunga, B. Delahunt, L. Egevad et al., "Pleomorphic giant cell carcinoma of the urinary bladder: an extreme form of tumour dedifferentiation," *Histopathology*, vol. 68, no. 4, pp. 533–540, 2016.

[5] B. A. Alexiev, J. C. Papadimitriou, T. C. Chai, E. Ramos, P. N. Staats, and C. B. Drachenberg, "Polyomavirus (BK)-associated pleomorphic giant cell carcinoma of the urinary bladder: a case report," *Pathology Research and Practice*, vol. 209, no. 4, pp. 255–259, 2013.

[6] J. H. Shanks, A. Chandra, L. McWilliam, and M. Varma, *Dataset for tumours of the urinary collecting system (renal pelvis, ureter, urinary bladder and urethra)*, The Royal College of Pathologists, London, United Kingodom, 2013.

[7] W. D. Travis, E. Brambilla, A. P. Burke, A. Marx, and A. G. Nicholson, *WHO Classification of Tumours of the Lung, Pleura, Thymus and Heart*, International Agency for Research on Cancer, Lyon, France, 2015.

[8] D. Baydar, M. B. Amin, and J. I. Epstein, "Osteoclast-rich undifferentiated carcinomas of the urinary tract," *Modern Pathology*, vol. 19, no. 2, pp. 161–171, 2006.

[9] A. Lopez-Beltran, V. Henriques, R. Montironi, A. Cimadamore, M. R. Raspollini, and L. Cheng, "Variants and new entities of bladder cancer," *Histopathology*, vol. 74, no. 1, pp. 77–96, 2019.

[10] K. Klopfer, B. Delahunt, M. Adamson, and H. Samaratunga, "The value of uroplakin III in distinguishing variants of primary bladder urothelial carcinoma from malignancy metastatic to the urinary bladder," *Anticancer Research*, vol. 34, no. 11, pp. 6779–6784, 2014.

[11] H. Kimura, Y. Uemura, Y. Megumi, M. Tachibana, and S. Fukuzawa, "A case Of cT3bN2M0 pleomorphic giant cell carcinoma of the bladder without recurrence after neoadjuvant chemotherapy and radical cystectomy for 4 Years," *Hinyokika Kiyo*, vol. 65, no. 9, pp. 377–380, 2019.

[12] M. Babjuk, M. Burger, E. M. Compérat et al., "European Association of Urology Guidelines on Non-muscle-invasive Bladder Cancer (TaT1 and Carcinoma In Situ) - 2019 Update," *European Urology*, vol. 76, no. 5, pp. 639–657, 2019.

# A Case of Localized Prostate Cancer Associated with Polymyalgia Rheumatica with Marked Symptomatic Improvement after Robot-Assisted Radical Prostatectomy

**Makoto Kawase,[1] Keita Nakane,[1] Sanae Namiki,[1] Yasumichi Takeuchi,[1] Shota Ueda,[1] Kota Kawase,[1] Chie Nakai,[1] Shinichi Takeuchi,[1] Daiki Kato,[1] Manabu Takai,[1] Koji Iinuma,[1] Masayuki Fuwa,[2] Chiemi Saigo,[3] Tatsuhiko Miyazaki,[3] Hiroyuki Morita,[2] and Takuya Koie[1]**

[1]*Department of Urology, Gifu University Graduate School of Medicine, Japan*
[2]*Department of General Internal Medicine, Gifu University Graduate School of Medicine, Japan*
[3]*Department of Pathology, Gifu University Graduate School of Medicine, Japan*

Correspondence should be addressed to Keita Nakane; keitaco@gifu-u.ac.jp

Academic Editor: Fumitaka Koga

A 73-year-old man visited our hospital with chief complaints of fever of unknown origin and bilateral shoulder and hip joint pain. He was initially diagnosed with polymyalgia rheumatica (PMR). Although the patient was treated with prednisolone 15 mg/day, his PMR-related symptoms did not improve. Further examination was performed as the patient was suspected of having paraneoplastic syndrome. Assessment results showed prostate cancer without metastases. After undergoing robot-assisted radical prostatectomy, the patient's PMR-related symptoms dramatically improved. Hence, the prednisolone dose was decreased to 4 mg/day. PCa may have triggered the development of PMR through the activation of immune-mediated systemic inflammatory responses.

## 1. Introduction

Paraneoplastic syndrome (PNS) is an extremely rare disorder that occurs in <1% of all cancer patients [1]. A paraneoplastic phenomenon usually develops due to the following reasons: (a) biologically active substances aberrantly produced by the underlying neoplasm; (b) modulation of the immune system via autoimmunity, immune complex production, and immunosuppression; and (c) unknown causes [2]. Polymyalgia rheumatica (PMR) is a relatively common inflammatory rheumatological disorder that is frequently associated with a certain type of cancer such as PNS [3]. Recently, three studies have reported the association between PMR and cancer [4–6]. However, it remains unclear whether a true association exists between PMR and malignant diseases, including prostate cancer (PCa), or whether it is a coincidental existence of the two conditions [3]. Thus far, only four prostate cancer patients with PMR who had multiple metastases received androgen deprivation therapy, and their PNS-related symptoms eventually improved without steroid treatment [7, 8]. In this case report, a PCa patient with PMR underwent surgical treatment and showed improvements in PMR-related symptoms.

## 2. Case Presentation

A 73-year-old Japanese man was referred to our hospital due to complaints of fever of unknown origin and bilateral shoulder and hip joint pain. His symptoms had gradually progressed, and he experienced loss of walking ability, general malaise, and lethargy. He was diagnosed with PMR according to the 2012 Provisional Classification Criteria for

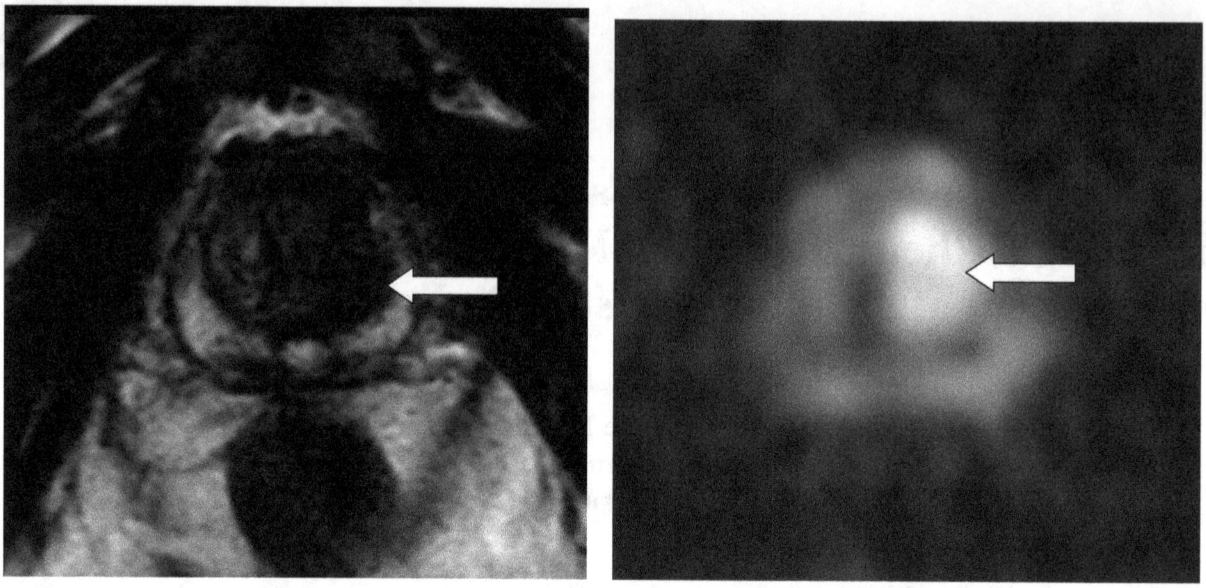

(a) (b)

FIGURE 1: (a) Magnetic resonance imaging showed a low-intensity area in the T2-weighted image (white arrow). (b) A high-intensity area in the diffusion-weighted image at the left transition zone (white arrow).

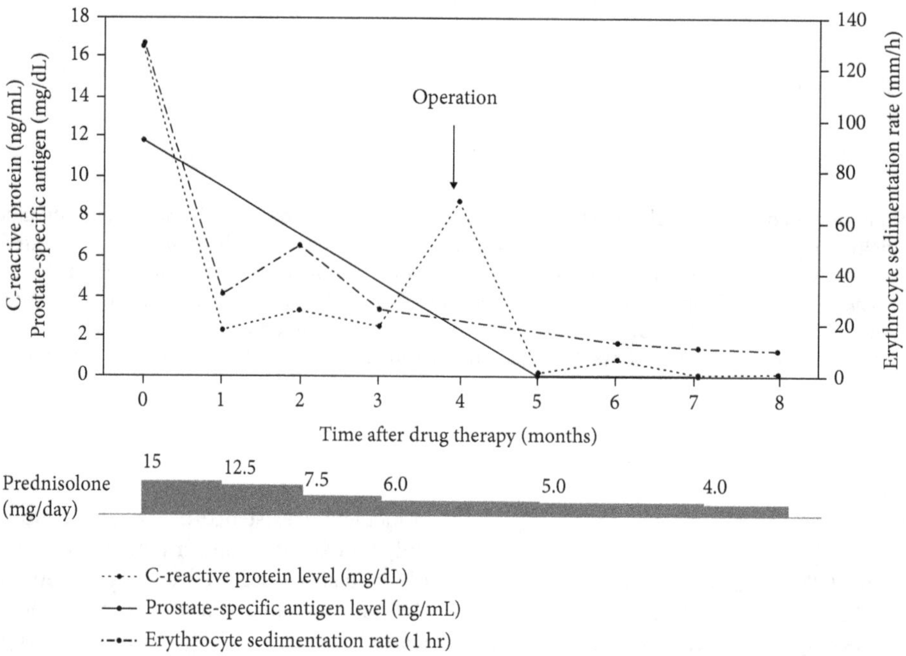


FIGURE 2: Clinical course and serum levels of an erythrocyte sedimentation rate, a C-reactive protein, and a prostate-specific antigen.

Polymyalgia Rheumatica [9]. He was treated with 15 mg/day prednisolone. Three months later, the patient's PMR-related symptoms did not improve. Thus, further examinations were performed as the patient was suspected of having PNS. He had a hemoglobin level of 8.0 g/dL (normal range: 13.7–16.8 g/dL), a leukocyte count of 16,140/$\mu$L (normal range: 3,300–8,600/$\mu$L), an erythrocyte sedimentation rate of 130 (1 h), and a C-reactive protein level of 16.54 mg/dL (normal level: <0.14 mg/dL). His renal, liver, and thyroid test results were normal. The serum prostate-specific antigen level increased to 11.852 ng/mL (normal level: <4.0 ng/dL). Magnetic resonance imaging revealed a low-intensity area in the T2-weighted image and a high-intensity area in the diffusion-weighted image at the left transition zone (Figures 1(a) and 1(b)). The patient was diagnosed with adenocarcinoma of the prostate with a Gleason score of 3 + 4 based on the results of the pathological examination of prostate biopsy specimens. Bone scintigraphy and chest and abdominal computed tomography showed absence of distant metastases and lymph node involvement. Hence, the patient was clinically diagnosed with localized PCa according to the staging system defined in the American

Joint Committee on Cancer Staging Manual [10]. Robot-assisted radical prostatectomy was performed. Histopathological findings showed presence of adenocarcinoma of the prostate with T2c stage, a Gleason score of 3 + 4, and a negative surgical margin. There were no neuroendocrine carcinoma components in the specimen. Four months after surgery, the patient's PMR-related symptoms dramatically improved, and he was able to walk without pain. The steroid dose was decreased to 4 mg/day (Figure 2).

## 3. Discussion

The association between cancer and PMR has been established in the following patients: first, patients with a rheumatic disorder, which is directly triggered by a tumor or its metastasis; second, patients with an established rheumatic condition who are at increased risk of specific malignancies; and third, patients with PNS [11]. Currently, PNS is recognized to be caused by antibody production [12] and aberrant hormone release or abnormal cytokine release due to the production of vascular endothelial growth factors [13]. PNS-related symptoms have an impact on several body systems, including the hematological, cutaneous, vascular, and neurological systems [14]. Although the exact cause of PNS in PCa remains unknown, most hypotheses suggest that inappropriate release of peptide hormones, biologic amines, or growth factors is the primary cause [15]. PNS caused by antibody production, aberrant hormone release, or abnormal cytokine is more frequently diagnosed in patients with prostate cancer, which contains small-cell carcinoma components than those of adenocarcinoma [15]. Nguyan et al. reported that interleukin-6 (IL-6) is a key mediator in several stages of the PCa pathogenesis, including initiation of prostate tumorigenesis, stimulation of tumor growth, induction of aggressive PCa phenotype, PCa progression to the castration-resistant state, promotion of tumor metastasis, and resistance to chemotherapy [16]. Although IL-6 may have an important role in the progression of PMR to PNS in patients with PCa, limited evidence suggests that PCa is commonly diagnosed with incident PMR [4].

According to a previous large cohort study, which enrolled 35,918 patients with PMR and giant cell arteritis (GCA) from Sweden using the Swedish Hospital Discharge Register, 3,941 patients (11.0%) were diagnosed with cancer [4]. Of these patients, 19.1% developed cancer within the first year after the diagnoses of PMR and GCA [4]. Moreover, PMR and GCA patients were frequently diagnosed with skin cancer and acute myeloid leukemia [4]. In 2013, using the General Practice Research Database, Muller et al. reported that older patients with PMR were more likely to be diagnosed with cancer within 6 months after the diagnosis of PMR [5]. Although these patients were treated with at least two different corticosteroid agents, data regarding patients' response to treatment were not available [5]. In a previous systematic review and meta-analysis including six studies, the pooled risk ratio of malignancy in patients with PMR and GCA compared with control patients was 1.14 (95% confidence interval: 1.05–1.22) [6]. The risk of malignancy appeared to be higher in the first 6–12 months after diagnosis [6]. However, the pooled risk ratio decreased to 8% and was not significant [6].

In this case, PCa may have triggered the development of PMR through the activation of immune-mediated systemic inflammatory responses caused by antibody production, aberrant hormone release, or abnormal cytokine. To our knowledge, this is the first case report to describe a PCa patient with PMR who underwent surgical treatment and showed improvements in PMR-related symptoms.

## References


[1] F. Graus, J. Y. Delattre, J. C. Antoine et al., "Recommended diagnostic criteria for paraneoplastic neurological syndromes," *Journal of Neurology, Neurosurgery, and Psychiatry*, vol. 75, no. 8, pp. 1135–1140, 2004.

[2] E. Sacco, F. Pinto, F. Sasso et al., "Paraneoplastic syndromes in patients with urological malignancies," *Urologia Internationalis*, vol. 83, no. 1, pp. 1–11, 2009.

[3] S. Muller, S. Hider, T. Helliwell, R. Partington, and C. Mallen, "The real evidence for polymyalgia rheumatica as a paraneoplastic syndrome," *Reumatismo*, vol. 70, no. 1, pp. 23–34, 2018.

[4] J. Ji, X. Liu, K. Sundquist, J. Sundquist, and K. Hemminki, "Cancer risk in patients hospitalized with polymyalgia rheumatica and giant cell arteritis: a follow-up study in Sweden," *Rheumatology (Oxford)*, vol. 49, no. 6, pp. 1158–1163, 2010.

[5] S. Muller, S. L. Hider, J. Belcher, T. Helliwell, and C. D. Mallen, "Is cancer associated with polymyalgia rheumatica? A cohort study in the general practice research database," *Annals of the Rheumatic Diseases*, vol. 73, no. 10, pp. 1769–1773, 2014.

[6] P. Ungprasert, P. Charoenpong, P. Ratanasrimetha, C. Thongprayoon, W. Cheungpasitporn, and P. Suksaranjit, "Risk of coronary artery disease in patients with systemic sclerosis: a systematic review and meta-analysis," *Clinical Rheumatology*, vol. 33, no. 8, pp. 1099–1104, 2014.

[7] I. Kane and S. Menon, "Carcinoma of the prostate presenting as polymyalgia rheumatica," *Rheumatology (Oxford) Carcinoma of the prostate presenting as polymyalgia rheumatica.*, vol. 42, no. 2, pp. 385–387, 2003.

[8] A. Emamifar, S. Hess, R. Gildberg-Mortensen, and I. M. Jensen Hansen, "Association of remitting seronegative symmetrical synovitis with pitting edema, polymyalgia rheumatica, and adenocarcinoma of the prostate," *Am J Case Rep*, vol. 17, pp. 60–64, 2016.

[9] B. Dasgupta, M. A. Cimmino, H. M. Kremers et al., "2012 provisional classification criteria for polymyalgia rheumatica: a European League Against Rheumatism/American College of Rheumatology collaborative initiative," *Arthritis and Rheumatism*, vol. 64, no. 4, pp. 943–954, 2012.

[10] M. K. Buyyounouski, P. L. Choyke, J. K. McKenney et al., "Prostate cancer - major changes in the American Joint Committee on Cancer eighth edition cancer staging manual," *CA: a Cancer Journal for Clinicians*, vol. 67, no. 3, pp. 245–253, 2017.

[11] V. Racanelli, M. Prete, C. Minoia, E. Favoino, and F. Perosa, "Rheumatic disorders as paraneoplastic syndromes," *Autoimmunity Reviews*, vol. 7, no. 5, pp. 352–358, 2008.

[12] E. Lancaster, "Paraneoplastic disorders," *Lifelong learning in neurology*, vol. 21, no. 2, pp. 452–475, 2015.

[13] H. Li, R. D. Altman, and Q. Yao, "RS3PE: clinical and research development," *Current Rheumatology Reports*, vol. 17, no. 8, p. 49, 2015.

[14] V. Durieux, M. Coureau, A. P. Meert, T. Berghmans, and J. P. Sculier, "Autoimmune paraneoplastic syndromes associated to lung cancer: a systematic review of the literature," *Lung Cancer*, vol. 106, pp. 102–109, 2017.

[15] J. K. Choi, W. J. Kim, and J. Y. Jeon, "Paraneoplastic sensorimotor polyneuropathy in prostatic adenocarcinoma: a case report," *Medicine (Baltimore)*, vol. 97, no. 15, article e0030, 2018.

[16] D. P. Nguyen, J. Li, and A. K. Tewari, "Inflammation and prostate cancer: the role of interleukin 6 (IL-6)," *BJU International*, vol. 113, no. 6, pp. 986–992, 2014.

# 30

# Ureteroarterial Fistula: A Diagnosis Which is not Always Black and White

**A. Haffar ,[1] T. Trump ,[2] A. A. Elbakry ,[2] K. McCluskey ,[3] M. W. Salkini ,[2] and A. Luchey [2]**

[1]*West Virginia University School of Medicine, West Virginia, USA*
[2]*Department of Urology, West Virginia University, West Virginia, USA*
[3]*Department of Interventional Radiology, West Virginia University, West Virginia, USA*

Correspondence should be addressed to A. Haffar; aihaffar@mix.wvu.edu

Academic Editor: Walid Farhat

Ureteroiliac artery fistulas are a rare, life-threatening condition that requires a high index of suspicion for prompt diagnosis. Presurgical diagnosis is challenging as this condition can lie hidden despite advanced imaging modalities. We present two cases of patients presenting with gross hematuria and exsanguination in the setting of a ureteroiliac artery fistula. These cases highlight the difficulties in timely diagnosis and treatment in a multidisciplinary team.

## 1. Introduction

A ureteroiliac artery fistula (UIAF) is a rare, life-threatening condition that can present suddenly with gross hematuria. Diagnosis is often delayed due to its insidious nature. The incidence of this condition has increased, secondary to risk factors such as pelvic radiotherapy, genitourinary surgery, chronic ureteral stenting, and peripheral arterial disease [1]. Despite its rarity, the diagnosis should be highly suspected when assessing patients with such risk factors due to the associated morbidity and mortality. We hereby present two cases of patients presenting with gross hematuria and exsanguination in the setting of a ureteroiliac artery fistula.

## 2. Case Presentation

*2.1. Case 1.* A 55-year-old female with a previous history of pelvic radiation and exenteration for cervical cancer presented with lower abdominal pain and gross hematuria from bilateral nephrostomy tubes and ileal conduit. She had a history of bilateral hydroureteronephrosis managed with chronic percutaneous nephroureteral stents. Of pertinence, she had a history of complicated UTIs, and her right nephroureteral stent was exchanged 2 weeks prior to presentation without complications.

On examination, the patient's abdominal pain was localized to the lower abdomen without radiation. She was noted to be afebrile with a heart rate of 97, respiratory rate of 18, and blood pressure of 129/83 mmHg. Hematuria from both nephrostomy tubes and ileal conduit was noted.

Initial workup was significant for anion gap metabolic acidosis with a pH of 7.10, $pCO_2$ of 19 mmHg, and a bicarbonate of 7.2 mEq/L. The patient was anemic with a hemoglobin of 8.1 g/dL. Blood urea nitrogen was found to be 37 mg/dL with a creatinine of 4.38 mg/dL, from a baseline creatinine of 3 mg/dL. The patient was initially managed empirically for a presumed urinary tract infection with intravenous piperacillin/tazobactam. CT imaging from an outside facility was unavailable but reportedly demonstrated an appropriate position of the bilateral nephroureteral stents. Ultrasound indicated bilateral hydronephrosis. Exchange of bilateral nephroureteral stents was scheduled for the following day. Later that evening, her hematuria had progressively worsened, with serial hemoglobin values dropping to 4.2 mg/dL, with associated hemodynamic instability. She was successfully resuscitated and stabilized with 4 units of blood, 1 unit of platelets, 1 unit of FFP, and 1 liter bolus of intravenous fluids. Upon repeat examination, frank hemorrhage was discovered at her left nephroureteral stent and the right nephroureteral stent demonstrated blood mixed with urine; despite this, the patient was asymptomatic. The CT abdomen and pelvis without contrast was performed and was negative. She was then taken for bilateral exchange of nephroureteral stents by interventional radiology. The left stent was removed first, and a significant amount of blood was noted along the stent tract, with an unknown source of the bleeding. Antegrade nephrostogram was performed, and a large fistula between the left ureter and the left common iliac artery was noted (Figure 1). In an attempt to control and tamponade the bleeding, a nephroureteral stent was placed. A rapid decision was made to perform a pelvic angiogram with stenting of the left common iliac artery. An 8 mm × 39 mm VBX covered stent was advanced and deployed in the midcommon iliac artery, with a follow-up angiogram showing no evidence of pseudoaneurysm, active bleeding, or fistula (Figure 2). The patient progressively improved postop with resolution of her acute kidney injury and was discharged 7 days postadmission. As of 6 months postoperatively from this procedure, the patient has been without further complications regarding the fistula. She continues to have regular exchange of her nephroureteral stents and has been without further hematuria.

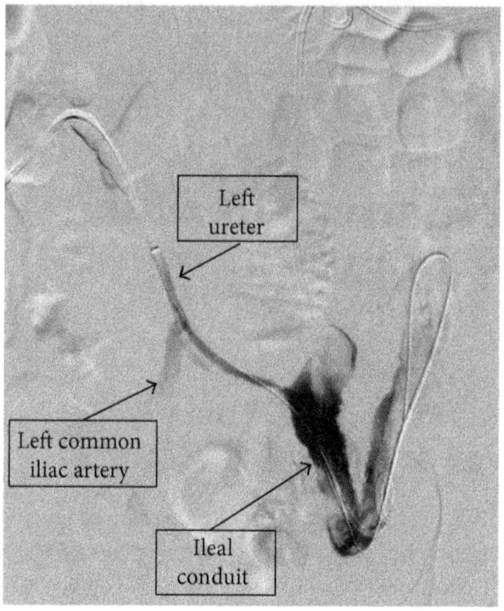


Figure 1: Left nephrostogram with contrast noted extravasating through the fistula tract from the left ureter into the left iliac artery.

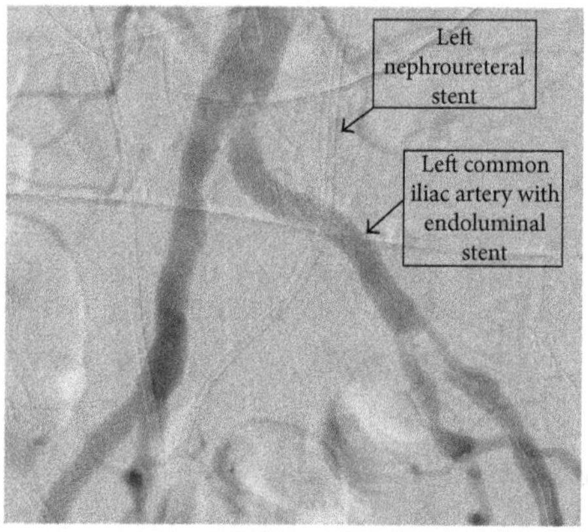


Figure 2: Arteriogram following endograft placement with no contrast exiting the arterial system. Left nephroureteral stent is noted traversing the location of graft placement highlighting the region of fistula formation.

*2.2. Case 2.* A 73-year-old female presented with shortness of breath, dizziness, and gross hematuria. She had a past medical history of cervical cancer requiring radiation and chemotherapy, chronic kidney disease stage IIIB, and chronic normocytic anemia. The patient has a history of left ureteral stricture with severe hydronephrosis managed with a chronic indwelling metal ureteral stent with regular exchanges for four years. She was initially planned to have a left nephrectomy 1 month prior to her presentation, but it was postponed due to a hemoglobin of 4 g/dl, requiring hospitalization at an outside facility. She reported that her stent was most recently exchanged 5 months prior to her presentation.

On examination, the patient was hemodynamically stable. Frank blood was found in her Foley bag without suprapubic tenderness. Of note, she had hemoglobin of 3.8 g/dL and her creatinine was 1.51 mg/dL. CT imaging with contrast was unable to demonstrate an active source of bleeding but did show severe left hydronephrosis and hydroureter as well as a segmental pulmonary embolus. Subsequent lower extremity Doppler imaging revealed multiple deep venous thrombi. She was initially managed with blood transfusions and continuous bladder irrigation. Interventional radiology was consulted for the placement of an IVC filter in the setting of pulmonary embolus with active bleeding prohibiting the start of anticoagulation. Arteriogram was done during the placement of the IVC filter but failed to demonstrate any evidence of ureterovascular fistula.

Two days later, after continued gross hematuria and sustained anemia, the patient was taken to the OR for cystourethroscopy with left retrograde pyelogram and left ureteral stent exchange. Cystoscopy did not reveal any obvious masses or lesions, but active bleeding was noted from the left ureteral orifice after removal of the ureteral stent. Subsequent left retrograde pyelogram did not reveal any obvious source for continued hematuria; in particular, this was negative for any obvious fistula involving the ureter. The left ureter was markedly dilated, and there were multiple large filling defects, likely clots from the upper tract bleed. A left 6 French × 24 cm Double-J silicone stent was placed under direct visualization. The decision was made to perform left renal artery arteriogram and left lumbar and pelvic angiography which again showed no renal vascular abnormalities or arterioureteral fistula. A decision was then made to embolize the left renal artery. Despite embolization, the patient still had continuous hematuria requiring CBI. Due to continued suspicion for ureteroiliac fistula, a decision was made to proceed with definitive management and perform robotic nephroureterectomy with excision of the ureteroiliac fistula.

The patient was taken to the operating room and positioned in a modified right lateral decubitus position. The procedure proceeded accordingly, and nephrectomy

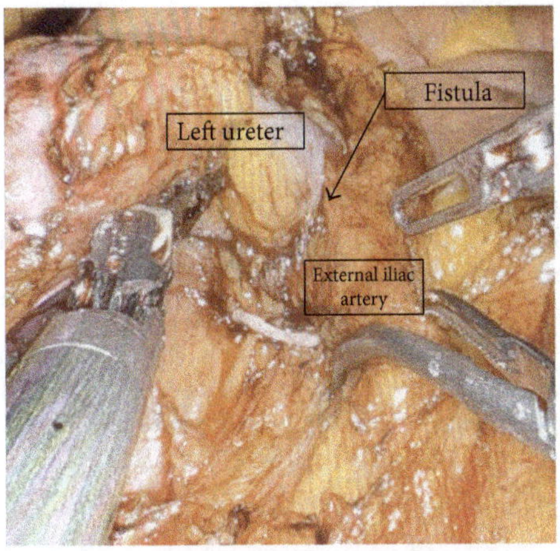


FIGURE 3: Left ureter raised with left bipolar forceps and small Hem-o-lok clip controlling the divided smaller vascular connection with a laparoscopic Satinsky clamp placed on the left external iliac artery proximal to the ureteroiliac fistula.

was completed uneventfully. At the stage of dissecting the ureter, it began to pulsate, indicating a possible ureteroiliac fistula. A small vessel directly communicating with the ureter and the left external iliac artery was identified and clipped with a Hem-o-lok and divided with good hemostasis (Figure 3). A much larger vessel was then identified inferiorly. An additional assistant port was placed, and a laparoscopic Satinsky clamp was used to clamp the external iliac artery. An attempt was made to dissect and divide the vascular connection with the ureter, but brisk bleeding was encountered. This proved to be very difficult to control robotically, and the decision was made to convert to open repair using a modified Gibson incision. Heavy bleeding was encountered, and the left common iliac artery was subsequently clamped which controlled active bleeding temporarily. The ureter was separated from the external iliac artery at the level of the fistula leaving a large defect of the fistula in the wall of the external iliac artery. Following temporization of the bleeding, vascular surgery was consulted, and they were able to suture the arteriotomy. With hemostasis maintained, the dissection of the distal left ureter was continued and clipped at the ureterovesical junction. A total of 8 units of packed red blood cells and 2 units of FFP were given with an estimated blood loss of 2500 mL.

Later that day, the patient was discovered to have faint left popliteal arterial pulse by Doppler with no pulse distally. The patient was taken back to the OR with vascular surgery for angiogram of the left lower extremity due to acute limb ischemia. Acute thrombosis was identified, and thrombectomy of the left common iliac artery and external iliac artery was performed, along with balloon angioplasty of the left common iliac artery and external iliac artery. A four-compartment fasciotomy was subsequently performed. During the course of her hospitalization, a total of 19 units of packed red blood cells, 4 units of FFP, and 2 units of cryoprecipitate were given. The patient progressively improved with resolution of her hematuria and was discharged to an inpatient rehabilitation facility. As of 4 months postoperatively, the patient has been without any adverse events. She had her IVC filter removed and was started on therapeutic anticoagulation without development of hematuria.

## 3. Discussion

A ureteroiliac artery fistula in the setting of ileal conduit is an exceedingly rare condition. They often occur in the setting of prior genitourinary surgery, chronic ureteral stenting, radiation therapy, and prior vascular pathology [2]. Additionally, pelvic lymphadenectomy has been proposed to render the vasculature more susceptible to fistula formation [3]. Despite the possibly lethal nature of this condition, the presenting symptoms are often innocuous. Although hematuria is the most common presenting symptom, and flank pain, urinary retention, and infection have also been described [4]. Ultimately, in a patient with a complicated genitourinary tract surgery/history presenting with hematuria and other equivocal symptoms, the physician's index of suspicion for UIAF should be heightened. Early involvement of vascular surgery/interventional radiology in the management is of paramount importance.

The principal difficulty in treating UIAF is diagnosing the condition in a timely manner, as no imaging modality is sensitive enough. CT, commonly done emergently in response to gross hematuria, has very low sensitivity and is rarely diagnostic [5]. Ureteroscopy can be performed and demonstrate pulsatile blood flow; however, in the setting of brisk bleeding, visualization could be difficult [5]. Angiography has even less sensitivity, as low as 23%-41% [6]. However, angiography with concurrent manipulation of a chronic nephroureteral stent was shown to improve sensitivity to 100% at one institution [6]. The sensitivity of provocative retrograde pyelogram was shown to be as low as 63%, which was demonstrated by our second case [7]. Ultimately, no single test will be perfectly diagnostic and will likely need to be reperformed.

Prior to advancements in endovascular techniques, open surgical repair was the predominant manner in which UIAF was treated and was considered the gold standard [8, 9]. However, this was often challenging as these patients have a complex history of genitourinary surgery, radiation treatment, and vascular pathology [10]. Furthermore, these patients were often not great surgical candidates due to their multiple comorbidities [10]. Despite this, open surgery is advantageous in its ability to treat UIAFs in scenarios with a high index of suspicion despite multiple nondiagnostic imaging tests, as proven in our second case [11]. In the current era, endovascular treatment is the preferred choice of intervention due to its minimally invasive nature, as well as its ability to maintain distal perfusion to the pelvis and lower extremities, and has shown to be successful in managing bleeding [2, 11]. Endovascular treatment typically consists of stent grafting with embolization. An early complication rate from endovascular treatment at a single institution was reported at 27%, consisting of graft infection, lower limb ischemia, stent graft thrombosis, and non-ST elevation myocardial infarction [4]. The most serious of which is graft infection, and some even consider infection or an unsterile environment to be a contraindication to endovascular treatment [5]. Unfortunately, due to the rarity and morbidity associated with this condition, the overall efficacy and complication rate are poorly studied. Long-term complications of both treatment modalities include lower extremity ischemia, renal loss, and recurrent hemorrhage [12]. The most common is lower limb ischemia with a prevalence of 67% with open repair vs. 50% from endovascular stenting [12]. Several studies have attempted to compare the outcome and complications between UIAF treatments with no clear advantage [9, 12]. We believe that these cases not only highlight the difficulty with managing this condition but also support endovascular management as the optimal management when feasible. Case 1 highlights successful endovascular management with minimal associated morbidity. Case 2 highlights some of the associated morbidity with an open surgical repair including both lower limb ischemia and increased blood loss. That being said, both approaches ultimately proved successful in the management of a life-threatening condition. Ultimately, it is apparent that treatment of a UIAF requires a multidisciplinary team of urologists, radiologists, and vascular surgeons.

## References

[1] H. Ishibashi, T. Ohta, I. Sugimoto et al., "Successful treatment of an aorto-ileal-conduit fistula with an endovascular stent graft: report of a case," *Surgery Today*, vol. 37, no. 4, pp. 305–307, 2007.

[2] A. Sukha and N. Smyth, "Fistula formation between the external iliac artery and ileal conduit following a radical cystoprostatectomy: a rare complication with prewarning signs of haemorrhage," *Case Reports*, vol. 2015, no. mar27 1, p. bcr2014208914, 2015.

[3] J. M. Beaugie, "Fistula between external iliac artery and ileal conduct," *British Journal of Urology*, vol. 43, no. 4, pp. 450–452, 1971.

[4] L. M. Hirsch, M. J. Amirian, S. G. Hubosky, A. K. Das, B. Abai, and C. D. Lallas, "Urologic and endovascular repair of a uretero-iliac artery fistula," *The Canadian Journal of Urology*, vol. 22, no. 1, pp. 7661–7665, 2015.

[5] S. Kurata, S. Tobu, K. Udo, and M. Noguchi, "Iliac artery-uretero-colonic fistula presenting as gastrointestinal hemorrhage and hematuria: a case report," *Journal of endourology case reports*, vol. 4, no. 1, pp. 1–4, 2018.

[6] G. Sarwal, S. Bidnur, E. C. Chedgy, and A. Kavanagh, "Case – Uretero-internal iliac artery fistula presenting with multiple negative angiographic studies," *Canadian Urological Association Journal*, vol. 12, no. 5, pp. E250–E252, 2018.

[7] L. Rittenberg, M. Nordsiek, D. Cahn, K. Zhang, N. Taylor, and P. Ginsberg, "Diagnosis and management of a challenging patient: ureteroarterial fistula," *Urology*, vol. 97, pp. e9–e10, 2016.

[8] L. Meecham, V. Koo, and P. H. Rajjayabun, "Uretero-iliac artery aneurysm fistula: a rare but fatal cause of haematuria," *Journal of surgical case reports*, vol. 2012, no. 8, pp. 16–16, 2012.

[9] G. Sachsamanis, K. Pfister, P. M. Kasprzak, W. Schierling, S. Denzinger, and K. Oikonomou, "Midterm Results after Open Surgical and Endovascular Management of Arterioureteral Fistula," *Annals of Vascular Surgery.*, vol. 73, pp. 280–289, 2021.

[10] T. Sasaki, T. Onishi, and A. Hoshina, "Fistula between the external iliac artery and the body of an ileal conduit," *International Journal of Urology*, vol. 18, no. 3, pp. 260-261, 2011.

[11] A. Crane, A. Rizzo, M. Gong, and S. Sivalingam, "Ureteroarterial fistula in a patient with an ileal conduit and chronic nephroureteral catheter," *Journal of Endourology Case Reports*, vol. 5, no. 2, pp. 64–67, 2019.

[12] J. A. Fox, A. Krambeck, E. F. McPhail, and D. Lightner, "Ureteroarterial fistula treatment with open surgery versus endovascular management: long-term outcomes," *The Journal of Urology*, vol. 185, no. 3, pp. 945–950, 2011.

# 31

# Conservative Management of the Duodenal Injury during Percutaneous Nephrostomy Placement: A Few and Far between Complications of the Urological Literature

**Aykut Colakerol,[1] Mustafa Zafer Temiz,[1] Mubarek Bargicho Adem,[2] Kamil Ozdogan,[3] Fatih Celebi,[3] Engin Kandirali,[1] and Ahmet Yaser Muslumanoglu[1]**

[1]*Department of Urology, Bagcilar Training and Research Hospital, Istanbul, Turkey*
[2]*Department of General Surgery, Urology Unit, St. Paul's Hospital Millennium Medical College, Addis Ababa, Ethiopia*
[3]*Department of General Surgery, Bagcilar Training and Research Hospital, Istanbul, Turkey*

Correspondence should be addressed to Mubarek Bargicho Adem; m.bargcho@yahoo.com

Academic Editor: David Duchene

Herein, we reported a duodenal perforation case as an intestinal injury during a percutaneous nephrostomy procedure. A 73-year-old woman with bilateral nephrostomy catheters was applied to the emergency service with right flank pain. Early in the day, her bilateral nephrostomy catheters had been changed. On physical examination, she had a defense and rebound at her right quadrant, and costovertebral angle tenderness was also positive. In the contrast-enhanced abdominal computed tomography scan, the right nephrostomy catheter was located in the second part of the duodenum, and the contrast agent did not leak into the peritoneum from the injury area. We decided on conservative management of the case with active surveillance using daily blood tests and physical examinations. The nephrostomy catheter in the duodenum was left to prevent fistula between the duodenum and the skin, and a new one was placed in the right kidney. The broad spectrum antibiotherapy regime was applied, and the patient was followed up closely. The catheter in the duodenum was removed on the 20th day, uneventfully, and the patient was discharged successfully on the 24th day with her permanent bilateral nephrostomy tubes. On the first follow-up, one month later, the patient had no active medical complaint.

## 1. Introduction

Percutaneous nephrostomy (PCN) is an interventional method of accessing the renal collecting system through the skin. It is a commonly used treatment approach in patients with urinary obstruction, especially when ureteral stent replacement is not possible [1, 2]. During the procedure, some major and minor complications can occur [1, 2]. Sepsis and massive bleeding are the most common major complications associated with PCN [2]. Intestinal complications are commonly associated with percutaneous nephrolithotomy, and to our knowledge, there is only one case with an intestinal complication in the form of duodenal perforation during PCN procedure without renal stone fragmentation [3]. Herein, after obtaining written informed patient consent, we report the second case of duodenal perforation as an intestinal injury during PCN.

## 2. Case Report

A 73-year-old woman with bilateral nephrostomy catheters was applied to the emergency service with right flank pain that started 10 hours prior after bilateral nephrostomy catheter replacement. She had a history of chronic kidney failure. She had been followed up with bilateral nephrostomy catheters for four years due to the bilateral ureteral stricture secondary to stone disease. Early in the day, her bilateral nephrostomy catheters had been changed under guiding assistance from ultrasound imaging. New nephrostomy placement was performed using the current tube tract instead of fresh stick/new site of nephrostomy tube placement. During the procedure, no signs of complication and unexpected events were recorded, and a day case hospitalization was provided for routine postprocedural monitoring. A few hours later, during physical examination, she had a defense and rebound at her right quadrant, and costovertebral angle tenderness was also positive. Body temperature and blood pressure were 36.7°C and 130/70 mmHg. Serum creatinine, hemoglobin, and C-reactive protein (CRP) levels were 2.43 mg/dL, 11.6 g/dL, and 90 mg/L, respectively. White blood cell count (WBC) was $14.9 \times 10^3$u/L. In the right nephrostomy bag, there was 800 cc fluid compatible with bilious fluid and small intestinal content. Subsequently, the patient underwent noncontrast-enhanced abdominal computed tomography (CT) scan to confirm the nephrostomy catheter placements. CT scan showed that the right nephrostomy catheter was located in the second part of the duodenum by piercing the right kidney. The patient's oral intake had been stopped, intravenous hydration and 2 × 1000 mg meropenem (Meronem, AstraZeneca BioPharma. Co., Macclesfield, UK) therapies had been started, and she consulted to the general surgery department which suggested oral and intravenous abdominal contrast-enhanced CT (CECT) imaging. In the CECT scan, the contrast agent did not leak into the peritoneum from the duodenal injury area (Figure 1). We decided on conservative management of the case with active surveillance using daily blood tests and physical examinations. The nephrostomy catheter was left in the duodenum to prevent fistula formulation between the duodenum and the skin, and a new one was placed in the right kidney.

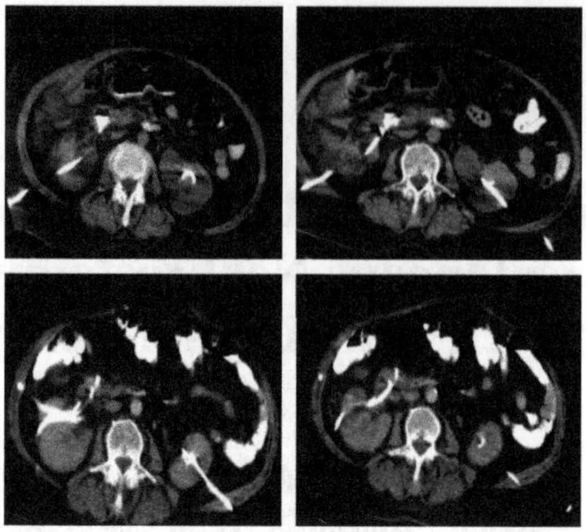

Figure 1: Oral and intravenous contrast-enhanced abdominal CT images. The right nephrostomy tube was located in the second part of the duodenum, and there was no leakage of contrast substance to the retroperitoneal site.

On the second day, a nasogastric tube was inserted and parenteral nutrition was started. The patient was stable, the creatinine level was increased to 2.7 mg/dL, WBC count was increased to $17.27 \times 10^3$ u/L, and CRP level was increased to 184 mg/L. The antibiotherapy regime was rearranged as intravenous injections of 3 × 1000 mg meropenem (Meronem, AstraZeneca BioPharma. Co., Macclesfield, UK), 2 × 1000 mg vancomycin (Vancomycin HCL DBL, Orna Pharma. Co., Istanbul, Turkey), and 3 × 500 mg metronidazole (Flagyl, Sanofi Pharma. Co., Kırklareli, Turkey) per day. Intravenous 1 × 40 mg proton pump inhibitor, pantoprazole (Pantpas, Takeda GmbH, Dingen, Germany), was also administrated daily. Daily outputs from catheters were about 1500 cc and 500 cc for nephrostomy tubes in the renal pelvis and in the duodenum, respectively. All blood parameters showed a gradual decrease during the conservative management. As mentioned above, the duodenal nephrostomy tube was not removed to prevent a new fistula tract formation between the duodenum and the skin during the three weeks. On the 20th day, the duodenal nephrostomy tube drainage was 50 cc. On the same day, the tube was retracted from the duodenal lumen to the retroperitoneal area near by the duodenal wall injury under direct endoscopic visualization in an attempt to avoid the potential retroperitoneal injury from possible leakage (Figure 2(a)). During the three-day follow-up of the retracted tube, no drainage was recorded and the tube was removed. During removal of the duodenal nephrostomy tube, oral contrast was given, and no signs of leakage to the retroperitoneal area were detected on fluoroscopy (Figure 2(b)). The period after the removal of the duodenal nephrostomy tube was uneventful. The serum CRP level exhibited gradual decrease and, finally, decreased to her basal value. Follow-up blood test results during the conservative management of the case are as shown in Table 1. The relatively higher basal CRP value was attributed to her chronic kidney disease because of no other additional signs of acute infection or severe disease. The patient was discharged successfully on the 24th day with her permanent bilateral nephrostomy tubes. On the first follow-up, one month later, the patient had no active medical complaint.

## 3. Discussion

The PCN procedure was firstly described by Goodwin et al. [4] in 1955, and then, it has become one of the most common urological procedures in clinical practice [2]. Because of the image-guided nature of the PCN procedure, commonly, it is smooth sailing. Safety and effectiveness of the procedure has been proven in the literature [5]. Technical success of the PCN is described as 93–99% [6]. Nevertheless, it is not a procedure that is free of complications. The general complication rate of PCN is approximately 10% [6]. Major complications such as septic shock and massive hemorrhage associated with PCN procedures are seen in about 4.5% of the cases [2]. Minor complications including catheter blockage, leaking, fracturing, and kinking of the catheter occur in 6.1% of the cases [2]. Rarely seen complications of the procedure are intestinal, pleural, and renal pelvic injuries with incidences of about 0.1-1% [3, 6].

Percutaneous renal procedures associated with damage to the gastrointestinal tract are extremely rare and most often seen in the colon. Only five cases of duodenal damage

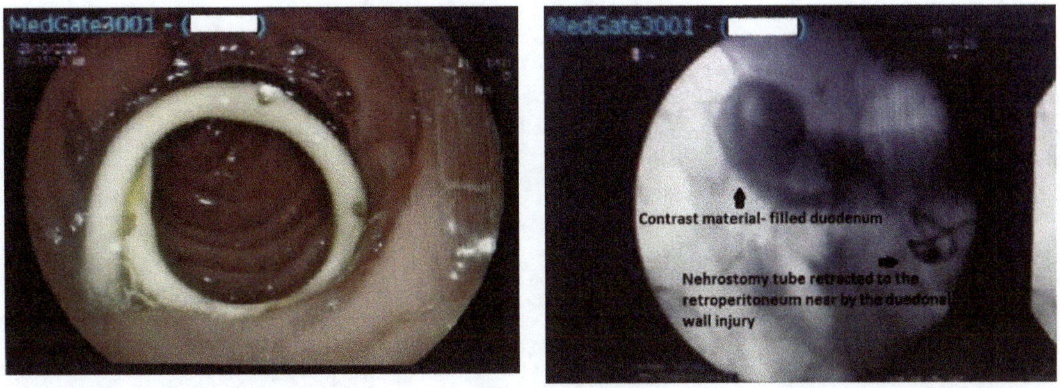


(a) (b)

FIGURE 2: (a) Nephrostomy catheter located in the part of duodenum. (b) During removal of the nephrostomy tube, oral contrast was given, and there was no sign of leakage to the retroperitoneal area.

TABLE 1: Serum CRP and creatinine levels and WBC count of the patient during the hospitalization. (On the third day, a second nephrostomy tube was replaced, and after 24 days of follow-up with a broad spectrum of antibiotics, the patient was discharged.)

| | Serum CRP levels (mg/L) | Serum creatinine levels (mg/dL) | WBC ($\times 10^3$ u/L) |
|---|---|---|---|
| Basal value (before the bilateral nephrostomy catheter replacement and duodenal injury) | 48 | 1.8 | — |
| Day 1 | 90 | 2.43 | 14.9 |
| Day 2 | 184 | 2.73 | 17.2 |
| Day 3 | 300 | 2.76 | 10.0 |
| Day 4 | 211 | 2.66 | 6.6 |
| Day 5 | 107 | 2.25 | 6.6 |
| Day 7 | 91 | 1.94 | 6.5 |
| Day 24 (discharged) | 47 | 1.8 | 5.1 |

CRP: C-reactive protein; WBC: white blood cell count.

associated with percutaneous procedures have been reported so far [7]. Moreover, all of them were specifically associated with percutaneous nephrolithotomy (PCNL), but one. To our knowledge, there is just one duodenal injury case during the PCN procedure, reported in 2019 [2, 3, 6]. Mehdi et al. [3] presented the first PCN-associated duodenal injury in a 45-year-old woman with emphysematous pyelonephritis who underwent PCN procedure. The authors diagnosed the duodenal injury with oral and intravenous abdominal CECT after bilious fluid drainage from the nephrostomy catheter. In the present case, similarly, the diagnosis of duodenal injury was made with CECT scan, after the suspicion of bilious fluid and small intestinal content output from the nephrostomy catheter, within 3 hours. The patient suffered from persistent lower back pain in the right side and vomiting as well.

Data about the management of duodenal injury after percutaneous renal procedures are very limited. With the present case, there are only two and four cases of duodenal injury after PCN and PCNL procedures, respectively, in the urological literature. Previous three cases associated with PCNL were managed with conservative approaches such as perinephric drainage, nasogastric tube, H2 antagonist, and total parenteral nutrition, whereas the other one was treated with laparotomy and primary suture repair [7]. The first case after PCN was similarly managed with open repair of the duodenal perforation [3]. In our case, we preferred the conservative management with parenteral nutrition and nasogastric tube and intravenous proton pump inhibitor and broad spectrum antibiotic administration. The absence of duodenal leakage and early placement of the second nephrostomy enabled the patient to be followed up stably. The conservative approach, instead of laparotomy with additional potential morbidity, turned out to be advantageous in the present case.

## References

[1] S. Lewis and U. Patel, "Major complications after percutaneous nephrostomy–lessons from a department audit," *Clinical Radiology*, vol. 59, no. 2, pp. 171–179, 2004.

[2] R. Turo, S. Horsu, J. Broome et al., "Complications of percutaneous nephrostomy in a district general hospital," *Turkish Journal of Urology*, vol. 44, no. 6, pp. 478–483, 2018.

[3] S. Mehdi, V. Singh, R. J. Sinha, and S. Pandey, "Concealed diagnosis of duodenal perforation in a patient with emphysematous pyelonephritis: the dilemma of air in the right perirenal space," *BML Case Reports*, vol. 12, no. 2, article e228629, 2019.

[4] W. E. Goodwin, W. C. Casey, and W. Woolf, "Percutaneous trocar (needle) nephrostomy in hydronephrosis," *Journal of the American Medical Association*, vol. 157, no. 11, pp. 891–894, 1955.

[5] W. E. A. Saad, M. Moorthy, and D. Ginat, "Percutaneous nephrostomy: native and transplanted kidneys," *Techniques in Vascular and Interventional Radiology*, vol. 12, no. 3, pp. 172–192, 2009.

[6] K. A. Hausegger and H. R. Portugaller, "Percutaneous nephrostomy and antegrade ureteral stenting: technique-indications-complications," *European Radiology*, vol. 16, no. 9, pp. 2016–2030, 2006.

[7] O. H. Dahril and A. Mustafa, "Duodenal perforation and a broken guidewire fragment inside the duodenum during supine percutaneous nephrolithotomy (PCNL) without adequate prior imaging: a case report," *Urology Case Report*, vol. 22, pp. 25–27, 2019.

# 32

# Minimally Invasive Robotic-Assisted Cystolithotomy in a Complicated Urinary Diversion: A Feasible and Safe Approach

A. Haffar,[1] C. Crigger,[2] T. Trump,[3] M. Jessop,[4] and M. W. Salkini[3]

[1]*West Virginia University School of Medicine, West Virginia, USA*
[2]*Johns Hopkins Children's Center, Baltimore, USA*
[3]*Department of Urology, West Virginia University, West Virginia, USA*
[4]*Benefis Health System Foundation, Great Falls, USA*

Correspondence should be addressed to A. Haffar; aihaffar@mix.wvu.edu

Academic Editor: Tun-Chieh Chen

Urinary diversion following radical cystectomy and neoadjuvant chemotherapy is the gold standard for the management of muscle-invasive bladder cancer. Urinary diversions are at an increased risk of urolithiasis as a result of various factors. Traditional surgical intervention has included open cystolithotomy which has given way to minimally invasive techniques as of late. We describe a case of a robotic-assisted cystolithotomy from a neobladder in a 54-year-old female patient with muscle-invasive bladder cancer. This is the first description of a robotic-assisted removal of a stone in an orthotopic neobladder. This approach has many advantages, especially in the removal of larger stones. Further study is needed to investigate the efficacy and success of this approach.

## 1. Introduction

The standard of care for muscle-invasive bladder cancer is neoadjuvant chemotherapy followed by radical cystectomy with bilateral pelvic lymph node dissection [1]. Urologists must discuss types of urinary diversions in detail preoperatively to maximize patient understanding and manage patient expectation postoperatively. Though different in their technique, ileal conduits and orthotopic neobladders allow patients to recover their normal lifestyle after a cystectomy. Patients with neobladders often report better self-image and a more active lifestyle [2]. Despite the benefits of these urinary diversions, they can give rise to multiple complications. Urolithiasis is a known complication of urinary diversions, and there are many factors that can influence this process. The use of intestinal segments to create a urinary diversion can cause urolithiasis from continued bicarbonate loss in the urine, hyperoxaluria, urinary stasis, excessive mucus production, and the use of surgical staples in the construction of the neobladder [3, 4].

In patients who develop urolithiasis, surgical management has traditionally involved open cystolithotomy, transurethral, and percutaneous approaches. While the merits and drawbacks of each are open to debate, a delicate balance exists—minimizing treatments to ensure a stone-free rate without compromising the reconstructed bladder. Despite improvements in robotics, a robotic approach has not been widely adopted. In what follows, we describe a robotic approach for the removal of calculus from a reconstructed bladder.

## 2. Case Presentation

A 54-year-old female was referred to an academic tertiary center's urology clinic for evaluation of bilateral hydronephrosis, recurrent urinary tract infections complicated by multiple instances of sepsis, a right ureteropelvic junction stone, and left renal abscess. Her urologic history is complicated by a history of muscle-invasive bladder cancer from 23 years prior status-post open cystectomy with subsequent undiversion without removal of neobladder. Her cystectomy and subsequent undiversion were both done at an outside institution, and the reason for not removing the neobladder at that time is unknown. She also has a history of tethered cord syndrome and neurogenic bowel with a colostomy. Bilateral nephrostomy tubes were placed, and she was treated for her abscess. After stabilizing, she underwent bilateral anterograde nephrostograms followed by bilateral antegrade ureteroscopy which revealed that her ureteroenteric anastomoses were patent bilaterally. Her ureteropelvic junction calculus was removed at this time. Imaging also demonstrated a 3.1 cm stone in her original neobladder which the patient elected to have removed (Figure 1). Her prior urologic infections were treated with outpatient IV Rocephin for a total of 6 weeks

The patient was taken to the operative suite for planned robot-assisted laparoscopic cystolithotomy with stone extraction. Under general anesthesia, the patient was placed in a dorsal lithotomy position. Preoperative cefazolin was administered. A Foley catheter was introduced into the conduit. A midline incision was made above the umbilicus, dissecting down to the peritoneum, and a 5/12 mm trocar was introduced via the Hassan technique. Two 8 mm trocars were placed 8 cm to either side of the camera trocar incision. A 5/12 mm assistant trocar was added lateral to the right robotic arm trocar. The patient was then placed in a steep Trendelenburg position, and the robot was docked. Multiple adhesions of the mesentery to the abdominal wall were lysed, allowing the colostomy and conduit to be easily identified. Initially, we believed the stone to be in the neobladder within the pelvis, so this was opened with monopolar cautery parallel to the blood supply, but the stone was not able to be visualized. We were then able to find the stone in the neobladder deeper in the pelvis, visible through the wall of the diversion. This area was opened, and the stone was able to be fully visualized. At the time of extraction, the stone was fractured inadvertently, likely due to the softer nature of the stone, requiring it to be removed in two pieces. The pieces were removed with the aid of an EndoCatch bag without the need to extend any fascial incisions. The neobladder was then closed in two layers using 3-0 Vicryl V-loc sutures, and a 15 Fr Blake drain was placed alongside the conduit. The catheter was then removed, and the trocar incisions were closed, terminating the procedure. Estimated blood loss was 50 mL. On admission, the patient's BUN was 31, and on the first postoperative day, it was 36. The patient tolerated the procedure well, and the postoperative course was uneventful with discharge occurring on the first postoperative day. JP creatinine on the first postoperative day was negative, and the patient was discharged the same day. She was discharged on DS bactrim BID for 10 days. The drain remained in place at discharge due to higher output and for monitoring of the closure. The output remained less than 50 cc/day per patient documentation and was removed without incident at her 2-week postoperative follow-up, where the patient denied any complaints. She reported consistent urine output from her urostomy with occasional mucous. The patient visited the ED approximately 5 weeks postop with concerns for constipation from her colostomy and at that point was found to have urinalysis concerning for UTI and started on Levaquin for 7 days. CT imaging from 4 weeks postop showed a 3.1 × 2.5 cm calculus within the neobladder lumen along with mild bilateral hydronephrosis similar to her preoperative imaging.

## 3. Discussion

Urolithiasis of urinary diversions is a rare complication with variable incidence rates depending on the type of diversion—13.4% of patients with ileal conduits were found to have an upper tract stone, while only 4.5% developed conduit stones [5]. However, only 3-9% of patients with an orthotopic neobladder using the Paduan technique form stones [3]. Studer et al. reported no neobladder stones in 482 patients when followed for 20 years [6]. Yet, the Kock pouch technique was found to have an incidence of up to 43%; this illustrates the importance that urinary diversion construction technique can have on complication rates [3]. As evidenced by the quick production of a new calculus, preventing stone recurrence is crucial when treating patients with diversions. Prevention relies on enhanced pouch drainage and correcting underlying metabolic abnormalities like acidosis, hyperoxaluria, and hypocitraturia [5].

Treatment of diversion stones typically involves endoscopic procedures as this is currently considered the safest method compared to open surgical procedures. However, a large stone will require extensive manipulation in the urethra, possibly jeopardizing the sphincter [7]. For this reason, others have described great success with endoscopic percutaneous cystolithotomy and adopted this approach as their preferred technique [8].

Regardless of the surgical approach utilized, the balance between optimizing stone-free rates without compromising the reconstructed bladder and limiting surgical procedures is a pressing consideration for both the patient and physician. This first description of a robotic-assisted approach for stone removal in a reconstructed bladder highlights the benefits of this technique. In addition to the many well-known benefits inherent to robotics such as 3-dimensional visualization, greater degrees of freedom in hand movements, accelerated recovery, and lower complication rates, the robotic approach specifically enabled success in our case. This patient had prior abdominal surgeries as outlined including a cystectomy with neobladder and subsequent undiversion to an ileal conduit. Given the complexity of the patient's anatomy and prior abdominal surgical history, we offered a minimally invasive approach in order to prevent an additional laparotomy incision and possible prolonged recovery associated with this approach. Obviously, this was approached with the understanding that as with any minimally invasive approach there is a chance of converting to open if the procedure cannot be safely carried out. Fortunately, this procedure was able to be conducted robotically. We believe that the main advantage of this approach was that the patient was able to be discharged on postoperative day 1 and avoided a prolonged hospital course that is typically associated with open incisions. We felt that using other approaches would not be ideal due to the high likelihood of requiring multiple procedures to address the large stone burden and difficult anatomy. The superior visualization and maneuverability afforded to us with this technique were superior to other minimally invasive techniques. While endoscopic percutaneous and transurethral

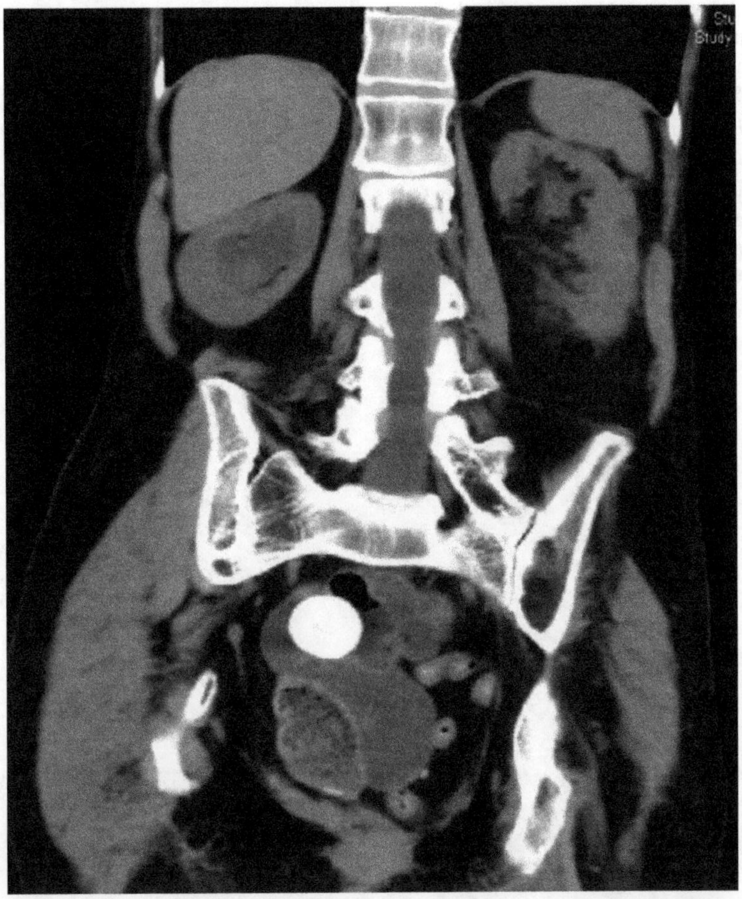

FIGURE 1: Computed tomography (coronal view) of abdomen and pelvis revealing the 3.1 cm calculus in question.

procedures are typically indicated for smaller bladder stones, open cystolithotomies are reserved for larger stones [9]. However, open cystolithotomies are also associated with longer recovery times, greater morbidity, and more rapid recurrence of bladder stones [10]. This case is an excellent illustration of the role robotic-assisted procedures may play in the removal of a urinary diversion stone.

In summary, robotic-assisted cystolithotomy is a modern approach to an old problem—allowing confident removal of calculi from reconstructed bladders that may be preferable in patients with history of prior surgery or complicated anatomy. We believe that in the setting of large stones that would be difficult to remove efficiently through a percutaneous approach, a robotic approach could be more advantageous. Particularly, we believe that stone removal through a minimally invasive approach, compared to the traditional open approach in the setting of prior abdominal surgeries, benefits the patient with faster recovery, potentially less blood loss, and likely shorter duration of hospital stay. Despite the advantages of minimally invasive endoscopic procedures, such techniques may prove difficult in altered anatomy as well as when removing larger stone burdens. Further evaluation is required to evaluate the place that this robotic approach has in challenging stone removal.

## References

[1] M. Babjuk, M. Burger, E. M. Compérat et al., “European Association of Urology guidelines on non-muscle-invasive bladder cancer (TaT1 and carcinoma in situ) - 2019 update,” *European Urology*, vol. 76, no. 5, pp. 639–657, 2019.

[2] A. Hobisch, K. Tosun, J. Kinzl et al., “Life after cystectomy and orthotopic neobladder versus ileal conduit urinary diversion,” *Seminars in Urologic Oncology*, vol. 19, no. 1, pp. 18–23, 2000.

[3] A. Tafuri, A. B. Porcaro, A. N. Ashrafi et al., “Multiple stones in neobladder: case report and literature review,” *Urologia Journal*, vol. 86, no. 4, pp. 216–219, 2019.

[4] S. Nguyen and C. Choi, “Neobladder stone,” *Journal of Medicine*, vol. 377, no. 10, p. 977, 2017.

[5] C. B. Anderson and J. M. McKiernan, “Surgical complications of urinary diversion,” *Urologic Clinics of North America*, vol. 45, no. 1, pp. 79–90, 2018.

[6] U. E. Studer, F. C. Burkhard, M. Schumacher et al., “Twenty years experience with an ileal orthotopic low pressure bladder substitute—lessons to be learned,” *The Journal of Urology*, vol. 176, no. 1, pp. 161–166, 2006.

[7] A. M. Moeen, A. S. Safwat, A. A. Elderwy, H. M. Behnsawy, M. M. Osman, and D. A. Hameed, “Management of neobladder complications: endoscopy comes first,” *Scandinavian Journal of Urology*, vol. 51, no. 2, pp. 146–151, 2017.

[8] A. Breda, M. Mossanen, J. Leppert, J. Harper, P. G. Schulam, and B. Churchill, "Percutaneous cystolithotomy for calculi in reconstructed bladders: initial UCLA experience," *The Journal of Urology*, vol. 183, no. 5, pp. 1989–1993, 2010.

[9] D. J. Hernandez, *Editorial comment: laparoscopic single port cystolithotomy using pneumovesicum*, SciELO Brasil, 2016.

[10] J. F. Donaldson, Y. Ruhayel, A. Skolarikos et al., "Treatment of bladder stones in adults and children: a systematic review and meta-analysis on behalf of the European Association of Urology urolithiasis guideline panel," *European Urology*, vol. 76, no. 3, pp. 352–367, 2019.

# 33

# Urothelial Carcinoma Recurrence in an Orthotopic Neobladder without Urethral or Upper Urinary Tract Involvement

**Chirag P. Doshi**,[1] **Guliz A. Barkan**,[2] **and Marcus L. Quek**[1]

[1]*Department of Urology, Loyola University Medical Center, Maywood, IL, USA*
[2]*Department of Pathology, Loyola University Medical Center, Maywood, IL, USA*

Correspondence should be addressed to Marcus L. Quek; mquek@lumc.edu

Academic Editor: Mohamed A. Ghoneim

We describe a case of a 71-year-old male with an isolated recurrence of urothelial carcinoma in an ileal neobladder without involvement of the upper urinary tract or urethra. He was diagnosed with high grade urothelial carcinoma involving a bladder diverticulum with associated carcinoma in situ. He underwent a radical cystectomy and orthotopic Studer ileal neobladder. On routine follow-up, 11 years following cystectomy, voided urine cytology was positive for high grade urothelial carcinoma. Further workup revealed normal upper urinary tracts, normal urethra, and a solitary lesion at the left anteroinferior wall of the neobladder. He subsequently underwent resection of the neobladder and conversion to an ileal conduit with pathology confirming the diagnosis of high grade urothelial carcinoma. Isolated recurrence of urothelial carcinoma within a neobladder without involvement of the upper urinary tract or urethra is rare. No guidelines exist regarding its management. Herein we present our management as well as the current literature published on this topic.

## 1. Introduction

The orthotopic ileal neobladder has become the preferred method of continent urinary diversion following radical cystectomy for bladder cancer. Urothelial carcinoma recurrence has been widely reported involving the urethra [1–3], upper urinary tract [4], or the ureteroenteric anastomosis [5–7]. However, isolated recurrences within the neobladder without concomitant disease in the remnant urothelium are exceedingly rare, with only 3 other case reports in the literature (Table 1). Here we present a patient with an isolated urothelial carcinoma recurrence in the neobladder 11 years after radical cystectomy.

## 2. Case Report

A 71-year-old gentleman who was diagnosed at age of 59 with high grade urothelial carcinoma involving a bladder diverticulum with associated carcinoma in situ underwent a radical cystectomy, prostatectomy, extended lymphadenectomy, and orthotopic Studer ileal neobladder. Pathology confirmed a high grade urothelial carcinoma arising in a right-sided diverticulum with extension into the perivesical fat and associated carcinoma in situ. There was no evidence of extension into the urethra or ureters and all surgical margins were negative. None of the 40 lymph nodes removed showed carcinoma (pathologic stage pT3aN0Mx). He underwent adjuvant chemotherapy (methotrexate, vinblastine, doxorubicin, and cisplatin), but only tolerated 2 cycles before discontinuing due to side effects. He continued to have surveillance imaging and follow-up every 6-12 months.

On routine follow-up, 11 years following cystectomy, voided urine cytology was positive for high grade urothelial carcinoma. Follow-up CT imaging showed normal upper tracts and interval development of focal mural thickening involving the left anteroinferior neobladder (Figure 1). He underwent a cystoscopy, which revealed a normal urethra, and a solitary lesion at the left anteroinferior wall of the neobladder. Biopsies of this mass revealed an invasive high grade urothelial carcinoma with focal squamous differentiation.

He subsequently underwent resection of the orthotopic neobladder and conversion to an ileal conduit.

TABLE 1: Cases of urothelial cell carcinoma recurrence in ileal neobladder.

| Paper | Patient age/sex | Recurrence site | Urethral recurrence | Upper tract recurrence | Treatment for recurrence |
|---|---|---|---|---|---|
| Kawamoto et al. [5] | 61y/M | Uretero-ileal anastomosis | No | Yes | Left nephroureterectomy, resection of neobladder, urethrectomy |
| Ide et al. [6] | 73y/M | Uretero-ileal anastomosis, urethral-neobladder anastomosis | Yes | Yes | Left nephroureterectomy, resection of neobladder, urethrectomy |
| Hadzi-Djokic et al. [7] | 65y/M | Uretero-ileal anastomosis | No | Yes | Right nephroureterectomy, partial resection of neobladder |
| Moore et al. [8] | 62y/M | Neobladder (multiple sites), urethral-neobladder anastomosis, urethra | Yes | No | Resection of neobladder, urethrectomy, creation of ileal conduit |
| *Yamashita et al. [9]* | *66y/M* | *Neobladder (multiple sites)* | *No* | *No* | *Transurethral resection + intravesical BCG* |
| *Cakmak et al. [10]* | *40y/M* | *Neobladder (multiple sites)* | *No* | *No* | *Transurethral resection* |
| *Cherbanyk et al. [11]* | *66y/M* | *Neobladder* | *No* | *No* | *Partial resection of neobladder* |
| *Present case* | *71y/M* | *Neobladder-left anterior wall* | *No* | *No* | *Resection of neobladder, creation of ileal conduit* |

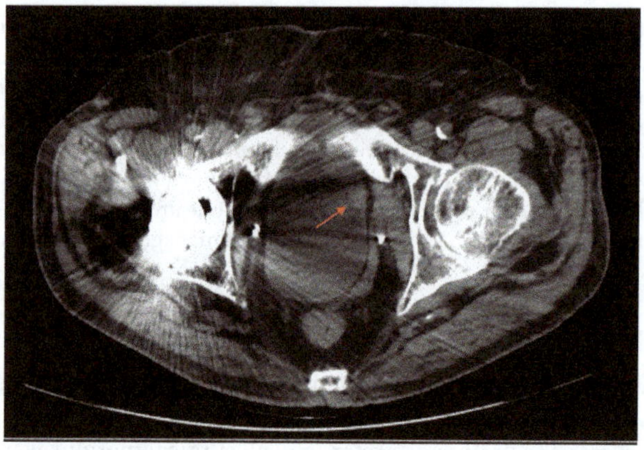

FIGURE 1: CT imaging with focal mural thickening involving the left anteroinferior neobladder.

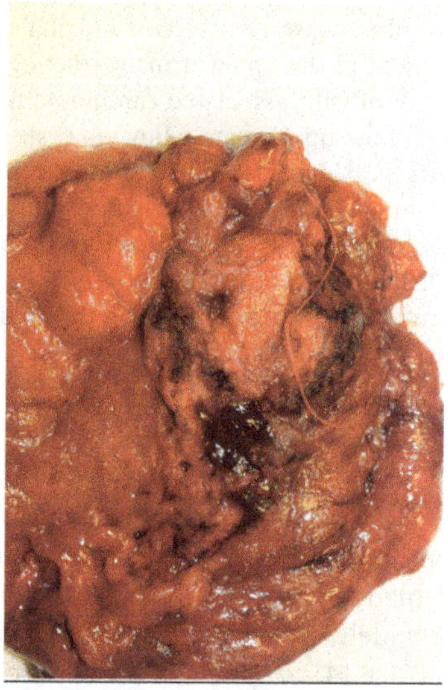

FIGURE 2: Gross pathology.

Intraoperatively, the mass involved the neobladder with possible extension into the pelvic sidewall and pubic bone periosteum. All gross disease was resected. Frozen section margins from pubic bone periosteum and urethra were negative. On gross examination of the final pathologic specimen, a 4.2cm x 2.3cm exophytic, friable mass was noted protruding into the neobladder lumen. Upon sectioning, this mass was noted to have variable depths of invasion, the highest being 9mm through the mucosa, submucosa, and serosa with involvement of the surrounding adipose tissue. Final pathology confirmed high grade urothelial carcinoma involving the neobladder and extending into the surrounding fat (Figures 2 and 3). No tumor was seen at the neobladder-urethral anastomosis and all surgical margins were negative.

## 3. Discussion

An isolated recurrence of urothelial carcinoma in an ileal neobladder without involvement of the upper tract or urethra is rare. To our knowledge, only 3 case reports have been previously published in the literature (Table 1) [9–11]. Patients may present with new hydronephrosis and gross hematuria or as in our case have an abnormal urine cytology. Management of the previously reported cases included transurethral resection in two and partial neobladder resections in the other.

The mechanism of local recurrence in the mucosa of the ileal neobladder is unclear. The development of recurrent solitary or multifocal tumors in the urinary tract is

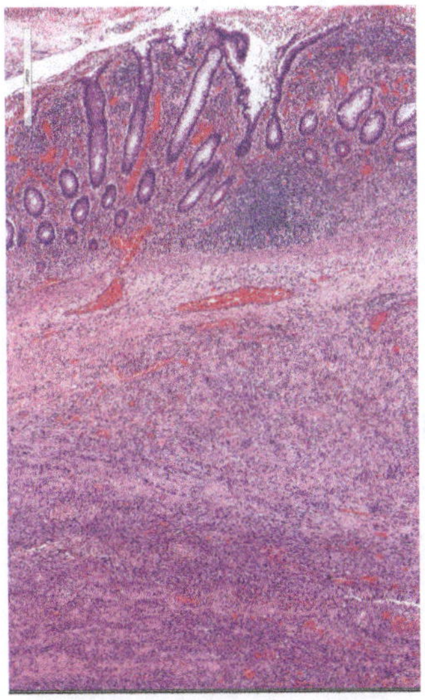

FIGURE 3: Microscopic pathology.

a well-known characteristic of urothelial cell carcinoma. After urinary diversion, recurrences have been reported to occur in the urethra [1–3], upper urinary tract [4], and ileal conduit [6], at the ureteroenteric anastomosis [5–7], as well as colonic mucosa of an ileocolonic neobladder [12]. Direct invasion and implantation are the two proposed hypotheses for urothelial carcinoma recurrence in any part of the urinary tract, including segments of bowel used for urinary diversion. Although some studies have provided evidence for the polyclonal origin of urothelial carcinoma, supporting the idea that multiple tumor recurrences might be the result of carcinogens in the urine, most molecular studies have favored the monoclonal origin, implicating an intraepithelial spread or intraluminal seeding as the source of multiple synchronous or metachronous urothelial tumors [12].

## 4. Conclusion

We report a rare case of urothelial carcinoma recurrence without involvement of upper tracts, ureteroileal anastomosis, or urethra, in an orthotopic ileal neobladder 11 years after radical cystectomy. Our patient underwent resection of the neobladder and conversion to an ileal conduit. At his most recent follow-up visit 3 months later, he continued to be without evidence of recurrence or metastasis. No guidelines exist regarding the management of urothelial carcinoma recurrence. Tumor recurrences have been reported up to 12 years from initial cystectomy, making it imperative that these patients have long-term follow-up.

## References

[1] U. E. Studer, H. Danuser, W. Hochreiter, J. P. Springer, W. H. Turner, and E. J. Zingg, "Summary of 10 years' experience with an ileal low-pressure bladder substitute combined with an afferent tubular isoperistaltic segment," *World Journal of Urology*, vol. 14, no. 1, pp. 29–39, 1996.

[2] J. P. Stein, P. Clark, G. Miranda, J. Cai, S. Groshen, and D. G. Skinner, "Urethral tumor recurrence following cystectomy and urinary diversion: clinical and pathological characteristics in 768 male patients," *The Journal of Urology*, vol. 173, no. 4, pp. 1163–1168, 2005.

[3] C. E. Iselin, C. N. Robertson, G. D. Webster, J. Vieweg, and D. F. Paulson, "Does prostate transitional cell carcinoma preclude orthotopic bladder reconstruction after radical cystoprostatectomy for bladder cancer?" *The Journal of Urology*, vol. 158, no. 6, pp. 2123–2126, 1997.

[4] S. Picozzi, C. Ricci, M. Gaeta et al., "Upper urinary tract recurrence following radical cystectomy for bladder cancer: a meta-analysis on 13,185 patients," *The Journal of Urology*, vol. 188, no. 6, pp. 2046–2054, 2012.

[5] B. Kawamoto, M. Honda, H. Iwamoto, S. Morizane, K. Hikita, and A. Takenaka, "Urothelial carcinoma recurrence at an ileal orthotopic neobladder and unilateral lower ureter after surgery," *Urology Case Reports*, vol. 9, pp. 27–29, 2016.

[6] H. Ide, E. Kikuchi, K. Shinoda, M. Mukai, and M. Murai, "Carcinoma in situ developing in an ileal neobladder," *Urology*, vol. 69, no. 3, p. 576.11, 2007.

[7] J. Hadzi-Djokic, T. Pejcic, V. Andrejevic et al., "Transitional cell carcinoma in orthotopic ileal neobladder 12 years after radical cystectomy," *Vojnosanit Pregl*, vol. 70, no. 11, pp. 1062–1064, 2013.

[8] C. D. Moore, K. A. Iczkowski, K. M. Blue, and C. B. Algood, "Urothelial carcinoma recurrence in ileal orthotopic neobladder: urethrectomy and creation of ileal conduit," *Urology*, vol. 69, no. 1, p. 184.e13, 2007.

[9] R. Yamashita, M. Matsuzaki, M. Niwakawa, and I. Ito, "Bacillus calmette-guérin treatment of urothelial carcinoma arising in the ileal neobladder after radical cystectomy," *International Journal of Urology*, vol. 21, no. 3, pp. 333-334, 2014.

[10] O. Cakmak, H. Tarhan, O. Celik et al., "Transitional Cell Carcinoma in Orthotopic Ileal Neobladder," *Case Reports in Urology*, vol. 2014, Article ID 218615, 3 pages, 2014.

[11] F. Cherbanyk, M. Prod'homme, E. Pezzetta et al., "Urothelial Carcinoma Recurrence in an Ileal Neobladder Nine Years after Primary Surgery with Muir-Torre Syndrome," *Case Reports in Urology*, vol. 2016, Article ID 4762514, 5 pages, 2016.

[12] M. Herawi, J. T. Leppert, G. V. Thomas, J. B. de Kernion, and J. I. Epstein, "Implants of noninvasive papillary urothelial carcinoma in peritoneum and ileocolonic neobladder: support for "seed and soil" hypothesis of bladder recurrence," *Urology*, vol. 67, no. 4, pp. 746–750, 2006.

# 34

# Emphysematous Pyelonephritis Caused by a Giant Fecaloma

**Mikael Abi Abdallah**,[1,2] **Nehme Raad,**[2] **Naim Yarak,**[1,2] **Jean Paul Noujeim,**[1,2] **and Antoine Noujeim**[2]

[1]*Division of Urology, Faculty of Medical Sciences, Lebanese University, Beirut, Lebanon*
[2]*Department of Urology, Lebanese Geitaoui Hospital, Beirut, Lebanon*

Correspondence should be addressed to Abi Abdallah Mikael; mikael.abiabdallah@hotmail.com

Academic Editor: David Duchene

Emphysematous pyelonephritis (EPN) is a gas-producing necrotizing bacterial infection that involves the renal parenchyma and perirenal tissue. It is a life-threatening condition that requires a high index of suspicion, an early diagnosis and an aggressive treatment. Rapid progression to septic shock may occur. We report, to the best of our knowledge, the first case of obstructive EPN caused by a giant fecaloma. The patient was successfully treated with percutaneous drainage and broad-spectrum antibiotics, in addition to fecaloma evacuation using fleet enemas and oral laxatives. This shows how fecal impaction, a common pathology in routine clinical practice, can cause some serious complications if left untreated, including extrinsic ureteral compression.

## 1. Introduction

Emphysematous pyelonephritis (EPN) is an uncommon acute gas-producing necrotizing bacterial infection that involves the renal parenchyma and its surrounding areas. It is a life-threatening condition that requires a high index of suspicion, especially in patients who do not respond to the routine management of pyelonephritis. Although it is most commonly seen in diabetic cases, it has also been reported in patients with urinary tract obstruction without diabetes mellitus (DM). EPN deserves special attention due to its considerable mortality rate [1, 2].

We present, to the best of our knowledge, the first case of obstructive EPN caused by a giant fecaloma in a patient known to have uncontrolled DM and a history of recurrent urinary tract infections.

## 2. Case Presentation

A 70-year-old male patient, nonsmoker, known to have hypertension, uncontrolled DM, Alzheimer's disease, benign prostatic hyperplasia and a history of recurrent urinary tract infections, presented to our emergency department with two days history of high grade fever and decreased level of consciousness. As reported by his family, he was complaining of abdominal distension and constipation since one week without any episode of vomiting. The patient has been recently treated for urinary tract infection with an unknown antibiotic that was intentionally stopped two days prior to his presentation to our department.

Upon arrival, vital signs showed a temperature of 39°C, heart rate of 98 beats per minute, blood pressure of 100/60 mmHg and a respiratory rate of 20 breaths per minute. The patient appeared obnubilated with a Glasgow Coma Scale (GCS) of 12. Physical examination was relevant for left-sided costovertebral angle tenderness, abdominal distension, and fecal impaction on digital rectal examination.

Initial laboratory tests were consistent with sepsis likely secondary to urinary tract infection with blood tests revealing a white blood cell count (WBC) count of 8,100/mm$^3$ with 76% granulocytes, hemoglobin of 10.4 g/dl, platelet count of 248 000/mm$^3$, creatinine level of 1.23 mg/dl, urea of 71 mg/dl, and CRP of 175. Urine analysis demonstrated 6 to 8 WBCs, 2 to 3 RBCs, positive nitrites, and numerous bacteria.

Urgent CT scan of the abdomen and pelvis revealed severe left hydronephrosis and hydroureter with the presence of gas in the left collecting system and left ureter (Figures 1 and 2). The aforementioned hydroureteronephrosis resulted from an

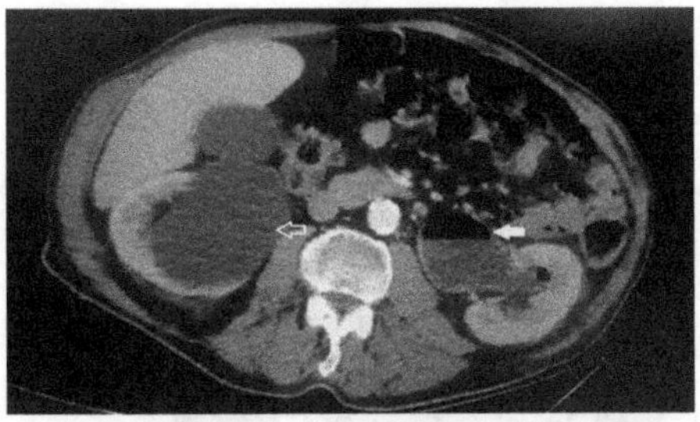

FIGURE 1: Computerized tomographic (CT) scan of the abdomen and pelvis. Left hydronephrosis with presence of air in the collecting system suggestive of left-sided emphysematous pyelonephritis (arrow). Right parapelvic cyst (empty arrow).

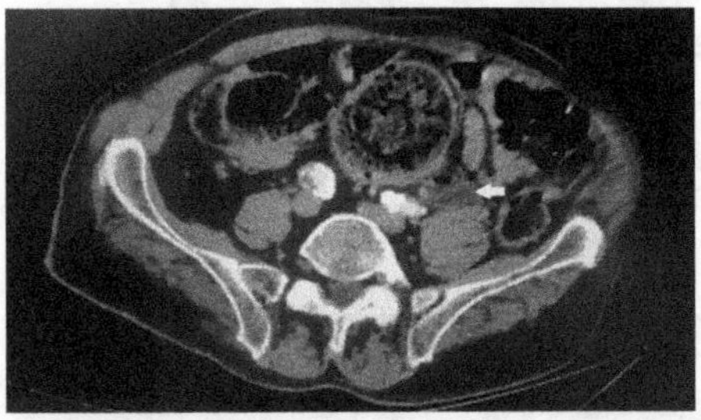

FIGURE 2: Computerized tomographic (CT) scan of the abdomen and pelvis. Left hydroureter with presence of intraluminal air (arrow).

extrinsic compression of the left pelvic ureter between an atherosclerotic external iliac artery and a giant fecaloma (Figure 3). It is noteworthy that the ureter distal to the level of obstruction was not dilated (Figure 4).

Urine and blood cultures were taken. Initial medical management consisted of intravenous fluids, broad-spectrum antibiotics (Meropenem and a single shot of Amikacin) and strict glycemic control. After failure of initial conservative measures of fecaloma evacuation by digital rectal examination and fleet enemas, an ultrasound and fluoroscopy-guided left percutaneous nephrostomy of 10 French (Fr) was inserted for drainage of the renal pelvis. Frank pus was aspirated, confirming a left pyonephrosis. An antegrade ureterogram was intentionally omitted in order to avoid any retrograde bacteremia in this septic patient.

A few hours following the nephrostomy insertion, the patient's confusion improved significantly. He became clinically and hemodynamically stable over the following days as the sepsis resolved. Oral laxatives and fleet enemas were given for fecaloma evacuation. Urine culture grew a multidrug-resistant Proteus Mirabilis. A follow-up noninjected CT scan was performed one week after the admission to document the resolution of the infection, the absence of renal abscesses and the resolution of the fecaloma (Figure 5). An antegrade ureterogram was performed showing a patent ureter with no intrinsic lesions (Figure 6); therefore the PCN was removed (in total nine days after patient's admission).

## 3. Discussion

Emphysematous pyelonephritis (EPN) is an uncommon acute gas-producing necrotizing bacterial infection that involves the

TABLE 1: EPN classification by Huang and Tseng.

| | |
|---|---|
| Class I | Gas in collecting system only |
| Class II | Parenchymal gas only |
| Class III-A | Extension of gas into perinephric space |
| Class III-B | Extension of gas into pararenal space |
| Class IV | EPN in solitary kidney or bilateral disease |

renal parenchyma and perirenal tissue. It is a life-threatening condition that requires a high index of suspicion, especially in diabetic patients who do not respond to the routine management of pyelonephritis. Up to 90% of patients with EPN have uncontrolled DM. Other reported risk factors include drug abuse, end-stage renal disease, immunosuppression, neurogenic bladder, alcoholism, and anatomic anomalies. EPN is more common in females, and a urinary tract obstruction is present in 25–40% of cases [1–3].

Causative organisms include *Escherichia coli (most common), Proteus mirabilis, Klebsiella pneumoniae, Enterococcus* species, and *Pseudomonas aeruginosa* [1]. These micro-organisms are responsible for the production of gas (hydrogen and carbon dioxide) via the fermentation of glucose and lactate, especially in patients with high tissue glucose level, impaired tissue perfusion and immunodeficiency [3, 4].

The most common clinical features include fever/chills, flank pain, nausea, vomiting, and dysuria. These symptoms and signs are nonspecific and cannot differentiate EPN from other upper urinary tract infections [1]. Crepitus in the lumbar region, if present, can provide an important clinical clue to the diagnosis of EPN [4]. The left kidney was found to be more frequently involved than the right one [5].

Based on the radiological findings, multiple classifications for EPN were published, the most recent being published in 2000 by Huang and Tseng (Table 1). It showed a correlation between the class of EPN and its clinical outcome [3].

EPN requires an urgent attention. Rapid progression to septic shock may occur [3]. Thrombocytopenia, acute renal failure, hypotension (systolic blood pressure <90 mmHg), as well as disturbance of consciousness were found to be associated with a poorer prognosis and higher mortality [1, 2].

Once the diagnosis of EPN is made with a CT scan confirming the presence of intrarenal gas, an aggressive resuscitation should be given including oxygen, intravenous fluids, acid-base correction, combination of two broad-spectrum antibiotics, along with strict glycemic control. Inotropic support should be considered to maintain a systolic blood pressure >100 mmHg [3].

The treatment of EPN is controversial. Until the late 1980s, the accepted treatment of EPN has been emergency nephrectomy together with antibiotic therapy. However, surgery is often poorly tolerated in EPN due to poor hemodynamic status, resulting in a reported mortality rate of 40–50% [3]. Significant advances in imaging modalities, antibiotics, and image-guided drainage have shifted the management of EPN from invasive surgery to more conservative nephron-sparing approaches: medical management (MM), with percutaneous drainage (PCD) when indicated [3, 4]. Mortality rates have improved since the 1970s,

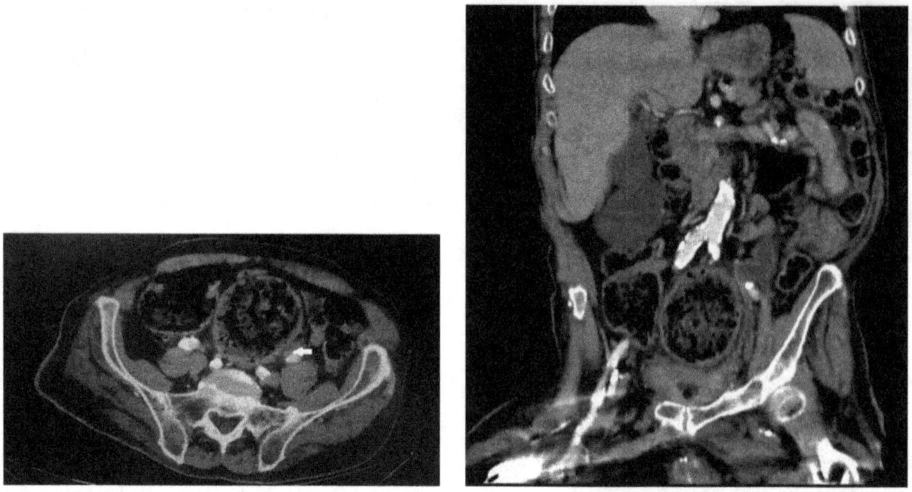

(a) (b)

FIGURE 3: Computerized tomographic (CT) scan of the abdomen and pelvis ((a): axial view, (b): coronal view). Extrinsic compression of the left midureter (arrow) between an atherosclerotic external iliac artery and a giant fecaloma.

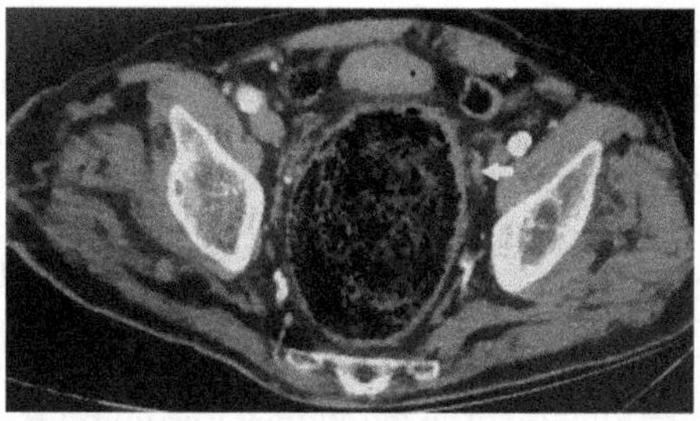

FIGURE 4: Computerized tomographic (CT) scan of the abdomen and pelvis. The left ureter (arrow) distal to the level of obstruction was not dilated.

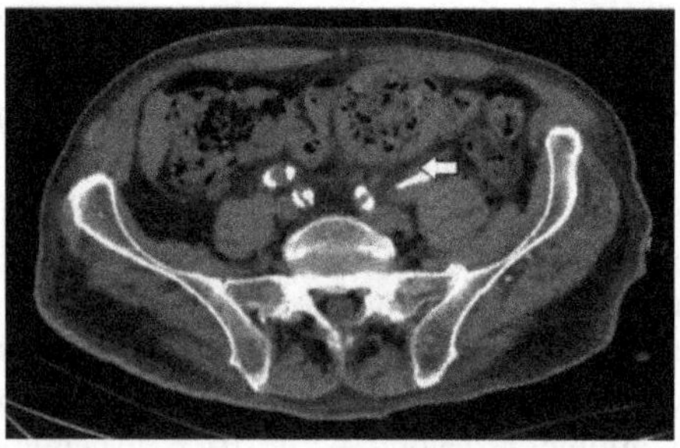

FIGURE 5: Follow-up noninjected computerized tomographic (CT) scan of the abdomen and pelvis. Resolution of the fecaloma and patency of the left ureter (arrow).

and MM plus PCD was found to be associated with the lowest mortality rate of 13.5% [6].

For localized EPN (classes 1 and 2), MM alone or combined with PCD provides generally a positive outcome. For extensive EPN (classes 3 and 4) with a benign course (0 or 1 risk factor), PCD combined with MM may be attempted first due to the high success rate (survival rate of 85%). PCD helps in the preservation of renal function in around 70% of cases. However, in patients with extensive EPN and a fulminant course (≥2 risk factors), MM plus PCD failed in 92% of cases

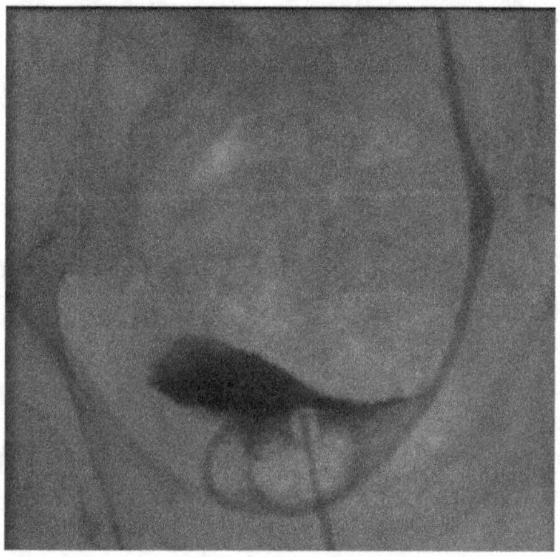

FIGURE 6: Antegrade ureterogram. Patency of the left ureter with absence of any intrinsic ureteral pathology.

and therefore nephrectomy should not be delayed in this setting (Figure 7). Patients who deteriorate or do not improve on conservative treatment require urgent nephrectomy (simple or radical/open or laparoscopic), with a reported mortality rate of 6.6% [2, 3].

A follow-up CT scan should be performed in patients on MM + PCD for EPN to evaluate the progression of the disease (formation of noncommunicating air-fluid collections) and the need for a more invasive treatment (nephrectomy) [7].

Our patient presented with a class I obstructive EPN (presence of gas in the collecting system only) caused by an uncontrolled DM and an extrinsic ureteral compression by a giant fecaloma. A conservative management (MM + PCD) was adopted as recommended with a favorable outcome.

## 4. Conclusion

Emphysematous pyelonephritis requires an early diagnosis and aggressive treatment. Mortality rates are high and rapid

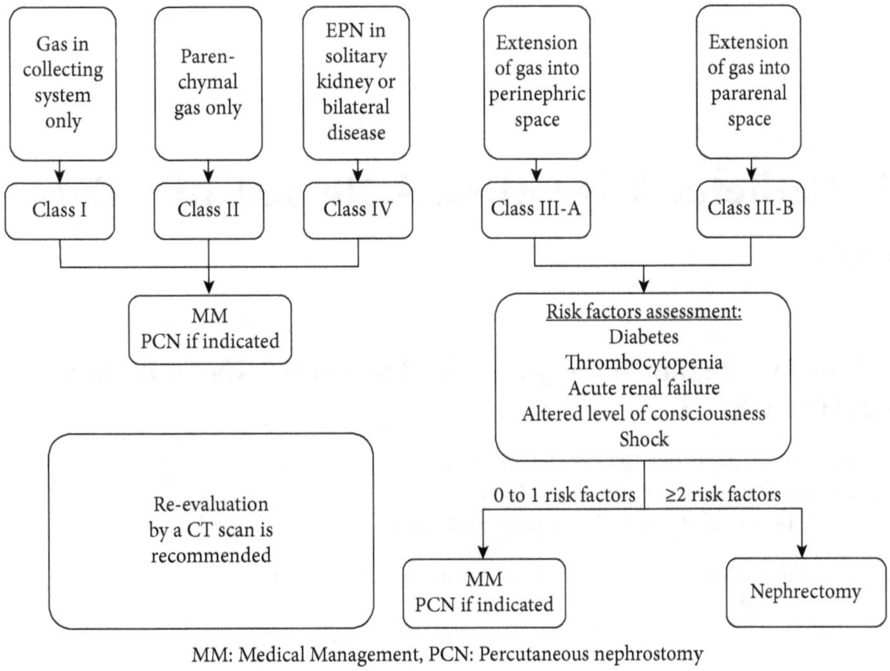


FIGURE 7: Management of EPN according to the classification of Huang and Tseng.

progression to septic shock may occur. Significant advances in image-guided drainage have shifted the management of EPN from invasive surgery to more nephron-sparing approaches. However, surgical intervention should not be delayed in patients with extensive disease or in those who do not improve on conservative treatment. This case report shows how fecal impaction, a common pathology in routine clinical practice, can cause some serious complications if left untreated, including extrinsic ureteral compression.

## References

[1] A. Strofilas, A. Manouras, and E. E. Lagoudianakis, "Aikaterini Kotzadimitriou Apostolos Pappas, Ioannis Chrysikos, and Evangelos Menenakos. Emphysematous pyelonephritis, a rare cause of pneumoperitoneum: a case report and review of literature," *Cases Journal*, vol. 1, no. 1, p. 91, 2008.

[2] J.-J. Huang and C.-C. Tseng, "Emphysematous pyelonephritis clinicoradiological classification, management, prognosis, and pathogenesis," *Archives of Internal Medicine*, vol. 160, no. 6, pp. 797–805, 2000.

[3] S. S. Ubee, L. McGlynn, and M. Fordham, " Emphysematous pyelonephritis," *BJU International*, vol. 107, no. 9, pp. 1474–478, 2011.

[4] R. A. Misgar, I. Mubarik, A. I. Wani, M. I. Bashir, M. Ramzan, and B. A. Laway, "Emphysematous pyelonephritis: a 10-year experience with 26 cases," *Indian Journal of Endocrinology and Metabolism*, vol. 20, no. 4, pp. 475–480, 2016.

[5] T. F. Imran, F. Yick, A. H. Qavi, S. Dhamotharan, and S. J. Sperber, "Emphysematous pyelonephritis with abscesses masquerading as an ordinary urinary tract infection," *American Journal of Infectious Diseases*, vol. 11, pp. 88–92, 2015.

[6] B. K. Somani, G. Nabi, P. Thorpe, J. Hussey, J. Cook, and J. N'Dow, "Is percutaneous drainage the new gold standard in the management of emphysematous pyelonephritis? Evidence from a systematic review," *Journal of Urology*, vol. 179, no. 5, pp. 1844–1849, 2008.

[7] M. T. Chen, C. N. Huang, Y. H. Chou, C. H. Huang, C. P. Chiang, and G. C. Liu, "Percutaneous drainage in the treatment of emphysematous pyelonephritis: 10-year experience," *Journal of Urology*, vol. 157, no. 5, pp. 1569–1573, 1997.

35

# Suprapubic Catheter Migration: A Review of a Rare Complication

**Amr Elmoheen**[1,2] **Mahmoud Saqr,**[1] **Waleed Salem**[1] **Khalid Bashir**[1,2] **and Ayman Hagras**[3]

[1]*Emergency Department, Hamad Medical Corporation, Qatar*
[2]*QU Health, College of Medicine, Qatar University, Qatar*
[3]*Urology Department, College of Medicine, Tanta University, Egypt*

Correspondence should be addressed to Amr Elmoheen; aelmoheen@hamad.qa

Academic Editor: Tun-Chieh Chen

*Background.* Suprapubic catheter migration to the vesicoureteral junction is an unusual complication, causing an obstruction that led to hydronephrosis and dilation of the pelvicalyceal system. *Case presentation.* A 30-year-old man with a suprapubic catheter (SPC) that was inserted one month before this current Emergency Department (ED) visit had severe left flank pain for 48 hours. The SPC was inserted in the context of urethral injury after falling astride. Point-of-Care Ultrasound (POCUS) showed a semifilled urinary bladder and moderate hydronephrosis on the left side. A computed tomography scan (CT scan) of the abdomen was performed and showed migration of the suprapubic catheter's tip into the left vesicoureteral junction, causing ureteral obstruction dilation of the ipsilateral pelvicalyceal system. The suprapubic catheter was changed in the ED, causing relief of symptoms, and the patient was referred to the urology department for follow-up. It was uneventful on the follow-up from the SPC clinic. *Conclusions.* This case report describes a rare complication of migration of the suprapubic catheter to the vesicoureteral junction causing acute ureteral obstruction and hydronephrosis.

## 1. Introduction

Suprapubic catheter drainage is a widely used urological procedure in patients with neurogenic bladder and acute retention of urine with failed urethral catheterization or in patients in whom the placement of a urethral catheter is contraindicated as urethral trauma [1]. The complication rate associated with cystotomy varies from 1.6 to 2.4% [2]. A poorly reported complication but with a significant impact on the quality of life of patients is catheter migration, which should be considered in patients with acute urine retention, obstructive urinary symptoms, low back pain, or impaired renal function [3]. This review describes an unusual complication of migration of the suprapubic catheter to the vesicoureteral junction, causing an obstruction that led to hydronephrosis and dilation of the left pelvicalyceal system.

## 2. Patient Information

A 30-year-old man with a suprapubic catheter (SPC) that was inserted one month before this current Emergency Department (ED) visit had severe left flank pain for 48 hours. The SPC was inserted in the context of urethral injury after falling astride. He did not report any fever, changes in urine coloration, nausea, vomiting, or diarrhea. The suprapubic catheter was changed five days before this current ED presentation, and the patient reported some resistance and difficulty during the exchange. Physical examination reveals only granulomatous tissue with pus in the suprapubic catheter port; however,

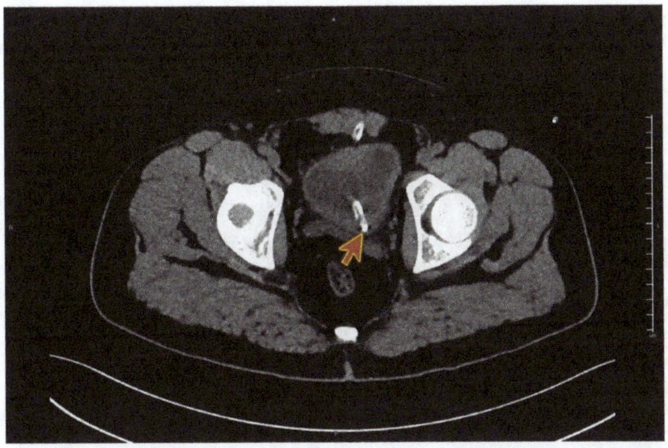

FIGURE 1: Computed tomography (CT) abdomen, axial view showing the tip of the suprapubic catheter inserted at the left ureterovesical junction (red arrow).

there is no pus in the catheter track. The rest of the general and systemic examination was within normal parameters.

## 3. Investigations

In order to rule out the presence of a urinary tract infection, a urine test was performed that reveals a high white blood cell count (28 $\mu$L). Laboratory tests reported leukocytosis (13900/$\mu$L), elevated absolute neutrophil count (10300/$\mu$L), hyponatremia (132 mmol/L), hypochloremia (93.0 mmol/L), and normal kidney function (creatinine, 77 $\mu$mol/L).

Bedside Point-of-Care Ultrasound (POCUS) showed a collapsed urinary bladder and moderate to severe hydronephrosis on the left side, and the balloon of the catheter in the bladder cannot be observed.

Computed tomography (CT) abdomen was performed, showing the tip of the suprapubic catheter inserted at the left ureterovesical junction causing obstruction the ureter (Figures 1 and 2) and moderate dilatation of the left pelvicalyceal system (Figure 3). This finding confirms the diagnosis of catheter migration.

## 4. Treatment

The emergency physician replaced the old suprapubic catheter with a new 16 Fr catheter. Its proper placement was confirmed by ultrasound, and a sample was taken for urine culture. After replacing the catheter, the patient drained 1200 mL of clear urine over 3 hours. At the time of home discharge, the patient was in good general condition and pain-free, and the catheter was draining clear urine. Outpatient treatment with ciprofloxacin 500 mg orally every 12 hours for seven days, paracetamol 1 gram orally every 8 hours for seven days, and outpatient follow-up with urology service were arranged.

## 5. Outcome and Follow-Up

After performing a combined cystourethrogram, that revealed short urethral stricture (less than 5 mm), a visualized internal urethrotomy was done after two weeks. During the cystoscopy, the left ureteral orifice was slightly dilated than the right one. The suprapubic catheter was removed, and an 18 Fr silicone urethral catheter was fixed. The patient had a regular follow-up with the urology outpatient services for three months. He did not report any new complications later on.

## 6. Discussion

The placement of a suprapubic cystotomy catheter is a frequent procedure used in urology, especially in patients with neurogenic bladder who require long-term bladder drainage. Suprapubic cystotomy is also indicated in cases of trauma or urethral pathology that prevent the placement of a transurethral catheter. The most frequent complications associated with cystotomy are bacteriuria, bleeding, and bladder stones [4]. Other complications such as intestinal perforation, enterocutaneous fistulas (ECF), neoplastic changes in the urinary bladder, and migration of the catheter into the ureter have also been reported [5, 6]. However, multiple meta-analyses have shown that bladder drainage using a suprapubic catheter is associated with a lower rate of complications compared to transurethral catheter drainage.

The migration of the suprapubic catheter to the vesicoureteral junction is a rare complication. The patients at greatest risk are those who have a permanent catheter and/or require long-term bladder drainage. This is because the bladder of these patients tends to contract, modifying the anatomical relationship between the bladder neck and the ureterovesical junction, which makes it easier for the catheter to enter the ureter. Furthermore, these patients require a regular change of the catheter; therefore, there is a greater probability that the catheter will inadvertently be inserted into the ureter. Patients with neurogenic bladder usually present ureterovesical reflux, which also predisposes to this complication [7].

In 1987, Borrero et al. reported a 35-year-old paraplegic man with suprapubic catheter migration diagnosed by intravenous venogram [8]. In 2010, Dangle Pankaj et al. described another case of suprapubic catheter migration to the left ureter that led to obstructive uropathy and hydronephrosis in a patient with a neurogenic bladder [9]. In 2011, Singh et al.

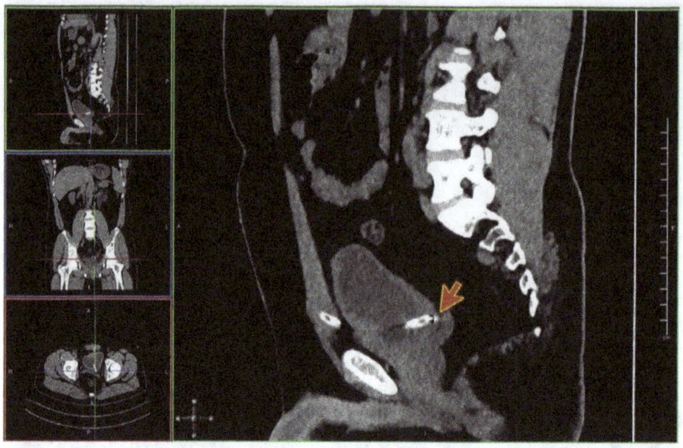

FIGURE 2: Computed tomography (CT) abdomen, sagittal view showing the tip of the suprapubic catheter inserted at the left ureterovesical junction (red arrow).

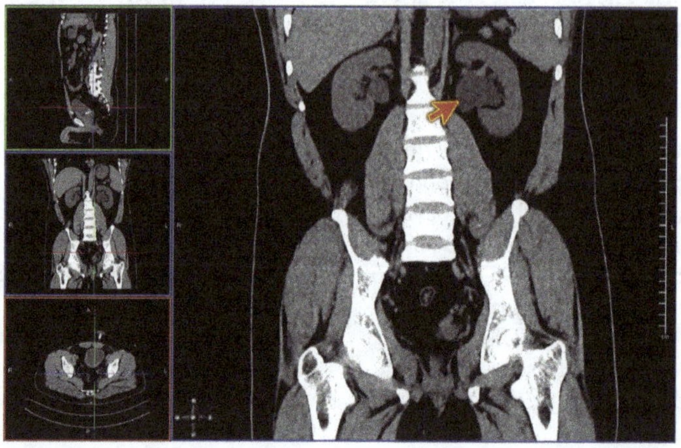

FIGURE 3: Computed tomography (CT) abdomen, coronal view showing moderate dilatation of the left pelvicalyceal system (red arrow).

defined a case of suprapubic migration due to a gaping ureteric orifice in a 27-year-old man with traumatic bulbomembranous urethral stricture [10]. In 2016, Luo et al. reported three cases of accidental suprapubic catheter placement at the vesicoureteral junction in patients with neurogenic bladder and/or voiding dysfunction [7]. In the same year, Shuaibin et al. reported on the case of an elderly male patient with senile dementia whose suprapubic catheter had migrated into a previously normal nongaping ureter [11].

This paper presents the case of a male patient, 30-year-old, with a history of urethral trauma (falling astride) that is managed by suprapubic catheter insertion one month before his current ED presentation to be prepared later for definitive management presented suprapubic heaviness and left flank pain for 48 hours. The diagnosis of catheter migration was confirmed by performing a computed tomography showing the tip of the catheter at the left ureterovesical junction, causing urinary flow obstruction, hydroureter, and ipsilateral hydronephrosis.

According to the cases reported so far, the diagnosis of catheter migration should be considered in a patient with long-term bladder drainage and/or urinary dysfunction who presents resistance when inflating the catheter balloon, urine leakage around the catheter or obstruction of the catheter, flank pain, urinary retention, and/or obstructive urinary symptoms.

Although most cases are reported in patients with a long-term catheter, we must bear in mind that inadvertent placement of the catheter in the ureter may occur at the first insertion.

Abdominal ultrasonography is a very useful tool to identify the catheter's location and its balloon. The computed tomography with contrast allows confirming the diagnosis of catheter migration and also allows evaluating the presence of complications such as ureteral rupture, hydronephrosis, and pyelonephritis. Patients who do not present with complications can be managed conservatively, repositioning or removing the catheter and treating urinary tract infection with antibiotics if present, as was done in this case.

## 7. Conclusion

In a patient with suprapubic cystotomy, urinary retention, hydronephrosis, flank pain, obstructive urinary symptoms, pericatheter urine leakage, or catheter blockage should make the diagnosis of catheter migration suspect. Point-of-Care

Ultrasound (POCUS) examination of the urinary bladder is very helpful in detecting the hydronephrosis, the empty bladder, and the position of the catheter balloon. Patients with neurogenic bladder or long-term bladder drainage are more prone to catheter migration. The suprapubic catheter must be securely anchored to prevent the migration of the catheter tip.

## Abbreviations

POCUS: Point-of-Care Ultrasound
CT: Computed tomography
ECF: Enterocutaneous fistulas
SPC: Suprapubic catheter
ED: Emergency Department.

## Additional Points

*Patient's Perspective.* I am delighted with the management I received during my suffering. I was in severe pain that I could not tolerate. I did not imagine that rare complications of my catheter would happen. I would like to appreciate the tireless efforts of the doctors and nurses who cared for me.

## Ethical Approval

The ethical approval is exempt from Medical Research Center at Hamad Medical Corporation, Qatar.

## Consent

Written informed consent to publish this information was obtained from the patient.

## Authors' Contributions

AE contributed to the manuscript writing, figures, and literature review. MS participated in treating physician and literature review. WS contributed to the manuscript writing. KB is the lead author and participated in the revision and literature review. AH contributed to the manuscript writing and literature review. All authors have read and approved the manuscript.

## References

[1] R. S. Ahluwalia, N. Johal, C. Kouriefs, G. Kooiman, B. S. I. Montgomery, and R. O. Plail, "The surgical risk of suprapubic catheter insertion and long-term sequelae," *The Annals of The Royal College of Surgeons of England*, vol. 88, no. 2, pp. 210–213, 2006.

[2] S. Nomura, T. Ishido, J. Teranishi, and K. Makiyama, "Long-term analysis of suprapubic cystostomy drainage in patients with neurogenic bladder," *Urologia Internationalis*, vol. 65, no. 4, pp. 185–189, 2000.

[3] K. Ananthakrishnan, R. Ayyathurai, J. K. Chiran, W. Islam, and V. Srinivasan, "An unusual complication of suprapubic catheter insertion," *The Scientific World Journal*, vol. 6, 2435 pages, 2006.

[4] H. K. Katsumi, J. F. Kalisvaart, L. D. Ronningen, and R. M. Hovey, "Urethral versus suprapubic catheter: choosing the best bladder management for male spinal cord injury patients with indwelling catheters," *Spinal Cord*, vol. 48, no. 4, pp. 325–329, 2010.

[5] R. J. Schaafsma, K. P. Delaere, and P. H. Theunissen, "Squamous cell carcinoma of suprapubic cystostomy tract without bladder involvement," *Spinal Cord*, vol. 37, no. 5, pp. 373-374, 1999.

[6] B. Adeyemo, S. Makovitch, and D. Foo, "A peculiar complication of suprapubic catheterization: recurrent ureteral obstruction and hydronephrosis," *The Journal of Spinal Cord Medicine*, vol. 36, pp. 166–169, 2013.

[7] R. Luo, S. L. Lee, F. C. Ng, and L.-T. Koh, "Inadvertent placement of a urinary catheter into the ureter: a report of 3 cases and review of the literature," *Asian Journal of Urology*, vol. 4, no. 4, pp. 256–261, 2017.

[8] G. O. Borrero, P. R. Miller, K. Vora, and C. A. Nepjuk, "Acute ureteral obstruction as a complication of suprapubic catheterization," *Urologic Radiology*, vol. 9, no. 1, pp. 171–173, 1988.

[9] P. P. Dangle, J. Tycast, E. Vasquez, B. Geary, and M. Chehval, "Suprapubic cystostomy: a bizarre complication of catheter migration causing ureteric obstruction," *Canadian Urological Association Journal*, vol. 4, no. 5, 2013.

[10] D. R. Singh, L. Sailo, N. B. Abraham, and N. Kekre, "An unusal complication of percutaneous suprapubic cystostomy," *Indian Journal of Urology*, vol. 2, pp. 179-180, 2001.

[11] W. Shuaibin, M. Haiqi, F. Qin, and Y. Haifeng, "An unusual complication of suprapubic catheter migration into the left ureter," *Urology Journal*, vol. 15, no. 3, 2018.

# Large Cell Neuroendocrine Carcinoma of the Bladder with Adenocarcinomatous Component

**Rami Halabi**,[1,2] **Maher Abdessater**,[1,2] **Johnny Boustany**,[1,2] **Anthony Kanbar**,[1,2] **Halim Akl**,[1,2] **Joey El Khoury**,[1,2] **Charbel El Hachem**,[1,2] **and Raghid El Khoury**[1,2]

[1]*Department of Urology, Notre Dame des Secours University Hospital Center (CHUNDS), Byblos City, Lebanon*
[2]*Faculty of Medicine and Medical Sciences, Holy Spirit University of Kaslik (USEK), Jounieh, Lebanon*

Correspondence should be addressed to Maher Abdessater; maher.abdessater@gmail.com

Academic Editor: Tun-Chieh Chen

Large cell neuroendocrine carcinoma (LCNC) is one of the rarest types of bladder cancer occurring in <1%. Either pure or mixed with another component, it remains one of the most aggressive types of bladder cancer. We report a case of LCNC of the bladder with an adenocarcinomatous component. The patient was a 64-year-old smoker male, who presented for the first time with dysuria and hematuria. A bladder tumor invading the anterior and right lateral bladder walls was discovered, without any secondary localizations. Tumor biopsy showed an LCNC with adenocarcinomatous components. The patient was treated by recurrent tumor resections, chemotherapy, and radiotherapy. No improvement was noted despite close follow-up and adequate treatment. Neuroendocrine bladder tumor is known to have an aggressive, rapid, and disadvantageous evolution. Multiple case reports were published so far, and a recent review was conducted in March 2020 by Sanguedolce et al. (2020). More cases are needed to establish the best management plan for this type of tumor.

## 1. Introduction

Bladder cancer (BC) is the 6th most frequent neoplasm in men and the 17th most frequent in women [1]. Its annual incidence increased from 430000 cases in 2012 to 550000 in 2018 [1, 2]. Lebanon was found to have the world's highest rate of BC [1]. According to the World Health Organization classification, more than 90% of BC are urothelial and around 5% are squamous cell carcinoma. The neuroendocrine bladder carcinoma is considered a rare variant (<1%) with highly aggressive potential. These tumors are divided into small cell neuroendocrine carcinoma, large cell neuroendocrine carcinoma, well-differentiated neuroendocrine tumor, and paraganglioma [2]. The small cell type is the most common, and the large cell neuroendocrine cancer type (LCNC) is the rarest. Less than forty cases of LCNC were reported so far in the literature. Only three cases had histological similarities to our case [3–5]. Management strategies are not yet studied prospectively [6, 7]. In this article, we report a case of LCNC with an adenocarcinomatous component.

## 2. Case Presentation

A 64-year-old heavy smoker male patient was admitted for the first time to our urology department for hematuria and dysuria. His past medical history was unremarkable. He had a transurethral resection of the prostate 5 years ago. He did not have any familial history of urothelial or bladder cancer. Physical examination and blood tests were normal. In the emergency room, an abdominal and pelvic ultrasound showed a thickening of the right lateral wall of the bladder with mild right side hydronephrosis (Figure 1). On cystoscopy, a large tumor was found on the anterior and right lateral walls of the bladder, with invasion of the bladder neck and the prostate. The anatomopathological study of the tumor showed a neoplastic proliferation of large malignant polygonal cells with dark, irregular nuclei and frequent mitosis. A second component made of cylindrical cells was also present. Muscular invasion was documented with multiple necrotic areas (Figure 2). Immunohistochemistry showed high positivity for CD56 marker and synaptophysin, minor

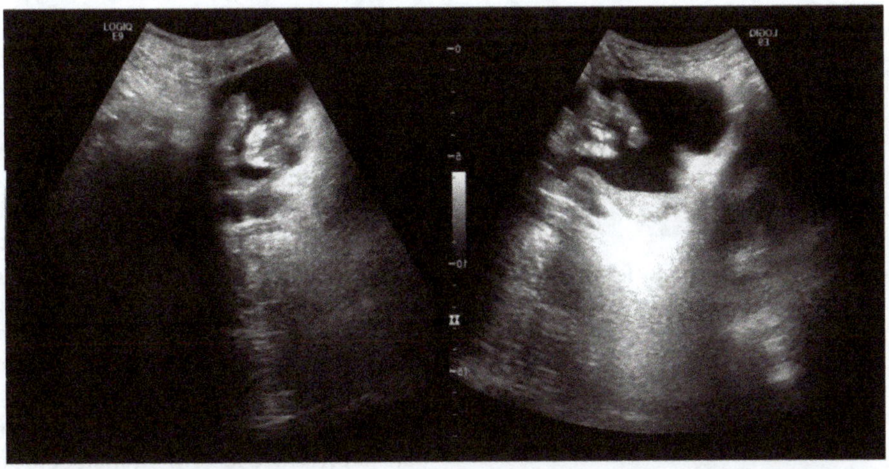

FIGURE 1: The first bladder echography showing a thickening of the right lateral wall.

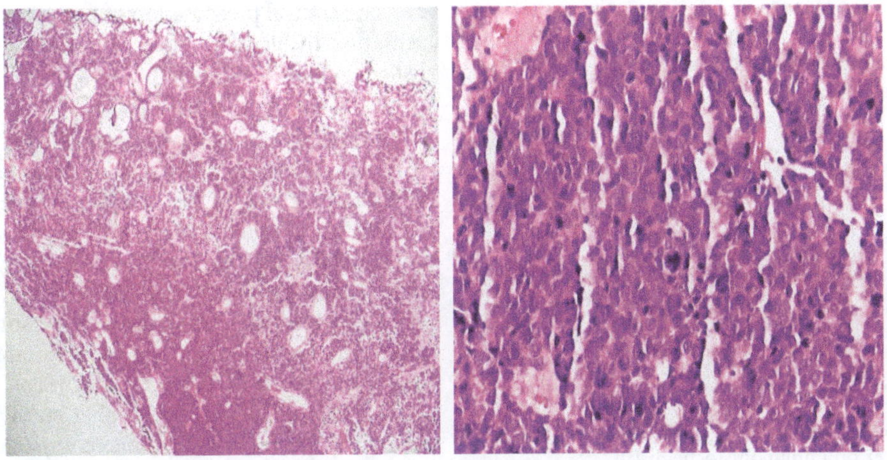

FIGURE 2: On the left: microscopic view of the bladder biopsy showing a proliferation of polygonal malignant cells and cylindrical cells with multiple necrotic areas; on the right: large polygonal cells with a dark and irregular nucleus and frequent metastases.

and heterogenic positivity for cytokeratin 7, and negativity for cytokeratin 20 and CDX2 (Figures 3–5). Overall, the histopathological study corresponded to LCNC with minor adenocarcinomatous component. Disease extension was assessed using computed tomography (CT) scan of the thorax, abdomen, and pelvis. A 6 × 3.5 cm mass of the anterior and right lateral walls of the bladder was identified, with diffuse infiltration of the perivesical fat and multiple necrotic iliac lymph nodes bilaterally (Figure 6). Neither visceral nor bone metastasis was identified. Initially, the patient refused the treatment and was lost to follow-up. Two months later, he was readmitted to the hospital for similar complaints and additional pelvic pain. Blood tests were normal. A new CT scan revealed an increase in the size of the tumor, occupying now the majority of the bladder lumen, a persistent right hydronephrosis, and no new secondary lesions. The tumor was resected again, until the appearance of the muscular layer of the bladder, and the patient was discharged after stabilization. A later PET CT confirmed the previous findings of locoregional disease (tumor of the bladder base with infiltration of the prostate gland and a diffuse metastatic bilateral iliac chain and retroperitoneal lymph nodes) and denied secondary lesions. The multidisciplinary team meeting decided for radiotherapy and chemotherapy using cisplatin and etoposide every 21 days. Four months later, after the completion of four cycles of chemotherapy, the patient underwent new assessment for disease extension (Figure 7). CT scan showed progression of the disease with the tumor occupying now the totality of the bladder lumen, infiltration of the anterior abdominal wall, and subcutaneous liquid collection measuring 33 × 36 mm. A similar left retrovesical mass of 60 × 38 mm along with multiple para-aortic and mediastinal lymphadenopathies with central necrosis was also found. A few months later, the patient died in the oncology department after recurrent admissions for different complications.

## 3. Discussion

Neuroendocrine carcinomas are most frequently seen in the pulmonary and gastrointestinal tracts. This type of tumor can be also found in the urinary tract. According to the literature, different types of neuroendocrine carcinomas of the

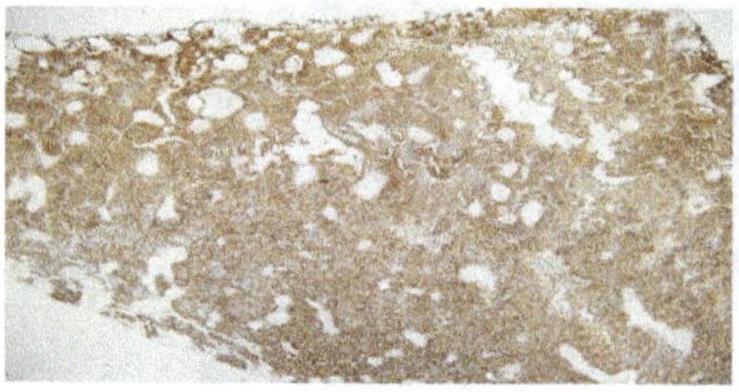

FIGURE 3: Malignant cells showing high positivity for CD56 marker on immunohistochemistry.

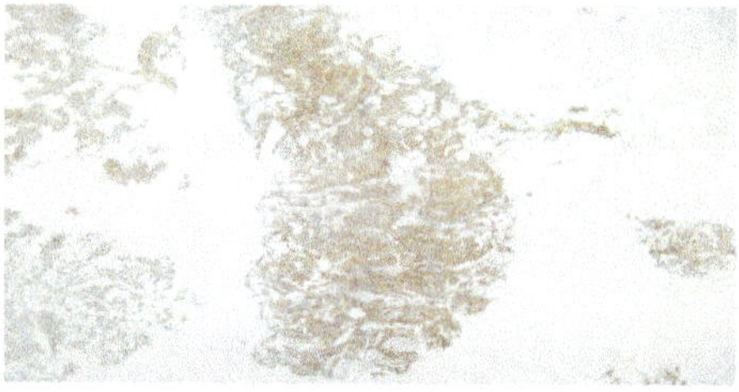

FIGURE 4: Malignant cells showing high positivity of synaptophysin marker on immunohistochemistry.

FIGURE 5: Malignant cells showing minor and heterogenic positivity for cytokeratin 7 marker on immunohistochemistry.

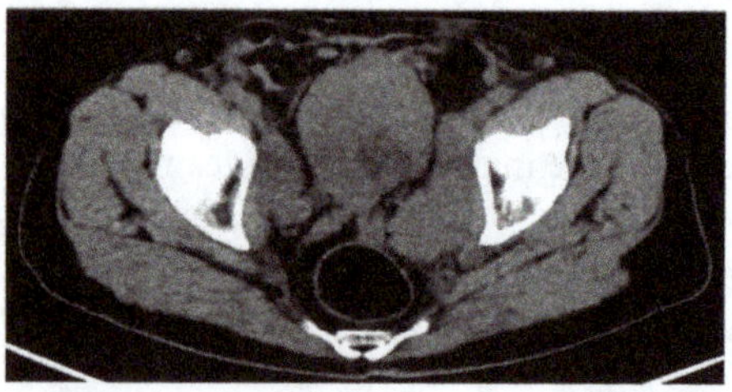

FIGURE 6: Pelvic scan showing a 6 × 3.5 cm mass of the anterior and right lateral wall of the bladder with diffuse infiltration of the bladder fat.

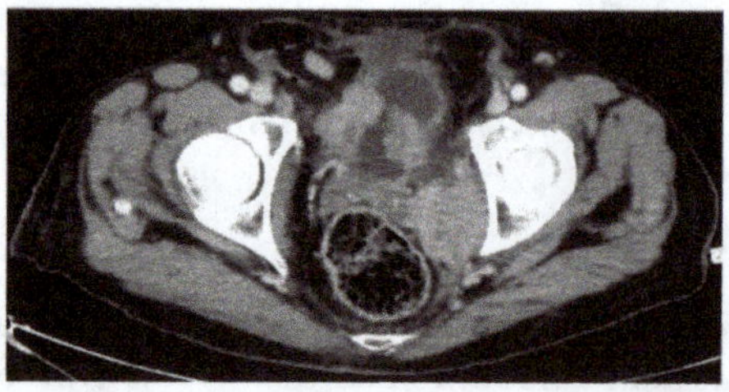

FIGURE 7: Pelvic scan showing the evolution of the bladder tumor.

bladder were described. The LCNC is the rarest type [8, 9]. It can present as a pure tumor, or in association with carcinosarcoma, adenocarcinoma or lymphoepithelioma-like carcinoma.

The first published case by Abenoza et al. had mixed histological features of LCNC and adenocarcinomatous cells. It was treated by a radical cystectomy and bilateral lymphadenectomy. The patient died 30 months after the surgery [9]. Subsequently, less than forty cases of pure and mixed LCNC were published [3, 4, 6–8, 10–21]. To our knowledge, only three cases showed similar histological characteristics to our case, with LCNC and adenocarcinoma components [7, 17, 22].

Only two of the published cases of LCNC were discovered from cutaneous or a brain metastasis [10, 13]. Our patient presented local infiltration of the prostatic gland with bilateral iliac and retroperitoneal lymph nodes. Although the latter was a frequent finding in the literature, the former has never been described [23].

The clinical presentation of our patient was a typical presentation of bladder cancer, similar to the previously published cases, in which hematuria was a frequent presentation [3–5, 7, 8, 12, 13, 17–19].

No guidelines were ever published concerning the treatment modalities of LCNC. A cisplatin-based chemotherapy consisted the base of the treatment strategies through literature. A multimodal therapeutic approach, using the combination of chemotherapy, radiotherapy, and radical or partial surgeries, has been reported [3, 4, 25, 27]. Dowd et al. reported after the treatment by surgical resection and adjuvant chemotherapy and radiotherapy, no recurrence at one year [4]. In their study in 2018 on thirty-five cases of LCNC, Niu et al. reported higher survival rates in patients treated by multimodal therapies compared to patients treated with a conservative treatment. They reported also that a platine-based chemotherapy was the most used option [28]. The management plan of our patient was similar to Dowd et al.'s plan. Our patient was managed by repetitive transurethral tumor resection of the bladder tumor, multiple cycles of cisplatin and etoposide chemotherapy, and radiotherapy.

Coelho et al. have stated in their case report and review that LCNC has a bad prognosis and is usually discovered in an advanced or metastatic stage [7]. A bibliographic review in 2011 by Martin et al. showed that the survival rate for all published cases concerning LCNC was 46.2% for a maximum follow-up of 20 months [23], which was the case of our patient.

## 4. Conclusion

Bladder tumor incidence is increasing nowadays. Neuroendocrine type is a rare one, with aggressive, rapid, and disadvantageous evolution. So far, we lack prospective studies concerning therapeutic strategies, and management is based on some previous published case reports.

## References


[1] J. Ferlay, M. Colombet, I. Soerjomataram et al., "Estimating the global cancer incidence and mortality in 2018: GLOBOCAN sources and methods," *International Journal of Cancer*, vol. 144, no. 8, pp. 1941–1953, 2019.

[2] J. Ferlay, I. Soerjomataram, R. Dikshit et al., "Cancer incidence and mortality worldwide: sources, methods and major patterns in GLOBOCAN 2012," *International Journal of Cancer*, vol. 136, no. 5, pp. E359–E386, 2015.

[3] E. Akdeniz, M. Bakirtas, M. S. Bolat, S. Akdeniz, and I. Özer, "Pure large cell neuroendocrine carcinoma of the bladder without urological symptoms," *Pan African Medical Journal*, vol. 30, pp. 1–4, 2018.

[4] K. Dowd, C. Rotenberry, D. Russell, M. Wachtel, and W. De Riese, "Rare occurrence of a poorly differentiated neuroendocrine tumor of the bladder," *Case Reports in Medicine*, vol. 2017, Article ID 4812453, 4 pages, 2017.

[5] S. Thota, G. Kistangari, H. Daw, and T. Spiro, "A clinical review of small-cell carcinoma of the urinary bladder," *Clinical Genitourinary Cancer*, vol. 11, no. 2, pp. 73–77, 2013.

[6] A. Bertaccini, D. Marchiori, A. Cricca et al., "Neuroendocrine carcinoma of the urinary bladder: case report and review of the literature," *Anticancer Research*, vol. 28, no. 2B, pp. 1369–1372, 2008.

[7] H. M. P. Coelho, B. A. G. J. Pereira, and P. A. S. C. Temido, "Large cell neuroendocrine carcinoma of the urinary bladder: case report and review," *Current Urology*, vol. 7, no. 3, pp. 155–159, 2013.

[8] K. H. Lee, S. B. Ryu, M. C. Lee, C. S. Park, S. W. Juhng, and C. Choi, "Primary large cell neuroendocrine carcinoma of the urinary bladder," *Pathology International*, vol. 56, no. 11, pp. 688–693, 2006.

[9] S. E. Mills, J. T. Wolfe, M. A. Weiss et al., "Small cell undifferentiated carcinoma of the urinary bladder. A light-microscopic, immunocytochemical, and ultrastructural study of 12 cases," *The American Journal of Surgical Pathology*, vol. 11, no. 8, pp. 606–617, 1987.

[10] W. J. Lee, C. H. Kim, S. E. Chang et al., "Cutaneous metastasis from large-cell neuroendocrine carcinoma of the urinary bladder expressing CK20 and TTF-1," *The American Journal of Dermatopathology*, vol. 31, no. 2, pp. 166–169, 2009.

[11] J. Wang, "Large cell neuroendocrine carcinoma of the urinary bladder: a pooled analysis," *Journal of Clinical Oncology*, vol. 32, article e15521, Supplement 15, 2014.

[12] H. Oshiro, K. Gomi, K. Nagahama et al., "Urinary cytologic features of primary large cell neuroendocrine carcinoma of the urinary bladder: a case report," *Acta Cytologica*, vol. 54, no. 3, pp. 303–310, 2010.

[13] A. Tsugu, M. Yoshiyama, and M. Matsumae, "Brain metastasis from large cell neuroendocrine carcinoma of the urinary bladder," *Surgical Neurology International*, vol. 2, no. 1, p. 84, 2011.

[14] M. Sroussi, M. Lorcet, M. P. Tardy et al., "Neuroendocrine carcinoma of the urinary bladder: a large analysis of the French GETUG consortium," *Annals of Oncology*, vol. 29, Supplement 8, pp. viii321–viii322, 2018.

[15] P. Dundr, M. Pesl, C. Povysil, I. Vitkova, and J. Dvoracek, "Large cell neuroendocrine carcinoma of the urinary bladder with lymphoepithelioma-like features," *Pathology, Research and Practice*, vol. 199, no. 8, pp. 559–563, 2003.

[16] Y. Li, J. E. Outman, and S. C. Mathur, "Carcinosarcoma with a large cell neuroendocrine epithelial component: first report of an unusual biphasic tumour of the urinary bladder," *Journal of Clinical Pathology*, vol. 57, no. 3, pp. 318–320, 2004.

[17] A. J. Evans, J. Al-Maghrabi, J. Tsihlias, G. Lajoie, J. M. Sweet, and W. B. Chapman, "Primary large cell neuroendocrine carcinoma of the urinary bladder," *Archives of Pathology & Laboratory Medicine*, vol. 126, no. 10, pp. 1229–1232, 2002.

[18] S. Hailemariam, A. Gaspert, P. Komminoth, P. Tamboli, and M. Amin, "Primary, pure, large-cell neuroendocrine carcinoma of the urinary bladder," *Modern Pathology*, vol. 11, no. 10, pp. 1016–1020, 1998.

[19] F. Alijo Serrano, N. Sanchez-Mora, J. Angel Arranz, C. Hernandez, and E. Alvarez-Fernandez, "Large cell and small cell neuroendocrine bladder carcinoma," *American Journal of Clinical Pathology*, vol. 128, no. 5, pp. 733–739, 2007.

[20] S. Akamatsu, S. Kanamaru, M. Ishihara, T. Sano, A. Soeda, and K. Hashimoto, "Primary large cell neuroendocrine carcinoma of the urinary bladder," *International Journal of Urology*, vol. 15, no. 12, pp. 1080–1083, 2008.

[21] V. Chong, J. Zwi, F. Hanning, R. Lim, and A. Williams, "A case of large cell neuroendocrine carcinoma of the bladder with prolonged spontaneous remission," *Journal of Surgical Case Reports*, vol. 2017, no. 5, pp. 1–4, 2017.

[22] P. Abenoza, C. Manivel, and R. K. Sibley, "Adenocarcinoma with neuroendocrine differentiation of the urinary bladder. Clinicopathologic, immunohistochemical, and ultrastructural study," *Archives of Pathology & Laboratory Medicine*, vol. 110, no. 11, pp. 1062–1066, 1986.

[23] I. J. Martin, D. G. Vilar, J. M. Aguado et al., "Large cell neuroendocrine carcinoma of the urinary bladder. Bibliographic review," *Archivos Españoles de Urología*, vol. 64, no. 2, pp. 105–113, 2011.

[24] L. Ghervan, A. Zaharie, B. Ene, and F. I. Elec, "Small-cell carcinoma of the urinary bladder: where do we stand?," *Medicine and Pharmacy Reports*, vol. 90, no. 1, pp. 13–17, 2017.

[25] M. L. Quek, P. W. Nichols, J. Yamzon et al., "Radical cystectomy for primary neuroendocrine tumors of the bladder: the university of southern California experience," *The Journal of Urology*, vol. 174, no. 1, pp. 93–96, 2005.

[26] Q. Niu, Y. Lu, S. Xu et al., "Clinicopathological characteristics and survival outcomes of bladder neuroendocrine carcinomas : a population-based study," *Cancer Management and Research*, vol. 10, pp. 4479–4489, 2018.

[27] F. Sanguedolce, B. Calò, M. Chirico, S. Tortorella, G. Carrieri, and L. Cormio, "Urinary tract large cell neuroendocrine carcinoma: diagnostic, prognostic and therapeutic issues," *Anticancer Research*, vol. 40, no. 5, pp. 2439–2447, 2020.

[28] H. Moch, P. A. Humphrey, T. M. Ulbright, and V. E. Reuter, "WHO classification of tumours of the urinary system and male genital organs," *World Heal Organ Classifcation Tumours*, vol. 70, pp. 106–119, 2016.

# 37

# A Rare Case of Urinary Tract Fungal Ball Leading to Fungemia and Bilateral Chorioretinitis

**Christopher Ferari, Chad Crigger, and Chad Morley**

*Department of Urology, West Virginia University School of Medicine, Morgantown, WV 26505, USA*

Correspondence should be addressed to Chad Crigger; chad.crigger@hsc.wvu.edu

Academic Editor: David Duchene

*Background.* Fungemia due to obstructive urinary tract fungal ball is exceedingly rare. These patients often have multiple predisposing conditions, including diabetes or antimicrobial exposure. While candiduria can be relatively common in this population, urinary tract fungal balls are a rare entity. Hospitalists should be aware of this rare complication in patients presenting with funguria. *Case Presentation.* We present a case of a 44-year-old male with type II diabetes, chronic hepatitis C secondary to injection drug use, and chronic kidney disease who developed a urinary tract fungal ball leading to fungemia and subsequent bilateral chorioretinitis, additionally complicated by emphysematous cystitis and pyelonephritis. Additional invasive treatment options beyond typical antifungals are often required in the case of urinary tract fungal ball, and in this case, bilateral nephrostomy tubes and micafungin were employed. Hospital course was complicated by *C. tropicalis* fungemia with subsequent bilateral fungal chorioretinitis on dilated fundus exam. This was effectively treated with cyclogyl and prednisolone drops along with bilateral voriconazole injections. Follow-up imaging and cultures showed resolution of fungemia, urinary tract masses, and chorioretinal infiltrates; however, recurrent polymicrobial UTIs continue to be an issue for this patient. *Conclusions.* Special multidisciplinary management is required in the treatment of urinary tract fungal balls with subsequent fungemia, including nephrostomy tubes, antifungal irrigation, ureterorenoscopy, and more powerful antifungals such as amphotericin B and 5-flucytosine. This management draws from a myriad of specialties, including urology, infectious disease, and interventional radiology. Additionally, the literature has demonstrated that only approximately half of patients with fungemia receive an ophthalmologic evaluation. Ophthalmologic and urologic cooperation is essential in the case of obstructive uropathy leading to fungemia as the obstructive uropathy must be relieved and these patients should receive a dilated fundus exam.

## 1. Introduction

Funguria is a common finding in hospitalized patients, most notably in the intensive care unit where patients often have multiple predisposing factors such as diabetes mellitus, indwelling catheters, and frequent antimicrobial exposure [1]. Studies have demonstrated a significant prevalence of candiduria in this population ranging from 1.6% to over 20% [2–4]. A urinary tract fungal ball, however, is rare in these patients. We report a case of emphysematous cystitis and pyelonephritis secondary to funguria originating from coexisting bladder and ureteral fungal balls leading to bilateral fungal chorioretinitis.

## 2. Case Presentation

A 44-year-old male with type II diabetes, chronic hepatitis C secondary to injection drug use, and chronic kidney disease presented to our facility as a transfer for suspected emphysematous pyelonephritis. This was initially demonstrated at an outside facility one month prior, at which time a left ureteral stent was placed. Symptoms at presentation included severe left flank and abdominal pain with pneumaturia, hematuria, fevers, and diarrhea. Immediate workup revealed a glucose of 647 mg/dL, hemoglobin A1c of 11.1%, and urine leukocytosis. Antibiotic therapy initially consisted of broad-spectrum meropenem 1 g and linezolid 600 mg,

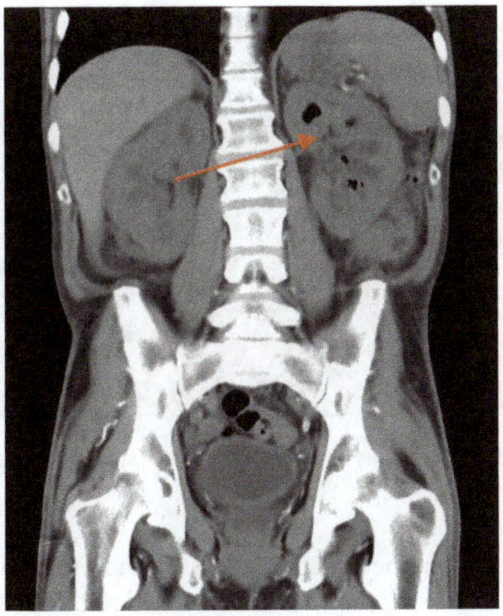

FIGURE 1: Coronal CT image showing evidence of emphysematous pyelonephritis (red arrow).

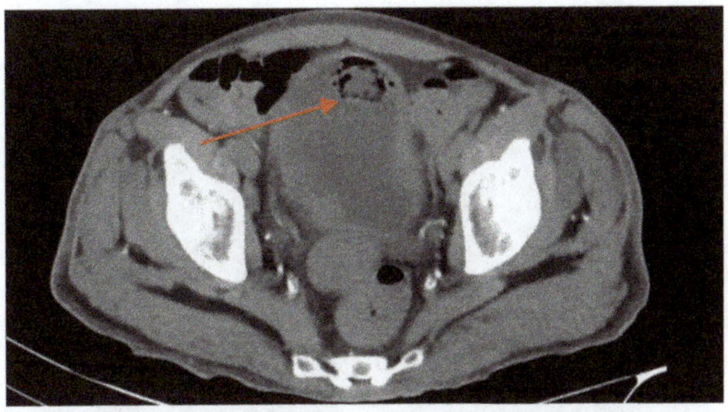

FIGURE 2: Transverse abdominal CT image showing evidence of bladder fungal ball with emphysematous cystitis (red arrow).

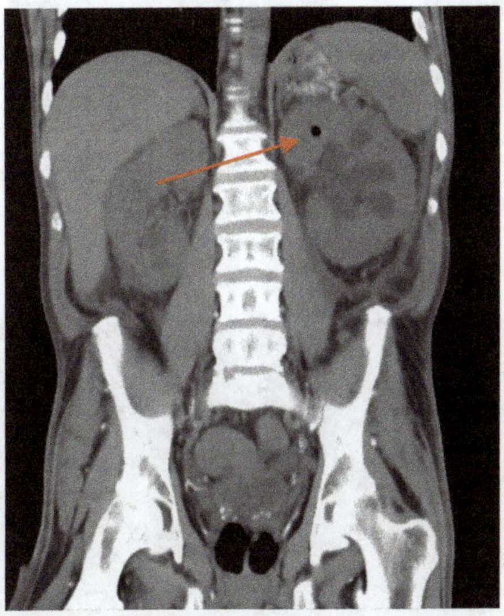

FIGURE 3: Coronal CT image showing evidence of diminished emphysematous pyelonephritis (red arrow) compared to Figure 1.

which was switched to fluconazole 200 mg and ertapenem 1 g per infectious disease (ID) recommendations after urine culture grew pan-sensitive *Candida tropicalis*. No bacteria were detected on urine culture.

Cross-sectional imaging revealed bilateral hydronephrosis with significant air in the left renal collecting system as well as concern for emphysematous cystitis with a lesion in the bladder (Figures 1 and 2). He was transferred to our facility 3 days later after repeat imaging showed decreased air in the left renal collecting system and the presence of a new hyperdensity in the left proximal ureter concerning for a fungal ball (Figures 3 and 4). Urine culture once again grew *C. tropicalis*, and antimicrobial therapy was changed to IV micafungin 100 mg. Again, no bacteria were detected on urine culture. Physical exam was noteworthy for bilateral flank pain and significant penile pain. He endorsed methamphetamine and marijuana use, and urine drug screen was positive for opiates and oxycodone.

Per urology recommendations, bilateral nephrostomy tubes were placed on the day of transfer and ID deescalated antifungals to fluconazole 200 mg. However, the patient's blood cultures grew *C. tropicalis* on day 3, which prevented his discharge at this time and prompted an escalation of antifungal therapy back to IV micafungin 150 mg. Ophthalmology was consulted per ID recommendations, and dilated fundus exam showed exudates suspicious for fungal chorioretinitis (Figures 5 and 6). Vision symptoms at this time included worsening of ongoing blurry vision as well as occasional black spots in his field of vision. Cyclogyl 1% and prednisolone 1% drops were started, with bilateral voriconazole 100 mcg intravitreal injections performed on day 6. The patient was discharged on day 11 in stable condition with bilateral nephrostomy tubes in place and a six-week course of PO voriconazole 200 mg bid.

Follow-up CT imaging one month after discharge showed resolution of emphysematous cystitis and pyelonephritis. Ophthalmology follow-up showed fading chorioretinal infiltrates. His recovery was complicated by an episode of *C. difficile* colitis three weeks after initial discharge, adequately treated with vancomycin. Since this discharge, the patient has had recurrent polymicrobial UTI issues, growing *Pseudomonas* and methicillin-resistant *S. aureus* (MRSA) on several occasions, some requiring readmission. At a future admission three months after discharge for nephrostomy exchange, nephrostomy cultures grew *Pseudomonas*, which was adequately treated. No further nephrostomy complications were encountered.

## 3. Discussion

Reports of a urinary tract fungal ball leading to separate findings of fungemia, emphysematous pyelonephritis and cystitis, and bilateral fungal chorioretinitis are rare in the literature [5–8]. This patient's urine cultures were negative for bacteria and positive for only *C. tropicalis*, which has been shown to be a gas producer in the literature [9]. We know that diabetes mellitus is a risk factor for

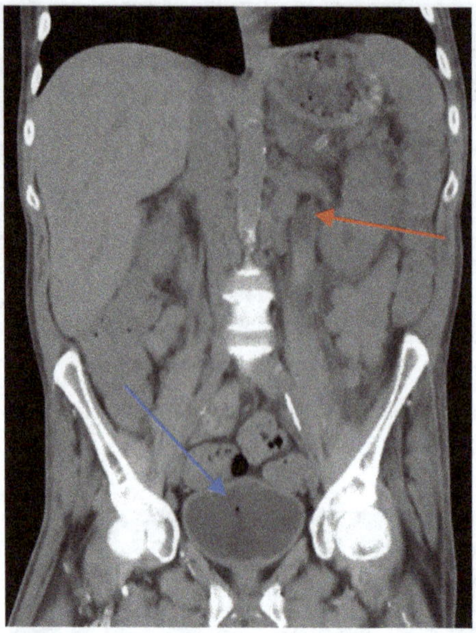

FIGURE 4: Coronal CT image showing evidence of ureteral fungal ball (red arrow) and emphysematous cystitis (blue arrow).

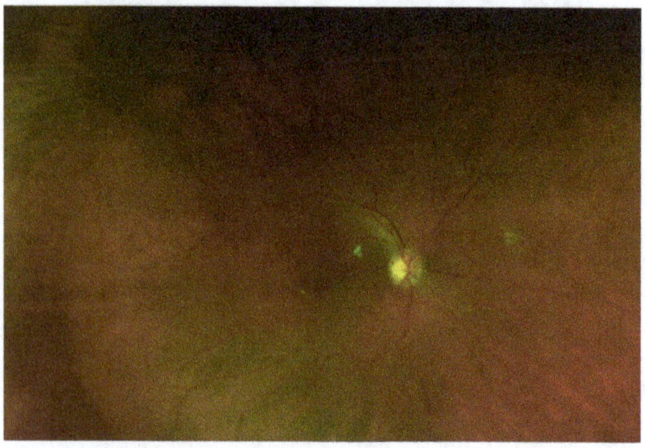

FIGURE 5: Right fundus showing exudates suspicious for fungal chrioretinitis.

emphysematous urinary tract infections [10, 11] and thus could have contributed to this patient's infection. In a retrospective review of patients with candidemia, only 51% of patients were evaluated by an ophthalmologist, of which evidence of ocular candidiasis was present in 12.5% [12]. It is clear that involvement of ophthalmology in cases of fungemia due to urinary tract fungal ball is critical, even with no ocular symptoms present. In lieu of typical first-line antifungals such as fluconazole, urinary tract fungal balls require special multidisciplinary management like nephrostomy tubes, antifungal irrigation, ureterorenoscopy, and more powerful antifungals such as amphotericin B and 5-flucytosine [5, 13–15]. Although chronic echinocandins are not thought of as good drugs for the urinary tract, there are case series and case reports of successful treatment of Candida species with micafungin while subsequently avoiding the toxicity of the previously mentioned antifungals such as amphotericin B [16–18]. Radiologic diagnosis of fungal balls is difficult as they can be mimicked by more common red herrings such as blood clots or inflammatory debris; however, an intraluminal defect coupled with air can be a clue [19].

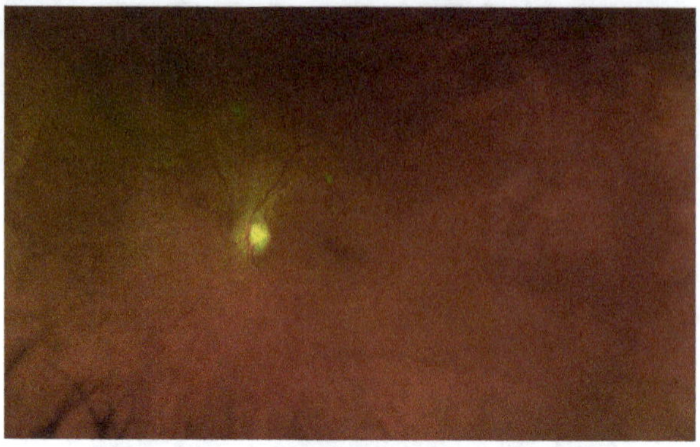

FIGURE 6: Left fundus showing exudates suspicious for fungal chrioretinitis.

One of our strengths in the treatment of this case included a relatively early ophthalmology consult in order to prevent future vision complications. An example of a limitation in our approach was the possible deescalation of antifungals too early, as blood cultures were subsequently positive. Hospitalists should be aware of the rare complications of funguria presented here and should not hesitate to involve urology, ophthalmology, and infectious disease specialists when concerning symptoms arise.

## Abbreviations

ID: Infectious disease
UTI: Urinary tract infection
MRSA: Methicillin-resistant *S. aureus.*

## Authors' Contributions

CF was the primary manuscript author and performed a literature search. CC was the secondary manuscript author and primary manuscript editor and participated in the patient's care. CM was responsible for the conception of the case report and participated in the patient's care.

## References

[1] J. D. Sobel, J. F. Fisher, C. A. Kauffman, and C. A. Newman, "Candida urinary tract infections–epidemiology," *Clinical Infectious Diseases*, vol. 52, supplement_6, pp. S433–S436, 2011.

[2] Z. He, Y. Liu, T. Wang, Y. Cheng, J. Chen, and F. Wang, "Candiduria in hospitalized patients: an investigation with the Sysmex UF-1000i urine analyzer," *PeerJ*, vol. 7, article e6935, 2019.

[3] M. Gharaghani, S. Taghipour, M. Halvaeezadeh, and A. Z. Mahmoudabadi, "Candiduria; a review article with specific data from Iran," *Türk Üroloji Dergisi/Turkish Journal of Urology*, vol. 44, no. 6, pp. 445–452, 2018.

[4] C. C. B. A. Kobayashi, O. de Fátima Lisboa Fernandes, K. C. Miranda, E. D. de Sousa, and M. do Rosário Rodrigues Silva, "Candiduria in hospital patients: a study prospective," *Mycopathologia*, vol. 158, no. 1, pp. 49–52, 2004.

[5] O. A. Abdeljaleel, I. Alnadhari, S. Mahmoud et al., "Treatment of renal fungal ball with fluconazole instillation through a nephrostomy tube: case report and literature review," *American Journal of Case Reports*, vol. 19, pp. 1179–1183, 2018.

[6] L. Wang, X. Ji, G.-F. Sun et al., "Fungus ball and emphysematous cystitis secondary to Candida tropicalis: a case report," *Canadian Urological Association Journal*, vol. 9, no. 9-10, pp. 683–E686, 2015.

[7] C. V. Comiter, M. McDonald, J. Minton, and S. V. Yalla, "Fungal bezoar and bladder rupture secondary to Candida tropicalis," *Canadian Urological Association Journal*, vol. 47, no. 3, pp. 439–441, 1996.

[8] J. Stein, S. Latz, J. Ellinger et al., "Fungaemia caused by obstructive renal Candida bezoars leads to bilateral chorioretinitis: a case report," *BMC Urology*, vol. 18, no. 1, p. 21, 2018.

[9] C. Suntara, A. Cherdthong, S. Uriyapongson, M. Wanapat, and P. Chanjula, "Comparison effects of ruminal Crabtree-negative yeasts and Crabtree-positive yeasts for improving ensiled rice straw quality and ruminal digestion using in vitro gas production," *Journal of Fungi*, vol. 6, no. 3, p. 109, 2020.

[10] D. A. El Rahman, G. Zanetti, M. Ferruti et al., "Emphysematous pyelonephritis in decompensated diabetes: a case report and review of the literature," *Archivio Italiano di Urologia e Andrologia*, vol. 83, no. 2, pp. 108–111, 2011.

[11] H. Yashima, M. Terasaki, H. Kushima, and T. Hirano, "Emphysematous cystitis in an elderly Japanese patient with type 2 diabetes mellitus," *Clinical Case Reports*, vol. 7, no. 3, pp. 585-586, 2019.

[12] A. Khalid, L. A. Clough, R. C. A. Symons, J. D. Mahnken, L. Dong, and A. J. Eid, "Incidence and clinical predictors of ocular candidiasis in patients with *Candida* fungemia," *Interdisciplinary Perspectives on Infectious Diseases*, vol. 2014, Article ID 650235, 6 pages, 2014.

[13] W. P. Tan, U. C. Turba, and L. A. Deane, "Renal fungus ball: a challenging clinical problem," *Urologia Journal*, vol. 84, no. 2, pp. 113–115, 2017.

[14] A. L. Alkalay, I. Srugo, C. Blifeld, M. S. Komaiko, and J. J. Pomerance, "Noninvasive medical management of fungus ball uropathy in a premature infant," *American Journal of Perinatology*, vol. 8, no. 5, pp. 330–332, 1991.

[15] M. Abuelnaga, S. Khoshzaban, M. Reda Badr, and A. Chaudry, "Successful endoscopic management of a renal fungal ball using flexible ureterorenoscopy," *Case Reports in Urology*, vol. 2019, Article ID 9241928, 4 pages, 2019.

[16] S. Grau, S. Luque, D. Echeverría-Esnal et al., "Urinary micafungin levels are sufficient to treat urinary tract infections caused by Candida spp," *International Journal of Antimicrobial Agents*, vol. 48, no. 2, pp. 212–214, 2016.

[17] S. Gabardi, S. Martin, M. Sura, A. Mohammed, and Y. Golan, "Micafungin treatment and eradication of candiduria among hospitalized patients," *International Urology and Nephrology*, vol. 48, no. 11, pp. 1881–1885, 2016.

[18] D. Lagrotteria, C. Rotstein, and C. H. Lee, "Treatment of candiduria with micafungin: a case series," *Canadian Journal of Infectious Diseases and Medical Microbiology*, vol. 18, no. 2, p. 150, 2007.

[19] G. Di Paola, A. Mogorovich, G. Fiorini, M. G. Cuttano, F. Manassero, and C. Selli, "*Candida* bezoars with urinary tract obstruction in two women without immunocompromising conditions," *The Scientific World Journal*, vol. 11, Article ID 549160, 1172 pages, 2011.

# Pathologic Complete Response to Neoadjuvant Nivolumab/Ipilimumab in a Patient with Metastatic Renal Cell Carcinoma

**Taylor C. Peak**[1] **Elena M. Fenu**[2] **Michael B. Rothberg**[1] **Christopher Y. Thomas**[3] **Ronald L. Davis**[1] **and Edward A. Levine**[4]

[1]*Department of Urology, Wake Forest Baptist Medical Center, Winston-Salem, NC, USA*
[2]*Department of Pathology, Wake Forest Baptist Medical Center, Winston-Salem NC, USA*
[3]*Department of Medical Oncology and Hematology, Wake Forest Baptist Medical Center, Winston-Salem NC, USA*
[4]*Surgical Oncology Service, Department of General Surgery, Wake Forest Baptist Medical Center, Winston-Salem, NC, USA*

Correspondence should be addressed to Edward A. Levine; elevine@wakehealth.edu

Academic Editor: Apul Goel

Nivolumab plus ipilimumab represents an effective combination of checkpoint inhibitors that can lead to a durable response with minimal toxicity in patients with metastatic renal cell carcinoma (mRCC). We present a case of a pathologic complete response to neoadjuvant nivolumab plus ipilimumab in a patient with a 13.9 cm left renal mass and significant retroperitoneal and iliac lymphadenopathy, classified as intermediate-risk mRCC. We discuss and review the literature on complete responses after systemic therapy and the ability to predict who has undergone a complete response in the face of residual radiographic evidence of disease.

## 1. Background

With the advent of targeted immunotherapy and checkpoint inhibitors, the treatment of metastatic renal cell carcinoma (mRCC) has undergone a paradigm shift. Only two decades ago, interleukin-2 and interferon alpha-2b were the only available options, both of which had only modest success with significant toxicity. The field has changed substantially since that time, first with tyrosine kinase inhibitors (TKIs) and now more recently with checkpoint inhibitors. In addition to advancements in targeted therapies, our understanding of prognostic factors has also progressed. The more recent International Metastatic Renal Cell Carcinoma Database Consortium (IMDC) prognostic criteria have been validated in the setting of targeted therapy and represent the most reliable tool to stratify patients for treatment [1, 2].

Of the checkpoint inhibitors developed, nivolumab represents one that has demonstrated remarkable clinical efficacy [3]. It is a monoclonal antibody that binds to and blocks the programmed cell death (PD-1) protein, preventing PDL-1 from binding and inactivating T cell activity. Ipilimumab, likewise, is a monoclonal antibody that targets cytotoxic T-lymphocyte-associated protein 4 (CTLA-4) [3]. By binding to this protein, it blocks the inhibitory signal that would otherwise turn off the cytotoxic activity of T lymphocytes. More recently with their proven role as first-line therapy for intermediate- and poor-risk mRCC, case reports are emerging that demonstrate that a complete response is possible. We report a case from our institution of a pathologic complete response to neoadjuvant nivolumab plus ipilimumab in a patient with mRCC and residual radiographic disease.

## 2. Case Presentation

The patient is a 66-year-old man with history of hypertension, stroke, and deep vein thromboses, who initially presented in October of 2018 with a cough that was subsequently evaluated with a CT of the chest. There was a 13.9 cm incidentally noted left renal mass concerning for renal cell carcinoma (Figure 1(a)). Upon further work-up, he was noted to have

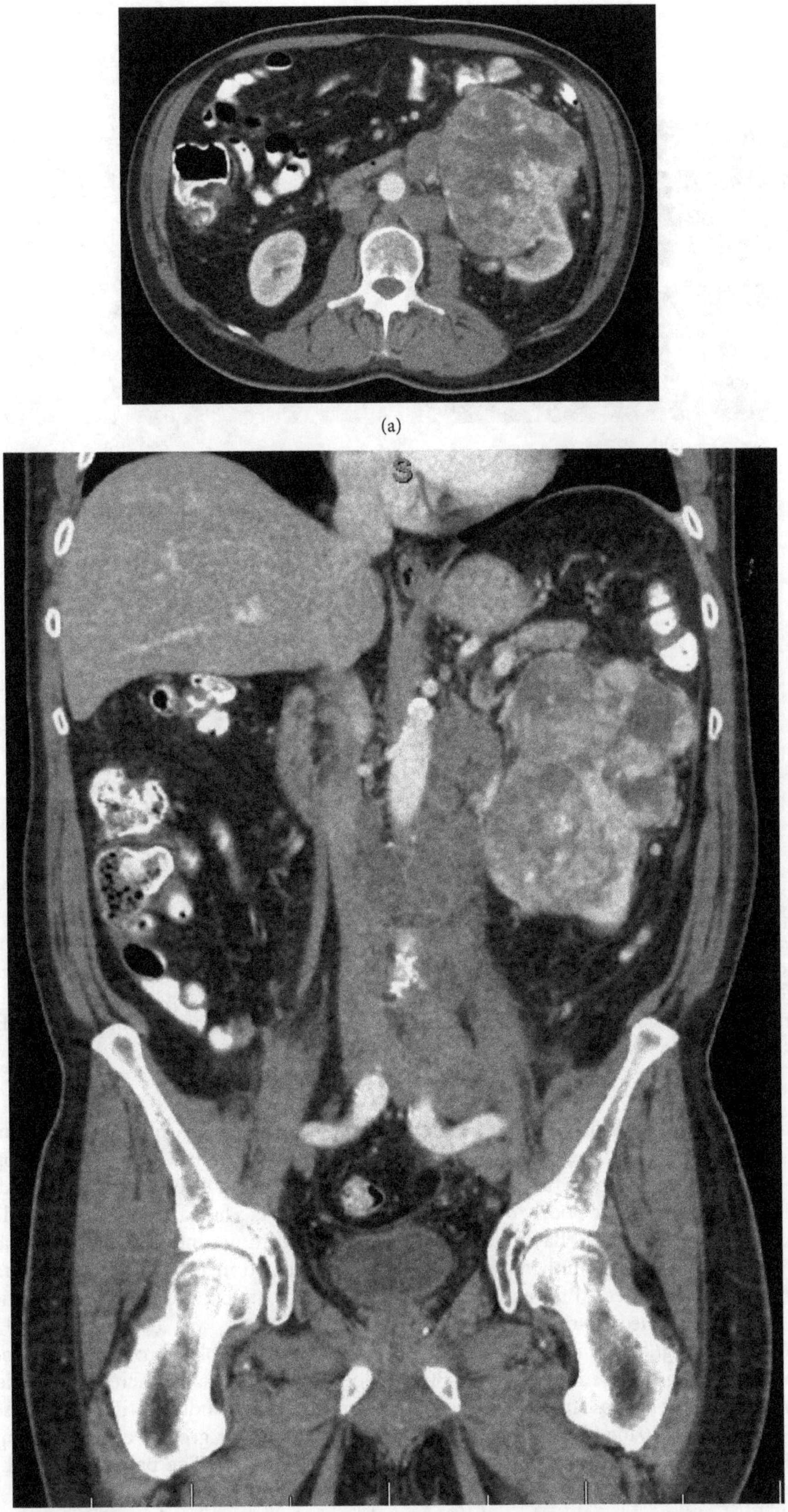

(a)

(b)

Figure 1: CT imaging prior to nivolumab/ipilimumab treatment: (a) axial imaging demonstrating the heterogeneously enhancing left renal mass; (b) coronal imaging demonstrating the enlarged retroperitoneal lymphadenopathy.

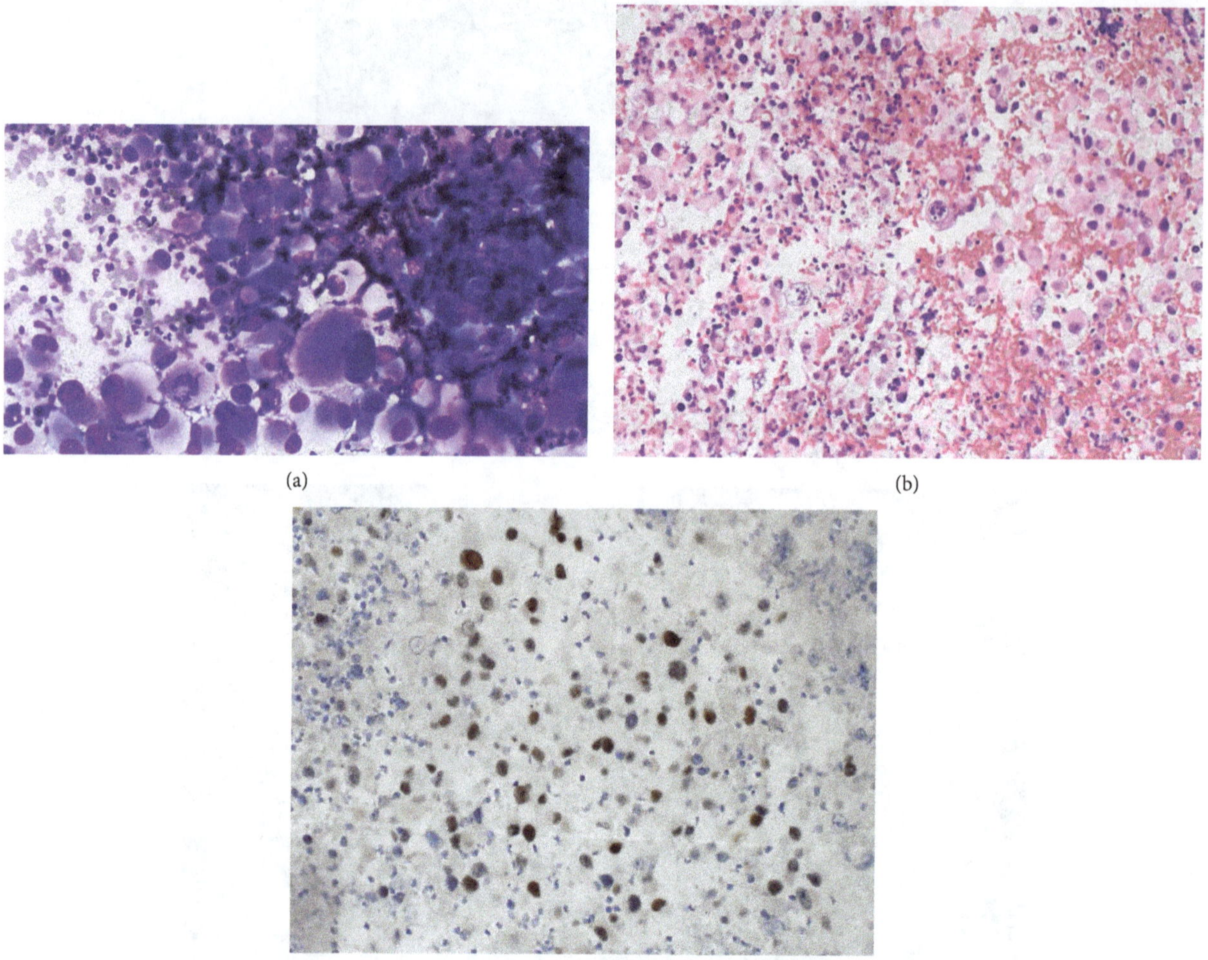

FIGURE 2: Fine needle aspiration from retroperitoneal lymph node biopsy. (a) Cytologic preparation (40x magnification) showing abundant large, pleomorphic tumor cells consistent with renal cell carcinoma. Small lymphocytes and neutrophils are present in the background for scale. (b) Cell block (20x magnification) demonstrating tumor cells with significant nuclear pleomorphism. Some cells have rhabdoid features with an eccentric nucleus and abundant eosinophilic cytoplasm. (c) PAX8 immunohistochemical staining is positive in the tumor cells, highlighting the renal origin.

significant retroperitoneal and iliac lymphadenopathy, the largest measuring 6.4 cm (Figure 1(b)). He underwent a biopsy of the retroperitoneal lymph nodes in November 2018 which was consistent with metastatic poorly differentiated renal cell carcinoma (Figures 2(a)–2(c)). Based on a performance status of <80% and eventual system therapy within one year of diagnosis, he was considered to have an IMDC risk score of 2, and as such intermediate-risk disease. He was started on nivolumab (3 mg/kg IV infused over 30 minutes) plus ipilimumab (1 mg/kg IV infused over 30 minutes) every three weeks for four cycles. This was followed up with a single agent nivolumab (240 mg IV infused) every 2 weeks for 12 cycles. There were no reported adverse events while on systemic therapy. Follow-up imaging revealed a significant decrease in disease burden with only subcentimeter retroperitoneal lymphadenopathy and shrinkage of the primary tumor to 9.5 cm (Figures 3(a) and 3(b)).

In October of 2019, the tumor was deemed surgically resectable. He was thus taken to the operating room for a complete resection. A midline laparotomy incision was used for the intraperitoneal approach. Intraoperatively, the tail of the pancreas and spleen were both fixed to the anterior surface of Gerota's fascia, thus requiring a distal pancreatectomy and splenectomy. Inferiorly, the descending mesocolon was found encased in the fibrotic mass, necessitating ligation of the inferior mesenteric artery and resection of the mesentery. The left kidney was eventually freed of its attachments through remarkably fibrotic tissue planes and removed, en bloc with the distal pancreas and spleen. Because of the immunotherapy-induced tissue response, there was no way of differentiating grossly enlarged lymph nodes from surrounding fibrosis. The patient did well postoperatively and was discharged on postoperative day nine. Pathology of the specimen returned as having no identifiable residual tumor present, with only extensive fibrosis, necrosis, chronic inflammation, hemorrhage, and edema (Figure 4). There was one renal hilar lymph node identified in the specimen, and it was negative for tumor as well. Immunotherapy was

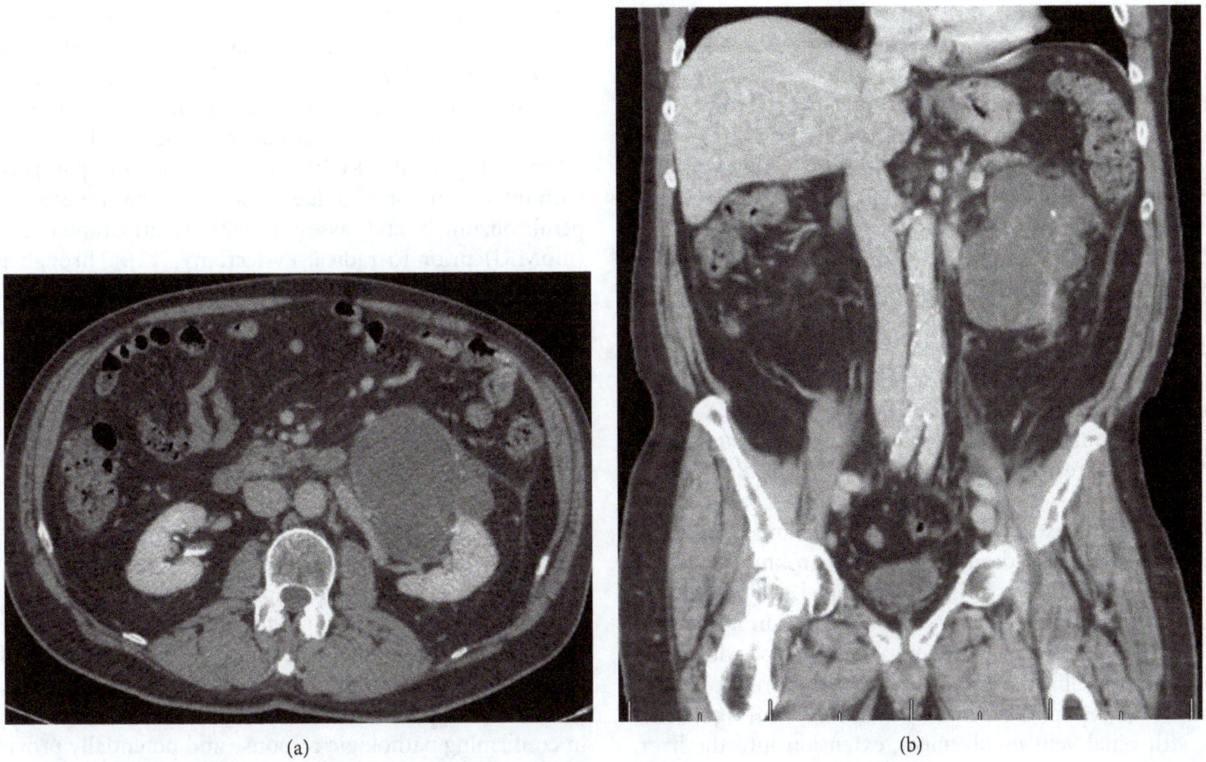

FIGURE 3: CT imaging after nivolumab/ipilimumab treatment: (a) axial imaging demonstrating significant decrease in size of the renal mass; (b) coronal imaging demonstrating resolution of the bulky retroperitoneal lymphadenopathy.

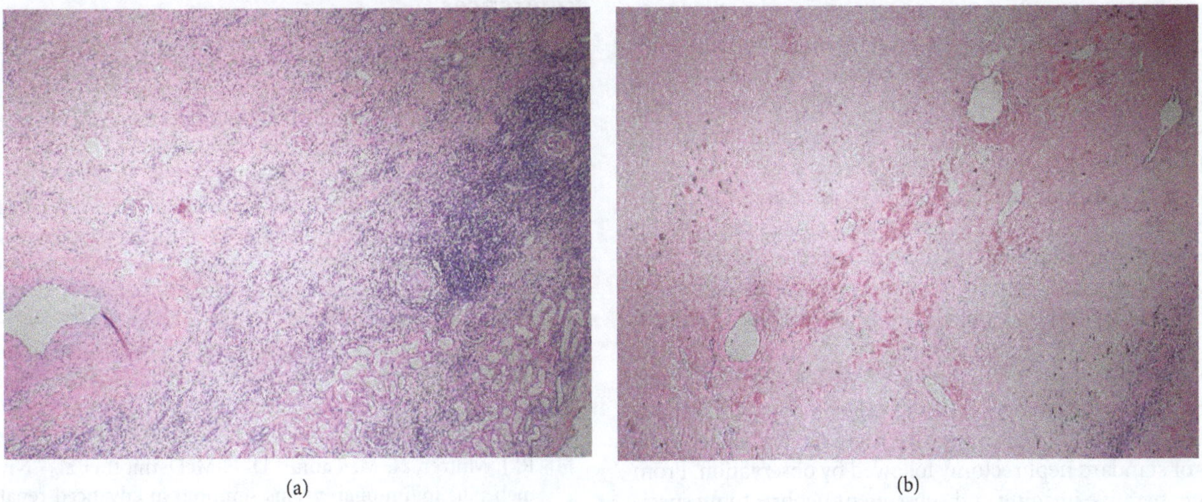

FIGURE 4: Final pathologic analyses of resected tumor specimen. (a) Resected tumor showing treatment effect (4x magnification). Large parts of the lesion are replaced by fibrosis with infiltrating lymphocytes. The relationship to normal viable kidney parenchyma is shown in the bottom right corner. (b) Resected tumor (4x magnification) demonstrating that the center of the lesion is entirely necrotic. No viable tumor cells remain.

discontinued after surgery. Follow-up imaging with CT chest, abdomen, and pelvis revealed no evidence of disease recurrence at 8 months postoperatively.

## 3. Discussion

Our case not only offers further support for the role of immunotherapy as first-line therapy for mRCC but also uniquely demonstrates that even a partial radiographic response may, in fact, represent a complete pathologic response at the time of radical nephrectomy. Obtaining such a response to systemic therapy has been an elusive goal for locally advanced or mRCC. The CheckMate 214 trial demonstrated that nivolumab plus ipilimumab led to improved overall survival in comparison to sunitinib in intermediate- and poor-risk patients with metastatic renal cell carcinoma

[4]. The objective response rate was 42% versus 20% ($p < 0.001$), and the *complete* response rate was 9% versus 1% for combination nivolumab/ipilimumab and single agent sunitinib, respectively. It is important to note, however, that unlike our patient who received immunotherapy in the neoadjuvant setting, over 80% of patients in the CheckMate 214 trial had already undergone a radical nephrectomy prior to receiving immunotherapy. Additionally, another 10% of patients in the trial had undergone radiotherapy. Therefore, the majority of patients with a complete response was based on radiographic evidence of disease regression. In contrast, the case presented here, in which there is only a partial radiographic response but subsequent complete pathologic response, represents a rare clinical entity.

There are only a few case reports demonstrating a complete pathologic response after neoadjuvant immunotherapy. In Shirotake et al., a patient with an 8.5 cm left renal tumor with multiple metastases to the brain, lung, and para-aortic lymph nodes progressed on pazopanib, everolimus, and axitinib, before starting fourth-line nivolumab [5]. This resulted in a complete response that was followed by surgical resection which found a pathologic complete response with tissue remarkable for fibrotic and lymphocyte-infiltrated tissues. Ikarashi et al. reported on a patient with a 9.7 cm right renal mass with renal vein involvement, extension into the liver, and multiple lung nodules [6]. She was started on nivolumab, and repeat imaging subsequently revealed resolution of the lung metastases and a response of the primary tumor. A radical nephrectomy and partial hepatectomy were performed, with pathology revealing no viable cancer cells. In Singla et al., the authors reported on a series of 11 patients with intermediate- or poor-risk disease who received neoadjuvant nivolumab or nivolumab plus ipilimumab and subsequently underwent nephrectomy [7]. Of these patients, only one was found to be pT0 on final pathology.

With mounting data that the new immune checkpoint inhibitors can lead to a complete pathologic response, it remains unclear if there are radiographic or histologic factors that could predict this prior to undergoing a nephrectomy. Further studies, such as the PROSPER trial (EA8143), may help determine which patients could avoid a radical nephrectomy and the associated morbidity. In this phase 3 study, patients with clinical stage ≥ T2 or node-positive RCC will be randomized to either perioperative nivolumab and nephrectomy or standard nephrectomy followed by observation. From the preoperative imaging and subsequent nephrectomy specimens in the treatment arm, clinicians might learn what factors predict a complete response.

This will undoubtedly be challenging as radiographic response patterns can be quite variable for tumors treated with immunotherapy. Specifically, immunotherapies can lead to a phenomenon known as "pseudoprogression," where there is initial radiographic progression followed by a response or stabilization [8]. Because the standard RECIST criteria would not apply to this tumor response pattern, other imaging modalities have been studied. 18F-FDG PET/CT scans, for example, have been shown to be highly accurate in predicting a response in patients treated with immunotherapy for metastatic melanoma and non-small cell lung cancer [9, 10]. Diffusion-weighted imaging may also hold promise as there is evidence that growing tumors demonstrate restricted diffusion because of high cellularity, whereas inflammation and necrosis tumors show increased diffusion because of prominent extracellular edema and decreased cellularity [11]. In the PURE-01 study, for example, patients with muscle-invasive bladder cancer were given neoadjuvant pembrolizumab and assessed with multiparametric MRI (mpMRI) prior to radical cystectomy [12]. Through their preliminary work, criteria were developed using mpMRI to accurately and reproducibly predict a complete pathologic response.

## 4. Conclusion

In conclusion, nivolumab plus ipilimumab remains the first-line therapy for patients with poor- or intermediate-risk mRCC. Even a partial radiographic response after therapy may actually represent a complete pathologic response that would obviate the need for cytoreductive surgery. However, until we have more data to confidently predict who is effectively cured in the face of residual disease on imaging, we must counsel patients on the role of cytoreductive surgery in confirming pathologic response and potentially providing improved survival.

## References

[1] D. Y. C. Heng, W. Xie, M. M. Regan et al., "Prognostic factors for overall survival in patients with metastatic renal cell carcinoma treated with vascular endothelial growth factor-targeted agents: results from a large, multicenter study," *Journal of Clinical Oncology*, vol. 27, no. 34, pp. 5794–5799, 2009.

[2] D. Y. C. Heng, W. Xie, M. M. Regan et al., "External validation and comparison with other models of the International Metastatic Renal-Cell Carcinoma Database Consortium prognostic model: a population-based study," *The Lancet Oncology*, vol. 14, no. 2, pp. 141–148, 2013.

[3] K. M. Hargadon, C. E. Johnson, and C. J. Williams, "Immune checkpoint blockade therapy for cancer: an overview of FDA-approved immune checkpoint inhibitors," *International Immunopharmacology*, vol. 62, pp. 29–39, 2018.

[4] R. J. Motzer, N. M. Tannir, D. F. McDermott et al., "Nivolumab plus ipilimumab versus sunitinib in advanced renal-cell carcinoma," *The New England Journal of Medicine*, vol. 378, no. 14, pp. 1277–1290, 2018.

[5] S. Shirotake, G. Kaneko, K. Nagata, M. Oyama, and K. Nishimoto, "Histological complete response with nivolumab for renal cell carcinoma with multiple metastases: a case report," *Molecular and Clinical Oncology*, vol. 10, no. 2, pp. 244–248, 2019.

[6] D. Ikarashi, Y. Kato, H. Katagiri et al., "Case of complete response to neoadjuvant therapy using nivolumab in a patient with metastatic renal cell carcinoma," *International Journal of Urology*, vol. 25, no. 6, pp. 630–632, 2018.

[7] N. Singla, R. Elias, R. A. Ghandour et al., "Pathologic response and surgical outcomes in patients undergoing nephrectomy following receipt of immune checkpoint inhibitors for renal

cell carcinoma," *Urologic Oncology*, vol. 37, no. 12, pp. 924–931, 2019.

[8] H. Wei, H. Jiang, and B. Song, "Role of medical imaging for immune checkpoint blockade therapy: from response assessment to prognosis prediction," *Cancer Medicine*, vol. 8, no. 12, pp. 5399–5413, 2019.

[9] S. Y. Cho, E. J. Lipson, H. J. Im et al., "Prediction of response to immune checkpoint inhibitor therapy using early-time-point $^{18}$F-FDG PET/CT imaging in patients with advanced melanoma," *Journal of Nuclear Medicine*, vol. 58, no. 9, pp. 1421–1428, 2017.

[10] K. Kaira, T. Higuchi, I. Naruse et al., "Metabolic activity by $^{18}$F–FDG-PET/CT is predictive of early response after nivolumab in previously treated NSCLC," *European Journal of Nuclear Medicine and Molecular Imaging*, vol. 45, no. 1, pp. 56–66, 2018.

[11] L. Qin, X. Li, A. Stroiney et al., "Advanced MRI assessment to predict benefit of anti-programmed cell death 1 protein immunotherapy response in patients with recurrent glioblastoma," *Neuroradiology*, vol. 59, no. 2, pp. 135–145, 2017.

[12] A. Necchi, M. Bandini, G. Calareso et al., "Multiparametric magnetic resonance imaging as a noninvasive assessment of tumor response to neoadjuvant pembrolizumab in muscle-invasive bladder cancer: preliminary findings from the PURE-01 study," *European Urology*, vol. 77, no. 5, pp. 636–643, 2019.

39

# Management of Intrauterine Device Migrated into the Bladder: A Case Report and Literature Review

A. K. Paré,[1] A. Ouattara,[1] D. Yé,[1] B. Kabré,[1] A. Bako,[1] B. M. Abubakar,[2] and T. Kambou[1]

[1]*Department of Urology, Souro Sanou University Teaching Hospital, Bobo-Dioulasso, Burkina Faso*
[2]*Department of Surgery, Federal Medical Center, PMB 02, Nguru, Yobe State, Nigeria*

Correspondence should be addressed to A. K. Paré; boupare@yahoo.fr

Academic Editor: Yankai Xia

Intrauterine device represents the most reversible method of contraceptive worldwide. Its insertion is a medical procedure not free from complication. We report a rare case of intravesical migration of a copper intrauterine device inserted 18 months earlier in a 28-year-old multiparous woman. The patient presented with irritative lower urinary tract symptoms, and she was managed endoscopically. This case underscores the role of cystoscopy in irritative lower urinary tract symptoms post IUD insertion.

## 1. Introduction

Intrauterine device (IUD) is the commonest method of reversible contraception worldwide. It is used by approximately 14% of women due to its efficacy, safety, and low cost. There are two types of IUD, the hormonal IUD which releases levonorgestrel and the copper IUD (TCu 380A) which releases copper ions [1], the last one being the most available form and constitutes the fourth choice of IUD by women in childbearing age in Burkina Faso [2]. IUD is not free from complications; in fact, complication such as IUD migration is one the gynaecologist's challenges [3]. IUD migration is commonly into the abdominal cavity; however, migration into the adnexa, iliac vein, and broad ligament has been reported [4]. Intravesical migration is a rare complication of IUD [5]. We present a case of intravesical migration of TCu IUD inserted 18 months earlier in a 28-year-old multiparous woman presenting with irritative lower urinary tract symptoms. The migrated IUD was retrieved endoscopically via cystoscopy.

## 2. Case Presentation

This was a 28-year-old woman presenting with 1-month history of mainly irritative lower urinary tract symptoms, characterized by urinary urgency and frequency. The patient had a history of copper IUD (TCu 380A) placed 18 months earlier for contraceptive purpose. There was a past history of haematuria 1 year prior to presentation which was intermittent and terminal associated with clot but no necroturia. Haematuria was spontaneously resolved by excessive water intake. There was a history of amenorrhea according to the patient for 1 year and condom use during sexual intercourse. The clinical examination revealed tenderness in the hypogastric region and moderate inflammation of urethral meatus. The gynaecological examination was normal. Urine microscopy and culture were done and were negative for the infection. Abdominal and pelvic ultrasound showed hyperechoic intravesical lesion (Figure 1) in keeping with IUD. The diagnosis of IUD migration into the bladder was made. Laboratory investigations found normal values for serum creatinine, haemoglobin, and write blood cells.

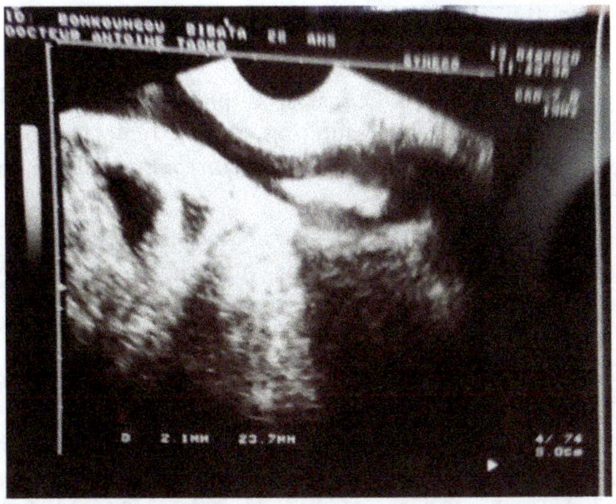

Figure 1: Hyperechoic image of intrauterine device in the bladder on pelvic ultrasonography.

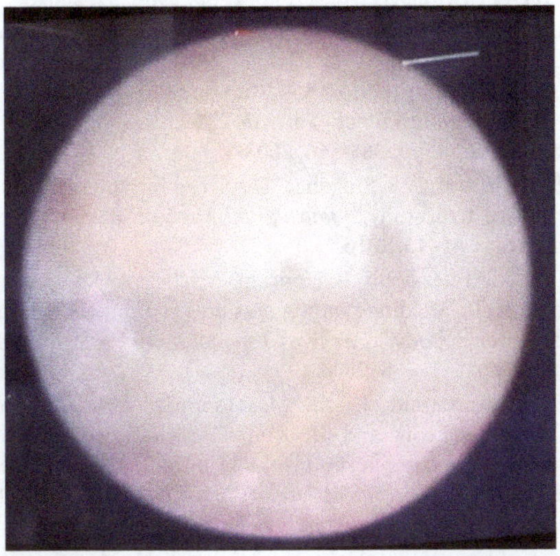

Figure 2: Cystoscopic vision of the intrauterine device with no damage to the bladder wall.

Cystoscopy was performed under local anaesthesia and antibiotic prophylaxis. The IUD was encrusted in the posterior bladder wall (Figure 2). The IUD was grasped with forceps and gently extracted (Figure 3) without any difficulty through the cystoscope (Figure 4). The postoperative management was uneventful. The patient was discharged the same day. She was seen 2 months post extraction with no any complaint. Pelvic ultrasound was done and was normal. Urine microscopy and culture were negative for the infection.

## 3. Discussion

Intrauterine device is the most popular method of reversible contraception in developing countries due to its efficiency and low cost [1, 2]. During the preinsertion counselling, patients are not often informed about rare complications such as intravesical migration of the device. Hence, IUD migration may lead to medicolegal issues [6].

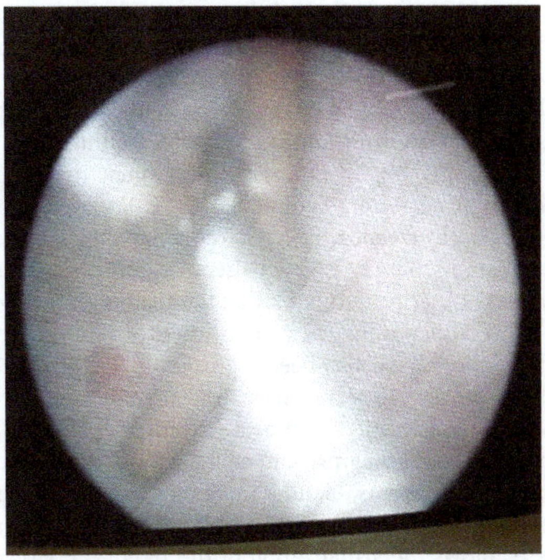

Figure 3: Intrauterine device grasped with forceps.

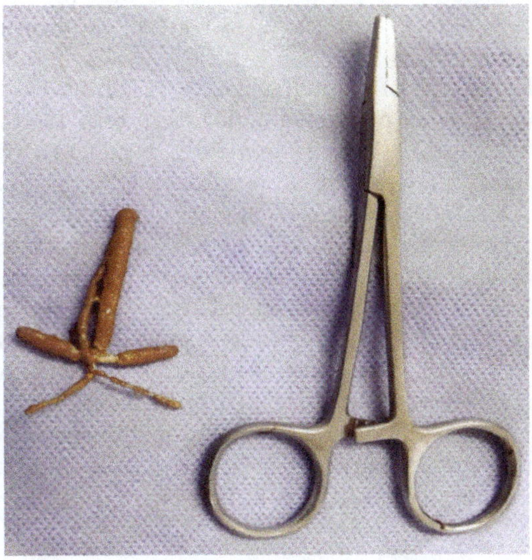

Figure 4: T-shaped intrauterine device completely extracted.

IUD migration into the structures adjacent to uterus is a rare complication with an estimated incidence of 1/1000 insertions [3]. The literature mainly mentions some case reports and case series [4–7]. Goyal et al. in India, in a study of 240 copper-bearing IUDs inserted during a 12-month period, had reported only 2 cases of migration, including intravesical migration [7]. This case is our first experience for a 5-year urology practice.

Its insertion is a medical procedure for which preinsertion counselling often mentions common complications such as spotting, heavy periods, pelvic pain, infection, and the possibility of pregnancy as well. However, complications such as IUD migration are rarely mentioned.

IUD migration usually occurs following partial or complete uterine perforation during insertion. This makes this complication commoner in scared myometrium from previous surgeries and misdiagnosed hypoplastic uterus, retroverted, or hyperanteverted uterus. The migration is aided by local inflammation caused by the copper IUD [1].

The clinical presentation of migrated IUD may be incidental discovery during routine evaluation without any previous symptoms [7]. In contrary, the patient may present with lower urinary tract symptoms (LUTS), mainly storage symptoms with urgency, urinary frequency, haematuria, or per vaginal discharge [8, 9]. Otherwise, urogenital fistula such as vesicouterine fistula may be the main presenting feature [10]. Bladder stones as complication of IUD migration into the bladder have also been reported causing obstructive (emptying phase) lower urinary tract symptoms, such as straining on micturition and acute retention of urine [11]. For the purpose of diagnosis, imaging, as well as endoscopy, may be required. Thus, bladder imaging can help to identify a foreign body in the bladder. Full bladder ultrasound, as in our case, allows the visualization of the IUD [12]. However, cystoscopy remains essential for a complete evaluation of the bladder. It may reveal the presence or absence of a foreign body such as calculus and also help in determining if the migration is partial or complete into the bladder [13]. A blue methylene test or cystography is often useful to rule out fistula.

The removal of the fully migrated IUD from the bladder is most often performed during cystoscopy [13], without difficulty in the cases seen early as in our case. In some cases, the removal is preceded by lithotripsy in the case of a calcified IUD. A cystotomy or even a laparotomy is sometimes necessary when an IUD migrated into the bladder and ascend into the ureter [14]. In some areas, herbal formula like Persian herbal recipe used to remove stones without open surgery (helped stone ejection or stone dissolution) [15]. In the case of a vesicouterine fistula, open surgery or laparoscopic surgery [16] remains the best treatment with an aim to close separately, both the bladder and uterine openings of the fistula, with or without preservation of the uterus.

## 4. Conclusion

IUD insertion is not a minor procedure. It requires regular monitoring to ensure its position. Serious complications such as intravesical migration are rare but are possible. Management is made easy with the aid of endoscopic evaluation and treatment.

## Ethical Approval

Ethical approval was obtained from the local ethical committee.

## Consent

Written consent was obtained from the patient for the publication of this case report and any accompanying images.

## References

[1] M. E. Ortiz and H. B. Croxatto, "Copper-T intrauterine device and levonorgestrel intrauterine system: biological bases of their mechanism of action," *Contraception*, vol. 75, no. 6, pp. S16–S30, 2007.

[2] R. L. Callahan, A. Brunie, A. C. L. Mackenzie et al., "Potential user interest in new long-acting contraceptives: results from a mixed methods study in Burkina Faso and Uganda," *PLoS One*, vol. 14, no. 5, p. e0217333, 2019.

[3] C. Varela, E. Siña, A. Rojas Astorga et al., "The walking IUDs," in *The gynecologists nightmare*, p. C-2334, ECR, 2017.

[4] A. Kallat, A. Ibrahimi, O. Fahsi et al., "Le dispositif intra-utérin: à propos d'une complication rare et revue de la littérature," *The Pan African Medical Journal*, vol. 27, p. 193, 2017.

[5] V. Ceccato, A. Boileau, M. Roblin, D. Tariel, D. Bon, and V. Estrade, "Migration intravésicale d'un dispositif intra-utérin. Stratégies d'exploration et modalités thérapeutiques," *Progrès en Urologie*, vol. 17, no. 2, pp. 256–259, 2007.

[6] L. Grimaldi, F. De Giorgio, P. Andreotta, M. C. D'Alessio, C. Piscicelli, and V. L. Pascali, "Medicolegal aspects of an unusual uterine perforation with multiload-Cu 375R," *The American Journal of Forensic Medicine and Pathology*, vol. 26, no. 4, pp. 365-366, 2005.

[7] S. Goyal and G. S. Snigdha, "Displaced intrauterine device. A retrospective study," *Journal of Medical Research*, vol. 2, no. 2, pp. 41–43, 2016.

[8] P. L. Martínez-Valls, B. Honrubia Vilchez, A. Rodríguez Tardido et al., "Voiding symptoms as presentation of an intravesical foreign body," *Archivos Españoles de Urología*, vol. 61, no. 7, pp. 781–785, 2008.

[9] D. Schwartzwald, U. M. M. Mooppan, M. Leon Tancer, G. Gomez-Leon, and H. Kim, "Vesicouterine fistula with menouria: a complication from an intrauterine contraceptive device," *The Journal of Urology*, vol. 136, no. 5, pp. 1066-1067, 1986.

[10] B. C. Ozgur, O. G. Doluoglu, H. Sarici, M. M. Sunay, M. A. Karagoz, and M. Eroglu, "S277: intrauterine device migration to two different localizations resulting in bladder stone and carrying the risk of vesicovaginal fistula," *European Urology Supplements*, vol. 13, no. 7, p. e1591, 2014.

[11] Y. Nouira, S. Rakrouki, M. Gargouri, Z. Fitouri, and A. Horchani, "Intravesical migration of an intrauterine contraceptive device complicated by bladder stone: a report of six cases," *International Urogynecology Journal*, vol. 18, no. 5, pp. 575–578, 2007.

[12] N. Peri and D. Graham, "Imaging of intrauterine contraceptive devices," *Journal of Ultrasound in Medicine*, vol. 26, no. 10, pp. 1389–1401, 2007.

[13] M. Vahdat, M. Gorginzadeh, A. S. Mousavi, E. Afshari, and M. A. Ghaed, "Cystoscopic removal of a migrated intrauterine device to the bladder; a case report," *Contraception and Reproductive Medicine*, vol. 4, no. 1, 2019.

[14] A. Van Ophoven and J. B. De Kernion, "Clinical management of foreign bodies of the genitourinary tract," *The Journal of Urology*, vol. 164, no. 2, pp. 274–287, 2000.

[15] A. Hosseinkhani, F. Tabatabaei, M. Mosaffa-Jahromi, and M. Pasalar, "Urinary bladder stone passing using Persian herbal recipe," *Journal of Evidence-Based Integrative Medicine*, vol. 23, pp. 1–4, 2018.

[16] N. N. Zhang, N. Zuo, T. S. Sun, and Q. Yang, "An effective method combining various endoscopes in the treatment of intravesical migrated intrauterine device," *Journal of Minimally Invasive Gynecology*, vol. 27, no. 3, p. 582, 2020.

# A Patient with Milky Urine: Nonparasitic Chyluria and Silver Nitrate Sclerotherapy

**M. Sivashankar and A. C. N. Nandasena**

*Department of Urology, Colombo North Teaching Hospital, Ragama, Sri Lanka*

Correspondence should be addressed to M. Sivashankar; shankarmegan1986@gmail.com

Academic Editor: Giorgio Carmignani

Chyluria has become a rare clinical presentation in Sri Lanka, which may have a direct correlation with the low prevalence of lymphatic filariasis following the use of diethylcarbamazine and albendazole mass drug administration (MDA) for five rounds between 2002 and 2006. Here we report a 50-year-old male who presented with milky urine and progressive weight loss, diagnosed as having nonparasitic chyluria. The patient was initially managed with a trail of diethylcarbamazine (DEC) 6 mg/kg/day for 21 days and a low-fat diet with an unsatisfactory response. Subsequent management with endoscopic instillation of 0.5% silver nitrate brought in him a quick response, which was maintained for a year. Endoscopic sclerotherapy is considered a safer, effective and a minimally invasive treatment option for symptomatic patients.

## 1. Introduction

The presence of intestinal lymph (chyle) in the urine is known as chyluria. From the etiological perspective, chyluria is classified into two types: parasitic and nonparasitic (1). The more common parasitic type is caused by Wucheraria Bancrofti and is found principally in filarial endemic areas, while the nonparasitic type has a variety of etiological factors falling under a broad category (2). Chyluria is still a symptom that urologists encounter, even though Sri Lanka has achieved filariasis eradication status according to WHO criteria (7). This clinical scenario aims to share our experience of a patient with nonparasitic chyluria following a lympho-urinary fistula of the left kidney, who has been treated successfully with endoscopic silver nitrate sclerotherapy.

## 2. Case Presentation

A 51-year-old male was admitted with a complaint of milky urine and significant weight loss (10 kg) for over four months. On further assessment, neither lower urinary tract symptoms nor a contact history of tuberculosis was observed. The patient was cachectic with a body mass index of 20.2 kg/m$^2$.

Macroscopically, urine appeared milky in colours (Figure 1(a)), and the analysis demonstrated severe proteinuria and a high triacylglycerides level of 370 mg/dl (standard 1-10 mg/dl). Chloroform test for chyluria was positive, whereas filarial IgM and IgG antibodies were negative. Imaging studies of the urinary tract, which included an ultrasound scan (KUB) and CT-urography, revealed no abnormality. During diagnostic rigid cystoscopy and ureterorenoscopy, egress of milky urine from the left ureter was observed (Figure 2). The retrograde pyelogram, performed subsequently, demonstrated a left-sided lympho-urinary fistula at the level of the renal pelvis (Figure 3).

Initially, he was managed with a low-fat diet and a trial of diethylcarbamazine 6 mg/kg/day for 21 days with an inadequate response. Persistent symptoms, despite initial management, encouraged us to change over to instillation therapy. 10 ml of 0.5% silver nitrate was instilled endoscopically to the left ureter via a 6 Fr ureteric catheter, and the procedure was repeated for another three cycles at 30 min intervals. Subsequently, bladder irrigation was continued for 12 hours, and cefuroxime was administered intravenously for three days. He had an uneventful recovery with complete clearance of urine over five days (Figure 1(b)) and was discharged later

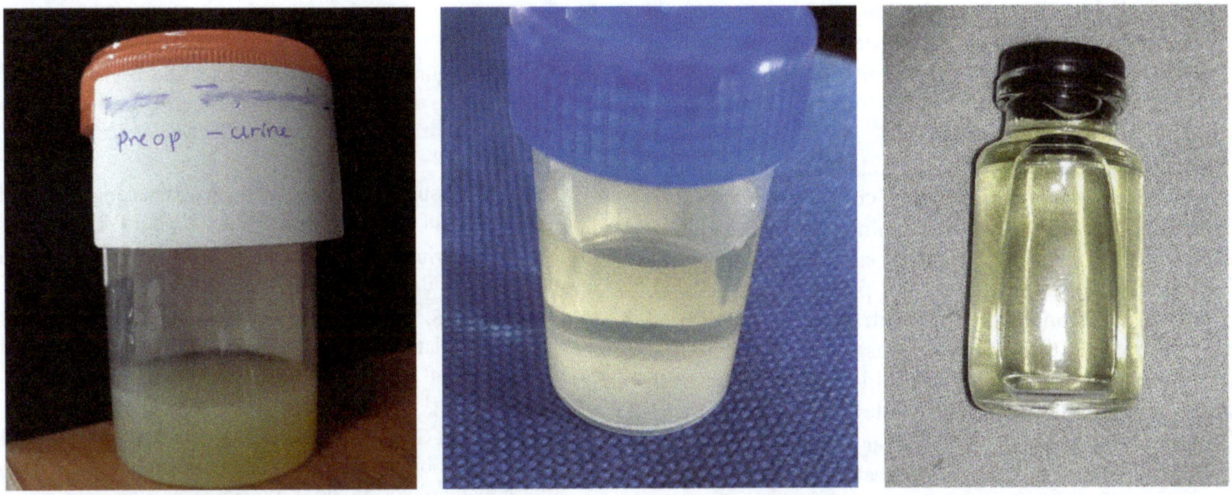


(a) (b) (c)

FIGURE 1: The color of urine samples prior and after the endoscopic sclerotheraphy, (a) prior to sclerotheraphy, (b) post surgery day 5, (c) one month after surgery.

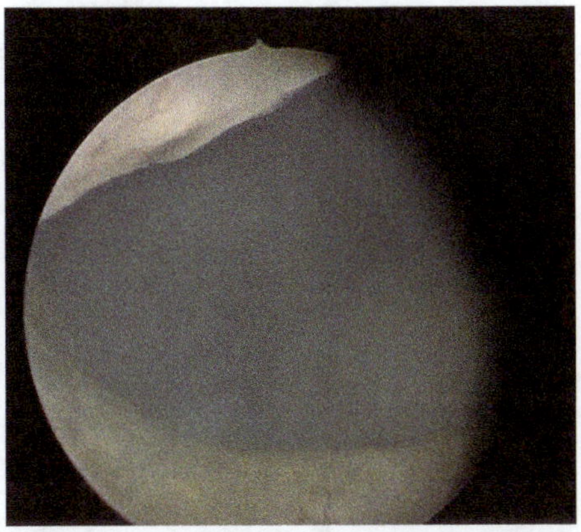

FIGURE 2: Cystoscopy view showing the chyluria.

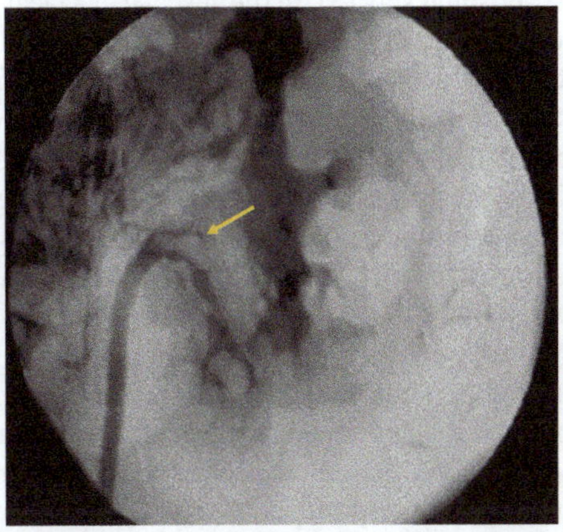

FIGURE 3: Left side retrograde pyelogram is showing the main lympho-urinary fistula at renal pelvis close to pelvic ureteric junction (marked by arrow).

on a low-fat diet. On routine follow up at one month, his urine was completely clear (Figure 1(c)), and a 3 kg increase in body weight was also observed. Follow up was carried out for twenty-two months with no recurrence of symptoms.

## 3. Discussion

Chyle is a milky fluid, rich in lymph and chylomicrons. Normally lymph flows through the intestinal lacteals to the cisterna chyle and the thoracic duct, which drain into the left subclavian vein. Although the pathogenesis of chyluria is not well described, two theories have been postulated: obstructive and regurgitative mechanisms for leakage of lymph into the urine (2). Commonly, leakage resulting from lympho-urinary fistula develops at the level of the renal pelvicalyceal system, but it can even occur at the level of the ureter and bladder (1).

Chyluria is confirmed by simple bedside chloroform or ether test, which extracts fat globules and forms an organic layer leaving the remaining urine clear. Sudan III test is also can be used to confirm fat globules in the urine. However, assessment of triglyceride levels in urine is by far the most accurate test to confirm chyluria when it is more than 15 mg/dl (1, 3).

Ascertaining the etiology, side, and the site of chyluria is an important part of the management. Usually, ultrasound scan (KUB) and computed tomogram imaging of upper tracts would fail to provide the necessary information decisive to the management of chyluria. However, it may reveal an uncommon, incidental primary cause helpful in the management of nonparasitic chyluria. Magnetic resonance imaging might show clusters of dilated lymphatic channels (1), and the necessity of such investigation should be individualized at the discretion of the attending clinician. Lymphangiography and Lymphoscintigraphy using 99 m Tc-nano colloid are capable of demonstrating the site of fistula, caliber, and the number of fistulous communications (6), hence can be described as important second-line investigations, while taking in to account its clinical value, cost and the availability (1, 6). Rigid cystoscopy examination helps in lateralizing chyluria by demonstrating chyle efflux from the ureteric orifice. Although less specific, retrograde pyelogram may be of help in identifying the site of leakage in the presence of chyluria before endoscopic sclerotherapy and during followup.

Symptomatic patients with severe chyluria and malnutrition need intervention rather than a conservative approach (1, 5). Endoscopic sclerotherapy is a minimally invasive treatment option for chyluria. Various types of sclerosant agents such as 0.1-1% silver nitrate, 0.2-5% povidone-iodine, 50% dextrose, 3% hypertonic saline and contrast media can be used for this purpose (1, 6). Initially, sclerosant induced chemical lymphangitis and oedema temporarily block the channels with eventual fibrosis to permanently occlude and close them (4, 5).

Sabinis (1992) pointed out 1% silver nitrate sclerotherapy as a safer and minimally invasive treatment option with a success rate of 82.25% (4). Dhabalia (2010) compared the efficacy of the 3-instillation regime with the 9-instillation regime of 1% silver nitrate in 60 patients with no significant difference in the success rate and concluded that a shorter regime is far better from the standpoint of cost-effectiveness and shorter hospital stay (5). In the absence of a clear consensus regarding the accepted regime, we instilled 10 ml of 0.5% silver nitrate, which was repeated three times in thirty-minute intervals without significant complications.

Sclerosant therapy has its drawbacks about side effects, out of which nausea, vomiting, flank pain, and haematuria are by far the commonest but transient (4, 5). However, high concentration silver nitrate therapy is known to cause dangerous and possibly fatal acute necrotizing ureteritis with obstructive uropathy (6).

10-40% of patients may develop recurrence following sclerotherapy requiring the procedure to be repeated (1). Those patients who develop recurrence within a short period are considered poor responders to repeat sclerotherapy (1). However, our patient was symptom-free for twenty-two months of followup in the clinic.

Failure of endoscopic instillation sclerotherapy requires a pyelo-lymphatic disconnection procedure as a final therapeutic option.

## 4. Conclusion

Chyluria is a rare clinical presentation demanding a high index of clinical suspicion, and symptomatic patients need surgical intervention to relieve symptoms. In this clinical scenario, the assumption of chyluria of nonparasitic origin is valid reasoning in accordance with the detection of the low prevalence of lymphatic filariasis in Sri Lanka and the announcement of the eradication of lymphatic filariasis based on WHO criteria (7). As a corollary, investigating for an uncommon primary cause for nonparasitic chyluria is quite relevant before labeling the condition as idiopathic. Endoscopic sclerotherapy considered a safer and more effective minimally invasive treatment option for severe symptomatic chyluria.

## References

[1] A. M. Abeygunasekera, K. Sutharshan, and B. Balagobi, "New developments in chyluria after global programs to eliminate lymphatic filariasis," *International Journal of Urology*, vol. 24, no. 8, pp. 582–588, 2017.

[2] D. Dalela, "Issues in etiology and diagnosis making of chyluria," *Indian Journal of Urology*, vol. 21, no. 1, pp. 18–23, 2005.

[3] Y. Tan, "Chyluria in non-filarial endemic areas: an internist's perspective," *BMJ Case Reports*, vol. 2017, 2017.

[4] R. B. Sabnis, S. V. Punekar, R. M. Desai, A. M. Bradoo, and S. D. Bapat, "Instillation of silver nitrate in the treatment of chyluria," *British Journal of Urology*, vol. 70, no. 6, pp. 660–662, 1992.

[5] J. V. Dhabalia, N. R. Pujari, V. Kumar, M. S. Punia, A. D. Gokhale, and G. Nelivigi, "Silver Nitrate Sclerotherapy for Chyluria: Evaluation for the Optimal Instillation Regime," *Urologia Internationalis*, vol. 85, no. 1, pp. 56–59, 2010.

[6] S. Sunder, R. Jayaraman, H. S. Mahapatra et al., "Analysis of case series of milky urine: a single center and departmental clinical experience with emphasis on management perspectives: a prospective observational study," *Urology Annals*, vol. 6, no. 4, pp. 340–345, 2014.

[7] R. U. Rao, K. C. Nagodavithana, S. D. Samarasekera et al., "A Comprehensive Assessment of Lymphatic Filariasis in Sri Lanka Six Years after Cessation of Mass Drug Administration," *PLoS Neglected Tropical Diseases*, vol. 8, no. 12, article e3281, 2014.

# 41

# Near-Miss Diagnoses of Solitary Bladder Tumors Highlight the Importance of Immunohistochemical Staining

**Van Schloegel, Syed M. Alam, Katie Dennis, Jeffrey Holzbeierlein, and John A. Taylor III**

*Department of Urology, University of Kansas Health System, 3901 Rainbow Boulevard, Kansas City, KS 66160, USA*

Correspondence should be addressed to John A. Taylor III; jtaylor27@kumc.edu

Academic Editor: Apul Goel

We report three cases of prostate adenocarcinoma appearing as bladder masses and misdiagnosed as muscle-invasive bladder cancer (MIBC). Patients were referred for consideration for radical cystectomy after initial pathological diagnosis suggested poorly differentiated bladder cancer. Pathological review of tissue samples and subsequent immunohistochemical (IHC) staining confirmed advanced prostatic adenocarcinoma. Systemic therapy for prostate cancer was then initiated. These cases highlight the importance of patient history, physical exam, and IHC staining in consideration of a bladder mass, as these patients may have been subject to undue morbidity and surgical intervention without accurate pathologic diagnosis.

## 1. Introduction

In 2020, prostate cancer and bladder cancer are expected to be diagnosed in 191,930 and 81,400 new patients, respectively [1]. Standard of care for a new bladder mass includes transurethral resection of bladder tumor (TURBT) for treatment, diagnosis, and initial staging. TURBT specimens appearing as poorly differentiated carcinomas, particularly from trigonal tumors, may be misdiagnosed as urothelial in origin without clinical suspicion and further evaluation. It is uncommon for invasive prostate cancer to present away from the trigone, and these tumors may be at even higher risk for misdiagnosis. This may lead to undue morbidity and mortality associated with systemic therapy and surgery for presumed bladder cancer. We describe three cases of near-miss diagnoses that emphasize the importance of appropriate IHC staining based on clinical suspicion and patient history.

## 2. Case Presentations

*2.1. Case 1.* An 83-year-old male presented with an enhancing posterior wall bladder mass identified on surveillance imaging for a known renal mass. A 1.5 cm enhancing posterior peripheral zone prostate nodule was also noted. Cystoscopy revealed a nodular tumor in the posterior bladder wall with diffuse erythematous papillary changes along the right lateral wall. TURBT was performed with initial pathology reported as poorly differentiated bladder cancer. Of note, this patient had a history of localized prostate cancer previously treated with radiotherapy at a separate institute eight years prior. Prostate-specific antigen (PSA) was 2.57 ng/mL just prior to TURBT, with a PSA nadir of 0.2 ng/mL approximately three years prior. As such, additional IHC staining for GATA3 and NKX3.1 was performed on the TURBT specimen. This revealed diffuse strong nuclear staining of NKX3.1 with GATA3 positivity only seen in benign surface epithelium supporting a diagnosis of prostatic adenocarcinoma (Figure 1). Appropriate therapy for prostate cancer was subsequently initiated.

*2.2. Case 2.* An 80-year-old male presented to his local urologist for worsening obstructive voiding symptoms. Flexible cystoscopy revealed a dense bladder neck contracture. The patient underwent transurethral incision of this contracture at which time abnormal papillary tissue was seen at the bladder neck. Transurethral resection of this tissue was reported as muscle-invasive urothelial carcinoma with squamous differentiation, prompting referral for radical cystectomy at

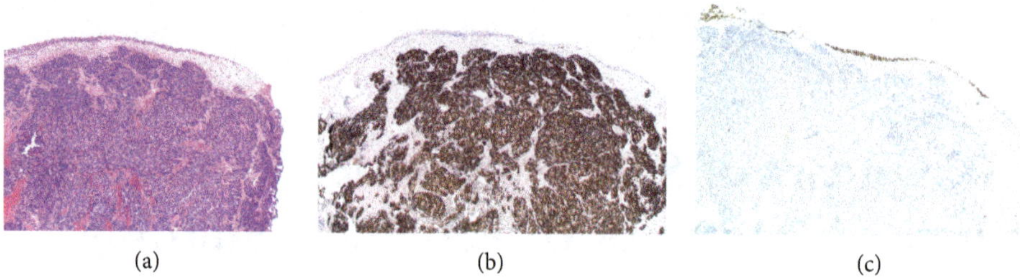

FIGURE 1: Negative GATA3 and positive NKX3.1 staining confirms prostatic adenocarcinoma. Low power view of the bladder tumor in (a) shows a normal urothelial mucosa and tumor beneath the urothelium, involving the submucosa. Underlying invasion of the muscularis propria was also present. (b) Strong diffuse nuclear staining with the immunohistochemical stain NKX3.1 was seen. Note the surface urothelium is negative. (c) The tumor cells are negative for the immunohistochemical stain GATA3, while the surface benign urothelium shows positive nuclear staining.

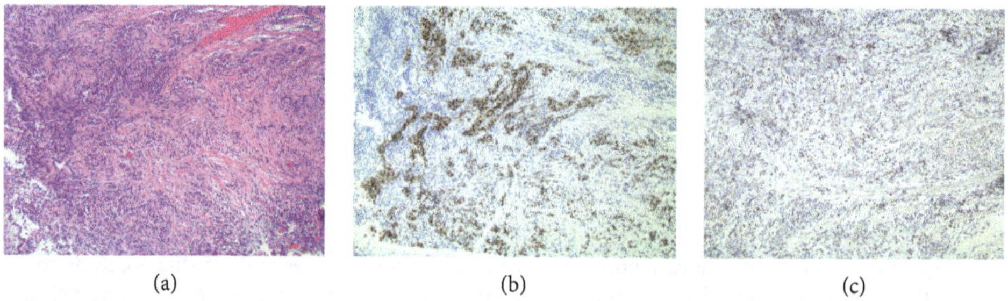

FIGURE 2: NKX3.1 distinguishes prostatic origin amidst significant cautery artifact. (a) Tumor cells can be seen infiltrating through smooth muscle tissue, which appear epithelioid, but otherwise show no distinguishing features. These tumor cells are in a background of inflammation and appear cauterized, making it difficult to classify based on morphology alone. (b) The immunohistochemical stain NKX3.1 shows strong nuclear positivity in the tumor cells. In contrast (c), the larger tumor cell nuclei are negative for the immunohistochemical stain GATA3 and only show nonspecific faint blushing of the cytoplasm. GATA3 is appropriately positive in an occasional small background of benign lymphocyte nuclei.

our institution. The patient was counseled on surgery for MIBC but on physical exam was found to have a nodular prostate. As such, the patient was scheduled for repeat TURBT. PSA was drawn and measured 179.91 ng/mL, prompting internal pathological review. Initial tissue samples revealed poorly differentiated tumor cells with muscular invasion. Staining for NKX3.1 and GATA3 showed strong nuclear positivity in the tumor cells while GATA3 was appropriately confined to benign lymphocyte nuclei, confirming a diagnosis of prostate adenocarcinoma (Figure 2). TURBT was deferred, and staging studies revealed multiple sclerotic osseous lesions consistent with metastatic disease. Appropriate treatment for metastatic prostate cancer was initiated.

*2.3. Case 3.* A 79-year-old male underwent TURBT at an outside institution for a sessile lesion located at the bladder neck. Initial pathological review suggested a diagnosis of muscle-invasive urothelial carcinoma. As such, he was referred to our institution for consideration for radical cystectomy. The patient was noted to have a history of prostate adenocarcinoma previously treated with external beam radiation therapy. Digital rectal exam was unremarkable, and he did not have evidence of biochemical recurrence up to that time. Given this history and the location of his tumor, IHC staining for prostate cancer markers was pursued and revealed poorly differentiated prostate cancer. After further counseling, he went on to receive androgen deprivation therapy.

## 3. Discussion

In any patient with a bladder mass, a biopsy is needed to determine the grade, stage, and tissue origin. In patients previously treated with radiation therapy for prostate cancer, the tissue can appear as poorly differentiated carcinoma making organ specific cancer diagnosis challenging. The location of the mass may correlate with tissue of origin, although this is not always the case, as in our patient with tumors distinctly away from the trigone/bladder neck. Here, we demonstrate the importance of appropriate IHC staining in bladder tumor samples to differentiate urothelial malignancy from invasive prostate adenocarcinoma.

A retrospective analysis by Liu et al. demonstrated that up to 3.1% of all prostate cancers may originally be misdiagnosed as bladder cancer, although the sample size in this study was small [2]. Misdiagnosed tumors in this report appeared on imaging as masses along the bladder neck and trigone. There is little data available on the locations outside of these regions of the bladder that may harbor prostate cancer. In a recent meta-analysis, Zhao et al. demonstrated that the hazard ratio for the development of bladder cancer after radiation for prostate cancer is approximately 1.6 [3]. In the setting of prior radiotherapy for prostate cancer, a high clinical suspicion for urothelial origin of bladder tumors may be warranted, but progression of the primary prostate cancer cannot be excluded.

Appropriate staining for prostate adenocarcinoma in these scenarios should include a panel of prostatic and urothelial markers, including PSA, NKX3.1, and GATA3. In a study by Mohanty et al. looking at high-grade prostate cancer of the bladder neck, PSA showed a sensitivity of only 25%, while NKX3.1 had a sensitivity of 100%. In this same study, both PSA and NKX3.1 showed 100% specificity with no false positives in urothelial carcinomas [4]. GATA3 has been shown to have a sensitivity of 80% as a urothelial marker in high-grade urothelial carcinoma and did not stain positive in any of the 38 high-grade prostatic adenocarcinoma samples in a study by Chang et al. [5]. The decision to pursue additional staining in the appropriate clinical context is key to avoiding the undue harm associated with misdiagnosis.

## 4. Conclusion

These cases emphasize the importance of a thorough history and physical exam in patients presenting with a new bladder mass. They also highlight the value of appropriate IHC staining of bladder tumor samples to distinguish prostatic and urothelial origin of malignancies in select patients, regardless of tumor location.

## Abbreviations

MIBC: Muscle-invasive bladder cancer
TURBT: Transurethral resection of bladder tumor
PSA: Prostate-specific antigen
IHC: Immunohistochemical.

## References

[1] F. Bray, J. Ferlay, I. Soerjomataram, R. L. Siegel, L. A. Torre, and A. Jemal, "Global Cancer Statistics 2018: GLOBOCAN Estimates of Incidence and Mortality Worldwide for 36 Cancers in 185 Countries," *CA: A Cancer Journal for Clinicians*, vol. 68, no. 6, pp. 394–424, 2018.

[2] R. Liu, X. Xie, Z. Zhang, and Y. Xu, "A retrospective study of prostate cancer cases mimicking urothelial cell carcinoma of the bladder," *European Journal of Medical Research*, vol. 18, no. 1, p. 36, 2013.

[3] S. Zhao, Q. Xie, R. Yang et al., "High prevalence of secondary bladder cancer in men on radiotherapy for prostate cancer: evidence from a meta-analysis," *Cancer Management and Research*, vol. Volume 11, pp. 587–598, 2019.

[4] S. K. Mohanty, S. C. Smith, E. Chang et al., "Evaluation of contemporary prostate and urothelial lineage biomarkers in a consecutive cohort of poorly differentiated bladder neck carcinomas," *American Journal of Clinical Pathology*, vol. 142, no. 2, pp. 173–183, 2014.

[5] A. Chang, A. Amin, E. Gabrielson et al., "Utility of GATA3 immunohistochemistry in differentiating urothelial carcinoma from prostate adenocarcinoma and squamous cell carcinomas of the uterine cervix, anus, and lung," *The American Journal of Surgical Pathology*, vol. 36, no. 10, pp. 1472–1476, 2012.

42

# Congenital Urethral Fistula: A Case Report and Literature Review

**Aamer Alghamlas,[1] Frédéric Auber,[1,2] and Yann Chaussy[1,2]**

[1]*Department of Pediatric Surgery, CHU Besançon, F-25000 Besançon, France*
[2]*Nanomédecine, Imagerie, Thérapeutique EA 4662, Université Bourgogne Franche-Comté, F-25000 Besançon, France*

Correspondence should be addressed to Yann Chaussy; yannchaussy@hotmail.com

Academic Editor: Apul Goel

Male congenital urethral fistula is an extremely rare condition. It is characterized by an abnormal opening of the ventral aspect of the penis. We report the case of a 1-month-old boy with congenital urethral fistula. We will describe the surgical technique, postoperative results, and literature review.

## 1. Introduction

Male congenital urethral fistula is an extremely rare condition [1–3]. It is usually an isolated anomaly but sometimes associated with genitourinary or anorectal anomalies [1, 3]. It is characterized by fistulisation of the penile urethra to the skin with a normal urethral meatus [3]. Sometimes, it can be confused with hypospadias [4]. We present the case of a 1-month-old boy with congenital urethral fistula associated with a genitourinary anomaly (right cryptorchidism).

## 2. Case Presentation

A 1-month-old male was referred to our center for penile anomaly discovered during a routine neonatal examination. The twin pregnancy was unremarkable, and he was born at 38 weeks of gestation (birth weight 2350 g). He had no previous history of circumcision, surgery, or trauma. The clinical examination at 1 month of age found a normal urethral opening at the tip of the glans, normal foreskin, localized hypoplasia of the corpus spongiosum, and skin on the ventral penis surface. There was no ventral chordee. There was initially an undamaged urethra visible through the corpus spongiosum and skin defect on the ventral aspect of the penile shaft (Figure 1). We found also a right cryptorchidism with the testis in the inguinal area. There was no anorectal anomaly. The parents noticed a bulge on the ventral penis through the skin defect during urination although the patient urinated from the normal urethral meatus at the tip of the glans. We suspected the diagnosis of incomplete congenital urethral fistula because there was a local defect of corpus spongiosum and skin adjacent to a preserved urethral wall. The abdominal ultrasound was normal.

At 1 month and 1 week of age, the parents noticed a rupture of the urethral wall and urination from both the normal urethral opening and the urethrocutaneous fistula. The clinical examination found an oval-shaped opening measuring approximately 1.5 cm in length and 0.5 cm in width (Figure 2).

Surgical correction was performed at the age of 6 months. After correction of the right cryptorchidism, testing of the distal urethra with a urethral dilator until 12 Fr demonstrated the absence of stricture; then, an 8 Fr Foley catheter was passed into the bladder. A longitudinal ventral incision circumscribing the fistula was performed. The penile shaft skin was ventrally degloved. We noticed a normal proximal and distal urethra surrounded by the corpus spongiosum. There was a large defect in the corpus spongiosum. The urethral plate was well developed. The urethroplasty was performed using a tubularization technique with a continuous 7.0 polydioxanone resorbable suture. The corpus spongiosum was then dissected in order to perform spongioplasty, covering the urethroplasty. The subcutaneous tissue was then used as an additional layer to cover sutures to limit the risk of fistula

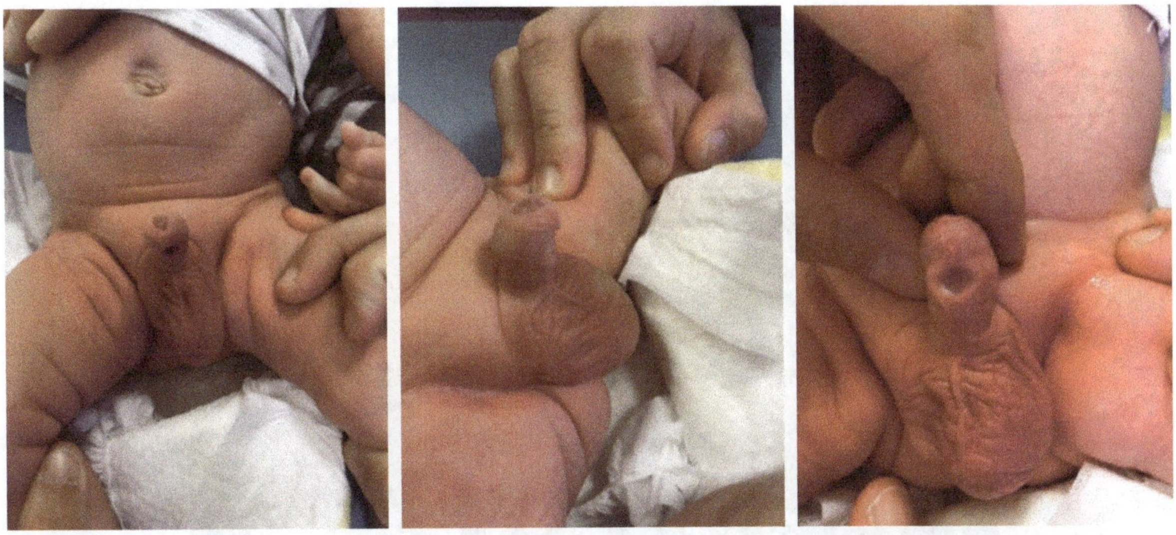

FIGURE 1: Clinical examination at the age of 1 month: an undamaged urethral wall with large corpus spongiosum and skin defect on the ventral aspect of the penis shaft. Associated right cryptorchidism.

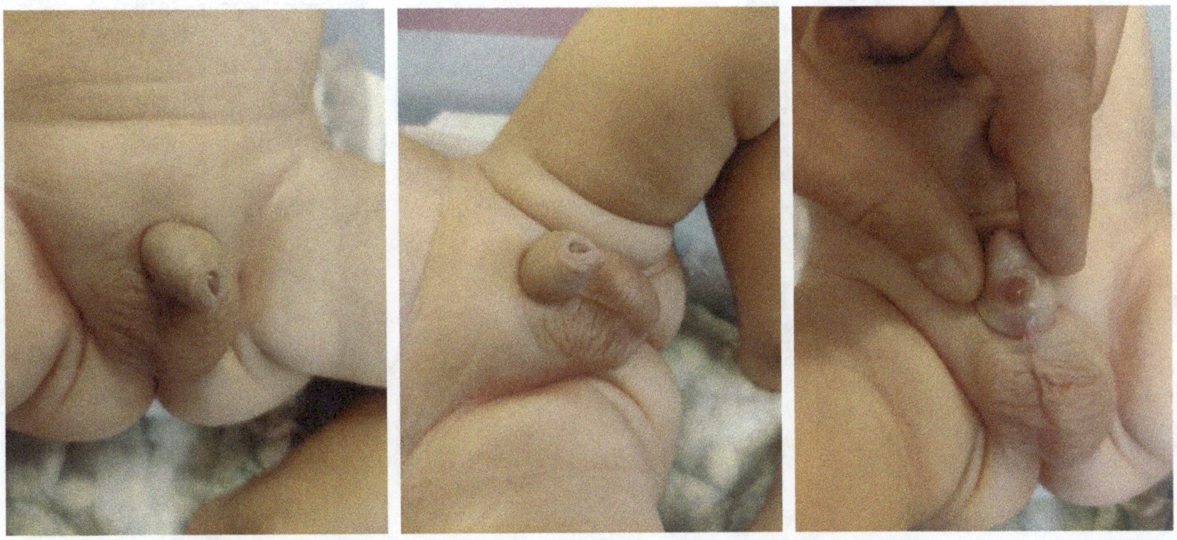

FIGURE 2: Clinical examination at the age of 3 months: urethrocutaneous fistula occurs after the rupture of the urethral wall. The patient is urinating from both the normal urinary meatus at the tip of the glans and the ventral urethrocutaneous fistula.

recurrence. Finally, the skin was longitudinally closed (Figure 3). The patient was discharged at day 2, and the Foley catheter was removed at day 6 on an outpatient basis.

Six months later, the patient had normal voiding without fistula recurrence. The parents had observed a normal stream via the urethral meatus without any leakage. The wound was completely healed without chordee and with good esthetic results (Figure 4). The right testis was located in the normal intrascrotal position.

## 3. Discussion

Congenital urethral fistula is a rare condition where an urethrocutaneous fistula occurs in the ventral aspect of the penis shaft with a normal urethral meatus. There are few reports of this congenital anomaly in literature [3]. The etiology and pathogenesis are uncertain, and several theories have been proposed. The male genitalia develop in a proximal-to-distal manner. As the penis forms from the elongation and enlargement of the phallus, the lateral walls of the urethral groove form from the ventrally located genital folds, which then fuse at the midline [5]. For Olbourne, fistulae located in the penile shaft probably reflect a focal or temporary defect in the urethral plate function. This would result in a complete defect or a partial deficiency of urethral fold fusion [2]. Another theory suggests that the misalignment of the glanular and penile urethra may explain the coronal type of congenital urethral fistula [1]. In addition, the anterior urethral

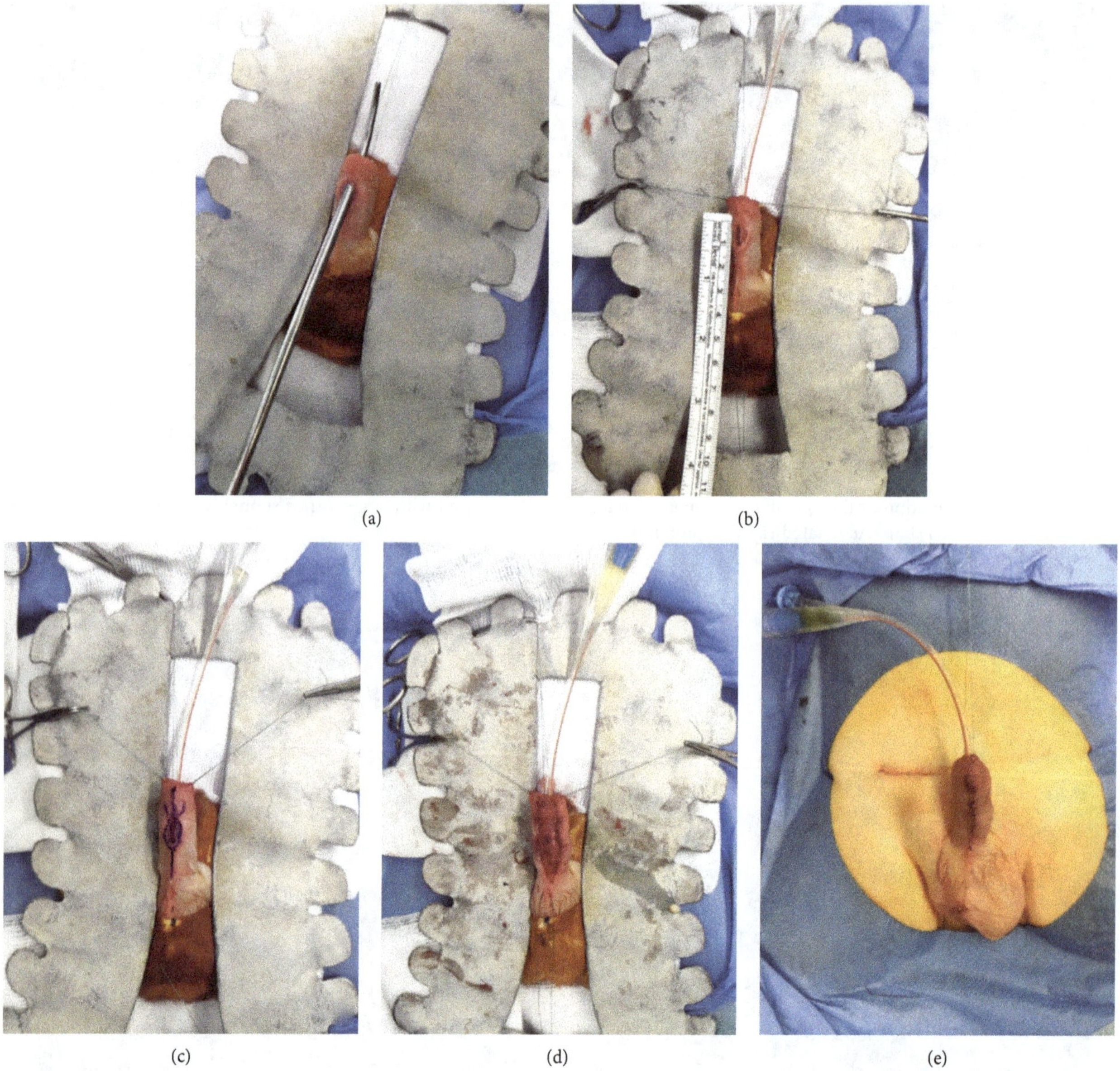

FIGURE 3: Surgical correction at the age of 6 months. Permeability of the distal urethra is tested with a urethral dilator until 12 Fr (a). An 8 Fr Foley catheter is inserted, and the congenital urethral fistula is measured (b). Drawing of skin incision (c). Primary fistula closure is performed by the tubularization technique, and spongioplasty is done to cover the urethroplasty (d). Final postoperative result (e).

fistula may be secondary to a blowout phenomenon of a urethral diverticulum. Consequently, this condition may lead to a defect in the corpus spongiosum or incomplete migration of the lateral spongy tissue of the inner genital folds with later erosion of the overlying skin [1, 6]. Our case supports this last hypothesis: the urethral wall was initially undamaged with a urethra bulging through the corpus spongiosum and skin defect during micturition. The pressure caused by the urinary stream led to the rupture of the thin urethral wall (which is not covered by corpus spongiosum) and subsequent urethrocutaneous fistula.

Congenital urethral fistula is usually an isolated disorder (with normal foreskin, normal urinary meatus, and no chordee). However, it can be associated with genitourinary anomalies (hypospadias-like characteristics, undescended testis, bifid scrotum, duplicated urethra, megalourethra, and penoscrotal transposition) or anorectal anomalies [1, 3]. Congenital anterior urethrocutaneous fistula is uncommon compared to posterior urethrocutaneous fistula which usually presents as a Y-type duplication of the urethra with anorectal atretic malformations [1]. It is important to differentiate between isolated congenital urethral fistula and urethral fistula with associated anomalies (particularly hypospadias-like anomalies or anorectal malformation) as the surgical treatment will be different.

The surgical approach to repair congenital anterior urethrocutaneous fistula depends on the type and size of a fistula. Primary fistula closure is considered if it appears that

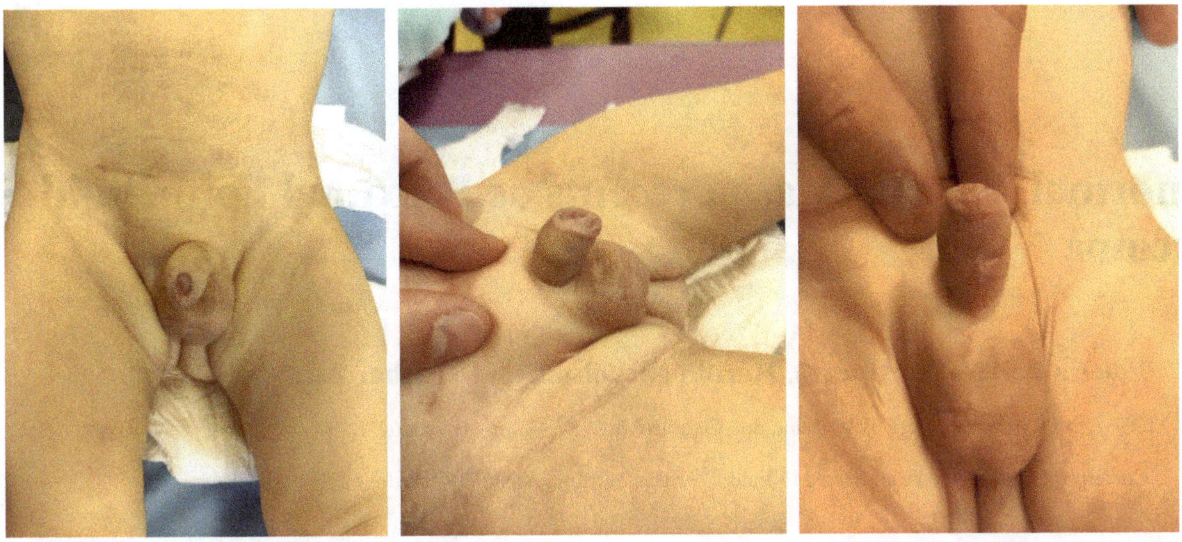

FIGURE 4: Postoperative results at 6 months: wound healing is complete without chordee and with a good esthetic outcome. The patient has normal voiding by urinary meatus without fistula recurrence.

the distal urethra and spongiosum are normally formed, as in our case. Thus, surgical correction requires circumscription of the fistula and closure in multiple layers, similar to a urethrocutaneous fistula after hypospadias repair [1, 5, 7]. Various techniques, depending on the size and location of the fistula, have been proposed to perform urethroplasties such as Thiersch-Duplay urethroplasty, turned-down flap urethroplasty, and pedicled island tube or onlay urethroplasty [3, 4]. When the congenital urethral fistula is associated with deficient distal urethra or spongiosum, chordee, or hypospadias, formal hypospadias repair is recommended [1, 7]. The functional and esthetic results are usually good with a low risk of fistula recurrence when the surgical technique is correctly chosen [1].

## 4. Conclusion

Congenital urethral fistula is a very rare condition. Careful diagnosis and exploration for associated anomalies are necessary for good management. The surgical approach depends on the type and size of a fistula, with usually very good functional and esthetic results.

## Authors' Contributions

Aamer Alghamlas wrote the first draft of the manuscript. Each author listed has seen and approved the submission of this version of the manuscript and takes full responsibility for the manuscript.

## Acknowledgments

We thank Ashley Ridley for her assistance for the preparation of this manuscript (language help).

## References

[1] A. A. Caldamone, S. C. Chen, J. S. Elder, M. L. Ritchey, D. A. Diamond, and M. A. Koyle, "Congenital anterior urethrocutaneous fistula," *The Journal of Urology*, vol. 162, no. 4, pp. 1430–1432, 1999.

[2] N. A. Olbourne, "Congenital urethral fistula. Case reports," *Plastic and Reconstructive Surgery*, vol. 57, no. 2, pp. 237–239, 1976.

[3] Y. Lin, C. Deng, and Q. Peng, "Congenital anterior urethrocutaneous fistula: a systematic review," *African Journal of Paediatric Surgery*, vol. 15, no. 2, pp. 63–68, 2018.

[4] A. Bhatnagar, V. Upadhyaya, and B. Kumar, "Congenital urethrocutaneous fistula: case report with review of literature," *Indian Journal of Plastic Surgery*, vol. 45, no. 3, pp. 563–565, 2012.

[5] L. S. Palmer and J. S. Palmer, "Management of abnormalities of the external genitalia in boys," in *Campbell-Walsh Urology*, A. J. Wein, L. R. Kavoussi, A. W. Partin, and C. A. Peters, Eds., pp. 3368–3379, Elsevier, Philadelphia, PA, eleventh edition, 2016.

[6] M. Campbell, *Clinical Pediatric Urology*, W.B. Saunders Co, Philadelphia, 1951.

[7] R. M. Shukla, B. Mukhopadhyay, K. C. Mandal, and S. S. Barman, "Congenital penile urethrocutaneous fistula: a rare anomaly and review of literature," *Urology Annals*, vol. 3, no. 3, pp. 161–163, 2011.

43

# Abnormal Adrenal Mass Presents as Proximal Epithelioid Sarcoma

**Valeria Pereira Martinez, Marilin Nicholson, and Trushar Patel**

*USF Health Morsani College of Medicine, 560 Channelside Drive, Tampa, FL 33602, USA*

Correspondence should be addressed to Valeria Pereira Martinez; valeria5@usf.edu

Academic Editor: Yankai Xia

Epithelioid sarcoma (ES) is a rare malignant mesenchymal neoplasm that accounts for less than one percent of all soft-tissue sarcomas. Only two cases of ES involving the adrenal gland were found after a literature review. We report a case of an 82-year-old female initially presenting with right flank pain who was subsequently found to have an incidental left adrenal mass on CT imaging. After appropriate diagnostic workup, the patient underwent surgical resection. A diagnosis of ES was made from the histopathological analysis. The characteristic findings of ES are epithelioid cells with rhabdoid morphology and moderate eosinophilic cytoplasm. Immunohistochemical findings are significant for positive staining for epithelial markers, cytokeratins, vimentin, and CD34, and loss of INI-1 stain. Due to the aggressive nature and limited data of ESs, the standard treatment continues to remain wide surgical excision.

## 1. Introduction

Epithelioid sarcoma (ES) is a malignant mesenchymal neoplasm that shows some level of epithelial differentiation [1–4]. It is a very rare sarcoma that accounts for less than one percent of all soft tissue sarcomas [1, 2]. There are two subtypes: classic and proximal [1–4]. The classic subtype presents more commonly in adolescents and young adults in distal extremities, whereas the proximal subtype tends to present in older adults in proximal soft tissue [1–4]. The cytomorphology of the proximal type tends to be higher grade than the classic type, and some of its malignant cells have a rhabdoid phenotype [1–4]. We report a case of proximal ES that is presented as an adrenal mass. This is the third reported ES presenting as an adrenal mass. The first reported primary adrenal ES was in 2017 by Alikhan et al. [3] and the second was in 2019 by Huang et al. [4].

## 2. Case Report

An 82-year-old female initially presented with right flank pain. The patient's past medical history was noncontributory. Family history was significant for breast, stomach, uterine, and colon cancer. The initial CT abdomen with and without contrast showed a 3.3 cm left adrenal indeterminate mass with an absolute and relative washout of 21.9% and 10.1%, respectively, which did not meet the washout criteria for an adrenal adenoma (Figure 1). Metabolic workup with a comprehensive metabolic panel, plasma metanephrines, and dexamethasone suppression test was all normal. The patient showed no signs of refractory hypertension or stigmata of Cushing's disease. Based on the negative metabolic workup and relatively small size of the adrenal mass, the patient was placed on active surveillance. A follow-up MRI, ten months later, showed significant enlargement of the left adrenal mass, which at the time measured $6.5 \times 5.1 \times 5.0$ cm (Figure 2). Repeat metabolic testing was again negative. Surgical treatment was recommended, and the patient underwent left open adrenalectomy. Laparoscopic/robotic adrenalectomy was not considered because of the suspicion of adrenal cortical carcinoma and the data that has been presented regarding the increased risk of peritoneal dissemination with laparoscopic surgery in these cases [5]. The intraoperative findings included limited access to the mass due to the proximity of

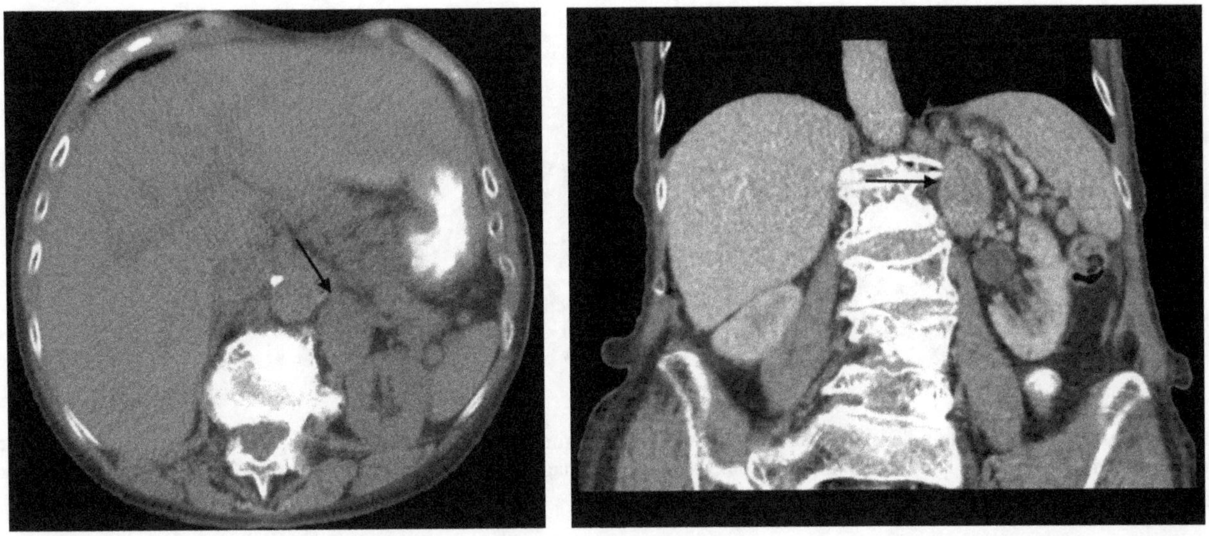

(a) (b)

FIGURE 1: Initial CT abdomen showed a 3.3 cm left adrenal indeterminate mass.

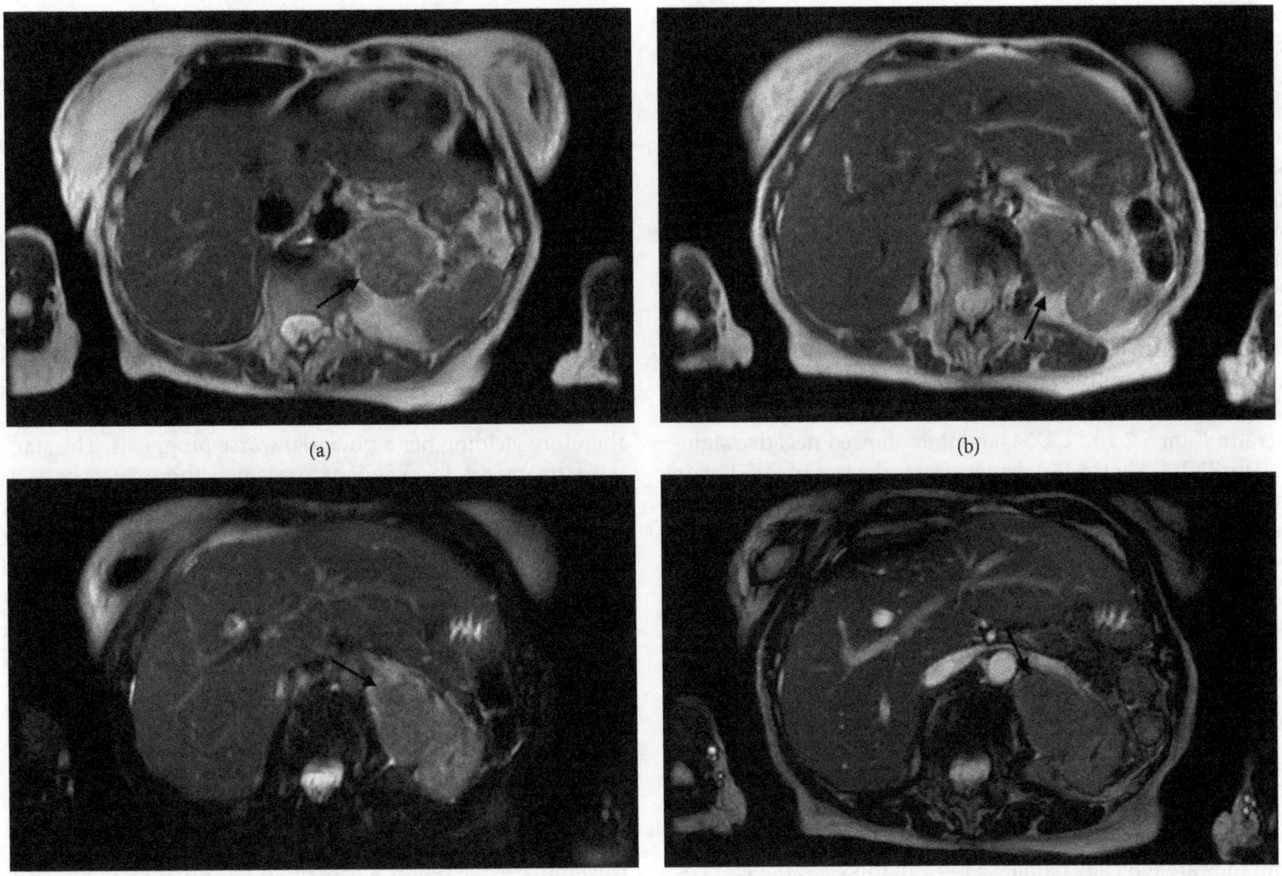

(a) (b) (c) (d)

FIGURE 2: Follow-up MRI, ten months later, showed significant enlargement of the left adrenal mass, measuring 6.5 × 5.1 × 5.0 cm.

the spleen and the mass being significantly involved with the renal hilum. To aid in access to the mass, a splenectomy had to be performed. The adrenal mass was densely adherent to the renal hilum, specifically the renal vein. After unsuccessful attempts to safely release the renal hilum, the decision was made to perform a nephrectomy, with the adrenalectomy and mass excision. The postoperative course was complicated by congestive heart failure exacerbation which was

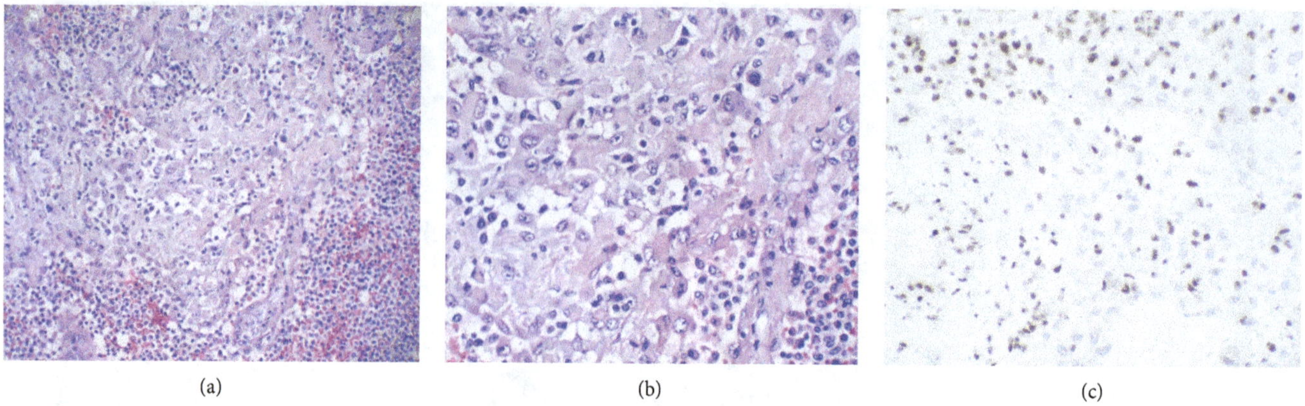

FIGURE 3: Immunohistochemical findings postresection. (a) Malignant epithelioid cells with moderate eosinophilic cytoplasm and rhabdoid features along with prominent lymphoid infiltrate (200x). (b) Higher magnification (400x). (c) Loss of INI-1 stain in neoplastic cells; background inflammatory cells stained positive with INI-1.

ultimately managed with diuretics. The remainder of the postoperative course was uneventful, and the patient was ultimately discharged on postoperative day 5. At four months post-op, the patient is doing well with a creatinine of 1.62. Follow-up imaging has been delayed due to the COVID-19 pandemic.

The pathologic analysis of the spleen found no diagnostic abnormalities, and the analysis of the left kidney was only significant for benign cysts. Macroscopic analysis of the resected specimen showed a well-defined, 7 cm tumor mass which was actually adjacent to the adrenal gland. One lymph node was analyzed and showed no malignancy. The microscopic analysis of the tumor showed malignant epithelioid cells with moderate eosinophilic cytoplasm and rhabdoid features (Figure 3). Prominent lymphoid infiltrate was associated with the tumor cells (Figure 3). Areas of tumor necrosis were also identified. The tumor cells stained positive for keratin Cam 5.2 and CD34, and they showed negative staining for INI-1. Figure 3(c) demonstrates the loss of INI-1 stain in neoplastic cells; background inflammatory cells stained positive with INI-1. Focal immunoreactivity for calretinin was identified. Additionally, the tumor cells stained negative for smooth muscle actin, desmin, myoD1, myogenin, S100, inhibin, synaptophysin, CD31, ERG, and D240. The diagnosis of ES proximal type was made.

## 3. Discussion

ESs are very rare neoplasms that tend to have an aggressive clinical course and tend to recur [1–4]. The size of ES neoplasms can get quite large with a median diameter of 4 cm, and they are typically painless [1–4]. In this case, the ES neoplasm presenting as an adrenal mass was an incidental finding and was quite large as well—measuring 6.5 × 5.1 × 5.0 cm. Differential diagnoses included adenoma or adrenocortical carcinoma. The diagnosis of ES is done with histopathology [2, 4]. ESs are composed of epithelioid cells with rhabdoid morphology and moderate eosinophilic cytoplasm, as was seen in our case [1–4]. The neoplastic cells in the proximal subtype tend to exhibit prominent nucleoli and vesicular nuclei [1–3]. Signs of chronic inflammation, such as the presence of lymphocytes, are also associated with ESs [1–3]. The common immunohistochemical findings are positive staining for epithelial markers, cytokeratins, vimentin, and CD34—which helps distinguish from carcinoma [1–4]. Other immunohistochemical findings are negative staining for CD31, nuclear INI1, and S100 [1–4]. In terms of prognosis, the reported probability of the recurrence of ES varies in the literature with a range from 34% to 87% and 30% to 50% for metastasis [1, 4]. The five-year survival rates reported also vary in the literature with a range of 49-75% depending on prognostic factors [1]. Factors that are associated with a worse prognosis for ESs are proximal and deep location, rhabdoid features, large size, older age, male sex, necrosis, and vascular invasion [1]. In our case, our patient has several of these negative prognostic factors: proximal and deep location, rhabdoid features, necrosis, large size, and older age, therefore yielding her a potential worse prognosis. The standard treatment for ESs that present without metastasis is wide surgical excision, and some patients receive adjuvant high-dose chemotherapy or radiotherapy to help prevent local relapse [1, 4]. Due to the tendency of relapse from ESs, follow-up after surgical excision is imperative. Our patient is currently 3 months from her surgical resection with no evidence of recurrence or metastatic disease on axial imaging. Based on the limited evidence of adjuvant therapy, we have continued her on active surveillance with repeat scans scheduled for 3 months post-op.

## 4. Conclusion

In summary, we report a case of an ES proximal type that is presented as an incidental adrenal mass. The diagnosis of ES is dependent on histopathology. The significant findings for ESs are epithelioid cells with rhabdoid morphology, moderate eosinophilic cytoplasm, positive staining for epithelial markers, cytokeratins, vimentin, and CD34, and loss of INI-1 stain in neoplastic cells. Due to the aggressive nature and limited data of ESs, the standard treatment continues to remain wide surgical excision.

## Acknowledgments

The authors thank Edward O'Neill, MD.

## References

[1] K. Thway, R. L. Jones, J. Noujaim, and C. Fisher, "Epithelioid sarcoma: diagnostic features and genetics," *Advances in Anatomic Pathology*, vol. 23, no. 1, pp. 41–49, 2016.

[2] Y. Zhang, F. Liu, Y. Pan, J. Liang, Y. Jiang, and Y. Jin, "Clinicopathological analysis of myxoid proximal-type epithelioid sarcoma," *Journal of Cutaneous Pathology*, vol. 45, no. 2, pp. 151–155, 2018.

[3] M. B. Alikhan, G. Pease, W. Watkin, R. Grogan, T. Krausz, and T. Antic, "Primary epithelioid sarcoma of the kidney and adrenal gland: report of 2 cases with immunohistochemical and molecular cytogenetic studies," *Human Pathology*, vol. 61, pp. 158–163, 2017.

[4] X. Huang, R. Nayar, and H. Zhou, "Primary adrenal gland epithelioid sarcoma: a case report and literature review," *Diagnostic Cytopathology*, vol. 47, no. 9, pp. 918–921, 2019.

[5] R. Autorino, P. Bove, M. De Sio et al., "Open versus laparoscopic adrenalectomy for adrenocortical carcinoma: a meta-analysis of surgical and oncological outcomes," *Annals of Surgical Oncology*, vol. 23, no. 4, pp. 1195–1202, 2016.

# 44

# A Case of Papillary Urothelial Neoplasm of Low Malignant Potential (PUNLMP) in Childhood

**Reza Abbasion**,[1] **Amir Jafarpisheh**,[2] **Paria Dehghanian**,[3] **and Mahdi Mottaghi**[4]

[1]*Department of Pediatric Urology, Faculty of Medicine, Akbar Hospital, Mashhad University of Medical Sciences, Mashhad, Iran*
[2]*Department of Urology, Faculty of Medicine, Mashhad University of Medical Sciences, Mashhad, Iran*
[3]*Pathology Department, Pediatric Pathologist, Akbar Children's Hospital, Iran*
[4]*Students Research Committee, Faculty of Medicine, Mashhad University of Medical Sciences, Mashhad, Iran*

Correspondence should be addressed to Mahdi Mottaghi; mmottaghi.3000@gmail.com

Academic Editor: Mohamed A. Ghoneim

Urothelial carcinoma (UC) of the bladder is exceedingly rare in the pediatric population. It commonly presents as isolated hematuria. Considering the age group, the physician's low index of suspicion causes a delay in diagnosis. We present a seven-year-old girl complaining of dysuria and painless, intermittent hematuria. She was misdiagnosed with urinary tract infection several times. Although the initial ultrasound showed no abnormality, the second ultrasound after one year detected the tumor. The confirmation and resection are simultaneously achieved by cystoscopy. We concluded that chemotherapy is unnecessary due to the tumor's low-grade nature and the absence of detrusor involvement. One-year follow-up showed no relapse.

## 1. Introduction

Urothelial carcinoma (UC) of the bladder is exceedingly rare in the pediatric population. The disease incidence is about 0.1-0.4% for patients younger than twenty years old [1]. It is the most common bladder tumor between 13 and 18 years [1, 2]. Based on a recent systematic review, only 243 patients were reported in the literature until February 2019. The male to female ratio is 2 : 1 for the pediatric population [1]. We report another case of pediatric UC, which was managed successfully with tumor resection and no chemotherapy.

## 2. Case Presentation

A seven-year-old Caucasian girl referred to our tertiary clinic complaining of dysuria and painless gross hematuria of a three-month duration. She experienced three dysuria episodes last year, but further evaluation showed normal findings on ultrasound and only microscopic hematuria on urine analysis. She was treated for urinary tract infection several times, with partial improvement of her symptoms. In the last episode, the dysuria accompanied gross hematuria for a three-month duration. Repeated ultrasound showed "polyploid, 20∗29 mm mass with vascular peduncle on the right side of the bladder trigone. Size and the cortical echo of both kidneys were normal."

Past medical history was unremarkable except for the urinary complaints mentioned. Her father was a heavy smoker who smoked in the house. He worked as a building painter and stocked chemical dyes at home. The only finding of physical examination was a mild suprapubic tenderness. Cystoscopy demonstrated a vegetative lesion on the right lateral aspect of the bladder. Transurethral resection of the bladder (TURB) was performed. Histological findings were "noninvasive papillary urothelial neoplasm composed of delicate and fused papillae lined by transitional cells with uniformly enlarged round to oval nuclei that show normal polarity and fine chromatin without visible nucleoli. The umbrella cells are present" (Figure 1). Thus, the pathology results confirmed the diagnosis of the papillary urothelial neoplasm of

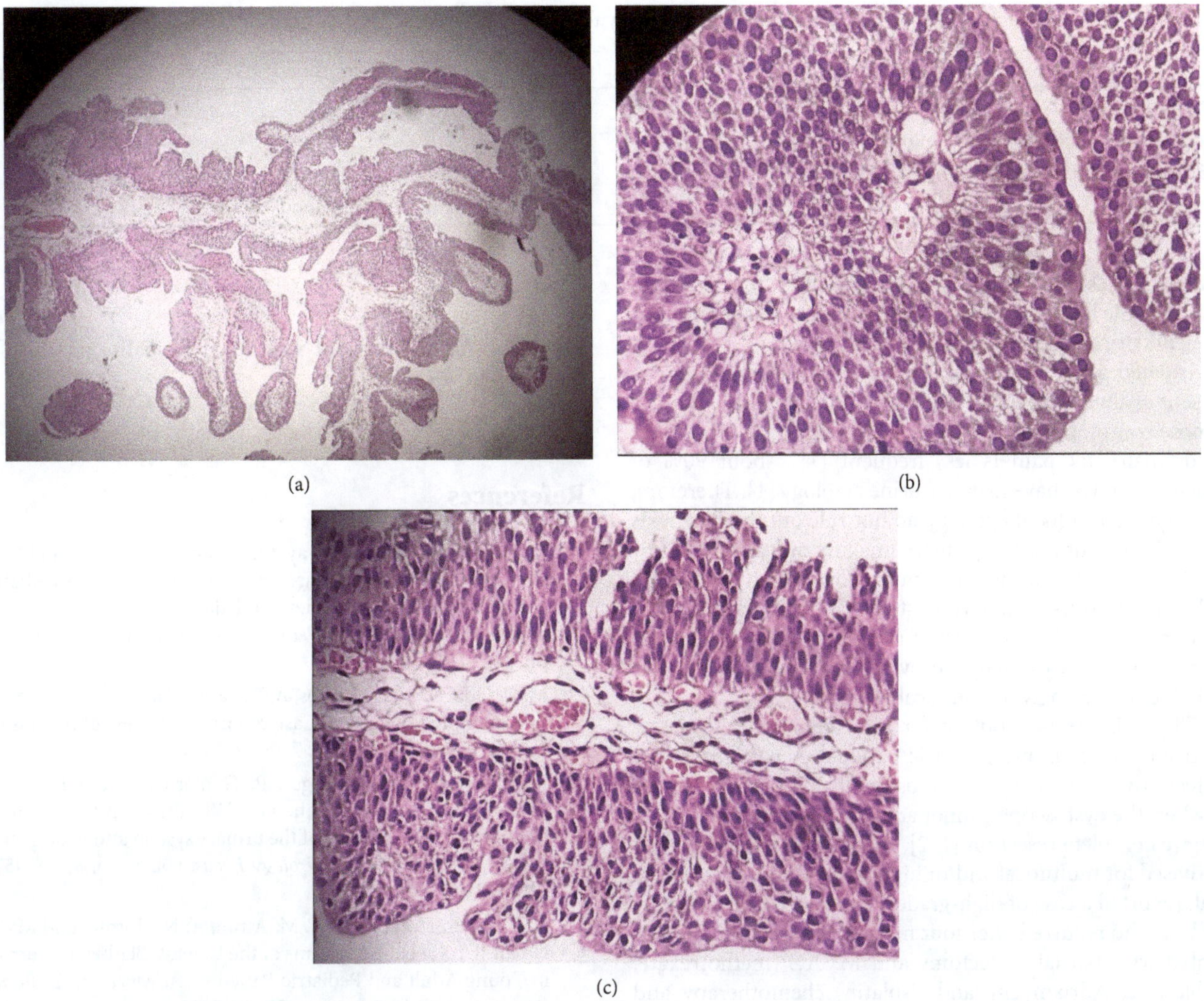

FIGURE 1: (a) Papillary urothelial neoplasm (H&E staining, low power field). (b, c) Low-grade noninvasive papillary urothelial carcinoma. The cytologic and architectural disorder is apparent with mild to moderate pleomorphism and scant mitotic figures (H&E staining, high power field).

low malignant potential (PUNLMP). Tumor margins were clear with no detrusor involvement. Therefore, the chemotherapy regimen did not use as a part of treatment. The follow-up performed with cystoscopy every 6 months plus urine analysis and cytology every three months. No sign of recurrence was detected after one year.

## 3. Discussion

Based on WHO 2016 system, the UC classified into three subtypes: (1) papillary urothelial neoplasms of low malignant potential (PUNLMP), (2) noninvasive low-grade papillary urothelial carcinoma (NILGC), and (3) noninvasive high-grade papillary urothelial carcinoma (NIHGC) [3]. Any involvement of detrusor muscle signifies high-grade tumors [3]. It is worth mentioning that T1 tumors (invasion to subepithelial connective tissue, no muscle invasion) might be classified as high grade when they extend beyond lamina propria, invade lymph vasculature, or metastasize. Thus, non-muscle-invasive tumors should evaluate carefully after tumor resection [3]. Pediatric UC in 93.4% of patients is low grade. In terms of staging, 86.4% are TaN0M0, 7.0% are T1N0M0, and only 4.1% have higher stages [1].

Previous reports of UC could only detect a risk factor in 13.2-30% of cases. The most significant risk factor is tobacco exposure, which is reported in 7.8% of pediatric patients [1]. Other probable risk factors are environmental toxins (aromatic amines of hair dyes, industrial solvents, rubber), cancer medications (cyclophosphamide), congenital bladder abnormalities, and cancer-predisposing conditions (like Costello syndrome, Li-Fraumeni, Retinoblastoma, Turner syndrome) [1, 4]. Paner et al. declared lower Cyclin D2 hypermethylation and p53 overexpression among less than 20 years old compared to the adult population [4]. Oda et al. proposed that mutations in KRAS, and BRAF genes are possible predisposing factors [2]. However, previous studies suggested a latency time for a substance to exert its carcinogenic effects; our patient's exposure to second-handed smoke and

TABLE 1: Follow-up strategy for low-grade pediatric UC.

| | Urine analysis | Ultrasound | Cystoscopy |
|---|---|---|---|
| 1st year after TURB every 3 months | + | + | + |
| 2nd year after TURB every 6 months | + | + | + |
| 3-5 years after TURB every 12 months | + | + | -/+ |
| After 5 years | Patient education about red flags. | | |

industrial dyes might cause a synergistic effect. It is hypothesized that the higher incidence after the age of 13 shows probable endocrine-related pathogenesis of UC.

Isolated gross hematuria is the most common symptom present in about 75-80% of patients [1, 2]. Painless hematuria is more common, followed by irritative symptoms. However, abdominal/flank pain is less frequent [1]. About 90% of patients with UC have negative urine cytology [1]. Therefore, the negative results of cytology do not rule out the diagnosis of UC. Ultrasound is the primary imaging modality with 85-100% sensitivity, although computed tomography (CT) and MRI were also used in several studies [1]. Considering the pediatric population and risk of radiation, MRI is preferred over CT scans. Cystoscopy provides a definitive diagnosis and able the urologist for surgical resection.

TURB is the best option for the treatment with a low recurrence rate among pediatric patients. A partial bladder cystectomy is an option for those with high-grade tumors or when the cystoscope cannot access the tumor margins to achieve complete resection [1, 2]. Intravesical chemotherapy is advised for multifocal and/or high-grade tumors [1]. Neogi et al. reported a case of high-grade T2b-stage UC in a 4-year-old boy who recurred after four months of resection. He was treated with partial cystectomy and MVAC (methotrexate, vinblastine, Adriamycin, and cisplatin) chemotherapy and remained tumor-free for six months [5]. Patients with high-grade tumors and stages higher than TaN0M0 were more likely to recur [1].

There is no reliable guideline to define how to follow the patients and for how long. Based on Rezaee et al. study, most of the recurrences detected within the first year after TURB. They also found that the longest duration between the TURB and recurrence was 32 months. Therefore, they advised following low-grade cases less aggressively after three years of TURB. The recommended follow-up strategy is shown in Table 1 [1].

## 4. Conclusion

Painless hematuria in children and younger adults rarely suggests malignancy. Nevertheless, physicians need a high index of suspicion to diagnose bladder malignancies in the early stages. Early use of noninvasive ultrasound in persistent or intermittent hematuria seems reasonable. Physicians should also note that cytology has limited diagnostic value for UC. Regarding a safe follow-up approach, low-grade tumors are unlikely to recure after three years. Therefore, lower use of cystoscopy after three years of TURB is more likely to lower the adverse effects.

## Consent

Written informed consent was taken from the parents for publishing the case.

## References

[1] M. E. Rezaee, C. M. Dunaway, M. L. Baker, F. J. Penna, and D. R. Chavez, "Urothelial cell carcinoma of the bladder in pediatric patients: a systematic review and data analysis of the world literature," *Journal of Pediatric Urology*, vol. 15, no. 4, pp. 309–314, 2019.

[2] M. H. Oda, D. V. dos Santos, A. K. Farias et al., "Bladder urothelial carcinoma in a child: Case report and review of literature," *Frontiers in Pediatrics*, vol. 7, 2019.

[3] E. M. Compérat, M. Burger, P. Gontero et al., "Grading of urothelial carcinoma and the new World Health Organisation classification of Tumours of the urinary system and male genital organs 2016," *European Urology Focus*, vol. 5, no. 3, pp. 457–466, 2019.

[4] G. P. Paner, P. Zehnder, A. M. Amin, A. N. Husain, and M. M. Desai, "Urothelial Neoplasms of the Urinary Bladder Occurring in Young Adult and Pediatric Patients," *Advances in Anatomic Pathology*, vol. 18, no. 1, pp. 79–89, 2011.

[5] S. Neogi, P. L. Kariholu, G. Dhakre, V. Gupta, N. Agarwal, and P. Bhadani, "Malignant Urothelial Carcinoma of Urinary Bladder in a Young Child: A Rare Case Report," *Urology*, vol. 81, no. 4, pp. 888–890, 2013.

# Repair of Inguinal Bladder Hernias Concomitant with Localized Prostate Cancer: A Case Report and Review of the Literature

**Kenichi Hata**[1], **Kazuhiro Takahashi**[1], **Takahiro Kimura**[2] **and Shin Egawa**[2]

[1]*Department of Urology, Atsugi City Hospital, 1-16-36, Mizuhiki, Atsugi City, Kanagawa-ken 243-8588, Japan*
[2]*Department of Urology, Jikei University School of Medicine, 3-25-8, Nishi-Shinbashi, Minato-ku, Tokyo 105-8461, Japan*

Correspondence should be addressed to Kenichi Hata; hataken1@jikei.ac.jp

Academic Editor: Apul Goel

This study reports two rare cases of inguinal bladder hernias accompanied by localized prostate cancers. They were treated with simultaneous repair of inguinal bladder hernias and open retropubic radical prostatectomy. Additionally, we performed a literature review on previous inguinal bladder hernias case reports. In this present study, the first patient was a 64-year-old man histopathologically diagnosed with prostate cancer; computed tomography for staging of prostate cancer revealed a "Pelvic Mickey Mouse Sign." The second patient was a 75-year-old man with right inguinal swelling that gradually increased in size for 30 years. He was referred to our department due to nocturia and urge incontinence. His prostate-specific antigen level was 4.17 ng/mL, and a transrectal prostate biopsy revealed prostate cancer. Preoperative imaging studies revealed a right hernia wherein most of the bladder slid beyond the inguinal channel filling the scrotum. Both patients underwent the Lichtenstein technique for inguinal bladder hernias simultaneously with retropubic radical prostatectomy using separate surgical incisions to avoid urinary contamination of the mesh. In our comprehensive review of patients who underwent inguinal bladder hernias surgical repair, there were 51 cases (50 males and 1 female). The mean patient age was 60.6 ± 12.3 years. Five cases demonstrating concomitant prostate cancer were observed. This present case report is the first to describe two patients who underwent surgeries for the simultaneous repair of inguinal bladder hernias and retropubic radical prostatectomy with separate surgical incisions. Supposedly, this simultaneous approach is suitable for concomitant inguinal bladder hernias and prostate cancer treatment.

## 1. Introduction

Inguinal bladder hernias (IBHs) have been reported for more than 100 years [1]. They occur in approximately 1–4% of all cases of inguinal hernias [2]. The frequency of occurrence has hardly changed over the years because of the difficulty in establishing diagnosis prior to hernioplasty. Less than 7% of IBHs are diagnosed preoperatively, and 16% of IBH cases are diagnosed postoperatively because of urinary leakage from wounds or sepsis owing to inadvertent bladder injuries during operation [3]. It is important to establish diagnosis before any surgical procedure to avoid life-threatening complications. Bisharat et al. recommended resection of the bladder if a bladder diverticulum, an incidental bladder tumor, or bladder necrosis is present in hernias or hernias neck is less than 0.5 cm in diameter [4]. Therefore, not only is preoperative diagnosis important but also operative strategy is. Notably, this importance becomes more pertinent when genitourinary malignant diseases coexist. Several IBH patients with genitourinary malignancies, such as bladder cancer and prostate cancer (PCa), have been reported [5–8]. However, patients who underwent a simultaneous repair of IBHs with radical retropubic prostatectomy (RRP) have not been previously reported. This study presents two patients who underwent repair of IBHs simultaneously with RRP. Additionally, we performed a literature review on IBH surgical procedures.

## 2. Case Presentation

This study was conducted in accordance with the Declaration of Helsinki (1964). All patients provided written informed consent and the study was approved by the responsible Ethical Committee.

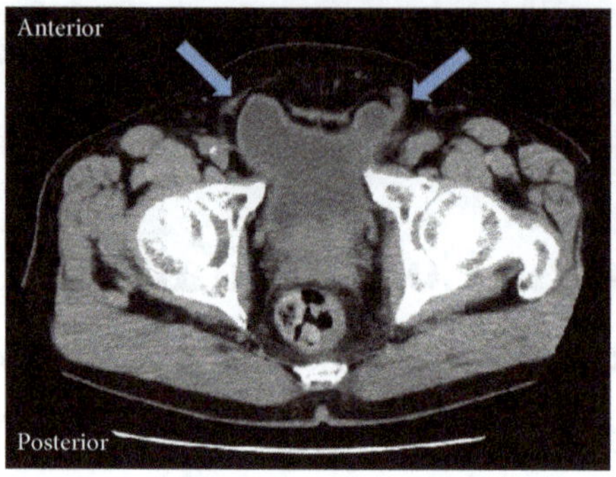


(a)

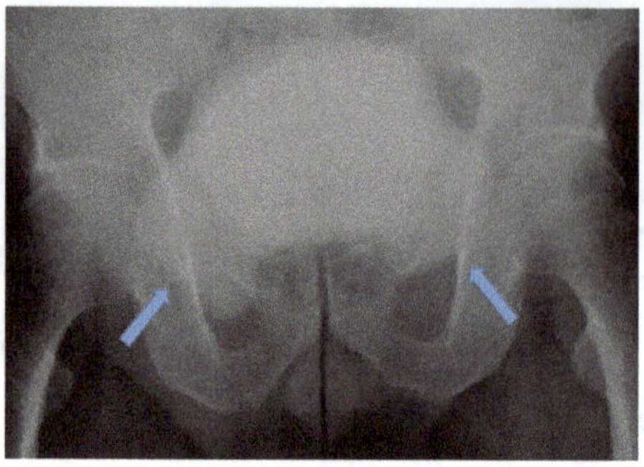

(b)

FIGURE 1: The images of case 1 showing the bladder in the right inguinal hernia. (a) Axial CT sections illustrate a small portion of the urinary bladder protruding into the bilateral inguinal canal with a "Mickey mouse"-like appearance. (b) Cystography shows the inverse "Mickey mouse".

*2.1. Case 1.* A 64-year-old man with prostate-specific antigen (PSA) of 25.29 ng/mL was referred to the Department of Urology, Atsugi City Hospital, Japan. He had a medical history of hypertension, diabetes mellitus, hypercholesterolemia, and epilepsy because of sequelae after a traffic accident. The patient reported no urinary symptoms or previous episodes of urinary retention. Physical examination was unremarkable. His body mass index was 26.01 kg/m$^2$. He underwent a transrectal prostate needle biopsy and was histopathologically diagnosed with PCa; the Gleason score was 4 + 5. Computed tomography (CT) for PCa staging incidentally revealed bilateral inguinal hernias with the bladder protruding anteroinferiorly on both sides without metastasis (Figure 1(a)). This yielded the appearance of a "Pelvic Mickey Mouse Sign," which Sagar et al. and Lichtenstein and Shulman described as an IBH phenomenon [9, 10]. Cystography showed the same "Mickey mouse" phenomenon with the bladder protruding into bilateral hernias mimicking the ears and the rest of the bladder resembling the face (Figure 1(b)) [9]. He underwent simultaneous RRP and IBH repair with the Lichtenstein technique (PerFix Light Plug; Bard Davol Inc., NJ, USA) [10]. First, radical prostatectomy was performed with extended pelvic lymphadenectomy in a lower abdominal longitudinal incision. The protruded bladder walls were smoothly replaced into their original positions. The operative field was sterilized a second time and covered with an antibiotic film. Second, bilateral inguinal hernia repairs were performed using bilateral inguinal incisions that extended medially to the pubis (Figures 2(a) and 2(b)). The surgery time was 434 minutes. His postoperative course was uneventful. The patient ambulated and ingested food on operative day 2. On postoperative day 7, Cystogram revealed no leakage or relapse of IBHs. Thereafter, bladder catheter was removed and intravenous 2 g cefotiam dihydrochloride twice daily was discontinued. Eventually, no relapse of IBHs or PCa occurred.

*2.2. Case 2.* A 75-year-old man with nocturia and urge incontinence was referred to the Department of Urology, Atsugi City Hospital, Japan. He experienced right inguinal painless swelling that gradually increased in size for 30 years. His medical history was unremarkable. A right scrotal mass was detected (20 cm in diameter). The mass was soft, non-transilluminated, and nonreducible without bowel sounds. His body mass index was 29.43 kg/m$^2$, and PSA level was 4.17 ng/mL. PCa was diagnosed with a transrectal prostate needle biopsy, and the Gleason score was 3 + 4. His CT, magnetic resonance imaging (MRI), and bone scintigraphy (BS) demonstrated a right IBH without metastasis (Figures 3(a)–3(c)). He was diagnosed with intermediate-risk PCa accompanied by the right herniation of the bladder. Simultaneous IBH repair and RRP were performed. During the operation, the bladder was squeezed out of the expanded inguinal neck (from 2 cm to 4 cm in diameter) and placed in its original position using a lower abdominal longitudinal incision. Subsequently, radical prostatectomy with pelvic extended lymph node dissection was performed. Finally, a right inguinal incision was made. The enlarged inguinal ring was repaired using a polypropylene mesh (Lichtenstein technique, PerFix Light Plug; Bard Davol Inc., NJ, USA) after concealment with the endopelvic fascia [9]. The operative time was 243 minutes. The patient ambulated and ingested food the next postoperative day. He received intravenously 2 g cefotiam dihydrochloride twice daily until the first postoperative Cystogram. The bladder catheter was removed after this postoperative normal Cystogram on postoperative day 7. The patient's postoperative course was uneventful, and the histopathological findings of the prostate revealed adenocarcinoma. Three months later, neither IBH relapse nor PCa recurrence was observed.

## 3. Discussion

IBH is defined as an acquired direct inguinal hernia with the bladder pulled into the hernia, together with a sheath of the peritoneum, which forms its sac. It can be classified into 3 types according to their relationships with the peritoneum [2]. Type I is a paraperitoneal hernia, with the extraperitoneal portion of the hernia lying along the medial wall of the sac. This is the most frequently observed IBH type, and it was noted in both cases. Type II is an intraperitoneal hernia, with the bladder completely covered by the peritoneum in the hernia sac. Type III is an extraperitoneal hernia, with the peritoneum remaining in the abdomen and the bladder herniating.

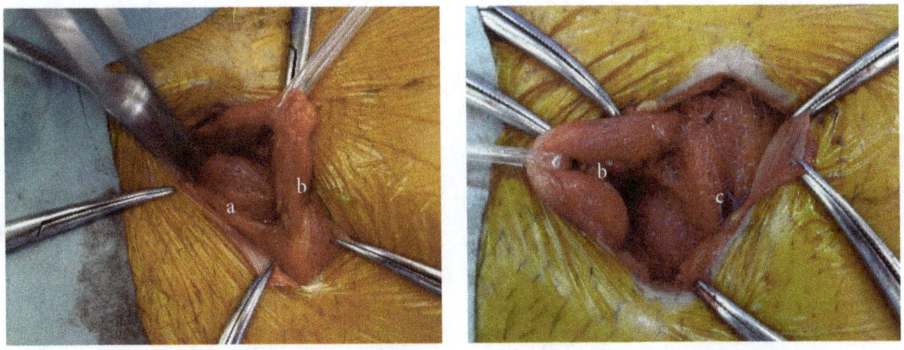


(a) (b)

Figure 2: Intraoperative appearance of the herniated bladder in case 1. (a) Herniated bladder. (b) Spermatic cord. (c) Polypropylene mesh.

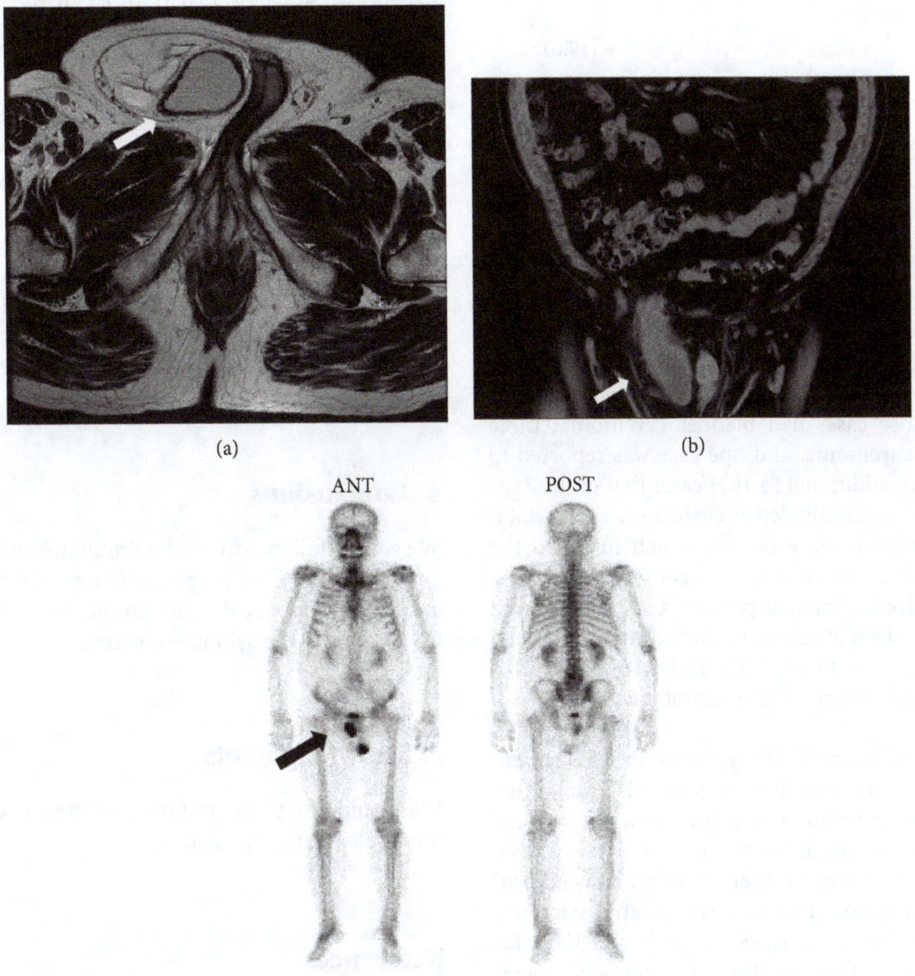


(a) (b) (c)

Figure 3: Images of case 2 showing the bladder in the right inguinal hernia. (a) Axial MRI image: the arrow indicates the IBH. (b) Coronal CT image: the arrow indicates the IBH. (c) BS image: the arrow indicates the IBH. BS: bone scintigraphy; MRI: magnetic resonance imaging; CT: computed tomography; IBH: inguinal bladder hernia.

Different factors can be associated with the pathophysiology of IBHs that include (i) bladder outlet obstruction (e.g., benign prostatic hyperplasia and bladder neck or urethral strictures), (ii) obesity, and (iii) decreased bladder tone and weakness of the pelvic musculature, which occur in an aging population [2, 4, 11, 12]. In case 2, we hypothesized that the bladder wall gradually slid into the scrotal canal due to the progression of obesity and lower urinary tract symptoms (LUTs). However, the mechanism for IBH occurrence was unclear in case 1.

As small IBHs are generally asymptomatic, preoperative diagnosis of IBHs is difficult, and such hernias are commonly

TABLE 1: Demographics of 51 patients with inguinal bladder hernia.

| Age (ys. mean ± SD, range) | 60.6 ± 12.3 (30-79) |
|---|---|
| Gender (%) | |
| Male | 50 (98.0) |
| Female | 1 (2.0) |
| Type of surgical incision ($n = 40$) (%) | |
| Single | 31 (77.5) |
| Dual | 3 (7.5) |
| Robot-assisted | 1 (2.5) |
| Laparoscopic | 5 (12.5) |
| Mesh implant ($n = 39$) (%) | |
| Use | 29 (74.4) |
| Nonuse | 10 (25.6) |
| Resection of the bladder (%) | |
| Yes | 9 (17.6) |
| No | 43 (82.4) |

diagnosed incidentally during surgery. Nevertheless, it is important for surgeons to be aware of IBHs because bladder injury during herniorrhaphy can unknowingly lead to infection, sepsis, or even death [12]. In contrast, large IBHs have the classical presence of LUTs such as two-stage micturition, frequency, urgency, nocturia, dysuria, and hematuria [6].

Oruc et al. reviewed a total of 116 patients with IBH in 2004 [12]. In their review, 13 cases (11.1%) showed malignancy. Nine of those cases had bladder carcinoma, three cases had prostate carcinoma, and one case was reported to have a neoplasm. An additional 51 IBH cases that underwent surgical procedures were evaluated after their review [4, 8, 11, 13–47]. In our comprehensive review, which included the two current cases, five cases showed concomitant PCa. One of these cases involved a Russian patient, and there was no detailed treatment information; two other cases were treated with hormone therapy for PCa [5]. To the best of our knowledge, this is the first report on the simultaneous repair of IBHs and RRPs.

In the review of 51 cases (Table 1), the mean ± SD patient age was 60.6 ± 12.3 years and there was only 1 female case. Most cases underwent repair of the IBH with an inguinal incision or an extended medial incision (77.5%). Only 6 cases underwent minimally invasive surgery (1 robot-assisted procedure and 5 laparoscopic procedures). In approximately three-fourths of the reviewed cases, a mesh was used for IBH repair. RRP is classified as a clean-contaminated operation according to the Centers for Disease Control and Prevention (CDC) because of contamination of the surgical field by urine [48]. In herniorrhaphy, incisions were classified from the lower midline incision for RRP, and polypropylene mesh was concealed from clean-contaminated wound. Choi et al. and Manoharan et al. mentioned that simultaneous repair of inguinal hernias during RRP was effective and technically feasible regardless of mesh usage. Similarly, two surgical options were indicated. The first was to make an additional inguinal incision and perform a classic hernioplasty. The second was to perform a preperitoneal hernioplasty with an incision. The possibility of complications related to urinary contamination was lower with the first option. However, the disadvantages associated with the first approach are a high likelihood of wound infection, increased discomfort and wound pain, long recovery time, increased operative time, and additional use of anesthesia [49, 50]. In these cases, the first option was selected because it strictly kept wounds separated and sterilized according to the preoperative design.

The bladder was resected in 18.0% of cases that underwent IBH surgery. Bisharat et al. suggested that bladder resection was indicated if a diverticulum, incidental tumor, or necrosis was present. In addition, it was also indicated for preventing bladder strictures that can occur if hernia neck was less than 0.5 cm in diameter [4]. In this case report, hernia necks were over 0.5 cm in diameter (approximately 3.0 cm and 2.0 cm in case 1 and case 2, respectively). No indications for bladder necrosis or ischemia were observed. Therefore, the bladders were entirely preserved by compressing them out through the expanded hernia rings.

The advantages of this approach involving simultaneous treatment of IBHs and localized PCa compared with the two-step procedure include the following: (i) compressing the bladder through the pelvis was more protective, smooth, and forceful than in groin incision; (ii) it allowed for an easy observation of the compressed bladder in the pelvis; (iii) swift actions were possible if it was necessary to resect bladder partially; and (iv) it prevented recurrence of IBHs during elective surgery.

## 4. Conclusions

We successfully performed a simultaneous treatment of IBHs and localized PCa through a safe repair of IBHs (using mesh) and RRPs. Supposedly, this simultaneous repair of IBHs and RRP with dual incisions is suitable.

## Acknowledgments

We would like to thank Editage (http://www.editage.jp/) for the English language editing.

## References

[1] H. J. Curtis, "A case of hernia of the bladder associated with an inguinal hernia, with reference to three other recent cases," *British Medical Journal*, vol. 2, no. 2219, pp. 69–71, 1903.

[2] L. G. Gomella, S. M. Spires, J. M. Burton, M. B. Ram, and R. C. Flanigan, "The Surgical Implications of Herniation of the Urinary Bladder," *Archives of Surgery*, vol. 120, no. 8, pp. 964–967, 1985.

[3] L. F. Watson, *Hernia, St*, Mosby Company, Louis CV, 1948.

[4] M. Bisharat, M. E. O'Donnell, T. Thompson et al., "Complications of inguinoscrotal bladder hernias: a case series," *Hernia*, vol. 13, no. 1, pp. 81–84, 2009.

[5] A. Sousa Escandon, M. Diaz Tie, F. Maceira Quintian, M. Armesto Fernandez, J. A. Lapena Villarroya, and C. Gonzalez Uribarri, "Inguinal bladder hernia in the adult," *Archivos Españoles de Urología*, vol. 52, no. 2, pp. 114–118, 1999.

[6] C. J. Das, J. Debnath, S. P. Thulkar, L. Kumar, and S. Vashist, "Transitional cell carcinoma in a herniated vesical diverticulum," *The British Journal of Radiology*, vol. 80, no. 957, pp. e227–e229, 2007.

[7] H. Pastor Navarro, J. Martinez Ruiz, P. Carrion Lopez et al., "Tumor inside an inguinoscrotal bladder hernia," *Archivos Españoles de Urología*, vol. 63, no. 6, pp. 471–476, 2010.

[8] A. Katsourakis, G. Noussios, C. Svoronos, M. Alatsakis, and E. Chatzitheoklitos, "Direct inguinal hernia containing bladder carcinoma: a case report and review of the literature," *International Journal of Surgery Case Reports*, vol. 5, no. 4, pp. 180–182, 2014.

[9] A. Sagar, S. Sabharwal, and N. S. Kekre, "Bilateral vesical inguinal hernia: a perineal 'Mickey mouse'," *Indian J Urol*, vol. 29, no. 2, pp. 154-155, 2013.

[10] I. L. Lichtenstein and A. G. Shulman, "Ambulatory outpatient hernia surgery. Including a new concept, introducing tension-free repair," *International Surgery*, vol. 71, no. 1, pp. 1–4, 1986.

[11] K. Moufid, D. Touiti, and L. Mohamed, "Inguinal bladder hernia: four case analyses," *Revista de Urología*, vol. 15, no. 1, pp. 32–36, 2013.

[12] M. T. Oruc, Z. Akbulut, O. Ozozan, and F. Coskun, "Urological findings in inguinal hernias: a case report and review of the literature," *Hernia*, vol. 8, no. 1, pp. 76–79, 2004.

[13] V. Gonzalvo Perez, R. Botella Almodovar, E. Canto Faubel, M. Gasso Matoses, B. Llopis Guixat, and A. Polo Peris, "Massive inguinal vesical hernia. Report of 3 cases," *Actas Urologicas Españolas*, vol. 22, no. 2, pp. 163–166, 1998.

[14] A. A. Wagner, P. Arcand, and M. H. Bamberger, "Acute renal failure resulting from huge inguinal bladder hernia," *Urology*, vol. 64, no. 1, pp. 156-157, 2004.

[15] R. Abaza, M. G. Rashid, and J. J. Sferra, "Obstructive uropathy from giant inguinal bladder and ureteral herniation," *Journal of the American College of Surgeons*, vol. 201, no. 2, p. 314, 2005.

[16] P. C. Fisher, B. K. Hollenbeck, J. S. Montgomery, and W. Underwood, "Inguinal bladder hernia masking bowel ischemia," *Urology*, vol. 63, no. 1, pp. 175-176, 2004.

[17] L. M. Minordi, P. Mirk, A. Canadè, and G. Sallustio, "Massive Inguinoscrotal Vesical Hernia Complicated by Bladder Rupture: Preoperative Sonographic and CT Diagnosis," *American Journal of Roentgenology*, vol. 183, no. 4, pp. 1091-1092, 2004.

[18] I. Sozen and J. Nobel, "Inguinal mass due to an external supravesical hernia and acute abdomen due to an internal supravesical hernia: a case report and review of the literature," *Hernia*, vol. 8, no. 4, pp. 389–392, 2004.

[19] S. Huerta, T. Fairbanks, and M. Cinat, "Incarcerated vesicoinguinal hernia presenting with gross hematuria," *Journal of the American College of Surgeons*, vol. 201, no. 6, pp. 992-993, 2005.

[20] A. Bernaerts, B. O. de Beeck, L. Hoekx, and P. M. Parizel, "Paraperitoneal indirect inguinal bladder hernia: MR demonstration," *Abdominal Imaging*, vol. 30, no. 6, pp. 685–688, 2005.

[21] M. Nicola and F. de Luca, "Bladder hernia," *Archivio Italiano di Urologia, Andrologia*, vol. 78, no. 2, pp. 77-78, 2006.

[22] A. Gurer, M. Ozdogan, N. Ozlem, A. Yildirim, H. Kulacoglu, and R. Aydin, "Uncommon content in groin hernia sac," *Hernia*, vol. 10, no. 2, pp. 152–155, 2006.

[23] M. A. Bjurlin, D. A. Delaurentis, M. D. Jordan, and H. M. Richter 3rd, "Clinical and radiographic findings of a sliding inguinoscrotal hernia containing the urinary bladder," *Hernia*, vol. 14, no. 6, pp. 635–638, 2010.

[24] J. N. Helleman, P. Willemsen, M. Vanderveken, J. Cortvriend, and P. Van Erps, "Incarcerated vesico-inguinal hernia: a case report," *Acta Chirurgica Belgica*, vol. 109, no. 6, pp. 815–817, 2016.

[25] B. Mahadevappa, S. C. Suresh, K. Natarajan, and J. Thomas, "Cystogram with dumbbell shaped urinary bladder in a sliding inguinal hernia," *J Radiol Case Rep*, vol. 3, no. 2, pp. 7–9, 2009.

[26] S. K. Mouli and E. Sabanegh Jr., "Acute vesicoinguinal hernia," *Urology*, vol. 75, no. 1, p. 73, 2010.

[27] K. H. Kim, M. U. Kim, W. J. Jeong et al., "Incidentally detected inguinoscrotal bladder hernia," *Korean Journal of Urology*, vol. 52, no. 1, pp. 71–73, 2011.

[28] M. K. Malhotra and Y. Kapoor, "Pre surgical evaluation of scrotal cystocele by conventional radiography (Cystogram)," *Niger J Surg*, vol. 18, no. 1, pp. 34–36, 2012.

[29] C. Ellimoottil, M. Ross, S. T. Hart, and J. Milner, "Unusual videourodynamic finding: massive scrotal cystocele," *Urology*, vol. 80, no. 5, pp. 53-54, 2012.

[30] S. Manfredelli, A. Zitelli, S. Pontone et al., "An inguinal bladder diverticulum case report of a rare finding in a recurrent inguinal hernia," *Annali Italiani di Chirurgia*, p. S2239253X12019810, 2012.

[31] E. M. Uchio, J. S. Calderon, and J. J. Hwang, "Laparoscopic repair of inguinal cystocele using cystoscopic light test," *Urology*, vol. 79, no. 3, pp. 725-727, 2012.

[32] J. Westera, J. Meyer, J. Reynolds, and A. Lambrianides, "Massive inguinoscrotal bladder hernia," *J Surg Case Rep*, vol. 2012, no. 5, p. 5, 2012.

[33] A. Karatzas, G. Christodoulidis, M. Spyridakis, C. Stavaras, E. Aravantinos, and M. Melekos, "A giant inguinoscrotal bladder hernia as a cause of chronic renal failure: a rare case," *International Journal of Surgery Case Reports*, vol. 4, no. 3, pp. 345–347, 2013.

[34] S. Hirasaki, M. Nishimura, Y. Ito, and T. Nagano, "Incidental detection of an inguinoscrotal urinary bladder hernia," *Internal Medicine*, vol. 52, no. 1, p. 165, 2013.

[35] H. K. Lee and J. Skarzynski, "Bladder herniation in inguinal hernia detected during bone imaging," *Clinical Nuclear Medicine*, vol. 11, no. 10, p. 740, 1986.

[36] A. Hamidi Madani, H. Mohammadi Nikouei, H. Baghani Aval, A. Enshaei, A. Asadollahzade, and S. Esmaeili, "Scrotal herniation of bladder: a case report," *Iran J Med Sci*, vol. 38, no. 1, pp. 62–64, 2013.

[37] J. P. McKay, M. Organ, S. Bagnell, C. Gallant, and C. French, "Inguinoscrotal hernias involving urologic organs: a case series," *Canadian Urological Association Journal*, vol. 8, no. 5-6, pp. 429–432, 2014.

[38] A. Khan, I. Beckley, B. Dobbins, and K. M. Rogawski, "Laparoscopic repair of massive inguinal hernia containing the urinary bladder," *Urol Ann*, vol. 6, no. 2, pp. 159–162, 2014.

[39] S. Vyas, N. Chabra, S. K. Singh, and N. Khandelwal, "Inguinal herniation of the bladder and ureter: an unusual cause of obstructive uropathy in a transplant kidney," *Saudi Journal*

*of Kidney Diseases and Transplantation*, vol. 25, no. 1, pp. 153–155, 2014.

[40] T. Kawaguchi, T. Itoh, K. Yoshii, and E. Otsuji, "Laparoscopic repair of a bilateral internal inguinal hernia with supravesical hernia - a case report," *International Journal of Surgery Case Reports*, vol. 14, pp. 108–111, 2015.

[41] A. Frenkel, A. Roy-Shapira, I. Shelef et al., "Inguinal Herniation of the Urinary Bladder Presenting as Recurrent Urinary Retention," *Case Reports in Surgery*, vol. 2015, Article ID 531021, 3 pages, 2015.

[42] M. Tarchouli, M. B. Ratbi, M. Bouzroud et al., "Giant inguinoscrotal hernia containing intestinal segments and urinary bladder successfully repaired by simple hernioplasty technique: a case report," *Journal of Medical Case Reports*, vol. 9, no. 1, 2015.

[43] L. N. Cetrulo, J. Harmon, J. Ortiz et al., "Case report of a robotic-assisted laparoscopic repair of a giant incarcerated recurrent inguinal hernia containing bladder and ureters," *Int J Med Robot*, vol. 11, no. 1, pp. 15–17, 2015.

[44] M. Ugur, N. Atci, C. Oruc, S. Akkucuk, and A. Aydogan, "Left inguinal bladder hernia that causes dilatation in the ureter," *Archives of Iranian Medicine*, vol. 19, no. 5, pp. 376–378, 2016.

[45] I. Zihni, A. Duran, and V. Soysal, "A rare cause of inguinal hernia: scrotal cystocele," *Ulus Cerrahi Derg*, vol. 32, no. 2, pp. 137–139, 2016.

[46] B. Cybulka, M. Podgorny, J. Rapela, and A. Wach, "Surgical trap of a routine procedure. Scrotal hernia with concomitant sliding of the urinary bladder–case report," *Polski Przeglad Chirurgiczny*, vol. 87, no. 11, pp. 587–591, 2015.

[47] R. D. Konik, P. Narh-Martey, and G. Bogen, "Recurrence of an inguinal hernia containing the dome of the bladder following laparoscopic repair with mesh: a case report," *International Journal of Surgery Case Reports*, vol. 25, pp. 218–220, 2016.

[48] A. J. Mangram, T. C. Horan, M. L. Pearson, L. C. Silver, and W. R. Jarvis, "Guideline for Prevention of Intravascular-Device-Related Infections," *Infection Control and Hospital Epidemiology*, vol. 20, no. 4, pp. 250–278, 1999.

[49] B. B. Choi, J. Steckel, G. Denoto, E. D. Vaughan, and P. N. Schlegel, "Preperitoneal prosthetic mesh hernioplasty during radical retropubic prostatectomy," *The Journal of Urology*, vol. 161, no. 3, pp. 840–843, 1999.

[50] M. Manoharan, P. Gomez, and M. S. Soloway, "Concurrent radical retropubic prostatectomy and inguinal hernia repair through a modified Pfannenstiel incision," *BJU International*, vol. 93, no. 9, pp. 1203–1206, 2004.

46

# Spontaneous Intraperitoneal Rupture of Bladder Diverticulum: A Rare Cause of Peritonitis

**Ahmed Ibrahimi,[1] Adil Kallat,[2] Idriss Ziani,[1] Hachem El Sayegh,[1] Lounis Benslimane,[1] and Yassine Nouini[1]**

[1]*Department of Urology A, Ibn Sina University Hospital, Faculty of Medicine and Pharmacy, Mohammed V University in Rabat, Rabat, Morocco*
[2]*Provincial Hospital Center of Azilal, Azilal, Morocco*

Correspondence should be addressed to Ahmed Ibrahimi; ahmed.ibrahimi@um5s.net.ma

Academic Editor: Apul Goel

Spontaneous rupture of acquired bladder diverticulum in an adult patient is an extremely rare pathological entity with only 15 cases reported in the available literature. Etiologies are dominated by bladder outlet obstruction, represented mainly by benign prostatic hypertrophy (BPH) in elderly men. Clinical presentation is nonspecific, leading to delayed diagnosis and treatment. Surgical management is the standard approach for intraperitoneal rupture of bladder diverticulum. The prognosis depends on the earliness of treatment, associated comorbidity, and the nature of underlying diseases. Herein, we report a rare case of a 65-year-old male patient, who presented a spontaneous rupture of a large acquired bladder diverticulum, secondary to acute urinary retention complicating benign prostatic hypertrophy. The diagnosis was suspected in the presence of generalized peritonitis associated with lower urinary tract symptoms (LUTS) and was confirmed accurately and promptly by a computed tomography (CT) of the abdomen and pelvis. The patient underwent a successful surgical excision of the diverticulum and bladder repair without delay. The postoperative course was uneventful, and he was discharged from the hospital without any complication.

## 1. Introduction

Spontaneous rupture of acquired bladder diverticulum in an adult patient is a very rare pathological entity; to the best of our best knowledge, only 15 cases have been reported in the literature, and we add case 16 [1–3]. A bladder diverticulum is a mucosal protrusion through the detrusor muscle defect, composed of urothelial lining without a muscular layer [2]. It is most often secondary to bladder outlet obstruction such as benign prostate hyperplasia, repetitive infections, and iatrogenic causes [2]. The nonspecificity of its symptoms can delay diagnosis and treatment and can lead to serious complications or even death [4]. Surgical management remains the standard approach for intraperitoneal bladder rupture [2, 3, 5, 6]. However, conservative management can be successfully performed in selected patients with favourable characteristics [1, 7].

Here, we report a rare case of spontaneous intraperitoneal rupture of bladder diverticulum secondary to an episode of acute urine retention complicating benign prostatic hypertrophy, described in a 65-year-old male patient with a history of untreated BPH, and which was successfully managed by a prompt diagnosis and surgical treatment. Through this report, we aimed to highlight this rare cause of acute peritonitis, as well as to discuss the different clinical, etiological, and therapeutic aspects of this surgical emergency.

## 2. Case Presentation

A 65-year-old man, with a history of benign prostatic hypertrophy (BPH) not followed for 2 years, without other medical complaints, was admitted to the emergency for acute urinary retention (AUR); he underwent urethral catheterization and returned home with alpha-blocker therapy, and two days later, he represented to the emergency department with diffuse acute abdominal pain, especially in the hypogastric region, nausea and vomiting, associated with generalized weakness and fever.

Physical examination of the abdomen revealed diffuse tenderness associated with muscle guarding and rebound pain especially in the hypogastric area, without distended urinary bladder; the digital rectal examination (DRE) was painful and found a firm and enlarged prostate gland. His temperature was 38°C, with blood pressure of 125/62 mmHg, heart rate of 94 beats/min, and respiratory rate of 17 breaths/min.

Laboratory testing revealed hemoglobin of 12.8 g/dL, platelet count of 520,000/mm$^3$, increase in serum urea of 0.73 g/dL and in serum creatinine of 27 mg/dL, with elevated of white blood cell (WBC) of 17,300/$\mu$L, and C-reactive protein (CRP) of 96.2 mg/dL. After conditioning, an intravenous antibiotic was administered, and a urinary catheterization had given 80 mL of cloudy urine, and the urine test strip was positive.

Ultrasonography (US) showed bilateral hydroureteronephrosis with empty bladder containing a small amount of urine and a large bladder stone; these findings are associated with the presence of a large full bladder diverticulum and a small amount of free peritoneal fluid. CT of the abdomen and pelvis without contrast (due to the kidney failure) confirmed the presence of a small amount of free fluid in the abdominal cavity, associated with massive fluid accumulation in the right anterolateral paravesical space, between the bladder and the anterior abdominal wall (Figures 1(b)–1(d), 2, and 3), and a ruptured large bladder diverticulum arising from the right superolateral wall of the urinary bladder (Figures 1(c) and 3) with bilateral hydroureteronephrosis (Figure 1(a)), large bladder stone (Figures 1(b), 1(d), and 2(b)) and enlarged prostate gland measuring 63 g (Figure 2). Clinical presentation and imaging findings lead to the diagnosis of acute peritonitis secondary to spontaneous intraperitoneal perforation of bladder diverticulum.

The patient was transferred to the operation theater, and an emergency midline laparotomy was performed, revealing an intraperitoneal rupture of a large bladder diverticulum which was located on the right superolateral wall of the bladder, with fluid collection around it, and free purulent fluid in the abdominal cavity; there was no evidence of pathologic lesions at the site of the injured diverticulum and peritoneum. A copious saline lavage of the peritoneal cavity was done, the diverticulum was excised, the bladder stone was removed, and the bladder defect was repaired in two layers with continuous 2/0 Vicryl sutures. Successful repair of the bladder defect was confirmed intraoperatively by the absence of leakage when filling the bladder, and a pelvic drain left in situ at the end of intervention.

The postoperative course was uneventful. The inflammatory markers and renal function showed decreases over the following days to reach its normal level. Cystogram performed at the eighth day showed a watertight bladder.

The patient was discharged from the hospital at the 10th day with an indwelling bladder catheter, and a transurethral prostatic resection (TUPR) was planned after 6 weeks.

## 3. Discussion

Urinary bladder ruptures are in most cases secondary to blunt abdominal trauma, pelvic fractures, or iatrogenic causes, and 96.6% of all cases of bladder ruptures are posttraumatic [8, 9]. A spontaneous, nontraumatic urinary bladder rupture is a very rare surgical emergency, with an incidence of 1 : 126,000 and a mortality rate of 47% [5].

Bladder rupture can be classified into intraperitoneal or extraperitoneal types depending on the defect location, which occurs usually in the bladder dome which is the weakest point of the bladder wall, causing an intraperitoneal bladder rupture [5, 10, 11]. Common predisposing factors for spontaneous bladder rupture are associated with either increased bladder pressure or decreased strength of the bladder wall or its combination [12]. In the available literature, only a few cases of spontaneous bladder rupture were reported; the common causes are malignancy, pervious pelvic radiotherapy, neuropathic bladder dysfunction, bladder inflammation or infection, bladder outflow obstruction [4, 5, 10, 12], alcohol intoxication (binge drinking) [13], female pelvic organ prolapse, and postpartum [10]; it can be also associated with extravesical pathology such as appendiceal abscesses, tuboovarian abscesses, divertitular disease, or even surgical drain placed alongside the bladder [14], or in the rare cases secondary to ruptured congenital or acquired bladder diverticulum [1–3].

The clinical presentation is nonspecific, including painful abdominal distension, decreased urine output, and voiding complaints [2, 11], and in some cases, it can take on the appearance of acute peritonitis with sepsis, oliguria, and acute renal failure due to reabsorption of creatinine in the urinary ascites [5, 9]; this atypical presentation can delay diagnosis and treatment and lead to serious, life-threatening complications, especially in the case of spontaneous intraperitoneal rupture of bladder diverticulum [4]. In the present case, both bladder diverticulum and bladder stone associated to renal failure are the complications of BPH, and intraperitoneal bladder rupture seems to be the result of a combination of sudden increase in intravesical pressure due to AUR, and a decrease of the strength of the bladder wall due to bladder diverticulum.

Considering its rarity, the diagnosis should be suspected in the presence of the past urological history of risk factors suggestive of bladder rupture, associated with symptoms of acute abdomen. The positive diagnosis is based on CT cystography which remains the gold standard for the diagnosis, and it is most sensitive for detecting the presence of bladder perforation than ultrasound or conventional CT [15]. CT cystography compared to retrograde cystography is less invasive with comparable findings and has an additional advantage of exploration the whole abdominal cavity [15]. Ultrasound can also make the diagnosis by instillation of saline and air into the bladder [11]. Cystoscopy is not recommended but can be used to place the urethral catheter in the cases of urethral stricture or false passage [16]. In our case, retrograde cystography was not performed because of the urinary tract infection, CT scan without contrast allowed us to make the diagnosis, and the exam positivity is due to the

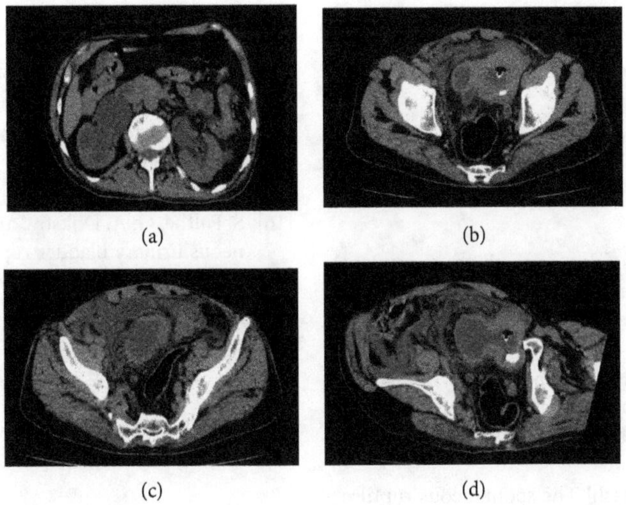

FIGURE 1: Axial view of CT scan showing (a) bilateral hydroureteronephrosis. (b, d) Empty bladder, associated to a large full bladder diverticulum, with bladder stone and bilateral ureteral dilation. (c) Small amount of free intraperitoneal fluid leaking from a defect in the bladder diverticulum wall.

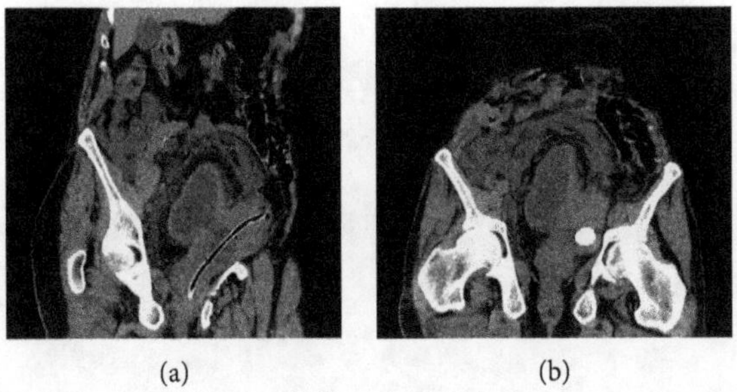

FIGURE 2: (a, b) Coronal oblique reconstruction of the CT scan showing collapsed bladder with a large diverticulum arising from the right superolateral bladder wall, with a large bladder stone and Foley catheter in place, associated to a small amount of free fluid in the peritoneal cavity and around the diverticulum, with an enlarged prostate gland.

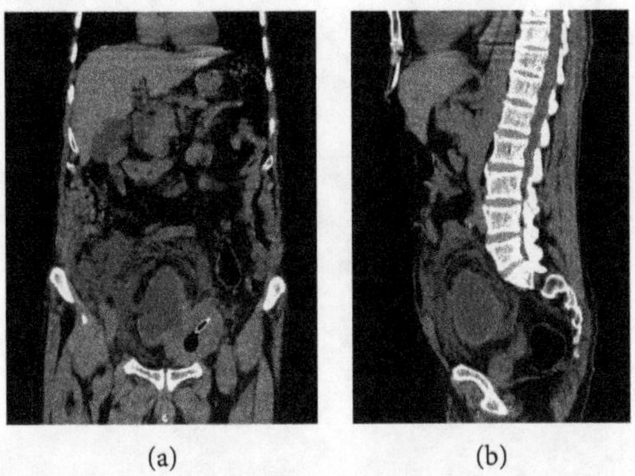

FIGURE 3: (a) Coronal reconstruction of the CT scan showing empty bladder with small amount of intra-abdominal fluid leaking from a ruptured large bladder diverticulum and perivesical fat infiltration. (b) Sagittal reconstruction of the CT scan showing a large full ruptured bladder diverticulum with fluid collection around it and ureteral dilation.

defect location which was not plugging during the radiological examination, and the large size of the diverticulum which was always filled with urine despite its perforation, probably because the diverticulum wall was not completely ruptured and because of the small size of the defect.

When diagnosed, treatment depends on type of bladder rupture as well as the presence of an underlying pathology which may require additional treatment [6]. Intraperitoneal rupture of a bladder diverticulum requires immediate surgical repair to avoid serious complications, it can be made by laparotomy or laparoscopically in selected patients [3], and it consists of exploring the whole abdominal cavity, excising the diverticulum, repairing the bladder defect, and draining the abdominal fluid [4, 8, 13, 14]. Conservative management without surgery can be successfully used in carefully selected patients with only urinary catheterization and antibiotics, with or without percutaneous peritoneal drainage [1, 4, 7].

After the acute episode, a special consideration must be given to the treatment of the associated diseases to prevent recidive. In our case, conservative management has not been attempted because of the presence of clinical and biological sepsis, and the presence of bladder stone requiring surgical treatment. The uneventful postoperative course without complication can be attributed to the prompt diagnosis and treatment and the absence of other associated pathologies.

## 4. Conclusion

Spontaneous intraperitoneal rupture of bladder diverticulum is a rare surgical emergency, and diagnosis should be suspected without delay in the presence of acute abdomen associated with lower urinary tract symptoms. Prevention requires better management of underlying pathologies and risk factors, and prompt and accurate diagnosis is the key for successful management.

## Authors' Contributions

All authors have read and approved the final version of the manuscript.

## References


[1] S. B. Oh and J. H. Ahn, "Successful conservative management of a spontaneous intraperitoneal rupture of bladder diverticulum in a critical patient," *Medicine (Baltimore)*, vol. 99, no. 7, article e19262, 2020.

[2] M. M. Britto, H. H. I. Yao, and N. Campbell, "Delayed diagnosis of spontaneous rupture of a congenital bladder diverticulum as a rare cause of an acute abdomen," *ANZ Journal of Surgery*, vol. 89, no. 9, 2019.

[3] O. Leahy and J. Grummet, "Splash! The spontaneous rupture of a bladder diverticulum: a rare cause of an acute abdomen," *ANZ Journal of Surgery*, vol. 83, no. 10, pp. 792-793, 2013.

[4] P. Qiao, D. Tian, and Q. Bao, "Delayed diagnosis of spontaneous bladder rupture: a rare case report," *BMC Women's Health*, vol. 18, no. 1, p. 124, 2018.

[5] X. Zhang, G. Zhang, L. Zhang, C. Sun, N. Liu, and M. Chen, "Spontaneous rupture of the urinary bladder caused by eosinophilic cystitis in a male after binge drinking: a case report," *Medicine (Baltimore)*, vol. 96, no. 51, article e9170, 2017.

[6] D. K. Sabat, P. K. Panigrahi, R. K. Sahoo, M. Acharya, and Sahu MCh, "Spontaneous puerperal extraperitoneal bladder wall rupture in young woman with diagnostic dilemma," *Journal of Family Medicine and Primary Care*, vol. 4, no. 4, pp. 601–603, 2015.

[7] C. Moreno-Alarcon, M. Rigabert-Montiel, P. Lopez-Cubillana, and G. Gómez-Gómez, "Conservative management is a reasonable option in intraperitoneal bladder rupture," *Archivos Españoles de Urología*, vol. 67, no. 9, pp. 788–791, 2014.

[8] R. Murata, Y. Kamiizumi, Y. Tani et al., "Spontaneous rupture of the urinary bladder due to bacterial cystitis," *Journal of Surgical Case Reports*, vol. 2018, no. 9, 2018.

[9] M. Wieloch, K. Bazylinska, and P. Ziemniak, "Spontaneous, idiopathic urinary bladder perforation - case report," *Polski Przeglad Chirurgiczny*, vol. 85, no. 12, pp. 727–729, 2013.

[10] A. Aber, S. A. Hyder, and V. Arumuham, "An unusual case of spontaneous bladder perforation with associated autodialysis of the ensuing urinary ascites," *Case Reports in Medicine*, vol. 2011, Article ID e145084, 2011https://www.ncbi.nlm.nih.gov/pmc/articles/PMC3226425/.

[11] N. Itoh and T. Kounami, "Spontaneous rupture of a bladder diverticulum: ultrasonographic diagnosis," *The Journal of Urology*, vol. 152, no. 4, pp. 1206-1207, 1994.

[12] T. Mitchell, S. Al-Hayek, B. Patel, F. Court, and H. Gilbert, "Acute abdomen caused by bladder rupture attributable to neurogenic bladder dysfunction following a stroke: a case report," *Journal of Medical Case Reports*, vol. 5, no. 1, p. 254, 2011.

[13] M. Muneer, H. Abdelrahman, A. El-Menyar, A. Zarour, A. Awad, and H. Al-Thani, "Spontaneous atraumatic urinary bladder rupture secondary to alcohol intoxication: a case report and review of literature," *American Journal of Case Reports*, vol. 16, pp. 778–781, 2015.

[14] J. L. Huffman, W. Schraut, and D. H. Bagley, "Atraumatic perforation of bladder: necessary differential in evaluation of acute condition of abdomen," *Urology*, vol. 22, no. 1, pp. 30–35, 1983.

[15] P. V. Quagliano, S. M. Delair, and A. K. Malhotra, "Diagnosis of blunt bladder injury: a prospective comparative study of computed tomography cystography and conventional retrograde cystography," *The Journal of Trauma*, vol. 61, no. 2, pp. 410–422, 2006.

[16] S. Palthe, G. A. Dijkstra, and M. G. Steffens, "A case of spontaneous urinary bladder rupture secondary to urinary retention due to an urethral stricture," *Urology Case Reports*, vol. 17, pp. 85–87, 2018.

# 47

# Growing Teratoma Syndrome: A Rare Outcome

**João Rebelo**,[1] **Francisco Moreira**,[2] **Margarida Morgado**,[1] **Ana Sofia Preto**,[1] **and António Madureira**[1,3]

[1]*Radiology Department, Centro Hospitalar Universitário de São João, Porto, Portugal*
[2]*Pathology Department, Centro Hospitalar Universitário de São João, Porto, Portugal*
[3]*Faculdade de Medicina da Universidade do Porto, Porto, Portugal*

Correspondence should be addressed to João Rebelo; rebelo.jmr@gmail.com

Academic Editor: Apul Goel

Growing teratoma syndrome is a rare condition described in both testicular and ovarian cancer. We present a case of a 26-year-old male with known mixed germ cell tumor which exhibited new and progressive secondary lesions during imaging surveillance, later to be histologically characterized as teratomas.

## 1. Introduction

Growing teratoma syndrome (GTS) was first reported by Logothetis in 1982, as a rare entity among patients with non-seminomatous germ cell tumors, characterized by growing masses developing during or after chemotherapy despite normal levels of tumoral biomarkers.

A close imaging surveillance is essential for early recognition of GTS, particularly in patients with risk factors, and because of the chemoresistant nature of GTS, there is a need to prevent further uneffective systemic therapy. Surgical resection is currently the gold standard for GTS treatment.

Although GTS typically has a good prognosis, regular follow-up is critical to detect malignant degeneration.

## 2. Case Report

A 26-year-old male was referred to our institution to study a potential mass of the right testicle, noted in the previous weeks on physical exam. The patient had no significant medical background or history of previous testicular trauma. A testicular ultrasound and serum tumoral biomarkers were ordered.

A testicular ultrasound was performed which showed an enlarged right testicle (estimated volume of 32 cc), presenting highly heterogenous parenchyma with multiple nodules, most of them hypoechogenic and demonstrating high vascularization. A right moderate hematocele was also present. Doppler analysis also showed bilateral varicocele (pampiniform plexus venous caliber above 3 mm), without significant reflux with Valsalva maneuvers. This finding precluded an abdominal ultrasound to exclude extrinsic causes for venous congestion. It revealed one superior retroperitoneal lymphadenomegaly with almost 4 cm on its major axis, associated with densification of its surrounding fat. Ultrasound findings suggested a testicular mass suspicious for malignancy with metastatic retroperitoneal lymph node (Figure 1).

A thoracoabdominopelvic computed tomography (CT) with IV contrast was performed for staging, confirming a retroperitoneal lateroaortic lymphadenomegaly and also finding a left supraclavicular lymphadenomegaly (2 cm of major axis). No other signs of secondary lesions were found (Figures 2 and 3).

A right orchidectomy was readily executed, and the histology revealed testicular involvement by mixed germ cell neoplasm associated with germ cell neoplasia in situ, with seminoma-type components, embryonal carcinoma type, and yolk sac type (Figure 4). At the time of the surgery, serum tumoral biomarkers such as alpha-fetoprotein (AFP -47.9 mg/dL (*N* 1-8 mg/mL)), chorionic gonadotropin (hCG -4.3 mUI/mL (*N* 0-4 mUI/L)), and lactate dehydrogenase (LDH -239 U/L (*N* 135-225 U/L)) were elevated (Figure 5).

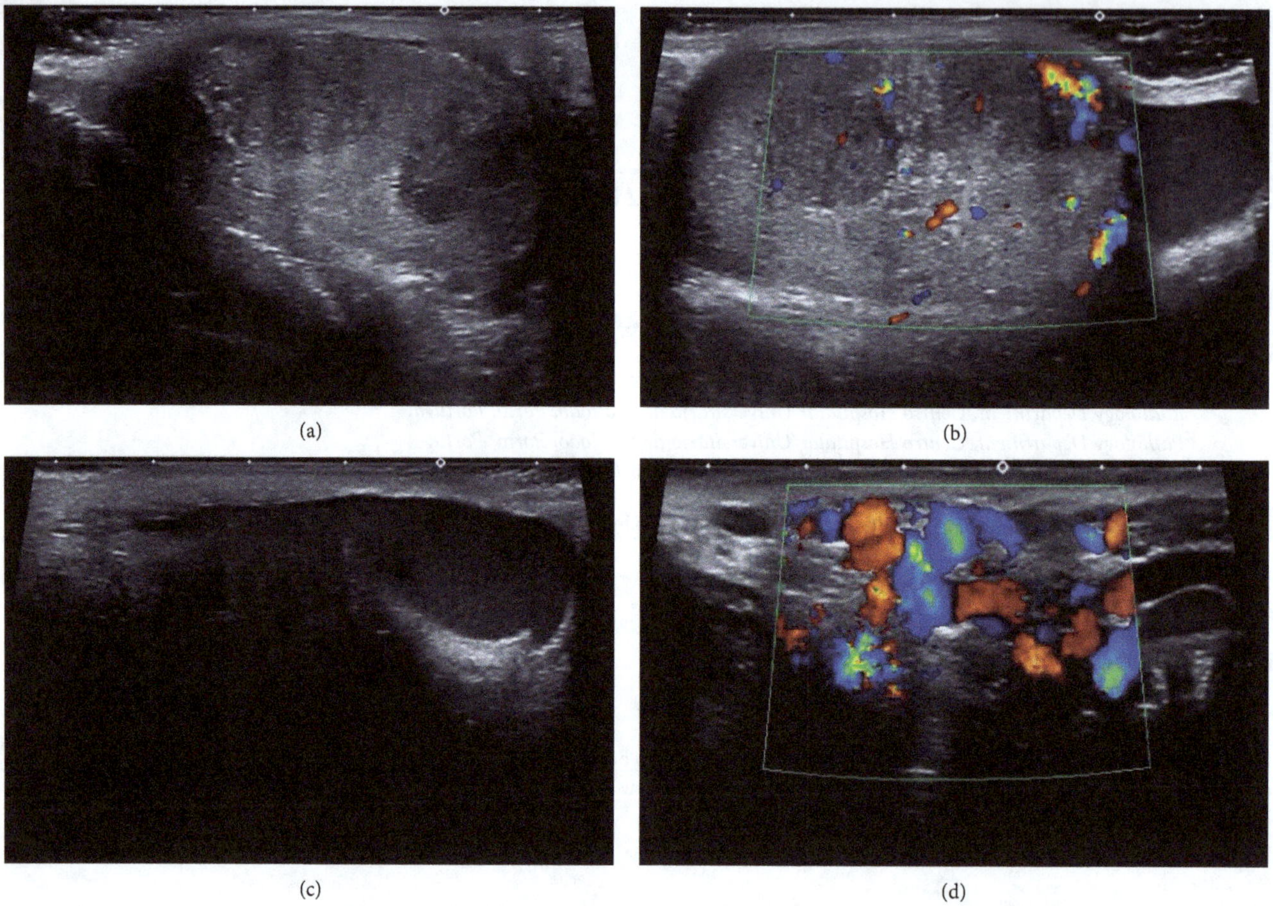

FIGURE 1: Ultrasound. (a–c) Enlarged right testicle (estimated volume of 32 cc) and a highly heterogenous parenchyma with multiple nodules, most of them hypoechogenic and demonstrating high vascularization. A right complex hydrocele, suggestive of an hematocele, is also seen. (d) Doppler analysis found bilateral varicocele without significant reflux with Valsalva maneuvers.

The case was presented and discussed on a multidisciplinary team conference, and chemotherapy with four cycles of bleomycin, etoposide, and cisplatin (BEP regimen) was chosen based on lymph node spreading.

At the beginning of chemotherapy, about 2 months after surgery, tumoral markers reached a maximum peak. Then, in the following two months, they finally decreased to normal values and remained normal until the present day (Figure 5).

On the other hand, follow-up CT imaging, performed about every 2 to 3 months, demonstrated increased number and larger cervical and retroperitoneal lymph nodes. Furthermore, it showed new mediastinal lesions with similar appearance—diffuse hypodensity—suggesting cystic/necrotic nature (Figures 6 and 7).

Five months postsurgery, when the chemotherapy regimen was completed, a microbiopsy was performed on a left cervical lymphadenomegaly (Figure 8). Since this lesion's histology was compatible with teratoma, and there was normalization of tumoral biomarkers and tumor growth during and after systemic chemotherapy after a significant reduction in tumor burden, the diagnosis of growing teratoma syndrome was suggested.

On the following multidisciplinary team meeting, excision of the cervical and retroperitoneal secondary lesions was proposed and the patient underwent cervical and retroperitoneal lymphadenectomies without major complications.

At 24 months of surveillance, tumoral biomarkers remained normal, and there were not new cervical or retroperitoneal secondary lesions to report on imaging. However, the mediastinal lesions persisted and showed slow size progression over time, but considering the known risks associated with their anatomical location, an active surveillance approach was decided. At the moment, the patient is compliant with the follow-up protocol without major events or complications associated.

## 3. Discussion

Growing teratoma syndrome (GTS) was first described by Logothetis in 1982, as a rare entity among patients with nonseminomatous germ cell tumors [1, 2]. It is characterized by growing metastatic masses despite appropriate systemic chemotherapy and normal serum markers. This condition remains poorly known, with most of the reports consisting of case series with few patients [1–5].

According to Logothetis, the diagnostic criteria of GTS were (a) normalization of elevated serum AFP and hCG, (b) tumor growth during or after systemic

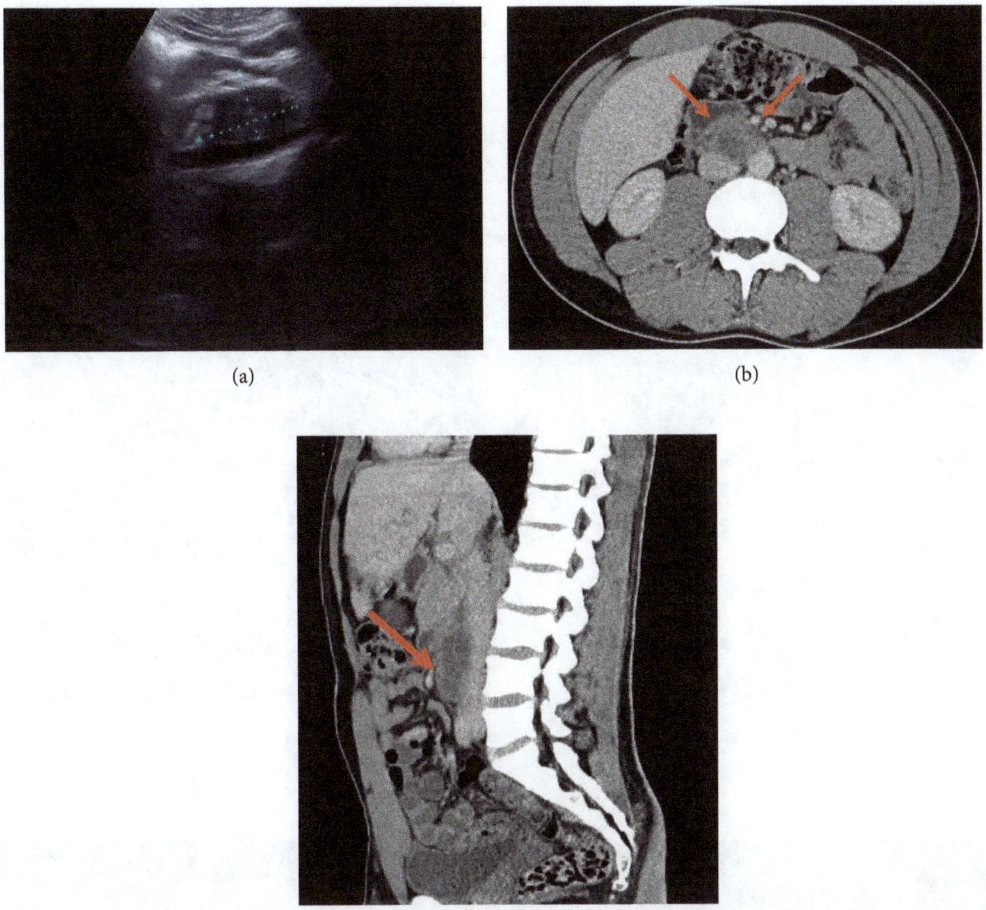

(a) (b) (c)

Figure 2: Ultrasound and CT. (a) Sagittal gray-scale abdominal ultrasound of the superior retroperitoneum, demonstrating a hypoechoic enlarged lymph node (between calipers). (b, c) Axial and sagittal contrast-enhanced CT abdominopelvic images showing the same enlarged lymph node (red arrows), on staging. Note the discrete fat stranding in the adjacent planes.

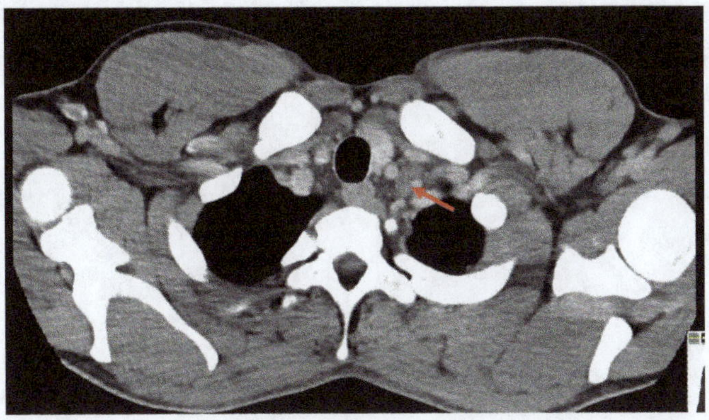

Figure 3: CT. Axial thoracic contrast-enhanced CT image at the thoracic inlet, showing a left supraclavicular lymphadenomegaly (red arrow).

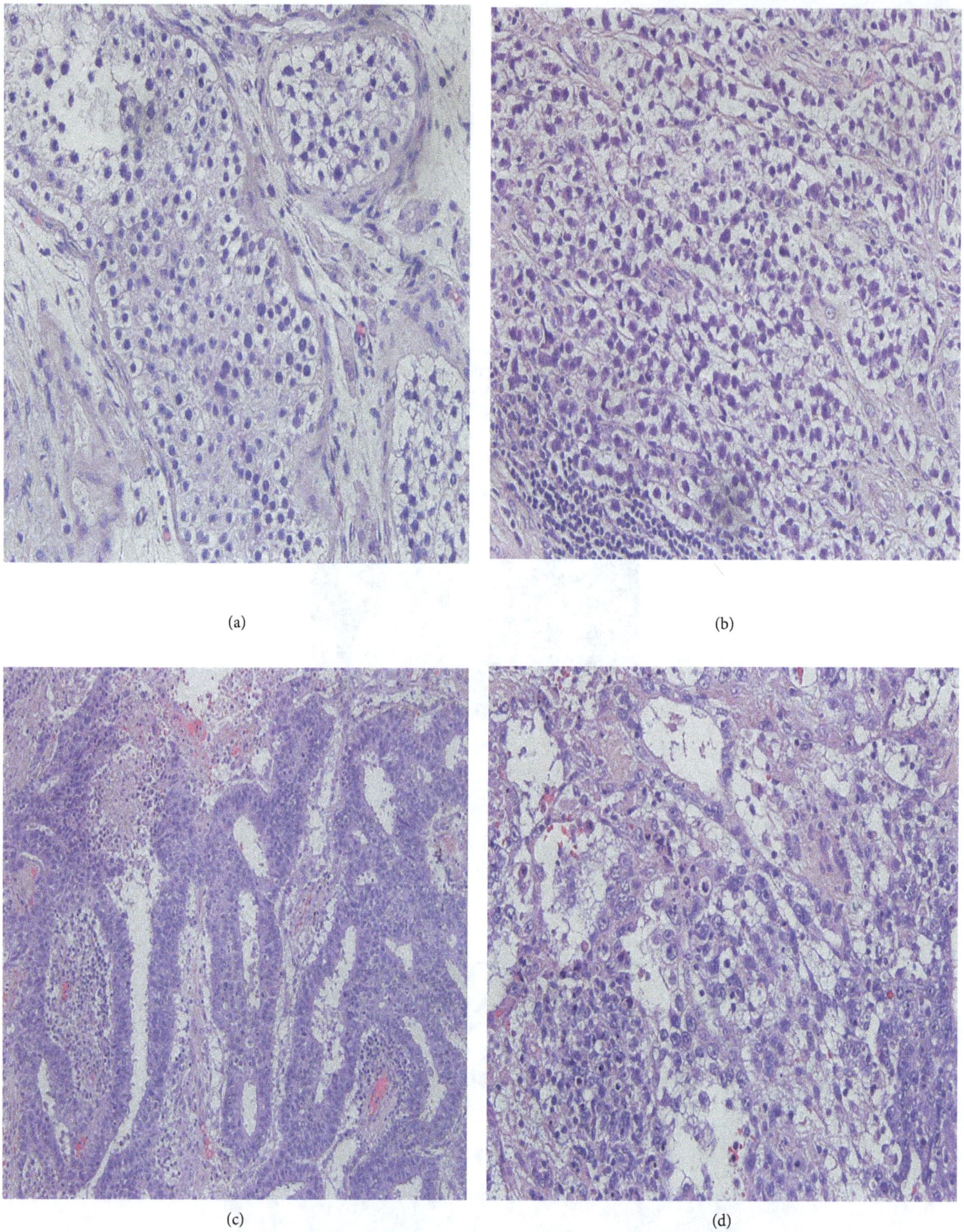


FIGURE 4: Testicular involvement by mixed germ cell neoplasm associated with germ cell neoplasia in situ (a, H&E 200x), with seminoma-type components (b, H&E 200x), embryonal carcinoma type (c, H&E 200x), and yolk sac type (d, H&E 200x).

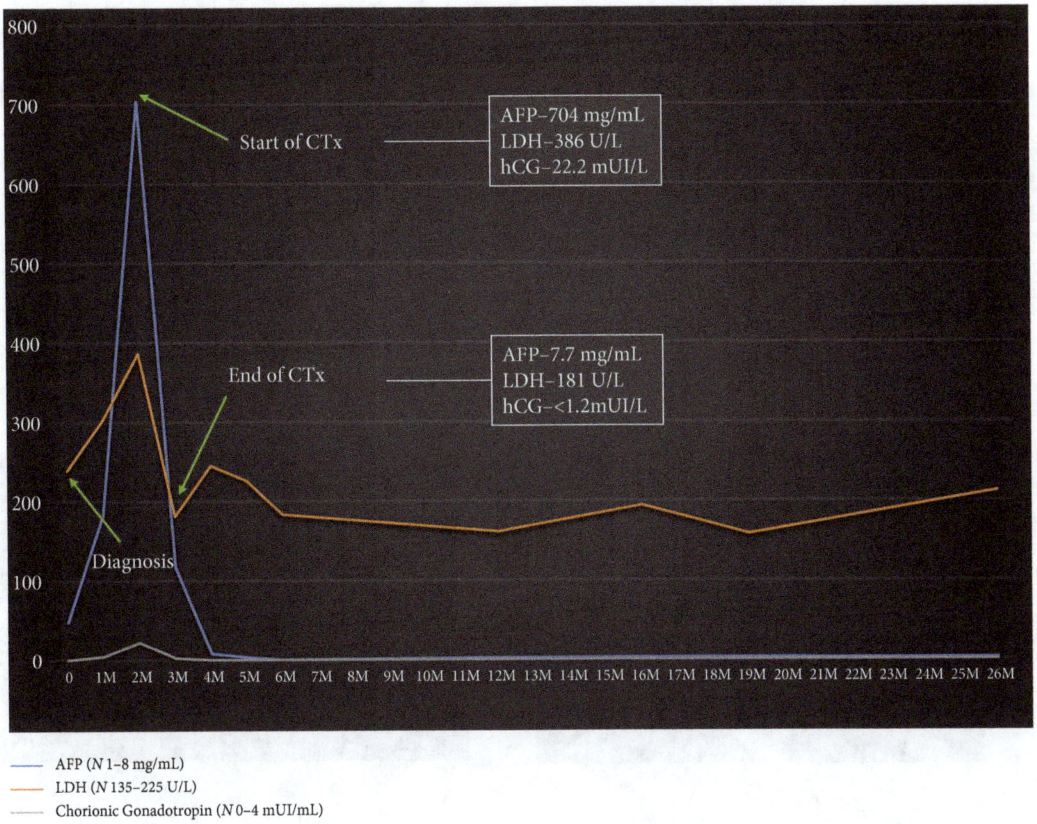


FIGURE 5: Evolution of tumoral biomarkers serum levels throughout patient follow-up, since diagnosis to the present day. AFP: alpha fetoprotein; LDH: lactate dehydrogenase; hCG: chorionic gonadotropin; CTx: chemotherapy.

chemotherapy, subsequently to a significant reduction in tumor burden or a disease-free interval, and (c) the exclusive histologicallypresence of mature teratoma in the resected specimen [6, 7].

GTS is now considered a condition related to both testicular and ovarian cancer (NSGCT), with a prevalence of about 1.9–7.6% in patients with testicular NSGCT [1, 7].

The most common site of involvement is the retroperitoneum, but it can be found in other locations such as the pelvis, chest, liver, or even in the cervical region as our case [3, 7].

GTS presentation is very variable regarding disease time course: during chemotherapy, after a large disease-free period, or after an initial reduction in size during chemotherapy, followed by regrowth [1, 7].

The etiology is still uncertain but there are two main hypotheses described in the literature based on the assumption that embryonal cells are pluripotent and that their origin results from differentiation of tumoral cells. One theory states that chemotherapy only cures the immature malignant cells but not the mature elements, which remain untreated and can transform into benign teratomatous elements. The other theory explains the transformation of a totipotent malignal germ cell into a benign mature teratoma by cell kinetics alterations stimulated by chemotherapy. There is still another lesser known hypothesis proposed by Hong et al., in which inherent and spontaneous differentiation of malignant cells into benign cells is pointed out as the cause of this pathology [4, 7–10].

Since this entity is rare, it is difficult to infer a statistically significant association between the primary pathology and the likelihood of GTS [1].

The most common risk factors include presence of mature teratoma in the primary tumor, incomplete resection after chemotherapy, no size reduction or even growth of metastatic lesions during chemotherapy, and presence of mature teratoma tissue in postchemotherapy residual masses [7, 11].

Among these mentioned risk factors, our patient presented with the two last ones.

However, according to recent studies, the only predictive factor associated with GTS syndrome seems to be cystic/necrotic lesions in the preoperative imaging as well as areas of low density on them at postchemotherapy CT scans compared to pretreatment images. Therefore, close imaging surveillance is crucial for early recognition of GST, particularly in patients with risk factors [1, 3, 11, 12, 13].

The residual masses of GTS do not demonstrate enhancement with 18-FDG PET (positron emission tomography) scans, which can be helpful in the differential diagnosis [14].

The chemoresistant nature of GTS makes additional cycles of chemotherapy ineffective; thus, early recognition is critical to prevent further systemic therapy and to allow for readily surgical planning. Surgical resection is currently the gold standard treatment for GTS. Despite the large tumor

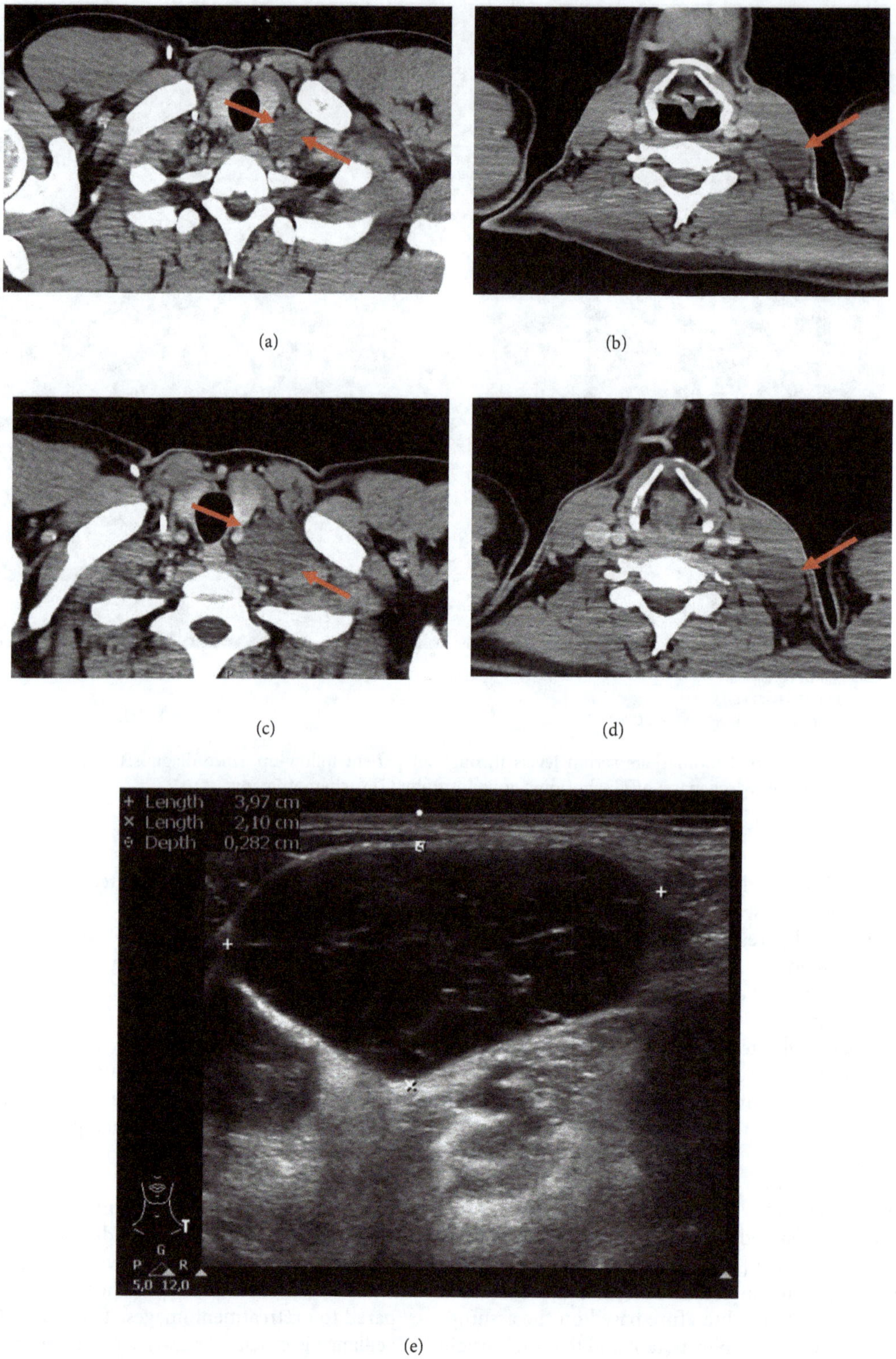


FIGURE 6: CT and ultrasound. Axial thoracic contrast-enhanced CT images at 2-month (a, b) and 5-month follow-up (c, d), showing progressive enlargement of left cervical lymph nodes with diffuse hypodensity (red arrows). (d) Ultrasound image of the same left cervical lymph node depicted on the CT images (a–d) at the microbiopsy, which showed mixed echogenicity, being primarily hypoechogenic with some echogenic septa.

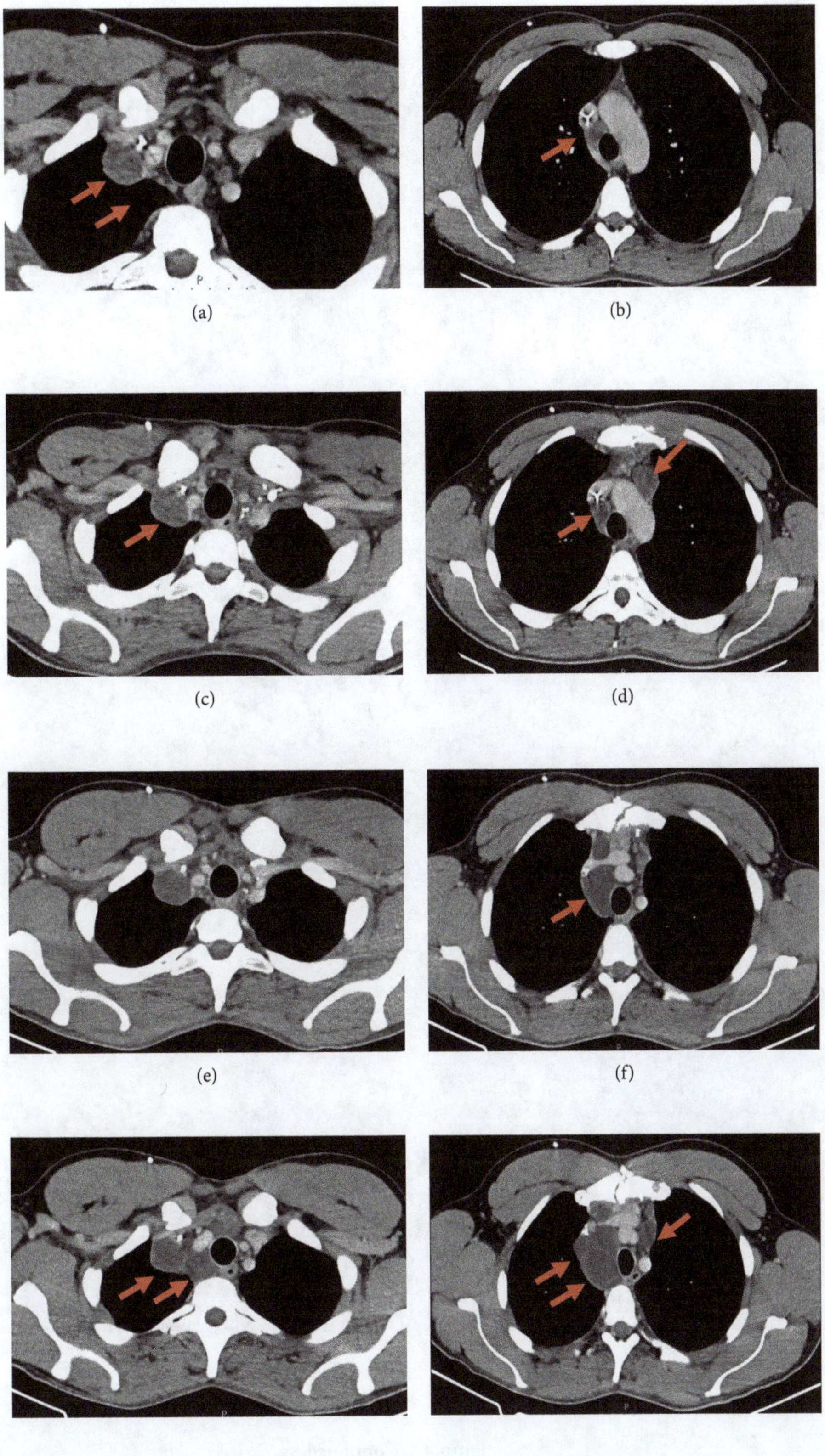

FIGURE 7: CT images. Axial thoracic contrast-enhanced CT images on two different mediastinal levels at 5-month (a, c), 7-month (c, d), 12-month (e, f), and 24-month (g, h) follow-up, depicting enlarging hypodense lymph nodes.

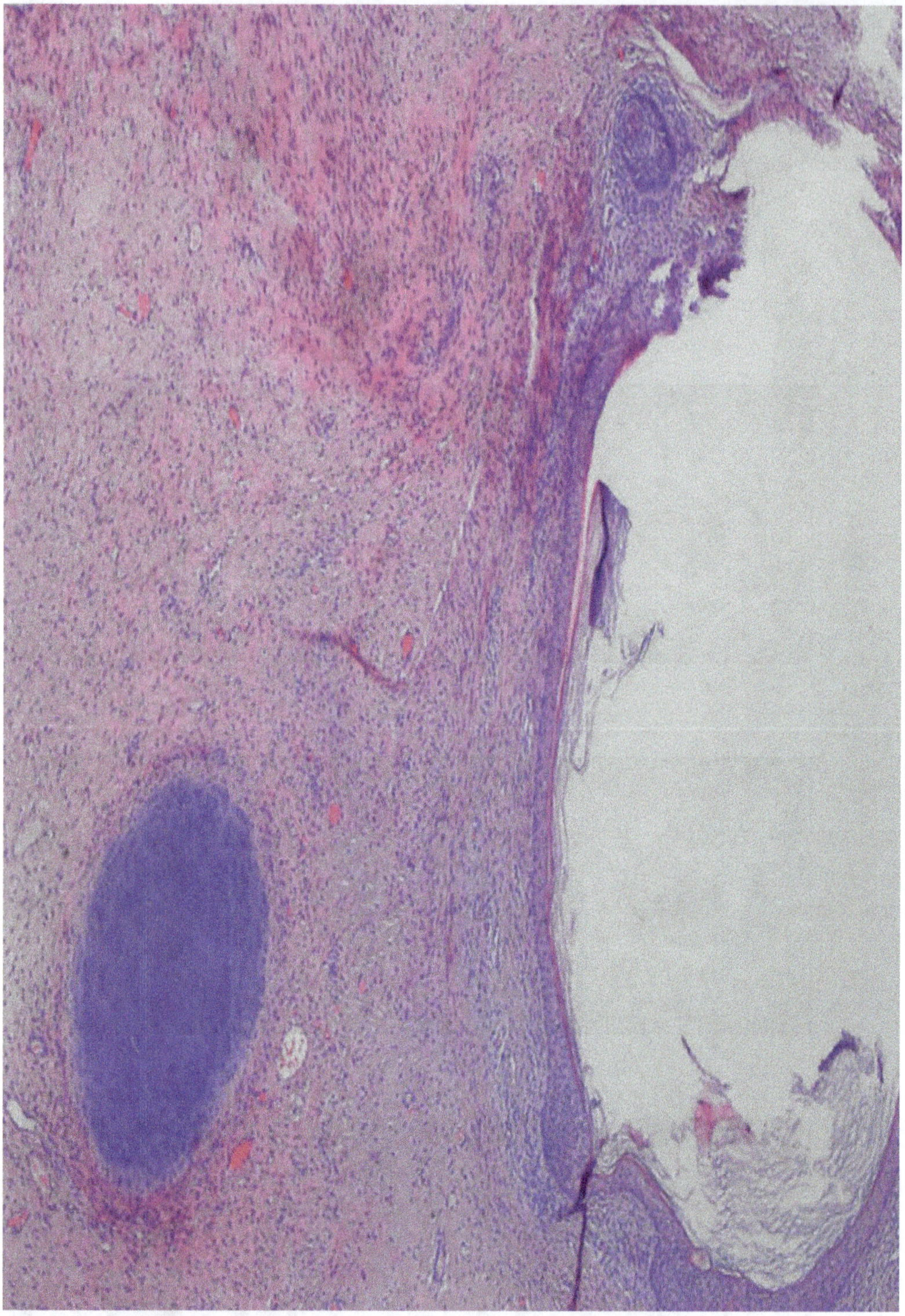

(a)

Figure 8: Continued.

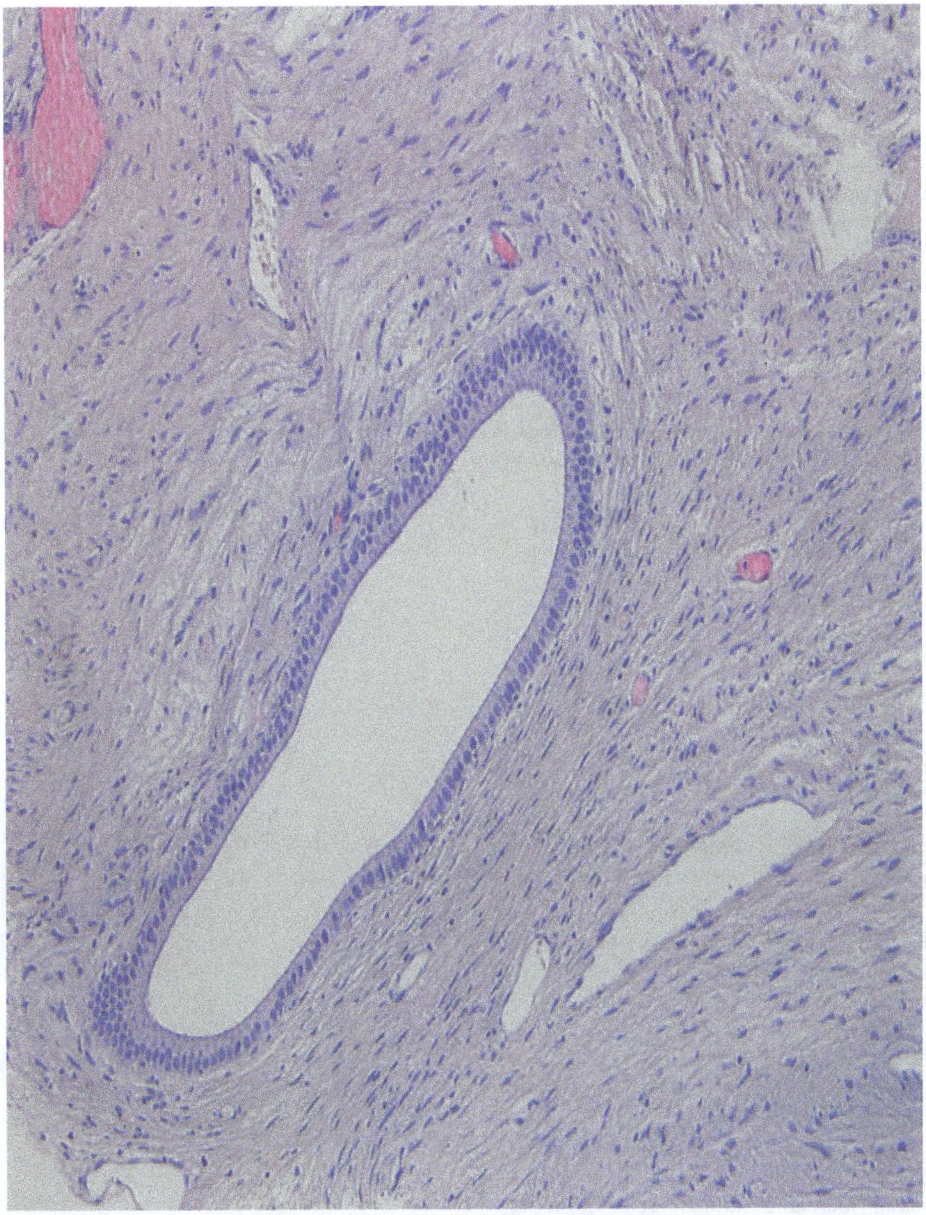

(b)

Figure 8: Lymph node metastases from germ neoplasia with characteristics of mature teratoma with components from the three germinal layers (a, b, H&E 100x).

burden, complete resection is reported to be often curative. Failure to promptly intervene leads to death from either compression of vital organs and/or subsequent malignant transformation [6, 7].

Giant GTS is a variant of this syndrome, with extensive retroperitoneal disease, defined as lesions with larger than 10 cm. Circumferential involvement of major vascular structures is often seen. Surgery is usually technically challenging but should not be disregarded [1].

Although GTS generally has a good prognosis, regular follow-up is critical, as malignant degeneration could occur. Imaging findings and tumor markers can suggest the presence of malignant lesions, but surgical excision or sampling of the lesions is mandatory to confirm the diagnosis and other di fferential diagnosis as incomplete response to chemotherapy or recurrent malignancy [4].

## 4. Conclusion

GTS is rare condition related to both testicular and ovarian NSGCT with generally good prognosis, but close imaging surveillance is crucial for early recognition, particularly in patients with risk factors. Surgery is the gold standard treatment.

## References

[1] D. J. Lee, H. Djaladat, N. N. Tadros et al., "Growing teratoma syndrome: clinical and radiographic characteristics," *International Journal of Urology*, vol. 21, no. 9, pp. 905–908, 2014.

[2] P. Paffenholz, D. Pfister, V. Matveev, and A. Heidenreich, "Diagnosis and management of the growing teratoma syndrome: a single-center experience and review of the literature," *Urologic Oncology*, vol. 36, no. 12, pp. 529.e23–529.e30, 2018.

[3] F. Priod, F. Lorge, M. Di Gregorio et al., "Recurrent masses after testicular cancer: growing teratoma syndrome. A case report and review of the literature," *Case Reports in Oncology*, vol. 10, pp. 910–915, 2018.

[4] W. Boukettaya, M. Hochlaf, Z. Boudagga et al., "Growing teratoma syndrome after treatment of a nonseminomatous germ cell tumor: a case report and a review of literature," *Urology Case Reports*, vol. 2, no. 1, pp. 1–3, 2014.

[5] K. A. Kesler, J. B. Patel, L. E. Kruter et al., "The "growing teratoma syndrome" in primary mediastinal nonseminomatous germ cell tumors: criteria based on current practice," *The Journal of Thoracic and Cardiovascular Surgery*, vol. 144, no. 2, pp. 438–443, 2012.

[6] N. Nassiri, A. Shah, and S. Daneshmand, "Growing teratoma syndrome of testicular origin," *Urology*, vol. 123, pp. 20–23, 2019.

[7] A. Scavuzzo, R. ZAR, N. R. Noverón, and R. MAJ, "Growing teratoma syndrome," *Case Reports in Urology*, vol. 2014, pp. 1–4, 2014.

[8] V. Gorbatiy, P. E. Spiess, and L. L. Pisters, "The growing teratoma syndrome: current review of the literature," *Indian Journal of Urology*, vol. 25, no. 2, pp. 186–189, 2009.

[9] W. K. Hong, R. E. Wittes, S. T. Hajdu, E. Cvitkovic, W. F. Whitmore, and R. B. Golbey, "The evolution of mature teratoma from malignant testicular tumors," *Cancer*, vol. 40, no. 6, pp. 2987–2992, 1977.

[10] J. Ponce de León Roca and H. Villavicencio Mavrich, "Growing teratoma syndrome," *Archivos Españoles de Urología*, vol. 53, no. 6, pp. 547–552, 2000.

[11] F. André, K. Fizazi, S. Culine et al., "The growing teratoma syndrome: results of therapy and long-term follow-up of 33 patients," *European Journal of Cancer*, vol. 36, no. 11, pp. 1389–1394, 2000.

[12] D. M. Panicek, G. C. Toner, R. T. Heelan, and G. J. Bosl, "Nonseminomatous germ cell tumors: enlarging masses despite chemotherapy," *Radiology*, vol. 175, no. 2, pp. 499–502, 1990.

[13] N. Aide, F. Comoz, and E. Sevin, "Enlarging residual mass after treatment of a nonseminomatous germ cell tumor: growing teratoma syndrome or cancer recurrence?," *Journal of Clinical Oncology*, vol. 25, no. 28, pp. 4494–4496, 2007.

[14] U. D. Ngabou, M. Dusaud, G. Boddaert, B. Grand, A. Houlgatte, and F. Pons, "Mediastinal localization of a growing teratoma syndrome: a case report," *Revue de Pneumologie Clinique*, vol. 70, no. 4, pp. 248–251, 2014.

# 48

# Surgical Management of Giant L2 Adrenal Neuroblastoma in Adult Male

**Bikash Bikram Thapa**,[1] **Sanjay Yadav**,[1] **Sujit Pant**,[2] **Pratik Rajkarnikar**,[3] **and Pankaj Mandal**[3]

[1]*Department of Surgery, College of Medicine, Nepalese Army Institute of Health Sciences, Nepal*
[2]*Department of Radio Diagnosis, College of Medicine, Nepalese Army Institute of Health Sciences, Nepal*
[3]*Department of Pathology, College of Medicine, Nepalese Army Institute of Health Sciences, Nepal*

Correspondence should be addressed to Bikash Bikram Thapa; bikashbikram.thapa@naihs.edu.np

Academic Editor: Mohamed A. Ghoneim

Neuroblastoma is an embryonal malignancy that arises from neural crest cells. Adult adrenal neuroblastoma is a rare disease, and less than 100 cases were reported in the literature. Adult neuroblastoma commonly presents with abdominal (retroperitoneal) lump and pain. A 35-year-old male patient presented with a giant (20 cm × 17 cm × 12 cm) nonfunctional left adrenal mass. He underwent en-bloc surgical excision of the left adrenal gland along with the left kidney. Histopathological examination revealed adrenal neuroblastoma (stage 2B, L2). We present here the surgical management of the rare adult adrenal neuroblastoma.

## 1. Introduction

Neuroblastoma (NB) is the most common extracranial solid malignancy in children that account for 15% of the cancer mortality [1]. Median age at diagnosis is 17 months, and only 2% of cases are found in patients above 10 years [2]. Less than 100 cases of adult neuroblastoma were reported in literature since it was first reported on 1957 by a Dutch physician [3–5]. Patients usually present with abdominal mass, pain, and other constitutional symptoms like fever, high blood pressure, flushing, and paraneoplastic syndrome [6]. There is no standard treatment protocol for adult neuroblastoma. Adults have lower tolerance to the treatment with low five-year overall survival rate (36% in adult vs 85% in infant) [7].

## 2. Case Report

A 35-year-old male with history of neurocysticercosis under medication presented to the surgery department with left upper abdominal pain and lump of one-week duration. The pain was acute in onset, dull aching type, intermittent, and severe enough to disturb daily activities. He was non-smoker, non-alcoholic, normotensive, and non-diabetic with no family history of malignancy. His body mass index was 25.3 kg/m$^2$. Clinical examination revealed a palpable mass in the left hypochondrium extending 7 cm below the left costal margin that was firm, smooth, and nontender.

The computed tomography with contrast (CECT) of the chest and abdomen-pelvis (Figure 1(a)) showed a well-defined multilobulated mass lesion measuring 16 × 13 × 16.5 cm with heterogeneous enhancement. The left suprarenal gland was not visualized separately. The mass lesion was abutting and displacing the pancreas, spleen, and left kidney. The lobulated mass was extending across the midline abutting and displacing the abdominal aorta, renal vessels, and encasing the left renal artery (Figure 1(a)). The complete blood count, renal function test, and liver function test were within the normal limit. The serum and blood metanephrines were in the normal limit; 36.1 pg/ml

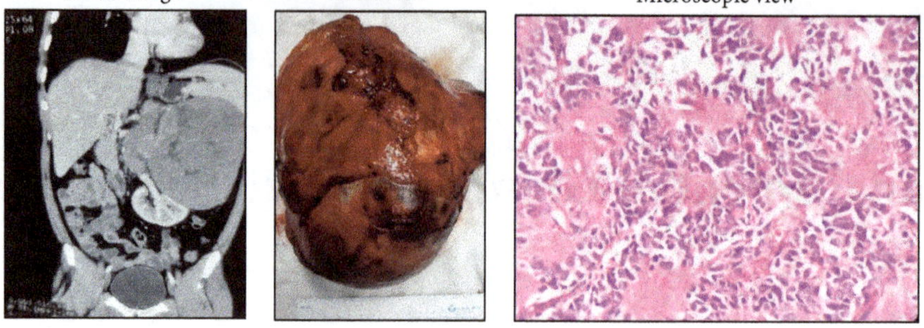


(a) CECT image (b) Gross view (c) Microscopic view

FIGURE 1: Left adrenal neuroblastoma.

and 74.29 μg/day, respectively. Serum cortisol and aldosterone were normal. Patient was managed with en-bloc left adrenalectomy, left nephrectomy, and paraortic lymph node dissection through left subcostal hockey stick incision under epidural-general anesthesia. The left renal vessels were completely encased, and abdominal aorta was partially encased by the lymph nodal mass. The surgery last for 210 minutes with blood loss of approximately 300 ml. The patient was discharged on postoperative day 7. Gross histopathology examination of the surgical specimen (Figure 1(b)) revealed adrenal mass of size 20 × 17 × 12 cm. Microscopic examination showed small round blue tumor cells arranged around the central area filled with neurofibrillary processes giving rosette appearance—Homer-Wright rosettes (Figure 1(c)). Tumor cells were differentiating with low mitotic index, and the margins were negative. The hilar lymph node (6/6) was positive for malignancy. Kidney margins were negative for malignancy. We could not perform Metaiodobenzylguanidine (MIBG)scan postoperatively due to lack of facility inside the country. However, the technetium bone scan was negative for bone metastasis. Patent was counseled by a clinical oncologist regarding adjuvant therapy but choose to continue follow-up. The CECT scan done 6 months postsurgery was normal.

## 3. Discussion

Neuroblastoma consists of a group of neuroblastic tumors (neuroblastomas, ganglineuroblastomas, and ganlioneuromas) that originate from neural crest cells. It is exclusively the disease of childhood. The incidence rate is 60% before the age of one year drops to 10% at age of 14 years. The incidence rate for patients aged over 30 years is 0.2 cases per million inhabitants per year [8]. Out of the 112 adult neuroblastoma patients reported from M.D. Anderson cancer center in 2014, there were 48% L1, 27% L2, and 14% M diseases [9].

The clinical presentation of neuroblastoma depends on the tumor's location, local invasion, and metastasis. The head and neck region, central nervous system, chest cavity, and abdominal cavity are most common primary sites of adult neuroblastoma. About 50% of the abdominal neuroblastoma is adrenal in origin [4, 9, 10]. Retroperitoneal neuroblastoma of size as big as 25 × 12 × 18 cm was reported in literature [11]. Our patient had stage 2B adrenal neuroblastoma based on the international neuroblastoma staging system (1990) [12]. According to the international neuroblastoma risk group staging system [13], he had L2M0 disease (locoregional disease involving the left renal pedicle with no metastasis).

Management of neuroblastoma requires a multimodality approach that includes surgery, radiotherapy, high-dose chemotherapy with stem cell rescue, and Iodine131-MIBG therapy [5, 9]. A retrospective study on stage I and II adult neuroblastoma (age group > 12 years) showed 83% 5-year overall survival (OS) after multimodality treatment. Surgery remains the choice of treatment for the local control of the disease [5]. We performed open transperitoneal adrenalectomy because of the size of the tumor and extent of the local spread. Laparoscopic adrenalectomy is gaining wider popularity over open adrenalectomy (then gold standard) since early 90s. A Cochrane review published on 2018 found no difference on overall early and late complications between intraperitoneal and retroperitoneal laparoscopic adrenal surgery [14].

Guidelines suggest laparoscopic adrenalectomy for malignant adrenal tumor with size less than 6 cm [15]. Number of studies had cautioned about the poor oncological outcome of the laparoscopy adrenal surgeries. However a meta-analysis reported a comparable outcome between the open and laparoscopic approaches in the management of adrenal malignancy [16, 17]. Laparoscopic excision of adrenal neuroblastoma (5 to 8 cm) has been successfully performed in recent years [4, 18]. The robot-assisted laparoscopic approach has added advantages over the laparoscopic approach for the management of the adrenal tumors due to its three-dimensional magnified vision and dexterity [19].

There is lack of standard treatment guidelines in the adult population due to rarity of the disease. The Surveillance, Epidemiology, and End-Results registry (SEER) database had a total of 181 adult neuroblastomas from 1973 to 2010. In those cohort of 181 adult (18-60 years) neuroblastomas, L1 and L2 diseases had better progression-free survival (PFS) and overall survival (OS) with the combination of surgery and radiation than surgery alone [8]. Adjuvant chemotherapy had no added benefit in progression-free survival (PFS) in adult L1 and L2 neuroblastomas [9]. Patient age at diagnosis, stage, histology, tumor grade, MYCN oncogene status, chromosome 11q status, and DNA ploidy are important prognostic factors for neuroblastoma [5, 9]. In recent days, attention has been given to miRNA (microRNA) and its relationship with the molecular pathogenesis of neuroblastoma that has important implications in the diagnosis, prognosis, and miRNA-based therapy for neuroblastoma [20].

## 4. Conclusion

Adult adrenal neuroblastoma of this size is the first of its kind in literature. Surgical management in L2 adrenal neuroblastoma is advised for local control of the disease. Minimal invasive surgery is a new standard for adrenal tumor. Multimodality treatment can offer long-term favorable oncological outcome in adult neuroblastoma. The treatment outcome is multifactorial. Larger and longer study series of the adult neuroblastoma can guide us through the challenges posed by the rarity of the disease.

## Consent

Informed written consent was received from the patient.

## Authors' Contributions

All authors have equal contribution for case data collection, literature review, and manuscript writing.

## References

[1] M. T. Goodman, J. G. Gurney, M. A. Smith, and A. F. Olshan, "Sympathetic nervous system tumors," in *Cancer Incidence and Survival among Children and Adolescents*, p. 35, United States SEER Program, 1975-1995," National Cancer Institute, Bethesda, 1999, 1975-1995.

[2] N. Esiashvili, M. Goodman, K. Ward, R. B. Marcus Jr., and P. A. Johnstone, "Neuroblastoma in adults: incidence and survival analysis based on SEER data," *Pediatric Blood & Cancer*, vol. 49, no. 1, pp. 41–46, 2007.

[3] F. De Meulemeester, "Adrenal neuroblastoma," *Maandschrift voor Kindergeneeskunde*, vol. 25, no. 11, pp. 389–402, 1957.

[4] H. Zhang and Z. Feng, "Adrenal neuroblastoma in an elderly adult: a case report and review of the literature," *Journal of Medical Case Reports*, vol. 13, no. 1, p. 284, 2019.

[5] M. G. Podda, R. Luksch, D. Polastri et al., "Neuroblastoma in patients over 12 years old: a 20-year experience at the Istituto Nazionale Tumori of Milan," *Tumori Journal*, vol. 96, no. 5, pp. 684–689, 2018.

[6] C. B. Golden and J. H. Feusner, "Malignant abdominal masses in children: quick guide to evaluation and diagnosis," *Pediatric Clinics of North Americ*, vol. 49, no. 6, pp. 1369–1392, 2002.

[7] L. M. Franks, A. Bollen, R. C. Seeger, D. O. Stram, and K. K. Matthay, "Neuroblastoma in adults and adolescents: an indolent course with poor survival," *Cancer*, vol. 79, no. 10, pp. 2028–2035, 1997.

[8] E. Rogowitz, H. M. Babiker, M. Kanaan, R. A. Millius, Q. S. Ringenberg, and M. Bishop, "Neuroblastoma of the elderly, an oncologist's nightmare: case presentation, literature review and SEER database analysis," *Experimental Hematology & Oncology*, vol. 3, no. 1, p. 20, 2014.

[9] H. J. Conter, V. Gopalakrishnan, V. Ravi, J. L. Ater, S. Patel, and D. M. Araujo, "Adult versus pediatric neuroblastoma: the M.D. Anderson cancer center experience," *Sarcoma*, vol. 2014, Article ID 375151, 6 pages, 2014.

[10] J. M. Maris, M. D. Hogarty, R. Bagatell, and S. L. Cohn, "Neuroblastoma," *The Lancet*, vol. 369, no. 9579, pp. 2106–2120, 2007.

[11] X. L. Wu, Y. J. Dai, G. Y. Sun et al., "Adult neuroblastoma in the retroperitoneum: a case report," *Medicine*, vol. 97, no. 51, article e13750, 2018.

[12] G. M. Brodeur, J. Pritchard, F. Berthold et al.et al., "Revisions of the international criteria for neuroblastoma diagnosis, staging, and response to treatment," *Journal of Clinical Oncology*, vol. 11, no. 8, pp. 1466–1477, 1993.

[13] T. Monclair, G. M. Brodeur, P. F. Ambros et al., "The International Neuroblastoma Risk Group (INRG) staging system: an INRG task force report," *Journal of Clinical Oncology*, vol. 27, no. 2, pp. 298–303, 2009.

[14] A. Arezzo, A. Bullano, G. Cochetti et al., "Transperitoneal versus retroperitoneal laparoscopic adrenalectomy for adrenal tumours in adults," *Cochrane Database of Systematic Reviews*, vol. 12, article CD011668, 2018.

[15] M. Fassnacht, W. Arlt, I. Bancos et al., "Management of adrenal incidentalomas: European Society of Endocrinology Clinical Practice Guideline in collaboration with the European Network for the Study of Adrenal Tumors," *European Journal of Endocrinology*, vol. 175, no. 2, pp. G1–G34, 2016.

[16] B. S. Miller, J. B. Ammori, P. G. Gauger, J. T. Broome, G. D. Hammer, and G. M. Doherty, "Laparoscopic resection is inappropriate in patients with known or suspected adrenocortical carcinoma," *World Journal of Surgery*, vol. 34, no. 6, pp. 1380–1385, 2010.

[17] G. Sgourakis, S. Lanitis, A. Kouloura et al., "Laparoscopic versus open adrenalectomy for stage I/Ii adrenocortical carcinoma: meta-analysis of outcomes," *Journal of Investigative Surgery*, vol. 28, no. 3, pp. 145–152, 2015.

[18] J. Ramsingh, H. Casey, and C. Watson, "Adult neuroblastoma: a rare diagnosis of an adrenal mass," *BML Case Reports*, vol. 12, no. 4, p. e228730, 2019.

[19] E. Mearini, R. Cirocchi, and G. Cochetti, "Robot-assisted surgery in urology: the show must go on," *Applied Sciences*, vol. 9, no. 5, p. 844, 2019.

[20] N. Aravindan, K. Subramanian, D. B. Somasundaram, T. S. Herman, and S. Aravindan, "Micrornas in neuroblastoma tumorigenesis, therapy resistance, and disease evolution," *Cancer Drug Resist*, vol. 2, pp. 1086–1105, 2019.

# Medullary Aplasia Revealing a Metastatic Prostatic Adenocarcinoma

**Idriss Ziani**, [1,2] **Ahmed Ibrahimi**, [1,2] **Omar Bellouki**, [1,2] **Youssef Zaoui**, [1,2] **Yasmine Laraqui Housseini**, [1,2,3] **Fouad Zouidia**, [1,2,3] **Hachem El Sayegh**, [1,2] **Lounis Benslimane**, [1,2] **and Yassine Nouini** [1,2]

[1] *Department of Urological Surgery "A", Ibn Sina University Hospital of Rabat, Rabat, Morocco*
[2] *Department of Anatomopathology and Cytology, Ibn Sina University Hospital of Rabat, Rabat, Morocco*
[3] *Faculty of Medicine of Rabat, Mohammed V University, Rabat, Morocco*

Correspondence should be addressed to Idriss Ziani; idrissziani20@gmail.com

Academic Editor: Tun-Chieh Chen

In this case report, we are reporting the case of a 68-year-old male patient who was admitted in our hospital for unintended weight loss, asthenia, and anorexia. Physical examination showed clinical signs of anemia such as pallor of skin and mucous membranes; hemodynamic parameters were normal. Complete blood count (CBC) analysis showed a pancytopenia with anemia, thrombocytopenia, and leukopenia. BM biopsy was performed, showing a malignant infiltration of bone marrow by a metastatic prostate cancer confirmed by immunohistochemistry. Prostate biopsy confirmed the diagnosis of acinar adenocarcinoma with Gleason score 8 (4 + 4), ISUP grade group 4. Our patient underwent chemical castration using LH-RH analogs in association with second-line hormone therapy by abiraterone acetate. The evolution was good on both the oncological and hematological levels.

## 1. Introduction

Prostate cancer is the second most frequently diagnosed cancer in men, with more than 1.2 million new cases worldwide and causing 3.8% of all deaths by cancer in men in 2018 [1].

The highest death rates were recorded in Central America (10.7 per 100,000 inhabitants), followed by Australia and New Zealand (10.2) and Western Europe (10.1) [2]. The 5-year relative survival rate for localized and regional prostate cancer is 100%, compared to 30.5% for metastatic cases [3]. Bones are common metastatic sites and can even be a form of revelation of advanced prostate cancer. [4].

However, metastatic invasion of the bone marrow remains exceptional in prostate adenocarcinoma [5]. This condition can lead to bone marrow failure involving one or more cell lines, which can cause pancytopenia when all the lines are affected. This condition can lead to serious complications and is linked to a poor prognosis [5]. Infiltration of the bone marrow by metastatic tumor cells can lead to bone marrow failure, resulting in hematologic abnormalities. When cancer cells invade healthy bone marrow, they replace hematopoietic stem cells, resulting in the depletion of several cell lines. Nieder et al. describe a typical pattern of anemia, thrombocytopenia, and increased mortality [5].

Although rare, cases of metastatic bone marrow invasion of prostatic adenocarcinoma often present with thrombocytopenia, whether or not associated with anemia [5].

We report a rare case of metastatic adenocarcinoma of the prostate with invasion of the bone marrow discovered in a bone marrow aplasia manifested by pancytopenia, which represents the particularity of our observation. Another peculiarity of our observation is the favorable response to second-line hormone therapy.

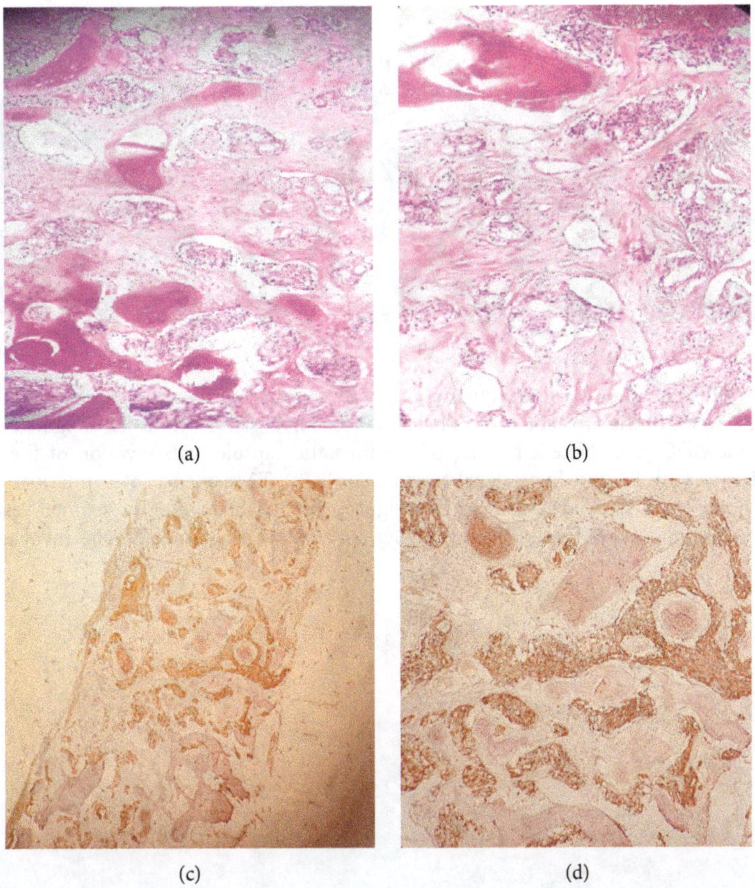

FIGURE 1: (a, b) Hematoxylin eosin (×100): medullary infiltration by an acinar adenocarcinoma of the prostate. (c) BOM immunohistochemistry: positive labeling of tumor cells by the anti-PSA G antibody (×40). (d) BOM immunohistochemistry: positive labeling of tumor cells by the anti-PSA G antibody (×100).

To our knowledge, this is the second observation reported in the literature relating to pancytopenia in metastatic prostate cancer.

## 2. Case Report

We report the case of a 68-year-old male patient with history of high blood pressure and hypercholesterolemia, who initially consults for an unintended weight loss estimated at 12 kg in 1 month, asthenia, and anorexia. The patient also reported bone pain in his pelvis.

Physical examination found a patient in poor general condition, with pallor of skin and mucous membranes and normal hemodynamic parameters. A CBC was performed showing white blood cell (WBC) count of 3,500 cells/mL (normal range: 4,000–11,000), platelets of 40,000 cells/mL (normal range: 150,000–450,000), and hemoglobin (Hb) of 5 g/dL (normal range: 13.0–17.0). Faced with this picture, a malignant hemopathy was suspected, after conditioning, of an emergency transfusion with units of red blood cells and platelets, in order to perform a bone marrow biopsy (OMB).

Pathology study showed malignant infiltration of the bone marrow. The tumor cells are medium sized with a thin cytoplasm. The nuclei are ovoid, finely nucleated, showing many figures of mitosis, these tumor cells probably suspect a prostatic origin, and immunohistochemical staining using prostate-specific antigen (PSA) confirmed the prostatic origin this metastatic invasion (Figure 1).

Rectal examination found hard prostate nodules. The PSA serum concentration was at 197 ng/mL.

A multiparametric MRI was performed. On T2-weighted (T2W) images, a PI-RADS V tumor focus in the left basal peripheral zone was detected (Figure 2).

A transrectal ultrasound guided biopsy of the prostate was performed and revealed an acinar adenocarcinoma with Gleason score 8 (4 + 4), ISUP grade group 4 occupying 20% of the biopsy surface on the left, and 10% on the right with perineural neoplastic invasion and invasion of the periprostatic tissue (Figure 3). Bone scan showed several secondary bone locations (Figure 4). Chest-abdomen-pelvis CT did not find any other visceral metastases.

Given the high metastatic volume, the multidisciplinary consultation meeting decided to perform chemical castration using LH-RH analogs in association with second-line hormone therapy by abiraterone acetate after a 15-day antiandrogen treatment to prevent "flare-up."

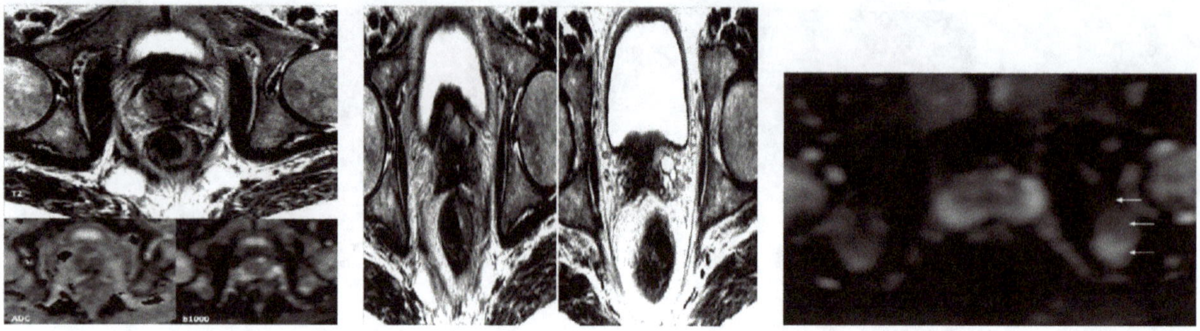

(a) (b) (c)

FIGURE 2: (a) Multiparametric MRI image showing a suspicious nodule with capsular intrusion and invasion of the rectal wall. Nodular image sitting at the level of the left CZ sector of the prostatic base in heterogeneous hyposignal on the T2-weighted images, in hypersignal B1000 diffusion with restriction on the ADC card. Note a rupture of the prostatic capsule with invasion of the left neurovascular strip and thickening of the rectal wall (isosignal T2 and hypersignal in diffusion). (b) T2 sequence of a multiparametric MRI of the prostate objectifying an invasion of the base of the seminal vesicles T2 hyposignal aspect of the base of the seminal vesicles denoting their invasion. (c) B1000 diffusion sequence of a multiparameter MRI objectifying an associated secondary bone involvement, with a heterogeneous aspect of the bone structure.

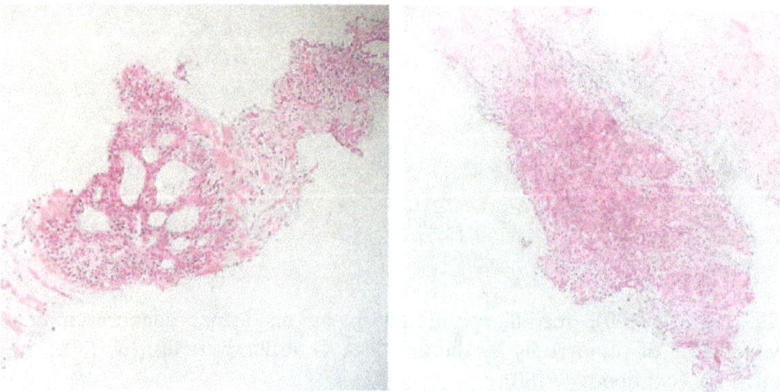

FIGURE 3: Hematoxylin eosin (×100): infiltration of the prostatic parenchyma by a grade 4 acinar prostatic adenocarcinoma 4.

Follow-up showed a platelet level of 70,000 cells/mL, and hemoglobin of 11 g/dL with normal WBC three months after treatment. PSA levels drop to 65 ng/mL at 3 months, and 43 ng/mL at 6 months.

## 3. Discussion

Prostate cancer is the second most common cancer in men, and it is the 5th leading cause of death worldwide [5, 16]. Metastatic forms of prostate cancer are linked to a highest rate of morbidity and mortality, and bones remain the most common metastatic site [6].

Depending on the extent of the metastatic lesion and its location in the bone, the consequences on the function of the bone marrow can be variable. Usually, it causes thrombocytopenia and anemia [4, 7]. In the literature, we find that thrombocytopenia and/or anemia are the most common consequences of bone marrow failure due to prostate cancer metastasis. Patients in this condition are reported to have poor prognosis [5, 8].

To our knowledge, pancytopenia due to medullary aplasia from a prostate cancer metastasis has only been reported once in the literature before our paper.

Jacho et al. reported "diffuse invasive carcinoma" as a type of bone metastasis in 1930 [9]. On the basis of this report, Hayashi et al. recommended the term "disseminated carcinomatosis of the bone marrow" (DCBM) with clinical pathological characteristics using the result of the count of diffuse metastases of the bone marrow of solid cancers in Japan in 1979 [9]. Gastric cancer accounts for >90% of all primary lesions, while prostate cancer accounts for only 3.7% [9].

Unfortunately, few data have been published in the literature on the prognosis and survival of the patient with a solid tumor with bone marrow metastases [5, 10].

The mechanism of damage to the bone marrow in case of bone metastases is based on fibrosis, necrosis, and osteoid formation resulting in damage to the hematopoietic function of the peripheral bone marrow.

Bone reactions in metastatic lesions are classified as osteoblastic, osteolytic, intertrabecular, or mixed metastases. Intertrabecular metastasis is a concept similar to DCBM. In the case of intertrabecular metastases, cancer cells are present between the bony trabeculae, and the bone cortex is preserved without destruction. Cancer cells replace bone cells and spread. Intertrabecular metastases are the initial

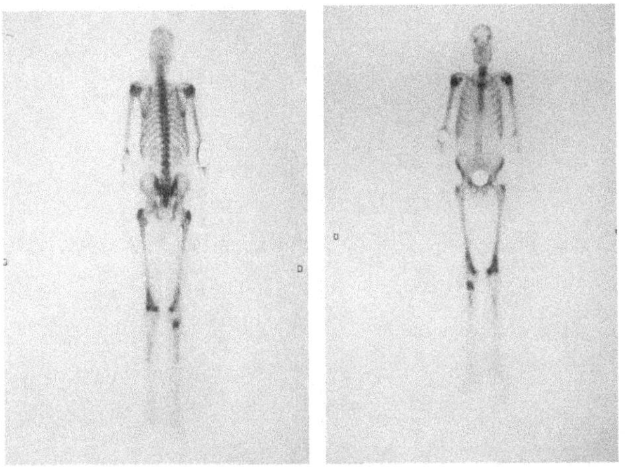

FIGURE 4: Objective bone scan of many secondary metastatic lesions.

presentation of bone metastases and can then progress to other patterns [5].

However, intertrabecular metastasis leads to DIC when it progresses without change. Older age, man, primary tumor necrosis, and advanced stage have been shown to be risk factors for CAD in solid tumors [9].

Chernow and Wallner recommend performing a bone scintigram and bone marrow biopsy, due to the high possibility of bone marrow metastasis if there are more than two findings among leukoerythroblastosis, platelet count < 100,000/$\mu$L, LDH > 500 IU/L, and/or bone pain [9].

Although thrombocytopenia in the context of metastatic disease is most often attributable to an actual invasion of the bone marrow by tumor cells, a review of the literature reveals a small number of cases in which an underlying immune component was suspected. Spivack et al. described 3 cases in which the patients presented both malignant epithelial tumors and a suspected ITP. Of these 3 patients, 1 had an adenocarcinoma of the prostate, and all 3 had isolated thrombocytopenia which responded to treatment with prednisone. Analysis of the bone marrow in the 3 patients showed no signs of replacement by metastatic tumor cells, contrary to the situation of our patient [11].

Contrary to our observation, Geenen et al. have previously shown that the white blood cell system does not appear to be affected in patients with metastatic prostate cancer [5].

Therapeutically, Nieder et al. who retrospectively analyzed 51 patients with anemia and thrombocytopenia by bone metastases, most of the patients (57%) were treated immediately with chemotherapy par by taxotere, and some patients also received second-line treatment with mitoxantrone. Most patients' survival was 2 to 3 years, but 4 patients were alive more than 5 years after detection of bone metastases [4].

Similarly in the 2nd case reported by Kunthur, the patient was treated from the start with a docetaxel chemotherapy with good progress [12].

Our patient was rather treated by a hormone therapy of 2 generations with a good evolution on the biological and oncological plan with a current decline of 12 months.

It should also be noted that androgen-deprivation therapy could lead to a decrease in hemoglobin, for example, an average reduction of 1.1 g/dL in the study by Curtis et al. [13]. Beer et al. observed an average decrease of 0.54 g/dL 3 months after the start of androgen-deprivation therapy [14]. However, the mean level increased in patients with a baseline level < 12 g/dL. A decrease after 3 months was independently associated with shorter survival and progression-free survival. Already in a previous study, the same group had described an association between anemia and shorter survival in men with newly diagnosed metastatic prostate cancer [15].

The delay in correcting anemia in our patient may be partly due to the treatment of hormone therapy.

The peculiarity of our observation, in addition to the fact that it is a rare case, is the response to second-generation hormone therapy, thus delaying chemotherapy.

## 4. Conclusion

Although bone metastases are common in prostate cancer, metastatic involvement of the bone marrow remains relatively rare and reflects an unfavorable course of the disease. The usual translation in the literature is an association between anemia and thrombocytopenia.

Our case has the particularity of reaching the 3 hematopoietic lines which led to aplastic anemia and pan cytopenia, the evolution was pretty good under second-line hormone therapy.

## References


[1] F. Bray, J. Ferlay, I. Soerjomataram, R. L. Siegel, L. A. Torre, and A. Jemal, "Global cancer statistics 2018: GLOBOCAN estimates of incidence and mortality worldwide for 36 cancers in 185 countries," *CA: A Cancer Journal for Clinicians*, vol. 68, no. 6, pp. 394–424, 2018.

[2] J. Ferlay, M. Ervik, F. Lam et al., "Global cancer observatory: cancer today. Lyon, France: International Agency for Research on Cancer," 2019 https://gco.iarc.fr/today, Accessed 02 February.

[3] "Cancer Stat Facts: Prostate cancer. National Cancer Institute," September 201 https://seer.cancer.gov/statfacts/html/prost .html. Accessed.

[4] C. Nieder, E. Haukland, A. Pawinski, and A. Dalhaug, "Anaemia and thrombocytopenia in patients with prostate cancer and bone metastases," *BMC Cancer*, vol. 10, no. 1, 2010.

[5] D. M. Betsch, S. Gray, and S. E. Zed, "A case of metastatic prostate cancer and immune thrombocytopenia," *Current Oncology*, vol. 24, no. 5, pp. 434–e436, 2017.

[6] M. N. Thobe, R. J. Clark, R. O. Bainer, S. M. Prasad, and C. W. Rinker-Schaeffer, "From prostate to bone: key players in prostate cancer bone metastasis," *Cancers*, vol. 3, no. 1, pp. 478–493, 2011.

[7] R. Khafagy, D. Shackley, J. Samuel, K. O'Flynn, C. Betts, and N. Clarke, "Complications arising in the final year of life in men dying from advanced prostate cancer," *Journal of Palliative Medicine*, vol. 10, no. 3, pp. 705–711, 2007.

[8] T. Hiroshige and Y. Eguchi, "Prostate cancer with disseminated carcinomatosis of the bone marrow: two case reports,"

*Molecular and Clinical Oncology*, vol. 7, no. 2, pp. 233–236, 2017.

[9] G. Pahouja, R. Wesolowski, R. Reinbolt et al., "Stabilization of bone marrow infiltration by metastatic breast cancer with continuous doxorubicin," *Cancer Treat Commun*, vol. 3, pp. 28–32, 2015.

[10] "Japanese Society of Medical Oncology, corp-author," in *Practical guideline of bone metastasis*, Nankodo Co., Ltd., Tokyo, 2015.

[11] M. Spivack, S. M. Brenner, M. J. Markham, E. L. Snyder, and D. Berkowitz, "Presumed immunethrombocytopenia and carcinoma," *The American Journal of the Medical Sciences*, vol. 278, no. 2, pp. 153–156, 1979.

[12] A. Kunthur, "A castrate-resistant metastatic prostate cancer patient with severe pancytopenia, successfully treated with docetaxel chemotherapy," *Journal of Oncology Pharmacy Practice*, vol. 26, no. 5, pp. 1254–1258, 2020.

[13] K. K. Curtis, T. J. Adam, S. C. Chen, R. K. Pruthi, and M. K. Gornet, "Anaemia following initiation of androgen deprivation therapy for metastatic prostate cancer: a retrospective chart review," *The Aging Male*, vol. 11, no. 4, pp. 157–161, 2009.

[14] T. M. Beer, C. M. Tangen, L. B. Bland et al., "the prognostic value of hemoglobin change after initiating androgen-deprivation therapy for newly diagnosed metastatic prostate cancer," *Cancer*, vol. 107, no. 3, pp. 489–496, 2006.

[15] T. M. Beer, C. M. Tangen, L. B. Bland, I. M. Thompson, and E. D. Crawford, "Prognostic value of anemia in newly diagnosed metastatic prostate cancer: a multivariate analysis of Southwest Oncology Group Study 8894," *Journal of Urology*, vol. 172, 6 Part 1, pp. 2213–2217, 2004.

# 50

# Skeletal Muscle Metastasis to Vastus Lateralis from a Urothelial Carcinoma: A Case Report and Review of its Diagnosis and Management

**A. M. Mainwaring, H. Wells, T. Banks, T. Ellul, and P. Bose**

*Department of Urology, Morriston Hospital, Swansea, UK*

Correspondence should be addressed to A. M. Mainwaring; anz1982@yahoo.co.uk

Academic Editor: Sigurdur Gudjonsson

Bladder cancer is a common genitourinary tract malignancy. Urothelial carcinoma is the most frequent type of bladder cancer and it commonly metastasises to lymph nodes, bone, lung and liver by a haematogenous route. Skeletal metastases are very rare and are usually present in patients with advanced metastatic disease. We present an unusual case of a 71-year-old male with a urothelial carcinoma metastasis to the vastus lateralis muscle 3 months following a cystoprostatectomy for muscle invasive bladder cancer.

## 1. Introduction

Bladder cancer is the ninth most common cancer worldwide, with an estimated 430,000 new cases in 2012 [1]. Urothelial carcinoma (UC) is the commonest type of bladder cancer and greater than 60% of newly diagnosed urothelial carcinomas of the bladder are nonmuscle invasive [2]. However, 50–70% of tumours reoccur and 10–30% progress to muscle invasive disease within 5 years [3]. Bladder cancer metastases to skeletal muscle are very rare and only a small number of cases have been reported in the literature. We present a rare case of a skeletal muscle metastasis to the vastus lateralis muscle from a urothelial carcinoma of the bladder. The authors have obtained the patient's informed written consent for electronic and print publication of the case report.

## 2. Case Report

A 71-year-old male attended haematuria clinic in 2017 with a short history of painless visible haematuria that first occurred on holiday in Vietnam. He has a background of a skin melanoma of the right leg which was completely excised. An ultrasound scan of the bladder and flexible cystoscopy was performed which showed a large bladder tumour on the left bladder wall. A staging computed tomography (CT) scan of the thorax, abdomen, and pelvis was negative for metastases, only the bladder tumour was observed (Figure 1). A transurethral resection of the bladder tumour was performed which showed muscle invasive disease. He subsequently underwent 3 cycles of neoadjuvant chemotherapy (gemcitabine and cisplatin), followed by a radical cystoprostatectomy and ileal conduit urinary diversion. Histological analysis confirmed a high grade muscle invasive urothelial carcinoma of the bladder with perineural invasion (pT3aN0). Three months after his surgery, he attended a follow-up clinic complaining of a painful right hip and a swelling in his right thigh worse on flexion at the hip. There were no skin changes or neurovascular compromise to the limb. Clinical examination revealed a diffuse swelling in the lateral compartment of the thigh. An ultrasound of the right thigh revealed a $43\,\text{mm} \times 31\,\text{mm}$ hypoechoic, well circumscribed lesion within the fibres of vastus lateralis (Figure 2). A subsequent contrast enhanced magnetic resonance imaging (MRI) scan showed a $37 \times 36 \times 48\,\text{mm}$ lesion of altered signal intensity with limited central enhancement, suspicious of a skeletal muscle metastasis (Figure 3). He also developed bone metastases at the L3 vertebra and right pubic bone. An ultrasound guided biopsy of the right thigh lesion was identified as a poorly differentiated carcinoma with positivity for

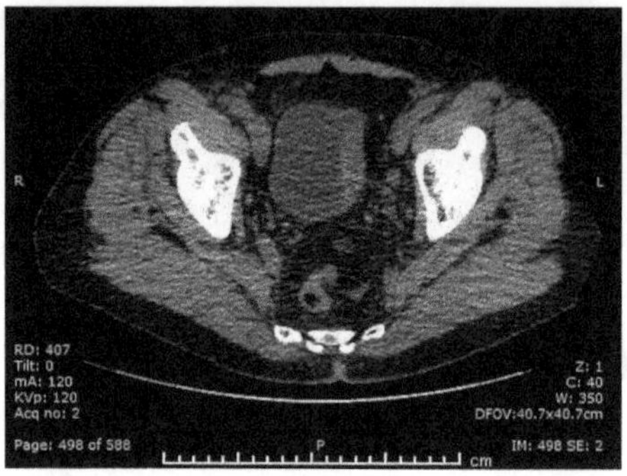


FIGURE 1: Computed tomography image of a bladder tumour on the left bladder wall.

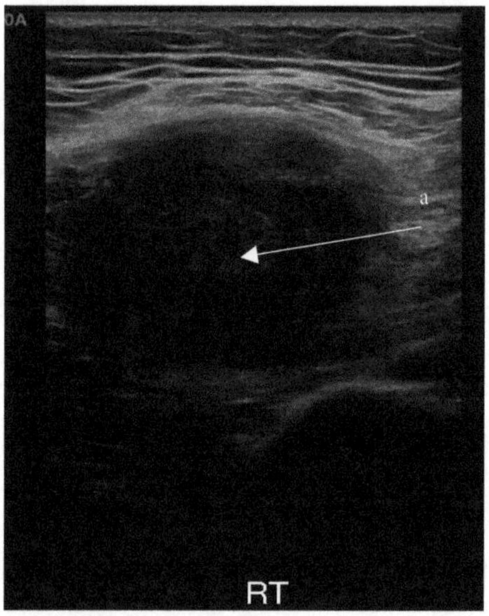


FIGURE 2: Ultrasound image of a mass in the right vastus lateralis muscle. a: Hypoechoic lesion in right vastus lateralis muscle.

pankeratin and cystokeratin 7 consistent with a urothelial carcinoma and confirming the diagnosis of skeletal muscle metastasis. He was referred to oncology and underwent 4 cycles of anti-PD-L1 monoclonal antibody immunotherapy (IV atezolizumab 1200 mg one dose per cycle) as part of a clinical trial. Despite better pain control and reduced right thigh swelling, follow up imaging suggested a slight increase in the size of the metastatic deposit in the thigh. He subsequently received a course of palliative radiotherapy to the lumbar spine, pelvis, and right thigh (20 Gy in 5 fractions at each site) followed by six 14 day cycles of IV paclitaxel chemotherapy (175 mg/m$^2$/day). The patient demonstrated partial remission as the skeletal muscle metastasis reduced in size to 22 × 34 × 52 mm (including an area of tumour necrosis) assessed by a repeat MRI scan in March 2018. However, the scan identified a new 53 × 40 × 18 mm subcutaneous UC metastasis over his left scapula which was fully excised, and the site was irradiated (20 Gy in 5 fractions). The patient continues to make good progress and he is mobile and self-caring. His disease to date has remained stable on follow up imaging and he is currently under CT surveillance.

## 3. Discussion

The commonest type of bladder cancer is UC accounting for over 90% of bladder tumours, 5% are squamous cell carcinomas and fewer than 2% are adenocarcinomas [4]. The commonest sites of metastases from bladder cancer are lymph nodes, bone, lung, liver and peritoneum [5]. Other unusual metastatic UC sites include the brain, skin and pericardial effusion have been reported [6–8]. Skeletal muscle metastases (SMM) are rare, despite muscle constituting up to 50% of total body mass and having a substantial blood supply [9]. Multiple factors have been hypothesised that limit the risk of metastatic spread to skeletal muscle. These protective factors include muscle pH, muscle contractility, alterations in oxygenation, and lactic acid accumulation that may reduce risk of metastatic tumour development [10, 11]. Magee and Rosenthal [12] reported that skeletal muscle trauma may increase the propensity for developing metastases within the affected muscle due to a change in muscle physiology that disrupts the previously described protective mechanisms. Other primary malignancies have been reported to metastasise to muscle such as the lung, kidney, stomach, pancreatic, colon and ovarian [13, 14]. The true incidence of muscle metastases may be underestimated. Autopsy studies have reported a higher incidence of muscle metastases ranging from 0.8% to 16% [15]. The number of patients who harbour muscle metastases may be higher in advanced stages of disease but only a few survive their disease long enough to present with clinical signs and symptoms from the affected site [13].

Metastases to skeletal muscle from UCs are extremely rare and only a few cases have been reported in the English literature [9, 16–21]. Nagao et al. [14] reported a case of a gluteus maximus metastasis from an adenocarcinoma of the bladder. A large proportion (50%) of muscle metastases from a carcinoma are found in the lower extremity [13]. Nabi et al. [22] reported UC metastases in the adductor, psoas, and rectus abdominis muscles. To date, our case is the first report of a biopsy proven UC metastasis to the vastus lateralis muscle. In all of the reported cases including our own, the presenting features were of a localised, painful swelling within the affected muscle.

It is difficult to distinguish between a metastatic carcinoma to the muscle and primary soft tissue sarcoma based on clinical examination or imaging studies [13]. Imaging can be used to help identify SMM and guide tumour biopsy. The CT features of SMM have been described as low density, ring enhancing lesions by Nabi et al. [22]. Surov et al. [23] described 5 different types of SMM based on CT appearances: focal intramuscular masses with homogenous contrast enhancement (type I), abscess-like intramuscular lesions (type II), diffuse metastatic muscle infiltration (type III), multifocal intramuscular calcification (type IV), and intramuscular bleeding (type V). SMM may present similarly to an abscess, therefore clinical corroboration and a high index of suspicion is required to achieve an accurate diagnosis. MRI is superior to CT for imaging soft-tissue tumours [24]. Heterogenous iso-signal intensity in T1-weighted sequences and heterogenous hyperintense signal in T2-weighted sequences with or without adjacent bone invasion with localised swelling and pain have been identified as features of SMM on MRI

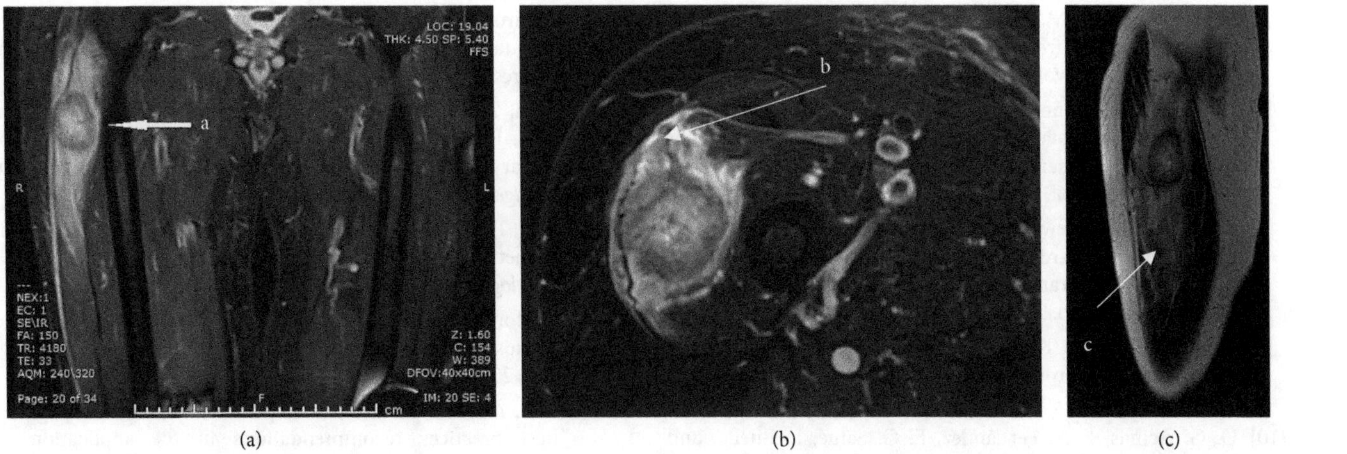


FIGURE 3: T2-weighted MRI images of the right thigh tumour. (a) Coronal image of the right thigh tumour. (b) Axial image of right thigh tumour and surrounding oedema. (c) Sagittal image of right thigh tumour with enhancing central element.

imaging [25]. Kashyap et al. [18] reported that F-18 FDG PET/CT scans could be useful to identify distant bladder cancer metastases. They observed intense FDG uptake in ring-enhancing lesions in multiple lower limb muscle groups suggestive of skeletal metastases from a primary bladder malignancy. However FDG is not specific for malignant cells and it also shows uptake in inflammatory/infectious sites, hence it is currently not recommended for routine imaging of soft tissue tumours [26]. Image guided biopsy of a suspected SMM is best to establish a diagnosis and hence, provide the most suitable treatment. Currently, there is no absolute immunohistochemistry marker or panel to confirm urothelial differentiation [27]. The uptake of immunohistochemical markers such as GATA3, S100P, CK7, CK20, HMCK, and p63 are suggestive of urothelial lineage of variant morphologies, whilst positivity for GATA3, CK20, p63, and either high molecular weight cytokeratin (HMCK) or cytokeratin (CK)5/6 can be useful in the differential diagnosis of urothelial carcinoma [27, 28].

Treatment of SMM is dependent on tumour location and the performance status of the patient. Chemotherapy, radiotherapy, and metastectomy are treatment options, usually performed for palliation of symptoms rather than with curative intent due to the likelihood of advanced malignant disease already present in the patient. Pretorius et al. [29] reported that 87% patients diagnosed with SMM had evidence of widespread metastatic disease. Patients presenting with a SMM have an average survival of less than 9 months and no more than 3 years after diagnosis, although there are reports of patients surviving up to 5 years after diagnosis [30]. Nabi et al. [22] reported in their series of UC SMMs patient survival was an average of 8 months (range 6–12 months), all 5 patients were treated with palliative chemotherapy and 2 patients also received palliative radiotherapy. Recent advances in immunotherapy have provided an additional treatment option for metastatic bladder cancer and since May 2016, 5 agents that target the programmed cell death 1 (PD-1) pathways have been approved for use following disease progression on platinum-based chemotherapy [31]. The SAUL trial, a multinational single-arm safety study of atezolizumab therapy for locally advanced or metastatic urothelial or nonurothelial carcinoma of the urinary tract for patients who had progressed during or after one to three therapies, has recently published its primary results. It showed that atezolizumab is tolerable and an effective treatment for urinary tract carcinoma, including patients with autoimmune disease and renal impairment [32]. These findings may provide a viable treatment option for this group of patients who may also have multiple co-morbidities, however the final results of the trial are awaited. Our patient received anti-PD-L1 monoclonal antibody immunotherapy, palliative radiotherapy and 6 cycles of chemotherapy. He continues to lead an active life and currently his disease burden is stable.

## 4. Conclusion

A skeletal muscle metastasis should be considered in patients with a history of urothelial malignancy who present with new muscle pain with or without swelling. MRI imaging together with tissue biopsy and a high index of clinical suspicion are the most useful methods of ascertaining a correct diagnosis.

## References

[1] S. Antoni, J. Ferlay, I. Soerjomataram, A. Znaor, A. Jemal, and F. Bray, "Bladder cancer incidence and mortality: a global overview and recent trends," *European Urology*, vol. 71, no. 1, pp. 96–108, 2017.

[2] H. Rubben, W. Lutzeyer, N. Fischer, F. Deutz, W. Lagrange, and G. Giani, "Natural history and treatment of low and high risk superficial bladder tumors," *Journal of Urology*, vol. 139, no. 2, pp. 283–285, 1988.

[3] A. M. Kamat, N. M. Hahn, J. A. Efstathiou et al., "Bladder cancer," *The Lancet*, vol. 388, no. 10061, pp. 2796–2810, 2016.

[4] D. S. Kaufman, W. U. Shipley, and A. S. Feldman, "Bladder cancer," *The Lancet*, vol. 374, no. 9685, pp. 239–249, 2009.

[5] A. B. Shinagare, N. H. Ramaiya, J. P. Jagannathan, F. M. Fennessy, M.-E. Taplin, and A. D. Van den Abbeele, "Metastatic pattern of bladder cancer: correlation with the characteristics of the primary tumor," *American Journal of Roentgenology*, vol. 196, no. 1, pp. 117–122, 2011.

[6] R. S. Anderson, A. M. El Mahdi, D. A. Kuban, and E. M. Higgins, "Brain metastases from transitional cell carcinoma of urinary bladder," *Urology*, vol. 39, no. 1, pp. 17–20, 1992.

[7] I. Agarwal, G. F. Bruney, C. Sands, G. Shirodkar, and M. Recine, "Cutaneous metastases from urothelial carcinoma of the bladder: a rare presentation and literature review," *West Indian Medical Journal*, vol. 63, no. 5, pp. 548–551, 2014.

[8] S. J. Fabozzi, J. R. Newton, R. P. Moriarty, and P. F. Schellhammer, "Malignant pericardial effusion as initial solitary site of metastasis from transitional cell carcinoma of the bladder," *Urology*, vol. 45, no. 2, pp. 320–322, 1995.

[9] S. W. Doo, W. B. Kim, B. K. Kim et al., "Skeletal muscle metastases from urothelial cell carcinoma," *Korean Journal of Urology*, vol. 53, no. 1, p. 63, 2012.

[10] O. G. Acinas, F. A. Fernández, E. G. Satué, L. Buelta, and J. F. Val-Bernal, "Metastasis of malignant neoplasms to skeletal muscle," *Revista Espanola de Oncologia*, vol. 31, no. 1, pp. 57–67, 1984.

[11] F. Mulsow, "Metastatic carcinoma of skeletal muscles," *Archives of Pathology & Laboratory Medicine*, vol. 35, pp. 112–114, 1943.

[12] T. Magee and H. Rosenthal, "Skeletal muscle metastases at sites of documented trauma," *American Journal of Roentgenology*, vol. 178, no. 4, pp. 985–988, 2002.

[13] C. L. Herring Jr., J. M. Harrelson, and S. P. Scully, "Metastatic carcinoma to skeletal muscle. A report of 15 patients," *Clinical Orthopaedics and Related Research*, vol. 355, pp. 272–281, 1998.

[14] E. Nagao, A. Nishie, K. Yoshimitsu et al., "Gluteal muscular and sciatic nerve metastases in advanced urinary bladder carcinoma: case report," *Abdominal Imaging*, vol. 29, no. 5, 2004.

[15] C. M. Pearson, "Incidence and type of pathologic alterations observed in muscle in a routine autopsy survey," *Neurology*, vol. 9, no. 11, pp. 757–757, 1959.

[16] M. Guidi, C. Fusetti, and S. Lucchina, "Skeletal muscle metastases to the flexor digitorum superficialis and profundus from urothelial cell carcinoma and review of the literature," *Case Reports in Urology*, vol. 2016, Article ID 2387501, 5 pages, 2016.

[17] I. Katafigiotis, A. Athanasiou, P. K. Levis et al., "Metastasis to sartorius muscle from a muscle invasive bladder cancer," *Case Reports in Medicine*, vol. 2014, Article ID 524757, 3 pages, 2014.

[18] R. Kashyap, B. R. Mittal, D. Chakraborty, A. Bhattacharya, and B. Singh, "Multiple skeletal muscle metastases in a case of transitional cell carcinoma of bladder detected by F-18 FDG PET/CT," *Nuclear Medicine and Molecular Imaging*, vol. 44, no. 4, pp. 297–299, 2010.

[19] L. Dell'Atti, "A rare metastatic myositis ossificans of obturator muscle secondary to urothelial carcinoma," *Rare Tumors*, vol. 7, no. 3, pp. 108–110, 2015.

[20] S. Ekici, H. Özen, G. Ö. Gedikoglu, and C. Aygü, "Skeletal muscle metastasis from carcinoma of the bladder," *Scandinavian Journal of Urology and Nephrology*, vol. 33, no. 5, pp. 336–337, 1999.

[21] J. G. Masters, J. A. Cumming, and P. Jennings, "Psoas abscess secondary to metastases from transitional cell carcinoma of the bladder," *British Journal of Urology*, vol. 77, no. 1, pp. 155–156, 1996.

[22] G. Nabi, N. P. Gupta, and D. Gandhi, "Skeletal muscle metastasis from transitional cell carcinoma of the urinary bladder: clinicoradiological features," *Clinical Radiology*, vol. 58, no. 11, pp. 883–885, 2003.

[23] A. Surov, M. Hainz, H.-J. Holzhausen et al., "Skeletal muscle metastases: primary tumours, prevalence, and radiological features," *European Radiology*, vol. 20, no. 3, pp. 649–658, 2010.

[24] A. M. Aisen, W. Martel, E. M. Braunstein, K. I. McMillin, W. A. Phillips, and T. F. Kling, "MRI and CT evaluation of primary bone and soft-tissue tumors," *American Journal of Roentgenology*, vol. 146, no. 4, pp. 749–756, 1986.

[25] Q. Li, L. Wang, S. Pan et al., "Skeletal muscle metastases on magnetic resonance imaging: analysis of 31 cases," *Współczesna Onkologia*, vol. 20, no. 3, pp. 242–250, 2016.

[26] D. Afonso and V. Mascarenhas, "Imaging techniques for the diagnosis of soft tissue tumors," *Reports in Medical Imaging*, p. 63, 2015.

[27] M. B. Amin, K. Trpkov, A. Lopez-Beltran, and D. Grignon, "Best practices recommendations in the application of immunohistochemistry in the bladder lesions," *The American Journal of Surgical Pathology*, vol. 38, no. 8, pp. e20–e34, 2014.

[28] G. P. Paner, C. Annaiah, C. Gulmann et al., "Immunohistochemical evaluation of novel and traditional markers associated with urothelial differentiation in a spectrum of variants of urothelial carcinoma of the urinary bladder," *Human Pathology*, vol. 45, no. 7, pp. 1473–1482, 2014.

[29] E. S. Pretorius and E. K. Fishman, "Helical CT of skeletal muscle metastases from primary carcinomas," *American Journal of Roentgenology*, vol. 174, no. 2, pp. 401–404, 2000.

[30] T. A. Damron and J. Heiner, "Distant soft tissue metastases: a series of 30 new patients and 91 cases from the literature," *Annals of Surgical Oncology*, vol. 7, no. 7, pp. 526–534, 2000.

[31] A. Tripathi and E. R. Plimack, "Immunotherapy for urothelial carcinoma: current evidence and future directions," *Current Urology Reports*, vol. 19, no. 12, p. 109, 2018.

[32] C. N. Sternberg, Y. Loriot, N. James et al., "Primary results from SAUL, a multinational single-arm safety study of atezolizumab therapy for locally advanced or metastatic urothelial or nonurothelial carcinoma of the urinary tract," *European Urology*, vol. 76, no. 1, pp. 73–81, 2019.

# 51

# Squamous Cell Carcinoma Developing from a Testicular Epidermal Cyst: A Case Report and Literature Review

**Ryo Kasahara,[1,2] Ryosuke Tajiri,[3] Kota Kobayashi,[1] Masahiro Yao,[2] and Kazuo Kitami[1]**

[1]*Department of Urology, Fujisawa City Hospital, 2-6-1 Fujisawa, Fujisawa City, Kanagawa Prefecture, Japan*
[2]*Department of Urology, Yokohama City University School of Medicine, 3-9 Fukuura, Kanazawa Ward, Yokohama City, Kanagawa Prefecture, Japan*
[3]*Department of Pathology, Fujisawa City Hospital, 2-6-1 Fujisawa, Fujisawa City, Kanagawa Prefecture, Japan*

Correspondence should be addressed to Ryo Kasahara; rk.ycu@hotmail.com

Academic Editor: Fumitaka Koga

A 50-year-old Japanese man with a two-year history of a painless right scrotal mass visited our hospital. Considering laboratory findings and computed tomography, the patient was diagnosed with an uncharacteristic testicular tumor. No metastases were present on radiographic study at the first visit. Emergent high radical orchiectomy was performed, and the tumor was identified as a squamous cell carcinoma (SCC) of a testicular epidermal cyst. He is alive without recurrence or metastasis six months after surgery. Testicular SCC is an extremely rare tumor. This is the third case of testicular SCC associated with an epidermal cyst in English literature.

## 1. Introduction

A large proportion of testicular cancers are seminomas, and most nonseminomas include embryonal carcinomas and yolk sac tumors [1]. We encountered a case of primary squamous cell carcinoma (SCC) of an epidermal cyst in the testis. Testicular SCC is extremely rare, except for metastasis from other primary lesions. Herein, we describe our experience with this case and review the relevant English literature.

## 2. Case Presentation

A 50-year-old Japanese man with a two-year history of a painless right scrotal mass visited our hospital. He was previously healthy and did not take any medications. His scrotal mass was elastic and hard and had no translucency. We palpated normal testis and epididymis in the contralateral scrotum.

We ordered blood laboratory examination and computed tomography (CT). Laboratory data were largely unremarkable and testicular tumor markers were not elevated (alpha-fetoprotein (AFP): 2.9 ng/mL; beta human chorionic gonadotropin (hCG): <0.1 ng/mL). CT revealed a testicular tumor with cystic structure in the right scrotum. The wall of the cystic structure was thickened and enhanced with contrast medium. The tumor size was 48 x 48 x 42 mm (Figure 1). Considering clinical and radiological findings, his scrotum mass was considered to be an uncharacteristic testicular tumor. CT showed no metastasis to lymph nodes or other organs.

Emergent high radical orchiectomy was performed. The operation time was 36 minutes and there was minimal bleeding. The resected tumor was cystic and filled with the brown pus-like fluid. He was discharged from our hospital on the second postoperative day.

The specimen was submitted for pathological examination. Hematoxylin-eosin staining revealed SCC developing from the cyst in the parenchyma of the testis (Figure 2). The neoplasm contained a cancer pearl and was consistent with typical SCC (Figure 3). The cyst did not have cutaneous appendages, bone, or cartilage; therefore, it was considered to be a simple epidermal cyst, not a dermoid cyst or teratoma. Intraepithelial carcinoma was present in the epidermal cyst. As a result, the tumor was considered a primary lesion, not a metastasis. An area of normal testicular parenchyma

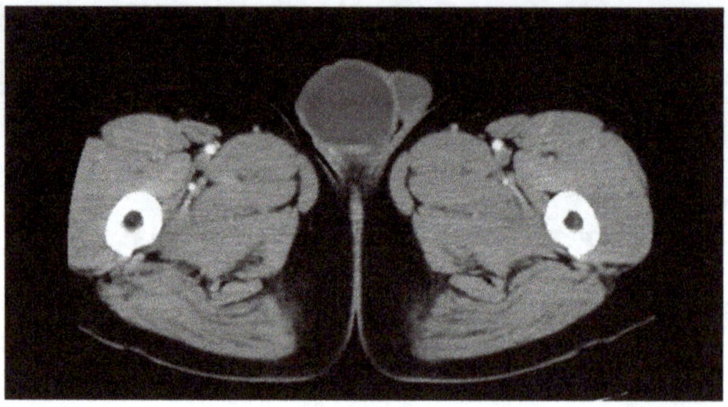

FIGURE 1: CT revealed a 48 x 48 x 42 mm cystic tumor. The wall of the cystic structure was thickened and enhanced with contrast medium.

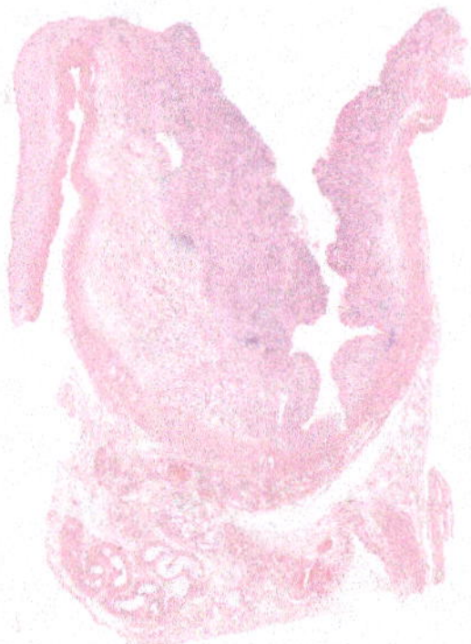

FIGURE 2: Loupe image of the tumor shows squamous cell carcinoma developing from the cyst in the parenchyma of the testis.

remained. The final diagnosis was SCC developing from a testicular epidermal cyst.

After discharge, he was followed up with CT and tumor marker (SCC). At six months after operation, SCC was within the normal range (1.1 ng/mL) and CT showed neither recurrence nor metastasis.

## 3. Discussion

Most primary testicular tumors are germ cell tumors, and primary testicular SCCs are very rare, with only three cases reported in the English literature [2–5].

The incidence of secondary (metastatic) testicular tumor has been reported as 0.06%, with origins including the lung, prostate, gastrointestinal tract, skin (melanoma), and kidney [2, 6]. We thought that this low incidence was, for the most part, the result of the blood-testis barrier and the scrotum, which keeps the testes at a low temperature. The blood-testis barrier is one of the tightest junctions in the human body and is composed of four different cells [7]. The scrotum, which works as a radiator, keeps the testes at a low temperature. These functions may make invasion and proliferation of metastatic tumor cells difficult. Furthermore, there are two case reports of testicular metastasis of SCC from the lung [8, 9]. Hence, it is important to determine whether the tumor is a primary tumor and other neoplasms should be excluded.

With regard to the diagnosis of testicular SCCs, it is common to suspect a malignant transformation of a teratoma

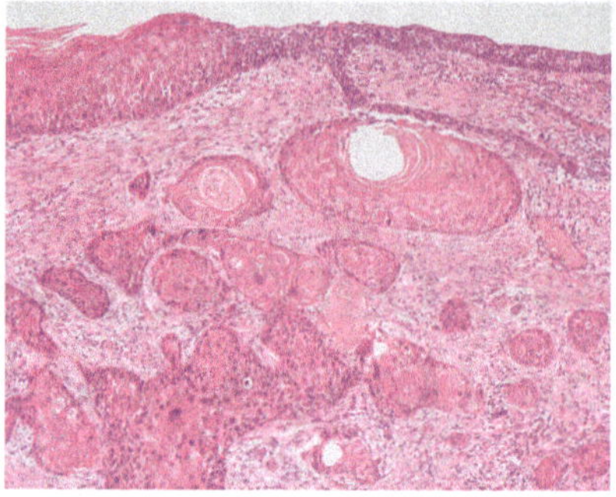

FIGURE 3: The neoplasm contained a cancer pearl which is consistent with typical squamous cell carcinoma.

or from other origins. In this case, the carcinoma developed from an intraepithelial tumor of the cyst, and the cyst did not have cutaneous appendages, bone, or cartilage. CT also revealed no other neoplastic lesions. From the abovementioned information, the tumor was diagnosed as a primary tumor that developed from an epidermal cyst.

Up to now, three cases of primary SCCs of the testis have been reported in the English literature [3–5]. Bryan et al. reported a case of a testicular tumor derived from the malignant transformation of an epidermal cyst [3]. Shih et al. described a case involving testicular SCC that arose from the malignant transformation of a hydrocele [4]. Kim et al. reported the case of a testicular tumor derived from the malignant transformation of an epidermal cyst [5].

Shah et al. collected 141 cases of testicular epidermal cysts [10], with patients aged from 3 to 77 years old. Ethnic grouping analysis revealed that testicular epidermal cysts were more common in white patients (92 patients) and 25 Japanese patients were included. Epidermal cysts of the testes account for less than 1% of all testicular tumors, are frequently benign, and have good prognoses. However, several cases demonstrated loss of heterozygosity for a certain chromosomal loci, supporting the possibility of neoplastic potential [10].

In general, squamous cell carcinogenesis has been thought to be related to chronic irritation and inflammation. However, with regard to testicular SCCs alone, it is unclear whether such mechanisms exist.

Due to its rarity, there are no guidelines or prognostic data available. However, as previously mentioned, epidermal cysts have the potential for malignant transformation. All SCC cases developing from epidermal cysts have been reported in patients over 50 years old [3, 5]. Therefore, there is the possibility that epidermal cysts in older patients may be complicated with neoplasm. Hence, it may be permissible to follow up older patients with epidermal cysts using SCC tumor marker and CT for several years.

We reported the third case of testicular SCC associated with an epidermal cyst in English literature.

## Acknowledgments

The authors would like to acknowledge Editage for English language editing.

## References


[1] C. La Vecchia, C. Bosetti, F. Lucchini et al., "Cancer mortality in Europe, 2000–2004, and an overview of trends since 1975," *Annals of Oncology*, vol. 21, no. 6, pp. 1323–1360, 2010.

[2] M. Nistal, P. Gonzalez-Peramato, and R. Paniagua, "Secondary testicular tumors," *European Urology*, vol. 16, no. 3, pp. 185–188, 1989.

[3] R. L. Bryan, S. Liu, J. Newman, J. M. O'Brien, and J. Considine, "Squamous cell carcinoma arising in a chronic hydrocele," *Histopathology*, vol. 17, no. 2, pp. 178–180, 1990.

[4] D.-F. Shih, J.-S. Wang, and H.-H. Tseng, "Primary squamous cell carcinoma of the testis," *The Journal of Urology*, vol. 156, no. 5, pp. 1772-1772, 1996.

[5] N. R. Kim, H. Y. Cho, S. J. Yoon, J. H. Park, and S. Y. Ha, "Primary squamous cell carcinoma in the testis: a case report," *Journal of Korean Medical Science*, vol. 25, no. 4, pp. 634–637, 2010.

[6] E. J. Pienkos and V. R. Jablokow, "Secondary testicular tumors," *Cancer*, vol. 30, no. 2, pp. 481–485, 1972.

[7] D. D. Mruk and C. Y. Cheng, "The mammalian blood-testis barrier: its biology and regulation," *Endocrine Reviews*, vol. 36, no. 5, pp. 564–591, 2015.

[8] D. A. Buck, R. H. Byrd, C. L. Holmes, and T. Pollock, "Testicular metastasis in a case of squamous cell carcinoma of the lung," *Case Reports in Oncology*, vol. 8, no. 1, pp. 133–137, 2015.

[9] M. A. Kaplan, M. Kucukoner, A. Inal et al., "Testicular mass: an initial sign of squamous cell carcinoma of the lung," *World Journal of Oncology*, vol. 3, no. 6, pp. 291–293, 2016.

[10] K. H. Shah, W. C. Maxted, and B. Chun, "Epidermoid cysts of the testis. A report of three cases and an analysis of four cases from the world literature," *Cancer*, vol. 47, no. 3, pp. 577–582, 1981.

# 52

# Use of SPY Elite Fluorescence Imaging in Creation of a Continent Urinary Diversion

**Ali Hajiran,[1] David Zekan,[1] Tyler Trump,[1] Dylan Dangerfield,[2] and Adam Luchey[1]**

[1]*Department of Urology, West Virginia University, Morgantown, WV 26505, USA*
[2]*Department of Urology, University of Tennessee Graduate School of Medicine, Knoxville, TN 37920, USA*

Correspondence should be addressed to David Zekan; dszekan@mix.wvu.edu

Academic Editor: Sigurdur Gudjonsson

The use of SPY Elite Fluorescence Imaging has recently grown popular among multiple surgical specialties, including colorectal, plastic, endocrine, ophthalmologic, and vascular surgery, due to its ability to quickly and accurately assess tissue perfusion and guide intraoperative decision making. To our knowledge, the use of SPY imaging in urologic reconstructive surgery has yet to be reported. We present a case in which SPY imaging was used intraoperatively to assess perfusion of an ileocecal anastomosis and a segment of bowel prior to creation of a continent urinary diversion following radical cystectomy.

## 1. Introduction

Inadequate tissue perfusion is a fundamental cause of early complications following surgery [1]. Historically, clinical judgment has been used as the primary means of evaluating tissue perfusion intraoperatively via palpation of pulses, assessing bleeding at cut edges, and observation of tissue color. However, this method is not always reliable. In many cases, more conclusive evaluation of tissue perfusion is desired intraoperatively in order to avoid the potentially devastating complications secondary to tissue ischemia. In urologic reconstructive surgery, ensuring adequate blood supply is critical in the creation of a continent urinary diversion. Failure to identify and address poorly perfused segments of bowel intraoperatively could lead to many devastating complications including anastomotic leak, breakdown, stricture or necrosis of the reservoir [2, 3].

Multiple modalities have been evaluated and used clinically in the past to assess tissue perfusion with mixed results. Use of the SPY Elite Fluorescence Imaging system, which utilizes indocyanine green (ICG) with laser angiography, has grown in popularity in ophthalmologic, plastic, endocrine, vascular, and colorectal surgeries. ICG injected intravenously allows for intraoperative assessment of visceral blood supply and bowel perfusion. This real time assessment allows for increased operative efficiency and assists in surgical decision-making [1]. In this case, we present the use of intraoperative laser angiography to aide in decision making while selecting bowel segment for use as a continent urinary diversion.

## 2. Case Presentation

A 61-year-old woman with high-grade nonmuscle invasive Ta urothelial carcinoma of the bladder presented to our clinic. The patient subsequently experienced recurrence of high-grade disease following two complete induction courses of intravesical BCG; therefore, we recommended proceeding with radical cystectomy. The patient agreed and requested creation of a continent urinary diversion.

We planned to perform an open radical cystectomy, extended pelvic lymph node dissection, and continent urinary diversion using the ascending colon, terminal ileum, and ileocecal valve as a continence mechanism (Indiana Pouch). Intraoperatively, the right colon was mobilized while carefully preserving the right colic and ileocolic arteries. A 12 cm segment of the distal ileum along with a 30 cm of cecum was harvested using a GIA stapler, while preserving the mesenteric blood supply. Bowel continuity was re-established by creating an ileocolic anastomosis using the GIA stapler. The SPY Elite Fluorescence system then was used to assess adequate perfusion of the anastomosis as well as the harvested bowel to be used for the urinary reservoir. This involved intravenous

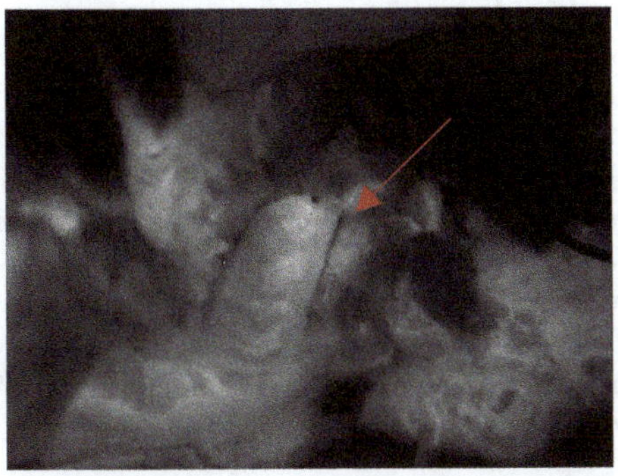

FIGURE 1: Intraoperative SPY Elite Fluoroscopy Imaging of well-perfused ileocecal anastomosis.

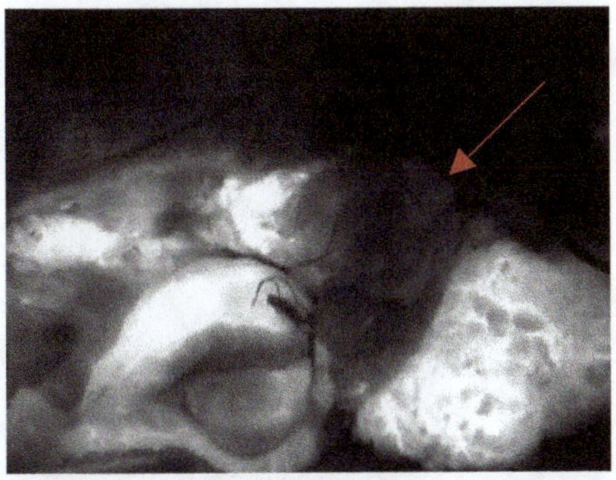

FIGURE 2: Intraoperative SPY Elite Fluoroscopy Imaging showing poorly perfused segment of ascending colon.

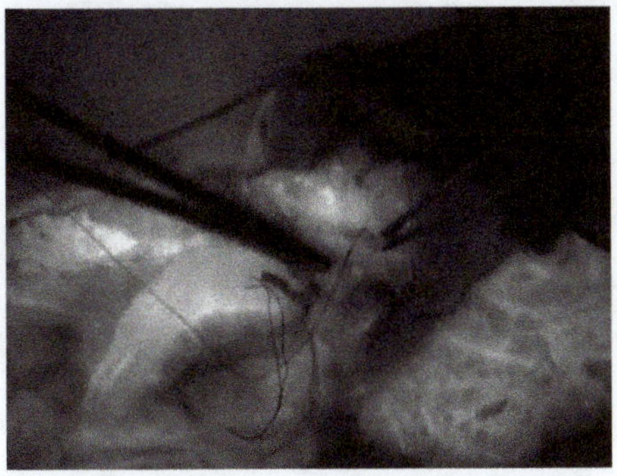

FIGURE 3: Intraoperative SPY Elite Fluoroscopy Imaging guiding marking of poorly perfused segment of ascending colon with a stitch.

injection of 1.25–5 mg of a 2.5 mg/mL indocyanine green solution followed by visualization using a laser diode array capable of illuminating a maximum field of $18.5 \times 13.5\ cm^2$. A device camera then captured these image sequences at a rate of 3.75–30 frames per second based on the desired recording time of 30 second up to a maximum of 4.5 minutes. Images were viewed on a high-definition monitor in real time in the operating room, allowing for immediate evaluation of tissue perfusion [1]. The anastomosis appeared to be well perfused (Figure 1); however, an approximately 3 cm segment of ascending colon demonstrated poor perfusion on SPY imaging (Figure 2). This segment of poorly perfused bowel was marked (Figure 3) and resected to ensure that it was not included in the urinary reservoir. The continent cutaneous urinary reservoir was then created without any complications. The remainder of the surgery was uneventful. The patient's hospital course was uneventful without complications and she was discharged home on post-operative day seven. She followed up three weeks post-operatively for pouchogram, which revealed appropriate filling with no contrast extravasation. Four months later, the patient reported that she was doing very well with no issues performing intermittent catheterization.

## 3. Discussion

Anastomotic leakage and breakdown are serious, potentially fatal complications known to occur in up to 5% of patients undergoing surgery requiring urinary diversion. Several factors can contribute to anastomotic breakdown including poor perfusion, prior radiation therapy, and use of bowel affected by chronic inflammation, among others. With regard to these factors, use of healthy, well-perfused bowel is critical to improving patient outcomes following anastomotic formation [2]. In this case, the authors implement the use of laser angiography to assess the perfusion and viability of bowel segment prior to selection for use in the ureteroenterostomy.

Intraoperative utilization of laser angiography has grown popular over the past decade with proven benefit to intraoperative decision-making and patient outcome in various fields, from mapping of the extrahepatic biliary tree in cholecystectomy to lymphatic mapping in sentinel lymph node biopsy [4]. The investigators in the PILLAR-II trial demonstrated a marked reduction in anastomotic leakage following colorectal surgery in those patients who had intraoperative laser angiography. The incidence of anastomotic breakdown in those who underwent laser angiography was 60% lower than in those who did not, including patients undergoing high-risk bowel anastomoses [5].

While there is sound evidence supporting the use of laser angiography to assist in bowel anastomosis, there is little literature addressing its utility in urologic surgery. Morozov et al. describe the use of SPY elite in lymph node dissection during radical prostatectomy, the identification of renal tumors during partial nephrectomy, and location of stricture during ureteroplasty [6]. Specifically, a majority of malignant renal growths (70%) demonstrated hypofluorescence on imaging, while the remaining group shows no difference in fluorescent uptake [7]. It has also been used in robotic partial nephrectomy to facilitate selective arterial clipping causing regional perfusion deficit directed specifically at a tumor [8]. Another small study demonstrated the benefit of laser angiography in the assessment of ureteral viability prior to ureteroileal anastomosis. In this study, 70% of patients required a segment of distal ureter to be removed prior to spatulation based on poor enhancement during laser angiography [9]. Similarly, Rother et al. demonstrate the utility of intraoperative laser angiography in renal transplant to assess allograft perfusion following implantation of the donor kidney [10]. The future of fluorescent imaging in urology is vast, with current developments describing the use of tumor markers such as prostate-specific membrane antigen with fluorescent tracers for intraoperative imaging in urologic oncology as well as diagnosis of shallow papillary bladder carcinoma and carcinoma in situ using fluorescent markers with high sensitivity and specificity [11, 12]. This case provides more supporting evidence of the benefits associated with the use of SPY technology in urology. This is the first case describing its use to aid in the formation of a successful neobladder.

## 4. Conclusion

The authors of the case described above present the use of laser angiography as an effective method to assist in selection of bowel for use during urinary diversion. We expect that this work will support fellow clinicians and researchers to explore laser angiography as a means for evaluating tissue viability. Further studies would be helpful in providing further support of low anastomotic leak and necrosis.

## References

[1] G. C. Gurtner, G. E. Jones, P. C. Neligan et al., "Intraoperative laser angiography using the SPY system: review of the literature and recommendations for use," *Annals of Surgical Innovation and Research*, vol. 7, no. 1, p. 1, 2013.

[2] S. B. Farnham and M. S. Cookson, "Surgical complications of urinary diversion," *World Journal of Urology*, vol. 22, no. 3, pp. 157–167, 2004.

[3] D. G. Holmes, J. B. Thrasher, G. Y. Park, D. C. Kueker, and J. W. Weigel, "Long-term complications related to the modified Indiana pouch," *Urology*, vol. 60, no. 4, pp. 603–606, 2002.

[4] M. Lavazza, X. Liu, C. Wu et al., "Indocyanine green-enhanced fluorescence for assessing parathyroid perfusion during thyroidectomy," *Gland Surgery*, vol. 5, no. 5, pp. 512–521, 2016.

[5] M. D. Jafari, S. D. Wexner, J. E. Martz et al., "Perfusion assessment in laparoscopic left-sided/anterior resection (PILLAR II): a multi-institutional study," *Journal of the American College of Surgeons*, vol. 220, no. 1, pp. 82–92, 2015.

[6] A. O. Morozov, Y. G. Alyaev, L. M. Rapoport et al., "Near-infrared fluorescence with indocyanine green for diagnostics in urology: initial experience," *Urologia Journal*, vol. 84, no. 3, pp. 197–202, 2017.

[7] S. Tobis, J. Knopf, C. Silvers et al., "Near infrared fluorescence imaging with robotic assisted laparoscopic partial nephrectomy: initial clinical experience for renal cortical tumors," *The Journal of Urology*, vol. 186, no. 1, pp. 47–52, 2011.

[8] M. A. Bjurlin, T. R. McClintock, and M. D. Stifelman, "Near-infrared fluorescence imaging with intraoperative administration of indocyanine green for robotic partial nephrectomy," *Current Urology Reports*, vol. 16, no. 4, p. 20, 2015.

[9] D. M. Freitas, T. Shin, N. Ahmadi et al., "PD38-02 utilization of indocyanine green fluorescence angiography prior to intracorporeal ureteroileal anastomosis following robotic radical cystectomy," *The Journal of Urology*, vol. 197, no. 4S, p. e739, 2017.

[10] U. Rother, A. Gerken, L. Karampinis et al., "Dosing of indocyanine green for intraoperative laser fluorescence angiography in kidney transplantation," *Microcirculation*, vol. 24, no. 8, p. e12392, 2017.

[11] N. S. van den Berg, F. W. van Leeuwen, and H. G. van der Poel, "Fluorescence guidance in urologic surgery," *Current Opinion in Urology*, vol. 22, no. 2, pp. 109–120, 2012.

[12] M. A. D'Hallewin, A. R. Kamuhabwa, T. Roskams, P. A. M. De Witte, and L. Baert, "Hypericin-based fluorescence diagnosis of bladder carcinoma," *BJU International*, vol. 89, no. 7, pp. 760–763, 2002.

# Successful Response of Pembrolizumab Rechallenge after Radiotherapy for a Patient with Bladder Cancer of Nonresponse of Pembrolizumab First Challenge

**Taro Ikeda,[1] Go Hasegawa,[2] Gen Kawaguchi,[3] Yohei Ikeda,[4] Noboru Hara,[1] and Tsutomu Nishiyama[1]**

[1]*Department of Urology, Uonuma Institute of Community Medicine, Niigata University Medical and Dental Hospital, Minamiuonuma, Niigata, Japan*
[2]*Department of Pathology, Uonuma Institute of Community Medicine, Niigata University Medical and Dental Hospital, Minamiuonuma, Niigata, Japan*
[3]*Department of Radiotherapy, Uonuma Institute of Community Medicine, Niigata University Medical and Dental Hospital, Minamiuonuma, Niigata, Japan*
[4]*Department of Diagnostic Radiology, Uonuma Institute of Community Medicine, Niigata University Medical and Dental Hospital, Minamiuonuma, Niigata, Japan*

Correspondence should be addressed to Tsutomu Nishiyama; nisiyama@med.niigata-u.ac.jp

Academic Editor: Fumitaka Koga

We report a patient with advanced bladder cancer in which the primary lesion and metastatic site disappeared following the pembrolizumab therapy rechallenge after radiotherapy for bladder cancer lesion of nonresponse of pembrolizumab first challenge. A 76-year-old man with advanced bladder cancer received three courses of the chemotherapy with gemcitabine and cisplatin combination; however, the chemotherapy was stopped because of adverse events. The patient started pembrolizumab therapy; however, the effect was not observed. Radiation therapy was given to the primary lesion and pelvic lymph node metastases for the purpose of local control of the lesions. Because the primary lesion was regrowth and para-aortic lymph node metastasis appeared, pembrolizumab therapy was resumed. Thereafter, the primary lesion and metastatic site disappeared.

## 1. Introduction

Although the treatments of advanced bladder cancer have made significant progress in recent years, most patients go on to have progressive disease and are still incurable [1]. We report a patient with advanced bladder cancer in which the primary lesion and metastatic site disappeared following the pembrolizumab therapy rechallenge after radiotherapy for bladder cancer lesion of nonresponse of pembrolizumab first challenge.

## 2. Case Report

A 76-year-old man was pointed out microhematuria and left hydronephrosis during treatment for rheumatoid arthritis at a nearby doctor and was referred to our hospital in April 2019. Cystoscopy showed a solid mass from trigonum to the posterior wall of the bladder, and bilateral ureteral orifices could not be confirmed. Contrast-enhanced computed tomography (CT) of the thoraco-abdomino-pelvis revealed bladder cancer with extramural invasion and left hydronephrosis and left renal urine extravasation due to left ureteral obstruction of exponential growth of bladder tumor (Figures 1(a) and 1(b)). Bladder magnetic resonance imaging (MRI) revealed bladder cancer with extramural invasion (Figure 1(c)). Bladder tumor biopsy revealed invasive urothelial cancer and high grade (Figure 2). With the diagnosis of left hydronephrosis and left renal urine extravasation due to left ureteral obstruction at the left ureteral orifice with

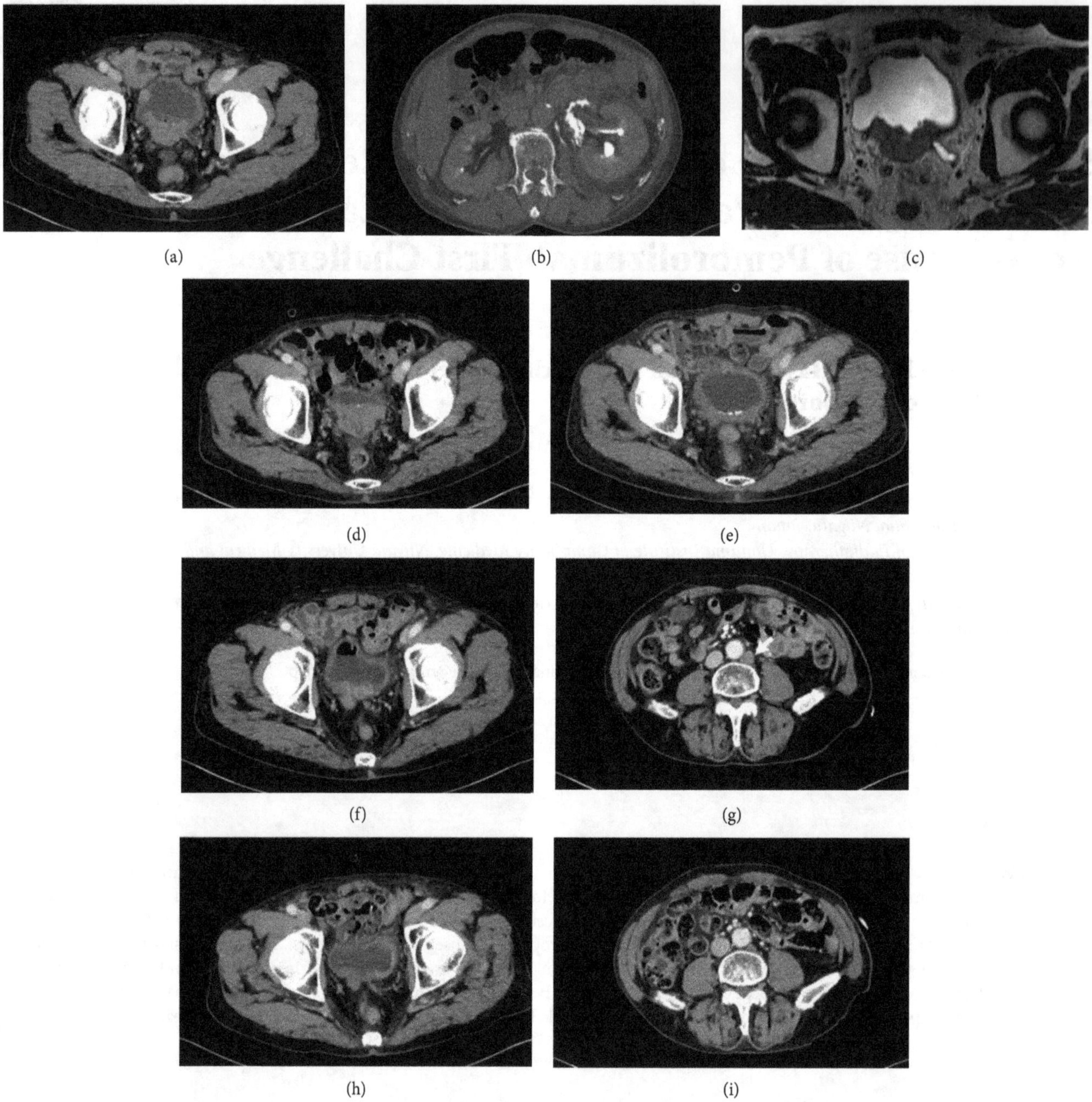

Figure 1: Imaging findings. (a) CT in April 2019 at diagnosis shows the extramural invasive tumor in posterior and trigonal bladder wall. (b) CT urography at diagnosis shows the leakage of contrast media because of extravasated urine. (c) MRI at diagnosis shows that the extramural invasive tumor in posterior and trigonal bladder wall is a low signal intensity on T2-weighted image. (d) CT in December 2019 at the discontinuation of pembrolizumab therapy shows growth in the primary lesion. (e) CT in June 2020 after radiotherapy shows diminished primary tumor in size. (f) CT in September 2020 three months following radiotherapy shows regrowth of the primary lesion. (g) CT in September 2020 three months following radiotherapy shows the emergency of para-aortic lymph node metastasis (arrow: para-aortic lymph node metastasis). (h) CT in February 2021 at the end of 8 doses of pembrolizumab therapy resumption shows significant reduction of the primary lesion. (i) CT in February 2021 at the end of 8 doses of pembrolizumab therapy resumption shows almost disappearance of para-aortic lymph node metastasis.

invasive bladder cancer, left nephrostomy was performed urgently. The patient underwent gemcitabine/cisplatin combination therapy (GC therapy) (70% dose in consideration for his age). The effect of three courses of GC therapy was stable disease. Continuing GC therapy was planned but was stopped because low-grade fever continued, and CT showed shadows in both lung fields. The patient started pembrolizumab therapy (pembrolizumab 200 mg intravenously, every 3 weeks) in September 2019 after confirming improvement in general condition and remission of shadows in both lung fields. The patient was noted to have a gastric ulcer after four courses of pembrolizumab therapy and discontinued

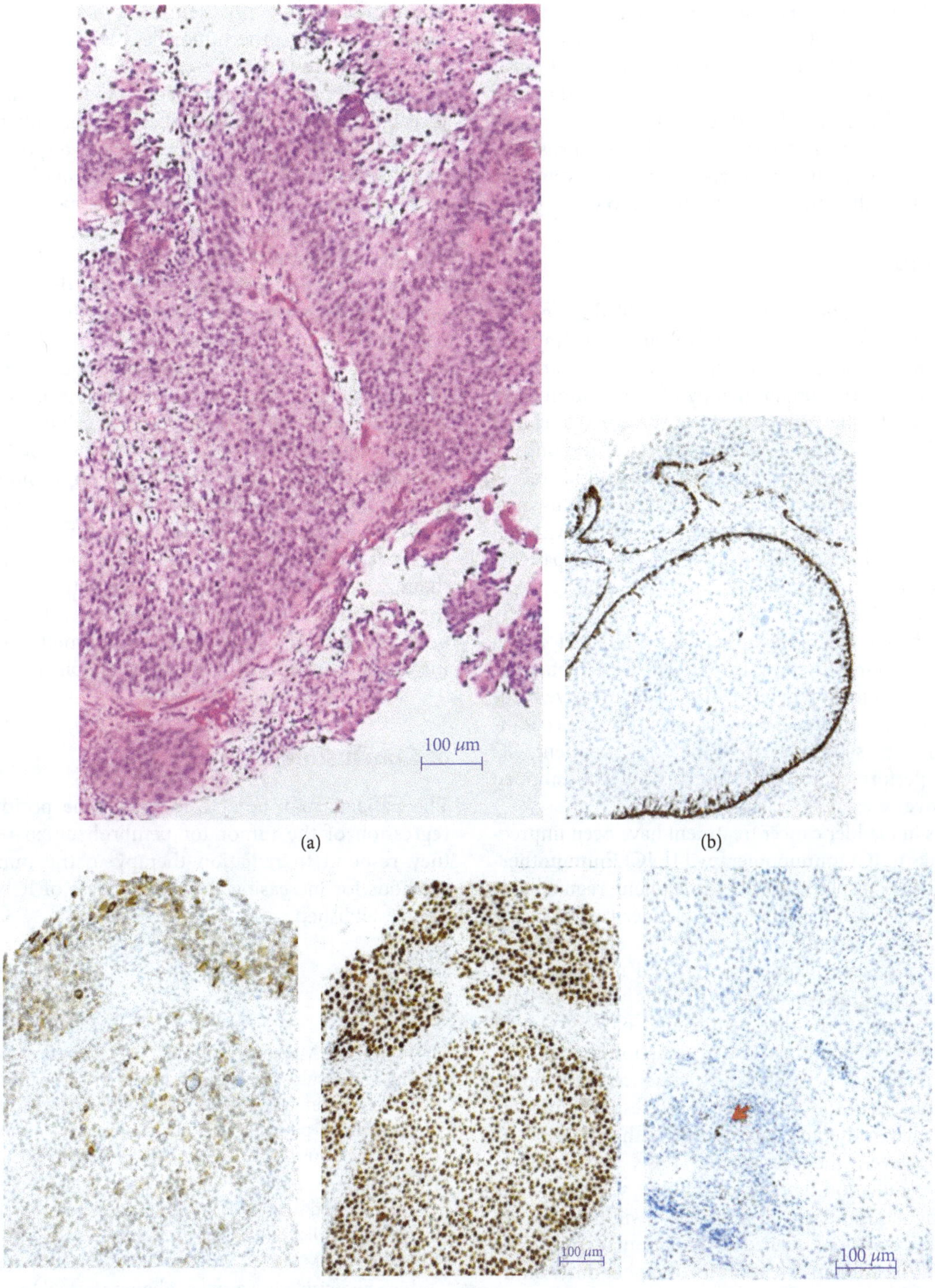


FIGURE 2: Pathological findings. Pathological findings revealed invasive urothelial carcinoma (UC) (luminal type UC, papillary, G2, high grade) (H&E stain (a)), CK5/6 negative (b), CK20 weak positive (c), GATA3 strong positive (d), and PD-L1 negative (red arrow: macrophage) (e).

pembrolizumab therapy due to regrowth in the primary lesion and the appearance of pelvic lymph node metastases in December 2019 (Figure 1(d)). The patient was found to have increased primary lesion and pelvic lymph node metastasis on CT in March 2020. The patient underwent radiotherapy (50.4 Gy with 28 fractions) on the primary lesion and pelvic lymph node metastasis site for the purpose of local control of the lesions. The primary lesion and pelvic lymph node metastasis site diminished in size after the radiotherapy (Figure 1(e)). The patient subsequently resumed pembrolizumab therapy due to regrowth of the primary bladder lesion and the appearance of para-aortic lymph node metastasis on CT in September 2020 (Figures 1(f) and 1(g)). At the end of eight doses of pembrolizumab therapy in February 2021, the primary lesion and para-aortic lymph node metastasis were significantly reduced and had maintained (Figures 1(h) and 1(i)). In May 2021, the patient was placed a ureteral stent in the left ureter, and the left nephrostomy catheter was removed. Immune-related adverse event due to pembrolizumab therapy has not been observed.

## 3. Discussion

We experienced a patient with advanced bladder cancer without any effect of the first pembrolizumab therapy in which the primary lesion and metastatic site disappeared by rechallenge of pembrolizumab therapy after radiation therapy was applied to the primary lesion. We could not find out a urothelial cancer case report of successful response of immune checkpoint inhibitor (ICI) rechallenge after radiotherapy, following discontinuation of ICI because of its ineffectiveness. Until now, almost all patients reported with ICI rechallenge after discontinuation of ICI were the patients experienced discontinuation of ICI due to the emergence of immune-related adverse events [2].

Platinum-based chemotherapy is the preferred initial approach for systemic therapy in patients with metastatic bladder cancer and most patients with muscle-invasive bladder cancer who will undergo a radical cystectomy in neoadjuvant chemotherapy setting [1, 3]. In the present patient, GC therapy was performed for three courses but was stopped because of adverse events.

Advances in bladder cancer treatment have been unprecedented thanks to ICI immunotherapy [4]. ICI immunotherapies continue to displace previous treatment regimens as first-line and second-line therapies in bladder cancer [4, 5]. ICI immunotherapies unfortunately are not effective in all patients with advanced bladder cancer, and many patients go on to have progressive disease. Various attempts have been made to improve the therapeutic effect of ICIs. One of the modalities is the combined use of radiation therapy [6]. Radiation therapy has been shown to enhance the priming and effector phases of the antitumor T-cell response rendering it an attractive therapy to combine with PD-1/PD-L1 inhibitors; however, the sequencing, dose, fractionation, and targets for radiation therapy are still investigations. The many ongoing clinical trials on the subject will help answer many practical questions related to radiation therapy. The abscopal effect has drawn attention for the phenomenon by which systemic antitumor responses are observed outside of the primary site of local irradiation [7]. It has been described in a number of different malignancies, including metastatic renal cell carcinoma, melanoma, and hepatocellular carcinoma. In the present patient, the primary lesion regrowth and new lesions appeared after irradiation, and the tumor shrank due to retreatment with pembrolizumab, which is unlikely to be the abscopal effect. Wu et al. demonstrated that the staining of PD-L1 was significantly linked with lower completed response rates, higher loco-regional failure rate, and reduced disease-free survival and lower survival with intact bladder for patients treated with definite completed chemoradiotherapy [8]. Radiation therapy may have been responsive well to the tumor because the tumor tissue was PD-L1 negative in the present patient.

There are mechanisms of action that have the potential to turn cold tumors into so-called hot and inflamed tumors, hence increasing the tumor's responsiveness to immunotherapy-increasing local inflammation, neutralising immunosuppression at the tumor site, modifying the tumor vasculature, targeting the tumor cells themselves, or increasing the frequency of tumor-specific T cells [9]. Radiation therapy for the purpose of local tumor disease control may have led to increasing inflammation in the tumor microenvironment. The present patient resumed pembrolizumab therapy due to regrowth of the primary bladder lesion and the appearance of para-aortic lymph node metastasis and by reference to an accumulating body of evidence showing the immunomodulatory role of radiation therapy and its increased efficacy when combined with immunotherapy. It is considered that the rechallenge of pembrolizumab therapy worked effectively for shrinkage of the regrowth of bladder tumor and the para-aortic lymph node metastasis after radiotherapy in the primary lesion. In the future, it is hoped that the mechanism of action of combination therapies centered on ICIs will be elucidated, and reliable methods for enhancing the effectiveness of ICIs will be established.

## 4. Conclusion

The patients may be able to expect the positive effect on regression of the tumor for pembrolizumab rechallenge if they respond to radiation therapy to the tumor. Reliable methods for increasing the effectiveness of ICIs will expect to be established.

## References


[1] H. von der Maase, L. Sengelov, J. T. Roberts et al., "Long-term survival results of a randomized trial comparing gemcitabine plus cisplatin, with methotrexate, vinblastine, doxorubicin, plus cisplatin in patients with bladder cancer," *Journal of Clinical Oncology*, vol. 23, no. 21, pp. 4602–4608, 2005.

[2] T. Bat, D. A. Buck, R. Nathan et al., "Advanced bladder cancer rechallenged with an immune checkpoint inhibitor: a case report," *Urology*, vol. 131, pp. 24–26, 2019.

[3] H. von der Maase, S. W. Hansen, J. T. Roberts et al., "Gemcitabine and cisplatin versus methotrexate, vinblastine, doxorubicin, and cisplatin in advanced or metastatic bladder cancer: results of a large, randomized, multinational, multicenter, phase III study," *Journal of Clinical Oncology*, vol. 18, no. 17, pp. 3068–3077, 2000.

[4] J. Bellmunt, R. de Wit, D. J. Vaughn et al., "Pembrolizumab as second-line therapy for advanced urothelial carcinoma," *The New England Journal of Medicine*, vol. 376, no. 11, pp. 1015–1026, 2017.

[5] T. Powles, S. H. Park, E. Voog et al., "Avelumab maintenance therapy for advanced or metastatic urothelial carcinoma," *The New England Journal of Medicine*, vol. 383, no. 13, pp. 1218–1230, 2020.

[6] M. Daro-Faye, W. Kassouf, L. Souhami et al., "Combined radiotherapy and immunotherapy in urothelial bladder cancer: harnessing the full potential of the anti-tumor immune response," *World Journal of Urology*, vol. 39, no. 5, pp. 1331–1343, 2021.

[7] Y. Abuodeh, P. Venkat, and S. Kim, "Systematic review of case reports on the abscopal effect," *Current Problems in Cancer*, vol. 40, no. 1, pp. 25–37, 2016.

[8] C. T. Wu, W. C. Chen, Y. H. Chang, W. Y. Lin, and M. F. Chen, "The role of PD-L1 in the radiation response and clinical outcome for bladder cancer," *Scientific Reports*, vol. 6, no. 1, article 19740, 2016.

[9] M. Ochoa de Olza, B. Navarro Rodrigo, S. Zimmermann, and G. Coukos, "Turning up the heat on non-immunoreactive tumours: opportunities for clinical development," *The Lancet Oncology*, vol. 21, no. 9, pp. e419–e430, 2020.

# 54

# Advanced Renal Pelvic Carcinoma Revealed after Treatment of a Staghorn Calculus by Endoscopic Combined Intrarenal Surgery

**Ichiro Tsuboi,[1,2] Yuki Maruyama,[2,3] Motoo Araki,[2,3] Nobuyoshi Ando,[1,2] Yasuhiro Nishiyama,[1,2] Ryoji Arata,[1,2] and Noriaki Ono[1,2]**

[1]*Department of Urology, Kochi Health Sciences Center, 2125-1 Ike, Kochi city, Kochi 781-8555, Japan*
[2]*Okayama Urological Research Group (OURG), 2-5-1, Shikata-cho, Kita-ku, Okayama 700-8558, Japan*
[3]*Department of Urology, Okayama University Graduate School of Medicine, Dentistry and Pharmaceutical Sciences, 2-5-1 Shikata-cho, Kita-ku, Okayama 700-8558, Japan*

Correspondence should be addressed to Ichiro Tsuboi; ichiro.tsuboi0810@gmail.com

Academic Editor: Imran Morhason-Bello

Renal pelvis carcinoma associated with staghorn calculus is a clinically rare condition. A 66-year-old man presented with flank pain due to an 8 cm complete staghorn calculus. We performed three lithotomies using endoscopic combined intrarenal surgery and carried out intraoperative biopsy. Histopathological examinations revealed a keratinized lesion. One month later, contrast-enhanced computed tomography showed an advanced renal pelvis carcinoma. These findings demonstrate that even an intraoperative biopsy may be insufficient to diagnose a renal pelvis carcinoma associated with a staghorn calculus. The possibility of RPCa developing when treating a long-standing staghorn calculus should therefore be kept in mind.

## 1. Introduction

Renal pelvic carcinoma (RPCa) associated with a staghorn calculus is a rare clinical condition, although it is well known that chronic irritation, inflammation, and infection from a long-standing renal stone can cause a RPCa [1, 2]. RPCa with a squamous cell carcinoma is an especially rare occurrence and accounts for only 0.5 to 0.8% of malignant renal tumors [3]. The preoperative diagnosis of urothelial carcinoma in patients with a staghorn calculus remains difficult even if computed tomography (CT) and urine cytology are performed [2]. Although intraoperative biopsies and urine cytology were not enough to diagnose due to the inflammation by the stone, they give us a chance of thinking about a possibility of malignancy. To our knowledge, there are no reports of RPCa being identified quickly within one month after endoscopic combined intrarenal surgery (ECIRS). We report a case of RPCa with a staghorn calculus, which possibly was disseminated by ECIRS.

## 2. Case Presentation

A 66-year-old man had been aware of left flank pain for 6 months prior to visiting his family doctor. The doctor carried out an X-ray of the kidney, ureter, and bladder and made a diagnosis of a staghorn calculus in the left kidney (Figure 1(a)). The patient was referred to our office for further examination and treatment. His previous medical history was a urinary tract stone 20 years ago. We performed no contrast-enhanced CT of the abdominal and pelvis, which revealed an 8 cm renal stone in the left renal pelvis (Figure 2). Urine tests showed hematuria and pyuria, but no bacteriuria, while the results of blood tests were unremarkable with a serum creatinine concentration of 0.95 mg/dL. We diagnosed a staghorn calculus in the functioning left kidney and attempted to perform an ECIRS, first establishing hydronephrosis using an occlusion catheter to puncture in order to make a percutaneous trocar nephrostomy easy. However, we were unable to insert the trocar, despite the left kidney

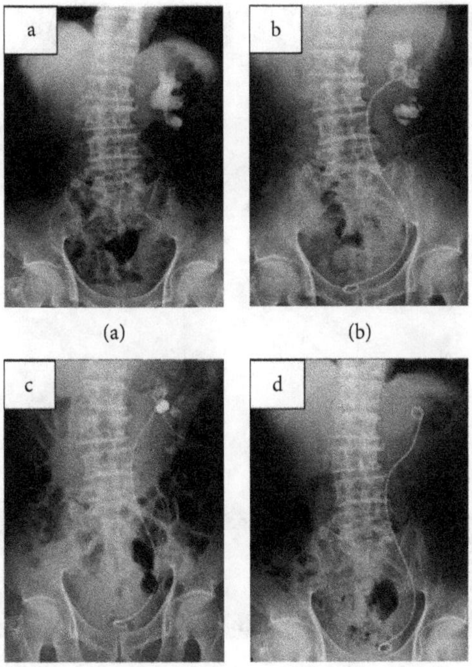


FIGURE 1: (a) A complete staghorn calculus of the left kidney (about 8 cm). (b) After the 1st ECIRS, a renal stone in the pelvis was removed. (c) After the 2nd ECIRS, most of the renal stone was removed. (d) After the last ECIRS, a stone-free state was achieved.

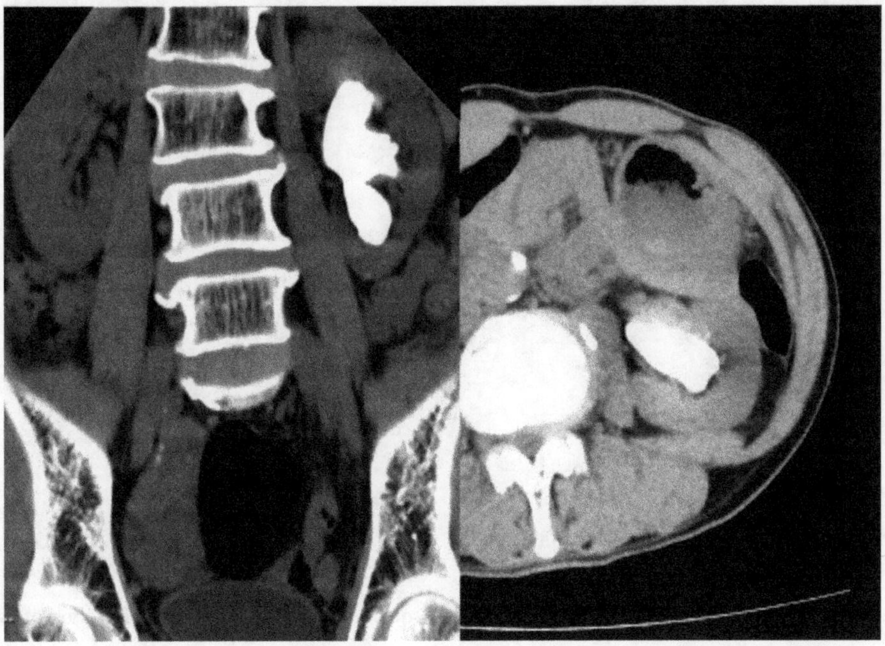

FIGURE 2: A complete staghorn calculus of the left kidney. The major diameter was about 8 cm. We could not identify the renal pelvic carcinoma retrospectively.

being punctured three times. A lithotripsy was only performed. Part of the left renal stone still existed, especially in the inferior calyx of the kidney (Figure 1(b)). Analysis showed the stone consisted of calcium phosphate. ECIRS was performed one month later, and we were able to insert the trocar at this time and carry out the procedure as planned (Figure 1(c)). Analysis of the stone showed it consisted of calcium oxalate (90%) and calcium phosphate (10%). At this time, we realized that the white fuzzy tissue was different from normal renal pelvic mucosa and therefore carried out urine cytology and a single targeted biopsy of the renal pelvic mucosa. Urine cytology identified squamous cells classified

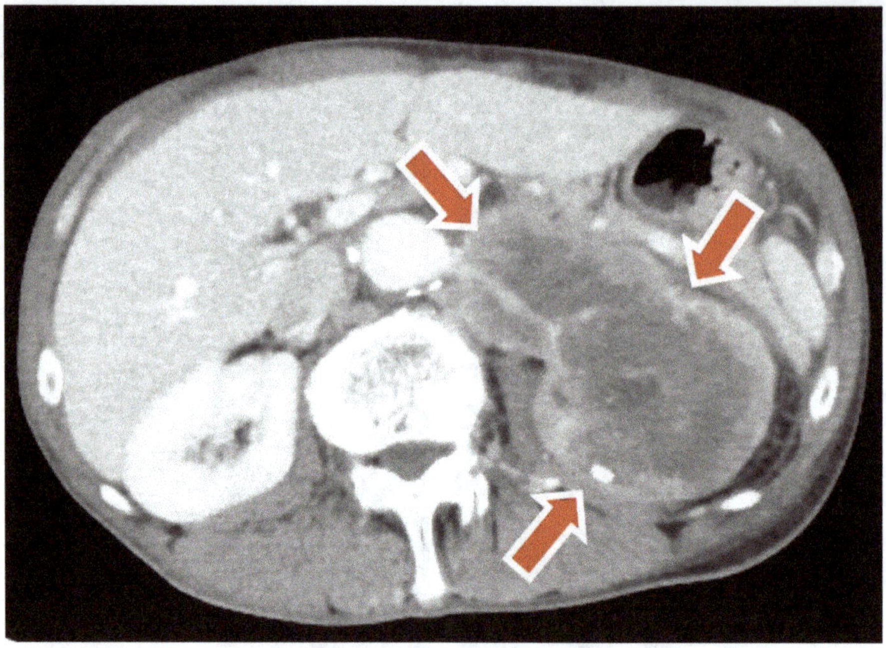

Figure 3: The renal tumor invaded the renal parenchymal and expanded about 10 cm. Lymph nodes can be seen expanded around the renal artery (red arrows). The clinical stage was classified as T4N1M0.

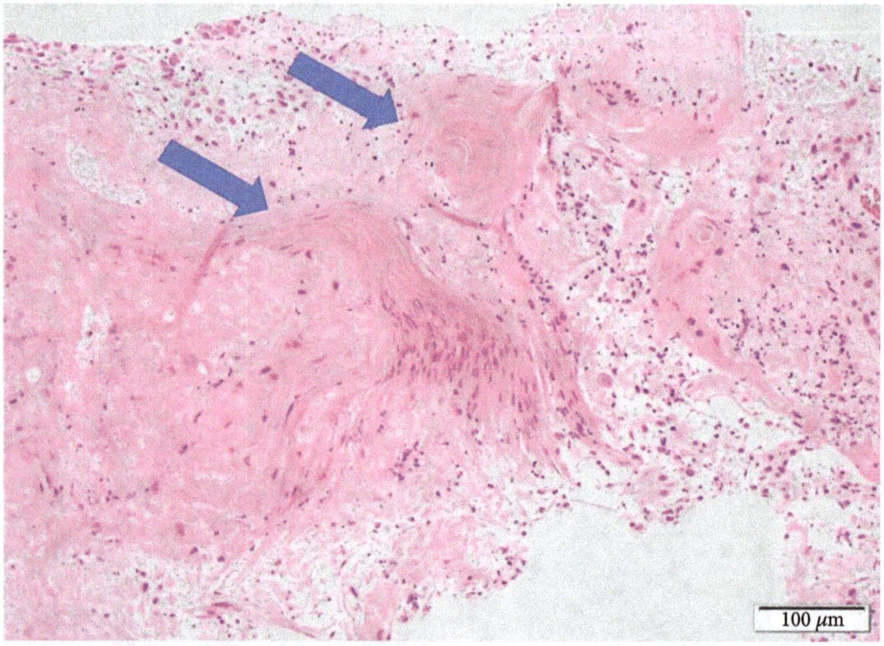


Figure 4: Urothelial carcinoma with squamous differentiation. Stratified squamous epithelium and keratinization of the lesion can be seen in some areas.

as class III. Histopathological examination showed a keratinized lesion and stratified squamous epithelium with atypical cells, although we were unable to determine whether these were malignant changes. ECIRS was performed and allowed the majority of the kidney stone to be removed (Figure 1(d)). One month after the last surgery, the patient complained of persistent left flank pain, with contrast-enhanced CT showing that almost all of the left kidney was invaded and replaced by a tumor. The tumor had expanded to around the left renal artery although there was no metastatic lesion (Figure 3). We performed a left renal biopsy because we suspected a renal cell carcinoma or RPCa. Histological examination revealed an invasive urothelial carcinoma with squamous differentiation and a clinical stage of T4N0M0 (Figure 4). We then performed two courses of neoadjuvant chemotherapy (cisplatin and gemcitabine). After

TABLE 1: Three cases of renal pelvic carcinoma with staghorn calculus, which was revealed after percutaneous nephrolithotomy.

| Authors [references] | Age | Sex | Duration after PNL | Location of spread | Histological examination | Treatment | Follow-up/ survival |
|---|---|---|---|---|---|---|---|
| Kim et al. [5] | 54 | Female | 1 mth | Nephrostomy of PCNL | SCC | Resection of the skin mass Radical nephrectomy | 12 mth/alive |
| Katz et al. [2] | 50 | Male | 2 wk | Lower pole of the kidney | UC | Radical nephrectomy Chemotherapy | 19 mth/death |
| Katz et al. [2] | 65 | Female | Inoperative | Diaphragm | UC with sarcomatoid | No | 2 mth/death |
| Tsuboi et al. [present report] | 66 | Male | 1 mth | Left kidney Para-aortic lymph node | UC with squamous differentiation | Chemotherapy | 3 mth/alive |

two courses of chemotherapy, CT showed stable disease. We judged that this chemotherapy was ineffective, and it is difficult to operate radical nephrectomy in this case. We started to administer pembrolizumab. After we performed 7 courses, CT showed progress disease. We stopped to administer pembrolizumab and started palliative treatment.

## 3. Discussion

RPCa with a staghorn calculus is a rare case and difficult to diagnose preoperatively, although intraoperative urine cytology and biopsy may indicate the possibility of a malignancy [2]. It was highly possible in our case that ECIRS disseminated the RPCa. This is the case of the advanced RPCa, which was revealed in one month after treatment of staghorn calculus by ECIRS.

A RPCa with staghorn calculus is a clinically rare case, although we, urologists, well know that a long-standing renal stone may cause malignancy because of chronic irritation, inflammation, and infection. Indeed, a retrospective study of more than 500 percutaneous nephrolithotomies (PCNL) showed three patients had RPCa that had not been diagnosed preoperatively. One patient who had a biopsy taken from suspicious looking tissue in the renal pelvis during PCNL was diagnosed with RPCa [2]. That report described difficulty diagnosing the RPCa by CT and urine cytology preoperatively. Our case showed that even intraoperative cytology and a biopsy did not confirm the diagnosis and was characterized by very early identification of the RPCa, leading us to suspect ECIRS had disseminated the tumor. Two cases of RPCa after PCNL have been reported although in these cases, PCNL had been performed 2 and 16 years earlier [4]. These cases should be distinguished from our case because we consider that there was no RPCa present when the PCNL was performed. On the other hand, Kim et al. reported a similar case of a 54-year-old woman who presented with a skin mass that surrounded the muscle tissue of the right flank. The patient had been treated for a right staghorn calculus by PCNL three months earlier. Histological examination of the skin mass showed an invasive well-differentiated squamous cell carcinoma. The PCNL had spread to surrounding tissues via the percutaneous nephrostomy track [5]. To our knowledge, there are only two similar reports (3 cases) in which RPCa appears to have been disseminated by PCNL (Table 1).

Preoperative urine cytology and CT should be performed to prevent spread of RPCa, even if there is the possibility of the false negative. In addition, we perform intraoperative urine cytology and a biopsy when we identify an abnormal renal pelvis mucosa. Because RPCa tends to be aggressive and invasive to renal tissues, it is likely a targeted and systematic renal biopsy during PCNL may contribute to an early diagnosis.

## 4. Conclusion

RPCa with a staghorn calculus is difficult to diagnose preoperatively. An intraoperative renal pelvis mucosa biopsy is not always useful to confirm the diagnosis of RPCa. The possibility of RPCa developing when treating a long-standing staghorn calculus should therefore be kept in mind.

## Abbreviations

CT: Computed tomography
ECIRS: Endoscopic combined intrarenal surgery
PCNL: Percutaneous nephrolithotomy
RPCa: Renal pelvic carcinoma.

## Authors' Contributions

All authors have read and approved the final version of the manuscript.

## References

[1] S. Holmäng, S. M. Lele, and S. L. Johansson, "Squamous cell carcinoma of the renal pelvis and ureter: incidence, symptoms, treatment and outcome," *The Journal of Urology*, vol. 178, no. 1, pp. 51–56, 2007.

[2] R. Katz, O. N. Gofrit, D. Golijanin et al., "Urothelial cancer of the renal pelvis in percutaneous nephrolithotomy patients," *Urologia Internationalis*, vol. 75, no. 1, pp. 17–20, 2005.

[3] M. K. Li and W. L. Cheung, "Squamous cell carcinoma of the renal pelvis," *The Journal of Urology*, vol. 138, no. 2, pp. 269–271, 1987.

[4] A. Jain, D. Mittal, A. Jindal et al., "Incidentally detected squamous cell carcinoma of renal pelvis in patients with staghorn calculi: case series with review of the literature," *ISRN Oncology*, vol. 2011, Article ID 620574, 6 pages, 2011.

[5] J. R. Kim, Y. B. Jeong, N. H. Lee, and S. I. Wang, "Squamous cell carcinoma of the renal pelvis presenting as an integumentary neoplasm of the flank: a case report," *Medicine*, vol. 98, no. 36, article e17049, 2019.

# 55

# Robot-Assisted Laparoscopic Adrenalectomy for Rare Myxoid Adrenocortical Carcinoma

**Grant Johnson**[1] **Kiran Thalody,**[2] **Umesh Kapur,**[3] **and Thai T. Nguyen**[4]

[1]*Franciscan Health Olympia Fields Hospital, Midwestern University, Downers Grove, IL, USA*
[2]*ROWAN SOM, Stratford, NJ, USA*
[3]*Comprehensive Pathology Services, Silvercross Hospital, New Lenox, IL, USA*
[4]*Advanced Urology Associates, Silvercross Hospital, New Lenox, IL, USA*

Correspondence should be addressed to Grant Johnson; gjohnson71@midwestern.edu

Academic Editor: David Duchene

*Background.* Surgical resection remains the standard treatment for adrenocortical carcinoma. Higher rates of local and peritoneal recurrence have been reported with the laparoscopic approach compared to open resection, although the evidence is limited. A dilemma occurs when tumors appear benign in nature, measure >5 cm, or when patients request a minimally invasive surgical approach. We describe the first reported case to date of successful robot-assisted laparoscopic adrenalectomy for myxoid variant adrenocortical carcinoma. *Case Presentation.* A 38 year old female presented with a large 8.0 cm enhancing left adrenal mass concerning for pheochromocytoma, given refractory hypertension and symptoms of palpitations and headaches. Functional work up was negative. The patient underwent robot-assisted laparoscopic left adrenalectomy after appropriate alpha and beta blockade. Histological sections demonstrated a cortical neoplasm with prominent myxoid changes consistent with myxoid adrenocortical carcinoma. The patient's symptoms resolved and serial imaging demonstrated no recurrence three and nine months, post-operatively. *Conclusion.* Myxoid adrenocortical carcinoma is a rare and aggressive entity best managed with surgical resection. Though open resection for invasive adrenal cancer remains the gold standard, minimally invasive approaches are being increasingly used, whether deliberately or not. We describe the first reported robot-assisted laparoscopic adrenalectomy for invasive myxoid adrenocortical carcinoma.

## 1. Introduction

Surgical resection remains the standard treatment for adrenocortical carcinoma (ACC). Open adrenalectomy has historically been used for large invasive tumors concerning for ACC, but laparoscopic adrenalectomy has been used for smaller lesions given potential advantages of decreased post-operative pain, shorter hospital stay, and faster recovery. Higher rates of local and peritoneal recurrence have been reported with the laparoscopic approach compared to open resection, although the evidence is limited. A dilemma occurs when tumors appear benign in nature, measure >5 cm, or when patients request a minimally invasive surgical approach. We describe the first reported case-to-date of successful robot-assisted laparoscopic adrenalectomy for myxoid variant ACC, a rare tumor of which only 42 cases have been reported worldwide.

## 2. Clinical History

A 38 year old female presented with a history of hypertension refractory to medical therapy. Given concerns for renovascular hypertension, she underwent abdominal ultrasound demonstrating a left adrenal mass. She was referred to urology for further work up and management. The patient denied any associated flank or abdominal pain, however, she did report experiencing palpitations and headaches with elevated blood pressure measurements. She denied diaphoresis, flushing, chest pressure, or visual disturbances. The patient denied any family history of Multiple Endocrine Neoplasia Syndrome (MEN) disorders, pheochromocytoma, or markedly elevated blood pressure. She had no personal history of diabetes or recent symptoms to suggest Cushing's syndrome. She denied any family history of adrenocortical carcinoma.

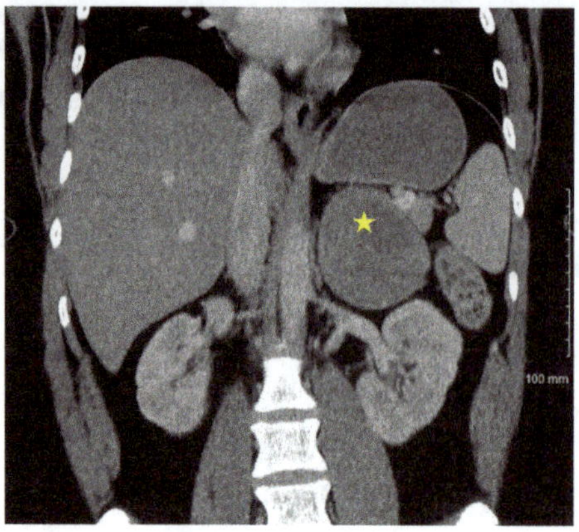


FIGURE 1: Contrast enhanced computed tomography imaging of abdomen, coronal view: left adrenal mass measuring 7.4 × 7.3 × 8.0 cm (star).

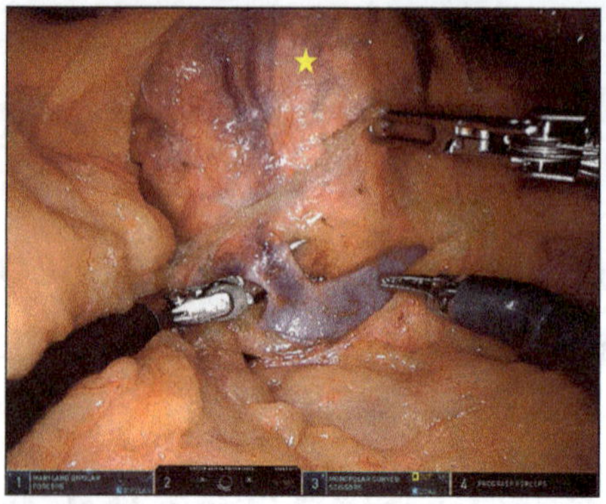

FIGURE 2: Left adrenal tumor (star) with exposed left renal and suprarenal vein during robot-assisted laparoscopic adrenalectomy.

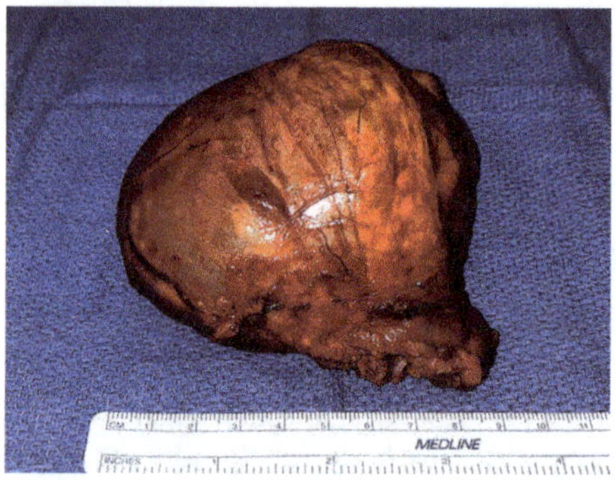


FIGURE 3: Surgically removed left adrenal tumor following robot-assisted laparoscopic adrenalectomy.

## 3. Physical Exam

She was noted to have a blood pressure of 170/100 mmHg without tachycardia. Body mass index was 36.8 kg/m$^2$. General appearance was normal without evidence of truncal obesity, moon facies, nuchal fat pad. Skin exam did not reveal violaceous striae or facial flushing. Cardiac, lung and abdominal exams were unremarkable without palpable mass or CVA tenderness. Neurologic and musculoskeletal exams were normal.

Laboratory evaluation demonstrated normal serum electrolytes, including normal serum potassium. She underwent work up for metabolic function of the adrenal lesion with normal serum catecholamines (norepinephrine 283 ng/mL, epinephrine <15 ng/mL, dopamine <30 ng/mL) and normal 24 urine collection for free serum cortisol (10.9 mcg/24 hr, 24 urine volume 1675 mL).

Imaging work up was performed including computed tomography (CT) scan with intravenous contrast revealing a large enhancing left adrenal mass measuring 7.4 × 7.3 × 8.0 cm with no washout on delayed imaging (Figure 1). Magnetic resonance imaging (MRI) of the abdomen with and without contrast, using Gadolinium (Gabobutrol) demonstrated a 7.4 × 7.4 × 8.0 cm heterogeneously T2 hyperintense and heterogeneously enhancing LEFT adrenal mass, highly suspicious for pheochromocytoma.

## 4. Diagnosis

Left adrenal mass measuring 8.0 cm in greatest dimension, suspected pheochromocytoma based on MRI characteristics, with negative functional work up. No biopsy was performed given underlying concern for pheochromocytoma.

## 5. Intervention

The patient underwent robot-assisted laparoscopic left adrenalectomy (Figures 2 and 3) after appropriate alpha blockade with phenoxybenzamine and beta blockade with propranolol. Three 8 mm robotic laparoscopic ports and one 12 mm assistant port were used, two along the midline and two in the left lower quadrant. A "T-incision" was made in the posterior peritoneum allowing inferomedial reflection of the splenic flexure. The adrenal vein was identified early, ligated with polymer locking clips then divided, after which the body was dissected away from the adrenal gland. The plane of dissection was taken outside of Gerota's fascia on all aspects except in the plane adjacent to the kidney, where perinephric fat was resected *en bloc* with the adrenal mass to ensure complete resection. As is our standard practice with all extirpative surgeries, the specimen was extracted intact using an impermeable laparoscopic bag through an extended port-site. The adrenal tumor measured 9.0 × 8.0 × 7.5 cm (260 grams). Histological sections showed a cortical neoplasm with prominent myxoid changes (Figure 4). Rare mitotic activity was identified (1/50 high-power field). No cytologic atypia or atypical mitoses were seen. Capsular invasion was present (entire capsule submitted for histological examination). Histologic diagnosis was reviewed and confirmed by an expert adrenal pathologist at a tertiary cancer center with experience in tumors of the endocrine systems.

## 6. Follow Up and Outcomes

Post-operatively, the patient developed dyspnea attributed to phenoxybenzamine and propranolol, and for which work up for myocardial and thrombotic causes were negative. She was

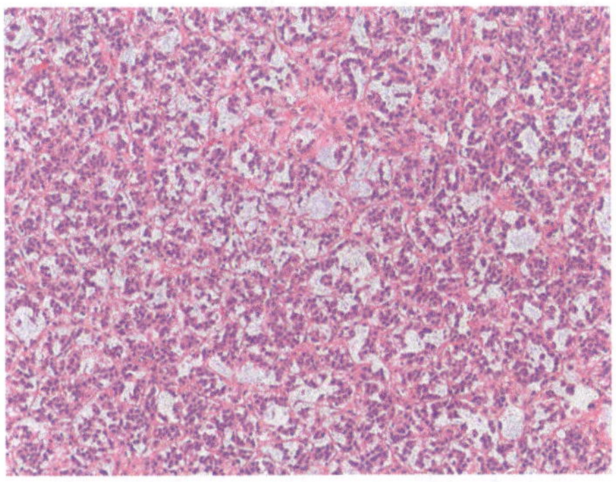

FIGURE 4: Adrenocortical carcinoma with myxoid background (H&E section, 100x).

weaned off her antihypertensive medications, and the dyspnea resolved. At one month follow up, her hypertension was resolved and she no longer required antihypertensive therapy. There was no evidence of recurrence on three and nine-month post-operative contrast enhanced CT imaging.

## 7. Discussion

Adrenocortical carcinoma is a rare malignancy of the adrenal cortex with an incidence of 0.7–2 cases per million per year [1]. Variants of ACC that have been identified to date include myxoid, sarcomatoid and oncocytic subtypes. At the time of this report, a PubMed search revealed that only 42 cases of myxoid adrenocortical carcinoma have been reported in the English literature [2]. Myxoid ACC is usually diagnosed in the fifth decade of life. While conventional adrenocortical carcinoma affects females more commonly than males, the myxoid variant has been found with an equal distribution among men and women.

To determine the functional status of a suspicious adrenal mass, laboratory screening is performed including basal cortisol, testosterone, estradiol, androstenedione, 17-hydroxyprogesterone, adrenocorticotropic hormone (ACTH), and urinary free cortisol level. Confirmatory testing can be performed as needed. Aldosterone and renin levels are recommended in patients with hypertension and/or hypokalemia. Our patient with myxoid ACC did not have any evidence of endocrine function on initial functional testing, however her presenting symptoms and the tumor characteristics on magnetic resonance imaging were concerning for pheochromocytoma. A biopsy was therefore not performed for fear of triggering a catecholamine crisis.

Myxoid ACC has a prognosis reported to be either similar or worse than that of conventional ACC. In one case review involving follow up of four patients with myxoid ACC, all four patients had a disease specific mortality between 11 and 69 months [3]. The Weiss scoring classification and Ki-67 classification system have been used to assist in determining ACC malignant potential and ACC prognostic value, respectively. However, myxoid variants of adrenocortical tumors are frequently malignant even in absence of mitotic activity and necrosis. In a recent report, 7 out of 14 patients with myxoid ACC died of disease even when these tumors were small and had few mitotic figures [4]. Therefore, the usual histologic criteria such as Weiss and New Helsinki cannot be used to reliably classify these tumors.

Because of the rarity of myxoid ACC there are no clear management recommendations. Treatment of conventional ACC is based on nonrandomized trials or retrospective cohort studies. Surgical resection is the only curative treatment for ACC, although the incidence of postoperative recurrence is high even in nonmetastatic disease, which is postulated to be caused by micrometastases at the time of surgery. Some retrospective studies have shown increased recurrence rates, faster time to recurrence and higher incidence of positive margins with laparoscopic adrenalectomy [2]. Robot-assisted technology for laparoscopic adrenalectomy has been used for both benign and incidentally malignant adrenal tumors for several years, however at the time of this manuscript, there has been no reported robot-assisted laparoscopic adrenalectomy for myxoid adrenocortical carcinoma in the literature to date. If a laparoscopic approach is used for large tumors and difficult dissection is encountered with concern for invasive tumor, a low threshold for conversion to open adrenalectomy should be maintained. Regardless of approach, wide resection is recommended to improve local recurrence rates. The preference of open over laparoscopic resection for large adrenal masses, in our opinion, is based on a relative paucity of data regarding laparoscopic efficacy rather than definitive evidence of inferiority of the laparoscopic approach. There have been significant advancements in laparoscopic instrumentation, techniques and surgeon experience since the early reports of laparoscopic adrenalectomy. The robotic approach provides increased dexterity than traditional pure laparoscopic adrenalectomy, albeit with a trade-off of losing haptic feedback. We ultimately decided, that the robotic approach was a feasible and safe technique in achieving oncologic success while conferring the potential benefits in post-surgical recovery.

Due to the high rates of recurrence, adjuvant chemotherapy in the form of mitotane can be considered, however the current data is limited to retrospective studies in higher risk patients. It is unclear if adjuvant mitotane therapy is beneficial in low to intermediate risk patients. The ADIUVO trial, with planned completion date in 2020, hopes to answer this question.

In general, post-operative management for conventional ACC includes surveillance CT imaging every three months for the first two years. Imaging intervals can be extended after two years and follow up is recommended for a minimum of ten years post resection [3]. If pre-operative functional studies were positive, then these should be monitored, post operatively. No specific follow up recommendations exist for myxoid ACC.

## 8. Conclusion

Myxoid adrenocortical carcinoma is a rare and aggressive entity managed with surgical resection. Though open resection for invasive adrenal cancer remains the gold standard according to most surgical associations, minimally invasive approaches are being increasingly used, whether deliberately or not [5]. We describe the first reported robot-assisted laparoscopic adrenalectomy for invasive myxoid adrenal cortical carcinoma. With further advancement in laparoscopic technology, we will likely see similar cases in the future, hopefully with excellent oncological outcomes. Regardless of approach, sound surgical principles, including wide resection and low threshold for open conversion due to difficult dissection or concern for malignancy, must be followed to ensure superior clinical outcomes for all patients.

## Abbreviation

ACC: Adrenocortical carcinoma.

## Acknowledgments

We would like to thank the University of Wisconsin Pathology Department for review and confirmation of histological diagnosis.

## References

[1] T. M. Kerkhofs, R. H. Verhoeven, J. M. Van der Zwan et al., "Adrenocortical carcinoma: a population-based study on incidence and survival in the Netherlands since 1993," *European Journal of Cancer*, vol. 49, no. 11, pp. 2579–2586, 2013.

[2] B. S. Miller, J. B. Ammori, P. G. Gauger, J. T. Broome, G. D. Hammer, and G. M. Doherty, "Laparoscopic resection is inappropriate in patients with known or suspected adrenocortical carcinoma," *World Journal of Surgery*, vol. 34, no. 6, pp. 1380–1385, 2010.

[3] A. Weissferdt, A. Phan, S. Suster, and C. A. Moran, "Myxoid adrenocortical carcinoma a clinicopathologic and immunohistochemical study of 7 cases, including 1 case with lipomatous metaplasia," *American Journal of Clinical Pathology*, vol. 139, no. 6, pp. 780–786, 2013.

[4] M. Papotti, M. Volante, E. Duregon et al., "Adrenocortical tumors with myxoid features: a distinct morphologic and phenotypical variant exhibiting malignant behavior," *The American Journal of Surgical Pathology*, vol. 34, no. 7, pp. 973–983, 2010.

[5] M. W. Ball, A. K. Hemal, and M. E. Allaf, "International consultation of urological disease and european association of urology international consultation on minimally invasive surgery in urology: laparoscopic and robotic adrenalectomy," *BJU International*, vol. 119, pp. 13–21, 2017.

# Nivolumab and Ipilimumab Combination Immunotherapy for Patients with Metastatic Collecting Duct Carcinoma

**Tetsuya Danno,[1] Shohei Iwata,[1] Fusako Niimi,[1] Sachi Honda,[1] Haruka Okada,[2] and Takeshi Azuma[1]**

[1]*Department of Urology, Tokyo Metropolitan Tama Medical Center, 2-8-29 Musashidai, Fuchu, Tokyo 183-0042, Japan*
[2]*Department of Pathology, Tokyo Metropolitan Tama Medical Center, 2-8-29 Musashidai, Fuchu, Tokyo 183-0042, Japan*

Correspondence should be addressed to Takeshi Azuma; tazuma-tky@umin.ac.jp

Academic Editor: Fumitaka Koga

Collecting duct carcinoma (CDC) is a rare, extremely aggressive form of renal cancer. Recently, immune checkpoint inhibitors (ICI), anti-programmed death-1 (PD-1) antibody, and anti-cytotoxic T lymphocyte-associated antigen 4 (CTLA-4) antibody were approved for use against metastatic renal cell carcinoma. We herein described two cases of metastatic renal collecting duct carcinoma treated with a combination immunotherapy consisting of nivolumab and ipilimumab. In the first case, which included a bone metastasis, the best response achieved was stable disease (SD) for one year. In the second case, which was accompanied by a lung metastasis, the best response achieved was a partial response. The outcome of these cases suggested that the combination of nivolumab and ipilimumab is effective against renal collecting duct carcinoma.

## 1. Introduction

Collecting duct carcinoma (CDC) is a rare form of renal cancer constituting fewer than 1% of renal cell carcinoma cases. CDC is extremely aggressive, with 40% of patients presenting a metastasis at the initial diagnosis. Because an effective, systemic therapy for metastatic CDC has not yet been established, the prognosis is poorer than that of clear cell carcinoma [1].

Azuma et al. published a prospective study of systemic therapy for CDC using a cisplatin-based regimen. However, the clinical benefits were limited, and the median survival time was less than 12 months. Targeted therapies have also had limited effect [1].

Recently, immune checkpoint inhibitors (ICI), anti-programmed death-1 (PD-1) antibody, and anti-cytotoxic T lymphocyte-associated antigen 4 (CTLA-4) antibody were approved as treatments for metastatic renal cell carcinoma (RCC). PD-1 and programmed death-1 ligand-1 (PD-L1) are expressed on T cells and cancer cells, respectively. Their interaction sends an inhibitory signal to T cells via PD-1 [2]. Cytotoxic T lymphocyte-associated antigen 4 (CTLA-4) is also expressed on CTLs and delivers an inhibitory signal to CTLs [3]. Using anti-PD-1 antibody or anti-CTLA-4 antibodies to block the interaction with their ligands can activate T cells against cancer cells.

Immunotherapy combining the anti-PD-1 and CTLA-4 antibodies has also been approved for the treatment of metastatic RCC. The anti-PD-1/anti-CTLA-4 antibody combination immunotherapy was more effective than anti-PD-1 antibody monotherapy. However, the efficacy of immunotherapies using ICI against CDC is unclear. We herein reported two cases which demonstrated the efficacy of the anti-PD-1/anti-CTLA-4 antibody combination immunotherapy against metastatic CDC.

## 2. Case Report

*2.1. Case 1.* A 75-year-old female patient with a left renal mass and bone metastases was referred to our institution. A biopsy of the left renal mass was performed, and pathological analysis revealed collecting duct carcinoma (CDC) (PAX8+,

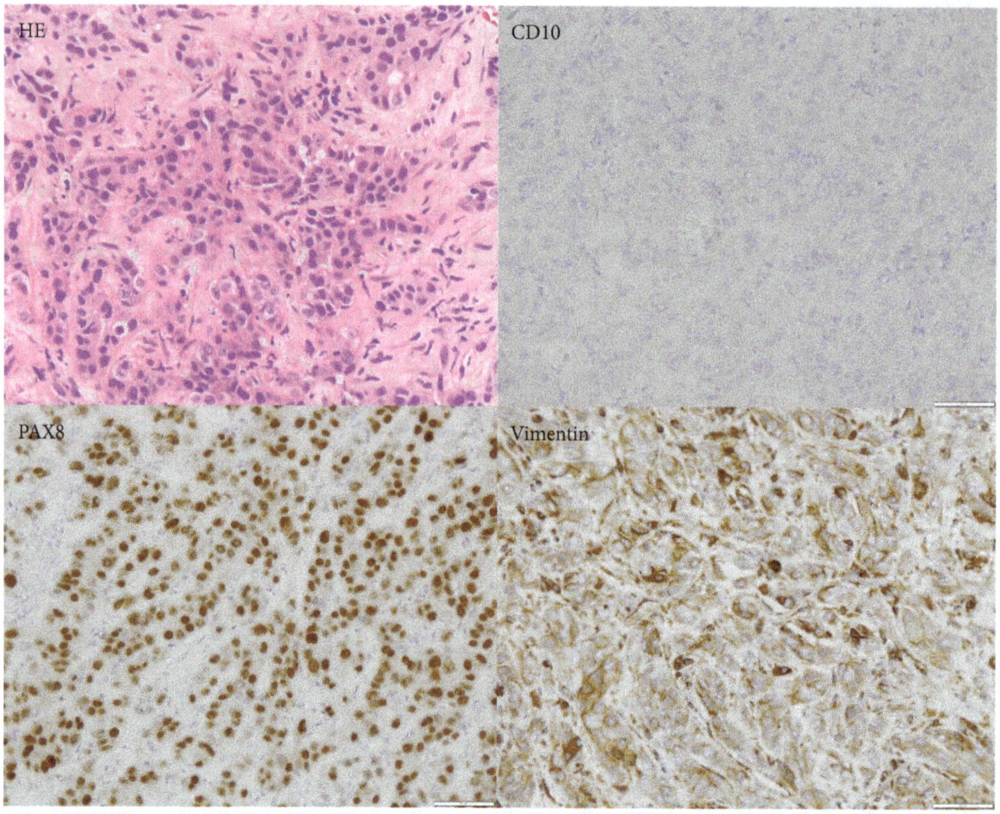


FIGURE 1: Hematoxylin and eosin staining and immunohistochemical staining of tissue from the renal biopsy in Case 1 (×400).

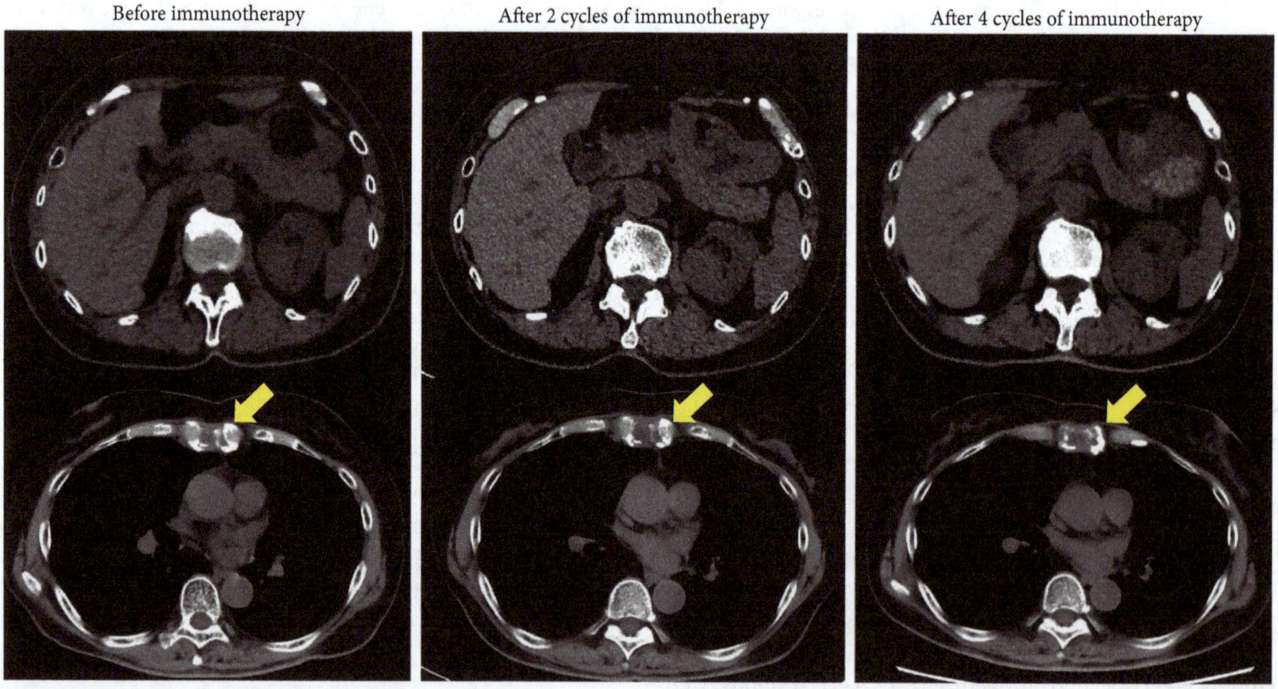


FIGURE 2: Computed tomography (CT) findings in Case 1. Abdominal CT showed no change in the right primary renal tumor or bone metastasis after four cycles of immunotherapy.

Vimentin+, and CD10-) (Figure 1) [4]. Based on the International Metastatic Renal Cell Carcinoma Database Consortium (IMDC) risk score, the prognostic risk was determined to be intermediate (<1 year since the diagnosis). Nivolumab and ipilimumab were administered four times every three weeks; then, nivolumab monotherapy was administered every two

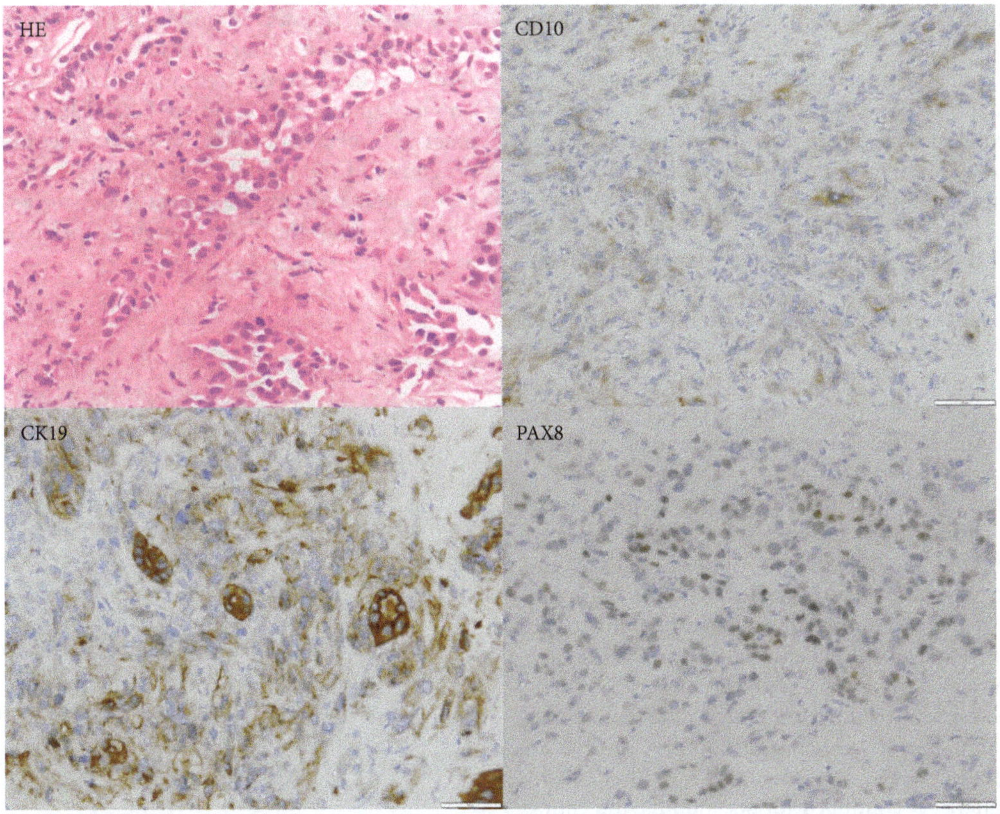


FIGURE 3: Hematoxylin and eosin staining and immunohistochemical staining of tissue from the renal biopsy in Case 2 (×400).

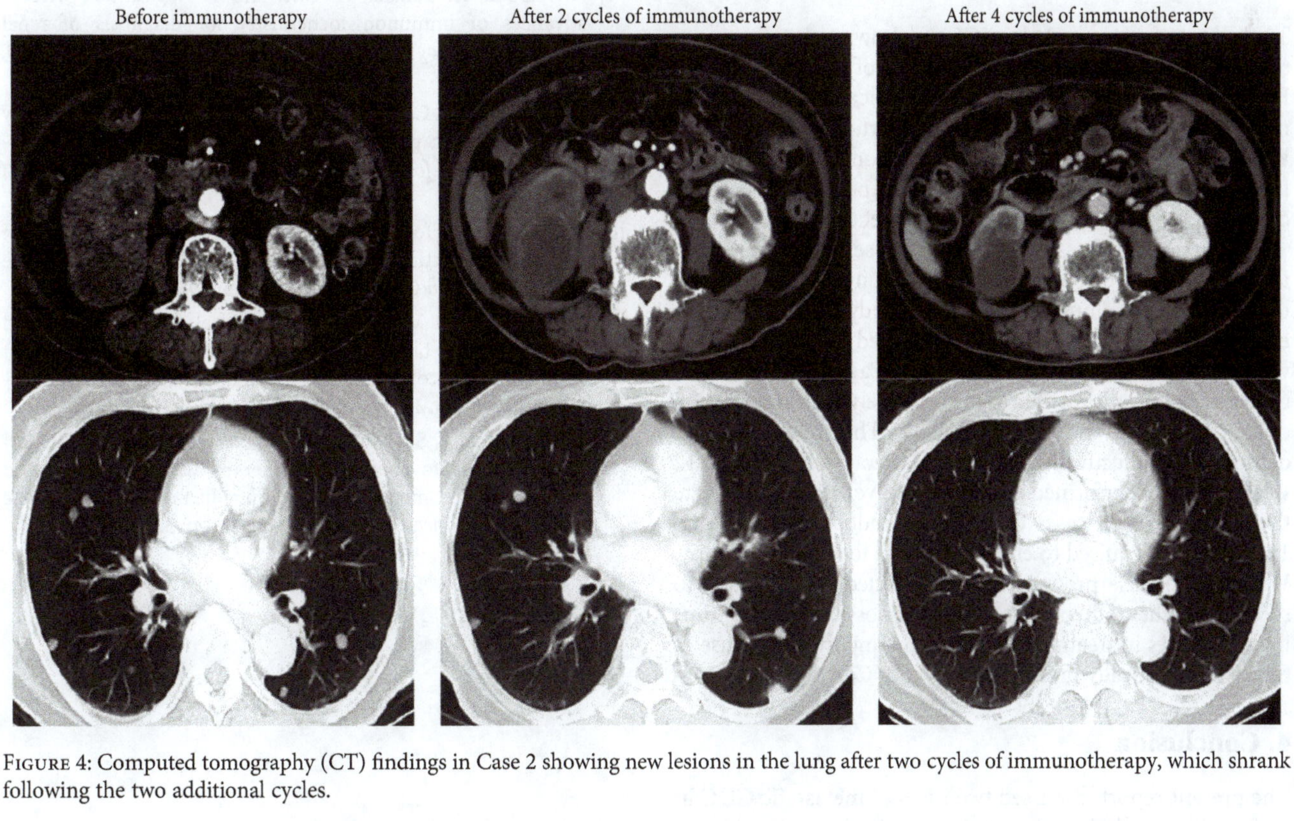


FIGURE 4: Computed tomography (CT) findings in Case 2 showing new lesions in the lung after two cycles of immunotherapy, which shrank following the two additional cycles.

weeks for maintenance. After completion of two cycles of the combination immunotherapy, computed tomography (CT) revealed a slight enlargement of the primary tumor and bone metastases but showed no change during the two additional cycles of the combination therapy or the nivolumab monotherapy (Figure 2). The best response achieved was stable disease (SD) lasting 23 months.

*2.2. Case 2.* A 79-year-old female patient had a right renal tumor and multiple metastases to the lungs and lymph nodes. Pathological analysis of a biopsy specimen of the right renal mass revealed CDC (CK19+, PAX8+, and CD10-) (Figure 3) [4]. Based on the International Metastatic Renal Cell Carcinoma Database Consortium (IMDC) risk score, her risk level was determined to be poor (neutrophilia, anemia, and duration < 1 year after diagnosis). Combination immunotherapy with nivolumab and ipilimumab was administered, and after two cycles, computed tomography (CT) revealed new bilateral lung lesions. After two additional cycles, all the tumors shrank markedly (Figure 4). However, the immunotherapy was unable to be continued due to rheumatoid arthritis development, an adverse event associated with the therapy. The best response achieved was a partial response (PR). The patient was followed up without treatment after four cycles of the combination therapy. After eight months, nivolumab was resumed because the lung metastases showed slight growth. Thereafter, SD continued for six months, indicating that the immunotherapy was able to suppress progression for 17 months.

## 3. Discussion

To the best of our knowledge, ICI was shown to be effective in treating five, previously reported cases of metastatic CDC. Four previous reports described the efficacy of nivolumab monotherapy, and only one study reported using the anti-PD-1 and CTLA-4 antibody combination immunotherapy [5–8]. The present study is the second report of the use of a combination immunotherapy against metastatic CDC.

In previous studies, two of five CDC cases were recurrences following a nephrectomy; one patient required a nephrectomy to reduce tumor volume. In the present study, the combination immunotherapy was promptly performed in both patients without performing a nephrectomy. In Case 2, there was no time for a nephrectomy due to the extremely swift progression of the cancer from the time of diagnosis. The previous reports demonstrated effectiveness of immunotherapy after four to 12 weeks. CT was performed every four to five weeks to evaluate the response. Both cases developed pseudoprogression, and 12 weeks was required to elicit a response to immunotherapy. Whenever disease progression was detected, we switched to second line chemotherapy as quickly as possible. Correct timing of changes in treatment is extremely important because of the characteristically rapid progression of CDC.

## 4. Conclusion

The present report discussed two cases of metastatic CDC in which PR and relatively long SD, respectively, were achieved by administering a combination of nivolumab and ipilimumab. To the best of our knowledge, the present report is the second to describe the treatment of CDC using a combination immunotherapy regimen. Establishing a standard treatment for metastatic CDC is crucial because of the poor prognosis of the disease. The findings of our study suggest that combination immunotherapy may be an effective treatment for metastatic CDC though further research is needed to verify the results.

## Consent

The patients provided written informed consent for the use of the details of their case in this case report.

## References

[1] T. Azuma, S. Yao, G. Zhu, A. S. Flies, S. J. Flies, and L. Chen, “B7-H1 is a ubiquitous antiapoptotic receptor on cancer cells,” *Blood*, vol. 111, no. 7, pp. 3635–3643, 2008.

[2] S. Dason, C. Allard, A. Sheridan-Jonah et al., “Management of renal collecting duct carcinoma: a systematic review and the Mcmaster experience,” *Current Oncology*, vol. 20, no. 3, pp. e223–e232, 2013.

[3] F. S. Hodi, S. J. O'Day, D. F. McDermott et al., “Improved survival with ipilimumab in patients with metastatic melanoma,” *New England Journal of Medicine*, vol. 363, no. 8, pp. 711–723, 2010.

[4] N. Kuroda, A. Tanaka, C. Ohe, and Y. Nagashima, “Recent advances of immunohistochemistry for diagnosis of renal tumors,” *Pathology International*, vol. 63, no. 8, pp. 381–390, 2013.

[5] V. S. Koshkin, P. C. Barata, T. Zhang et al.et al., “Clinical activity of nivolumab in patients with non-clear cell renal cell carcinoma,” *Journal for ImmunoTherapy of Cancer*, vol. 6, no. 1, 2018.

[6] K. Mizutani, K. Horie, S. Nagai et al., “Response to nivolumab in metastatic collecting duct carcinoma expressing Pd-L1: a case report,” *Mol Clin Oncol*, vol. 7, no. 6, pp. 988–990, 2017.

[7] K. J. Rimar, J. J. Meeks, and T. M. Kuzel, “Anti-programmed death receptor 1 blockade induces clinical response in a patient with metastatic collecting duct carcinoma,” *Clinical Genitourinary Cancer*, vol. 14, no. 4, pp. e431–e434, 2016.

[8] K. Watanabe, T. Sugiyama, A. Otsuka, and H. Miyake, “Complete response to combination therapy with nivolumab and ipilimumab for metastatic collecting duct carcinoma of the kidney,” *Int Cancer Conf J*, vol. 9, no. 1, pp. 32–35, 2020.

# SARS-CoV-2 Infection as a Determining Factor to the Precipitation of Ischemic Priapism in a Young Patient with Asymptomatic COVID-19

**Antonio Francesco Maria Giuliano,[1] Marco Vulpi,[2] Francesca Passerini,[1] Antonio Vavallo,[2] Anna Belfiore,[1] Saverio Forte,[2] Vincenzo Ostilio Palmieri,[1] and Pasquale Ditonno[2]**

[1]*Department of Biomedical Sciences and Human Oncology, Clinica Medica "A. Murri", Università degli Studi di Bari Aldo Moro Facoltà di Medicina e Chirurgia, Piazza Giulio Cesare n°11, 70124 Bari, Bari, Italy*
[2]*Department of Emergency and Organ Transplantation, Urology and Andrology Unit II, Università degli Studi di Bari Aldo Moro Facoltà di Medicina e Chirurgia, Piazza Giulio Cesare n°11, 70124 Bari, Bari, Italy*

Correspondence should be addressed to Antonio Francesco Maria Giuliano; drgiuliano.a@gmail.com

Academic Editor: Fumitaka Koga

COVID-19 is a disease characterized by respiratory distress, systemic inflammation, multiple organ dysfunction and coagulation disorders, chiefly pulmonary embolism, and deep venous thrombosis. In this case report, we discuss a peculiar case of ischemic priapism in a 36-year-old patient with asymptomatic COVID-19 and no other plausible causes of thrombophilia and/or alternative causes of priapism, as well as discussing possible explanations for such remarkable findings and comparing them to analogous cases recorded in literature. The patient was unsuccessfully treated via cavernous blood aspiration and required several shunting procedures, with no further recurrences and negative testing for pulmonary embolism, deep venous thrombosis, and other causes of thrombophilia.

## 1. Introduction

The current SARS-CoV-2 pandemic constitutes one of the most intense challenges faced by medicine in contemporary times. This novel coronavirus infection causes a unique form of disease (COVID-19) characterized by respiratory distress, systemic inflammation with multiple organ dysfunction, pulmonary embolism, and deep venous thrombosis [1]. Priapism is defined as a prolonged penile erection originating without any concurrent sexual stimulation, persisting for more than 4 hours and despite orgasm [2]. Conventionally, priapism is classified as ischemic, nonischemic, and stuttering, according to the underlying vascular lesions and clinical presentation: ischemic priapism is considered a medical emergency due to potentially irreparable damage leading to erectile dysfunction with fibrosis of the corpora cavernosa.

In this paper, we present an atypical case of priapism occurring in a patient with asymptomatic SARS-CoV-2 infection, whose peculiarities might offer further clarification of the possible role of SARS-CoV-2-induced systemic inflammation and hypercoagulability in the onset of this urologic emergency.

## 2. Case Presentation

A 34-year-old man was admitted to our unit complaining a 36-hour history of painful erection without sexual stimulation; one month prior to admission, the patient tested positive for SARS-CoV-2 infection via nasopharyngeal swab and had since been completely asymptomatic, save for persistent anosmia. The patient denied any history of pharmacological treatment or substance abuse and further questioning revealed no known risk factors for priapism; vital signs at admission were

TABLE 1: Key laboratory tests at admission. MCV: mean cellular volume; ESR: erythrocyte sedimentation rate; CRP: C-reactive protein; n/a: not applicable.

| | Patient | Laboratory standard |
|---|---|---|
| Erythrocytes ($\times 10^6/\mu L$) | 3.07 | 4.54-5.78 |
| Leukocytes ($\times 10^3/\mu L$) | 8.61 | 3.7-9.7 |
| Hemoglobin (g/dL) | 9.3 | 13.3-17.2 |
| Hematocrit (%) | 26.9 | 38.9-50.9 |
| MCV (fl) | 87.4 | 81.2-94 |
| Neutrophils (%) | 68.9 | 42.9-78.4 |
| Eosinophiles (%) | 4 | 0.3-6.2 |
| Basophiles (%) | 0.5 | 0.3-1.3 |
| Lymphocytes (%) | 20.9 | 14.1-45.8 |
| Monocytes (%) | 5.7 | 3.3-9.2 |
| Platelets ($\times 10^3/\mu L$) | 363 | 179-373 |
| Urea (mg/dL) | 28 | 15-38 |
| Bilirubin (mg/dL) | 0.32 | 0.2-1 |
| Glucose (mg/dL) | 95 | <100 |
| Glycated hemoglobin (mmol/mol) | 36 | 20-42 |
| Prothrombin time (INR) | 1.01 | n/a |
| Fibrinogen (mg/dL) | 429 | 200-400 |
| Activated partial thromboplastin time (ratio) | 0.89 | <1.20 |
| D-dimers ($\mu g/L$) | 5855 | <500 |
| Homocysteine (mmol/L) | 21.7 | 3.2-10.7 |
| Antithrombin III (%) | 116 | 80-130 |
| ESR (mm/h) | 69 | 1-15 |
| CRP (mg/L) | 37.5 | <2.9 |
| Presepsin (pg/mL) | 351 | 20-200 |
| IL-6 ($\mu g/L$) | 76.4 | 0-7 |
| Procalcitonin (ng/mL) | 1.19 | 0-0.05 |

TABLE 2: Arterial and penile blood gas analysis. n/a: not applicable.

| | Arterial blood gas | Cavernosal blood gas | Laboratory standard |
|---|---|---|---|
| pH | 7.51 | 7.47 | 7.35-7.45 |
| $pCO_2$ (mmHg) | 35 | 33 | 35-45 |
| $pO_2$ (mmHg) | 83 | 65 | 80-100 |
| $Na^+$ (mmol/L) | 135 | 139 | 135-150 |
| $K^+$ (mmol/L) | 3.1 | 2.7 | 3.4-5.0 |
| $Cl^-$ (mmol/L) | 103 | 111 | 98-107 |
| $Ca^{2+}$ (mmol/L) | 1.12 | 1.03 | 1.15-1.27 |
| Glucose (mg/dL) | 108 | 95 | 74-106 |
| Lactates (mmol/L) | 0.8 | 1.2 | 0.4-2.0 |
| P/F | 395 | 309 | >400 |
| $HCO_3^-$ (mmol/L) | 28.6 | 25.2 | 22-28 |
| Oxygen saturation (%) | 98.7 | 94.8 | >94% |
| $FiO_2$ (%) | 21 | 21 | n/a |

acceptable (BP: 165/85 mmHg, HR: 78 bpm, and body temperature 37°C). Low flow priapism was confirmed when cavernosal blood gas analysis showed hypoxia, hypercapnia, and acidosis. Two penile blood aspiration and intracavernous phenylephrine injection (diluted in normal saline to a concentration of 100–500 $\mu$g/mL and 1 mL given every 3–5 minutes, up to a maximum dosage of 1 mg) attempts proved unsuccessful, and a 14-G needle spongio-cavernosal shunt failed. Therefore, a bilateral T-shunt procedure was performed using a size 10 blade scalpel placed vertically through the glans until fully within the corpus cavernosum. The corpora-glandular shunt was completed by the retrograde insertion of a size 7 Hegar dilator into the distal end of each corpus cavernosum through the original glandular incision and blood evacuation by manual compression of the penis sequentially from a proximal to distal direction. The patient never required supplemental oxygen for the entirety of his hospital stay. A contrast-enhanced chest and pelvis CT scan and a lower extremity venous Doppler study were performed, with no signs of parenchymal involvement or pulmonary embolism nor any evidence of deep venous thrombosis, respectively. Further testing for other plausible causes of thrombophilia (such as factor V Leiden, antithrombin III deficiency, sickle-cell disease, hyperhomocysteinemia, and lupus anticoagulant) or alternative causes of priapism returned negative results. Penile tumescence gradually resolved during the next two days, and the patient was discharged on post-op day six, following complete remission of symptoms and with no need for anticoagulation.

At three-month follow-up, the patient reported complete erectile dysfunction with no further relapses of priapism; phosphodiesterase type 5 inhibitors were not prescribed since the patient underwent a shunting procedure. An inflatable penile implant was suggested but the patient asked to wait for some spontaneous improvement before undergoing surgery.

Key laboratory testing and blood gas analysis results are reported in Tables 1 and 2, respectively.

## 3. Discussion

Ischemic priapism is the most common form of this disease's presentation, a consequence of an obstruction of the penile venous outflow leading to a stasis of hypoxic blood within the corpus cavernosum akin to a proper compartment syndrome. In our patient, the clinical presentation with painful rigid erection, presence of dark, clotted blood at cavernosal blood aspiration, and blood gas analysis findings strongly supported ischemia-related priapism. SARS-CoV-2 infection has been associated to a unique set of coagulation changes collectively referred to as COVID-19-associated coagulopathy [3]: while the virus itself appears to have no intrinsic procoagulant activity, it has been hypothesized that a diffuse microangiopathy can be mediated via endothelial ACE2 receptors, disrupting natural antithrombotic pathways. A number of cytokines involved in the etiopathogenesis of COVID-19 have a well-known role in both inflammation and thrombosis: IL-6 in particular is linked to multiple such procoagulant pathways, purportedly through tissue factor expression on mononuclear cells [4]. Furthermore, available data heavily stresses IL-6's crucial role in COVID-19 pathophysiology [5] as well as in murine models investigating ischemic priapism [6].

Comparison with other literature reported cases of priapism in SARS-CoV-2-affected patients revealed several key differences: our patient's age and asymptomatic COVID-19 with an absence of known comorbidities seem to starkly contrast with the clinical profile noted in the three available reports, namely, older age, severe COVID-19, and admission to an Intensive Care Unit [7]. Notably, administration of anesthetics such as propofol and patient's exitus was recorded in two cases [8, 9]: previous case reports [10] suggest that propofol can cause ischemic priapism, with the work of Vesta et al. [11] confirming a strong association of propofol to priapism with rechallenge. In all three cases, priapism was managed conservatively or by intracavernosal injection of the sympathomimetic agents. Similarities between the reports however seem to corroborate the hypothesis of SARS-CoV-2 playing a role in promoting penile thrombosis regardless of COVID-19 severity and the onset of cytokine storms, both due to endothelial damage and through the prothrombotic action of cytokines, chiefly IL-6.

Our case, to our knowledge, represents the first report of priapism in mild COVID-19 without necessity of intubation and mechanical ventilation, managed by T-shunt procedure with potential permanent erectile dysfunction.

## 4. Conclusion

All data considered, priapism could represent a very rare yet plausible complication in the context of SARS-CoV-2 infection, regardless of symptoms, disease severity, patient's age, and concurrent risk factors. In particular, the role of a multidisciplinary evaluation involving emergency medicine, internal medicine, and urology specialists appears pivotal in ensuring swift detection and prompt, aggressive management of such an occurrence, since this condition is not commonly seen in clinical practice and may go unrecognized with potentially irreversible consequences. ACE2-induced microangiopathy and cytokine-activated thrombosis, especially IL-6-mediated, might be crucial in fully understanding the link between COVID-19 and thrombotic events, as well as potentially offering novel diagnostic and therapeutic approaches on the matter. Further data is auspicial in order to provide a clearer insight.

## Consent

Written informed consent was obtained from the patient, in accordance with the Declaration of Helsinki.

## Authors' Contributions

Writing—original draft was done by Dr. Antonio Francesco Maria Giuliano and Dr. Antonio Vavallo. Writing—review and editing was done by Dr. Marco Vulpi, Professor Vincenzo Ostilio Palmieri, and Professor Pasquale Ditonno. Validation was done by Dr. Anna Belfiore, Dr. Saverio Forte, Dr. Francesca Passerini, Professor Vincenzo Ostilio Palmieri, and Professor Pasquale Ditonno. Supervision was done by Professor Vincenzo Ostilio Palmieri and Professor Pasquale Ditonno. Dr. Antonio Francesco Maria Giuliano and Dr. Antonio Vavallo contributed to this manuscript in equal parts.

## References

[1] A. Gupta, M. V. Madhavan, K. Sehgal et al., "Extrapulmonary manifestations of COVID-19," *Nature Medicine*, vol. 26, no. 7, pp. 1017–1032, 2020.

[2] A. Salonia, I. Eardley, F. Giuliano et al., "European Association of Urology guidelines on priapism," *European Urology*, vol. 65, no. 2, pp. 480–489, 2014.

[3] J. M. Connors and J. H. Levy, "COVID-19 and its implications for thrombosis and anticoagulation," *Blood*, vol. 135, no. 23, pp. 2033–2040, 2020.

[4] M. Levi, J. Thachil, T. Iba, and J. H. Levy, "Coagulation abnormalities and thrombosis in patients with COVID-19," *The Lancet. Haematology*, vol. 7, no. 6, pp. e438–e440, 2020.

[5] S. Kaur, R. Bansal, S. Kollimuttathuillam et al., "The looming storm: blood and cytokines in COVID-19," *Blood Reviews*, vol. 46, p. 100743, 2021.

[6] E. Kölükçü, B. S. Parlaktaş, V. Kölükçü et al., "Protective effects of dexmedetomidine on ischaemia-reperfusion injury in an experimental rat model of priapism," *Andrologia*, vol. 53, no. 3, article e13985, 2021.

[7] M. Lamamri, A. Chebbi, J. Mamane et al., "Priapism in a patient with coronavirus disease 2019 (COVID-19)," *The American Journal of Emergency Medicine*, vol. 39, pp. 251.e5–251.e7, 2021.

[8] G. Lam, R. McCarthy, and R. Haider, "A peculiar case of priapism: the hypercoagulable state in patients with severe COVID-19 infection," *European Journal of Case Reports in Internal Medicine*, vol. 7, article 001779, 2019.

[9] M. L. Silverman, S. J. VanDerVeer, and T. J. Donnelly, "Priapism in COVID-19: a thromboembolic complication," *The American Journal of Emergency Medicine*, 2021.

[10] S. Senthilkumaran, S. Shah, N. B. Ganapathysubramanian, and P. Thirumalaikolundusubramanian, "Propofol and priapism," *Indian journal of pharmacology*, vol. 42, no. 4, pp. 238-239, 2010.

[11] K. S. Vesta, S. D. Martina, and E. A. Kozlowski, "Propofol-induced priapism, a case confirmed with rechallenge," *The Annals of Pharmacotherapy*, vol. 40, no. 5, pp. 980–982, 2006.

58

# Two Different Upper Tract Urological Malignancies on Either Side

**W. S. L. De Silva,[1,2] S. R. De Almeida,[2] G. D. B. J. Karunarathne,[2] A. A. S. Samarathunga,[2] K. M. C. S. Gannoruwa,[2] and J. A. S. B. Jayasundara[2]**

[1]*Postgraduate Institute of Medicine, University of Colombo, Sri Lanka*
[2]*District General Hospital, Nuwara Eliya, Sri Lanka*

Correspondence should be addressed to W. S. L. De Silva; supun85@gmail.com

Academic Editor: Claudio Simeone

*Introduction.* The genitourinary system is a recognized site for multiple primary malignant neoplasms even without syndromic anomalies. However, to the best of our knowledge, a case of upper tract urothelial carcinoma (UTUC) with contralateral renal cell carcinoma (RCC) is not reported in surgical literature so far. *Case Presentation.* A 52-year-old Sri Lankan male patient was found to have a right lower ureteric tumour and a left renal mass together upon investigating for painless visible hematuria. The right ureteric tumour measured 32 × 22 mm resulting in moderate hydronephrosis and cortical thinning of the right kidney, and the left renal mass measured 43 × 38 mm involving the lower pole. The biopsy of the right ureteric lesion revealed a high-grade transitional cell carcinoma with focal nested pattern and that of the left renal mass revealed a clear cell carcinoma. Right nephroureterectomy followed by a left partial nephrectomy was performed in six weeks' interval. The histology of both the resected specimens confirmed the biopsy findings. *Discussion.* A high-risk upper tract urothelial carcinoma such as the right ureteric tumour of this patient required a nephroureterectomy which makes the management of the contralateral renal cell carcinoma more complex. An adequate functional renal remnant was ensured after offering oncologically sound surgical treatment for both the malignancies of this patient. *Conclusion.* A UTUC when associated with a contralateral RCC poses challenges in patient management. The preservation of renal excretory function has to be considered as an important determinant in addition to oncologically sound surgical resection when managing complex cases of genitourinary malignancies involving both sides of the upper urinary tract.

## 1. Introduction

The phenomenon of multiple primary malignant neoplasms in nonsyndromic individuals was first described by Billroth way back in 1889 [1]. Moertel et al. detailed the criteria for the diagnosis of synchronous multiple primary malignancies (SMPM) later in 1961 [2]. The male genitourinary system (GUS) is considered as one of the commonest systems to harbor SMPM. Hence, the term synchronous primary urological cancer (SPUC) was coined by Qin et al. [3]. The knowledge about the behavior of each malignancy and the overall outcome of patients having SPUC is evolving. The overall prognosis of patients with SPUC is observed to be unfavorable to that of patients having a solitary urological malignancy, owing to the higher grade and the stage of tumours at presentation [3]. The management of patients with SPUC is challenging, especially when it involves the upper GUS because of the requirement to preserve an adequate functional renal remnant despite the advanced stage of the disease at presentation. We report a case of a high-risk upper tract urothelial carcinoma (UTUC) with a contralateral renal cell carcinoma (RCC) which required a patient-tailored management approach.

## 2. Case Presentation

A 52-year-old male was referred by the general practitioner for the management of an ultrasonographically detected left renal mass upon investigation for a single episode of frank

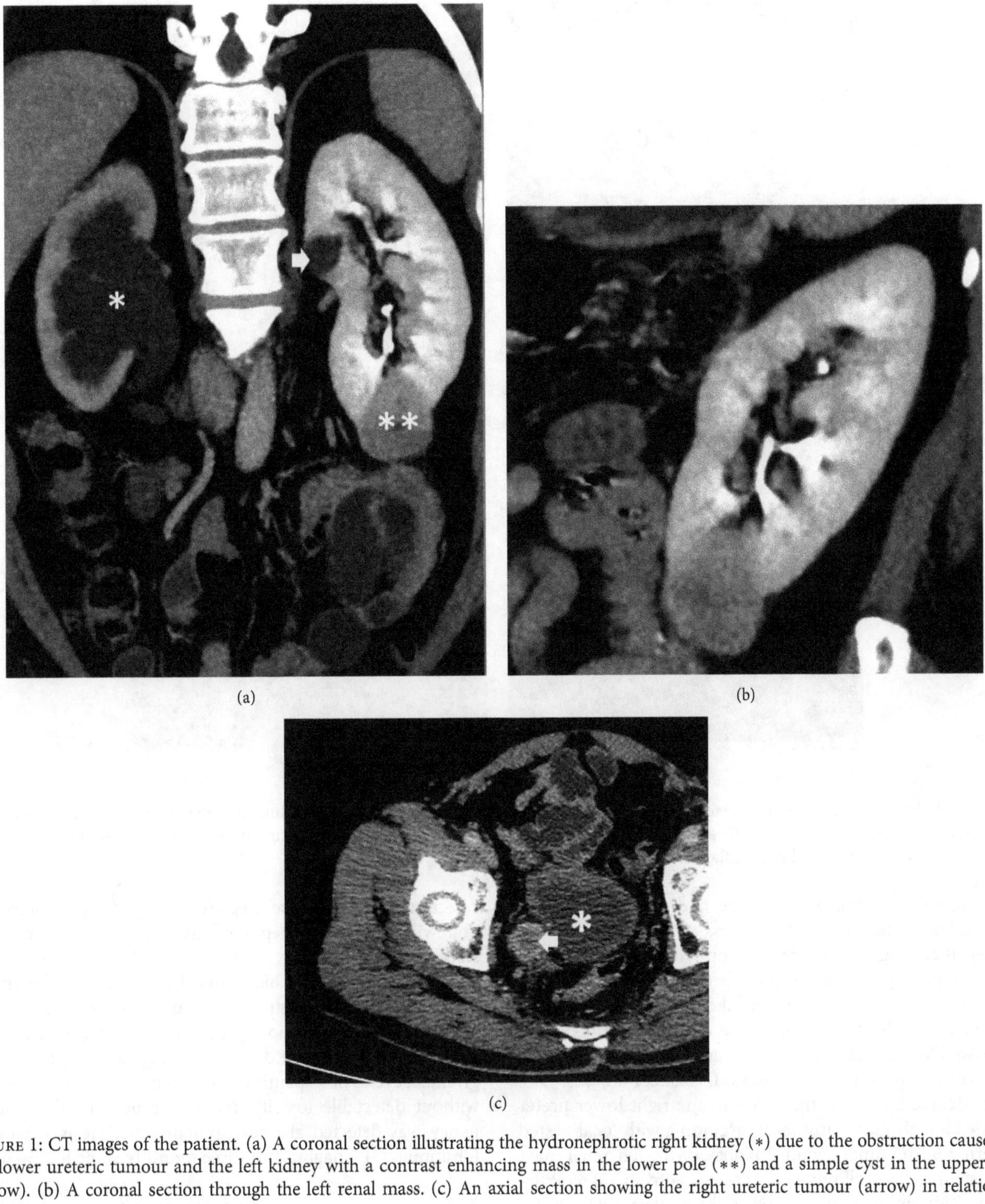

(a) (b) (c)

FIGURE 1: CT images of the patient. (a) A coronal section illustrating the hydronephrotic right kidney (*) due to the obstruction caused by the lower ureteric tumour and the left kidney with a contrast enhancing mass in the lower pole (**) and a simple cyst in the upper pole (arrow). (b) A coronal section through the left renal mass. (c) An axial section showing the right ureteric tumour (arrow) in relation to the posterior wall of the bladder (*).

hematuria. There was no history of loin pain, back pain, or lower urinary tract symptoms. He was a smoker (40 pack-years) but had no comorbidities. He had neither a personal history of malignancies elsewhere nor a history of cancer syndrome such as Lynch syndrome in the family. He had two subsequent bouts of frank hematuria in the preceding week and was admitted. No loin mass was palpable per-abdominally. The prostate gland was soft and not enlarged clinically, and the rest of the physical examination was unremarkable. The hemoglobin level on admission was 7.2 g/dl, and he was transfused accordingly. Other basic haematological and biochemical investigations were within normal limits. His baseline serum creatinine (S.Cr) was 0.9 mg/dl, and his serum prostate specific antigen level was 0.2 ng/ml.

The computerized tomographic urogram revealed an enhancing mass lesion measuring $32 \times 22$ mm in the right

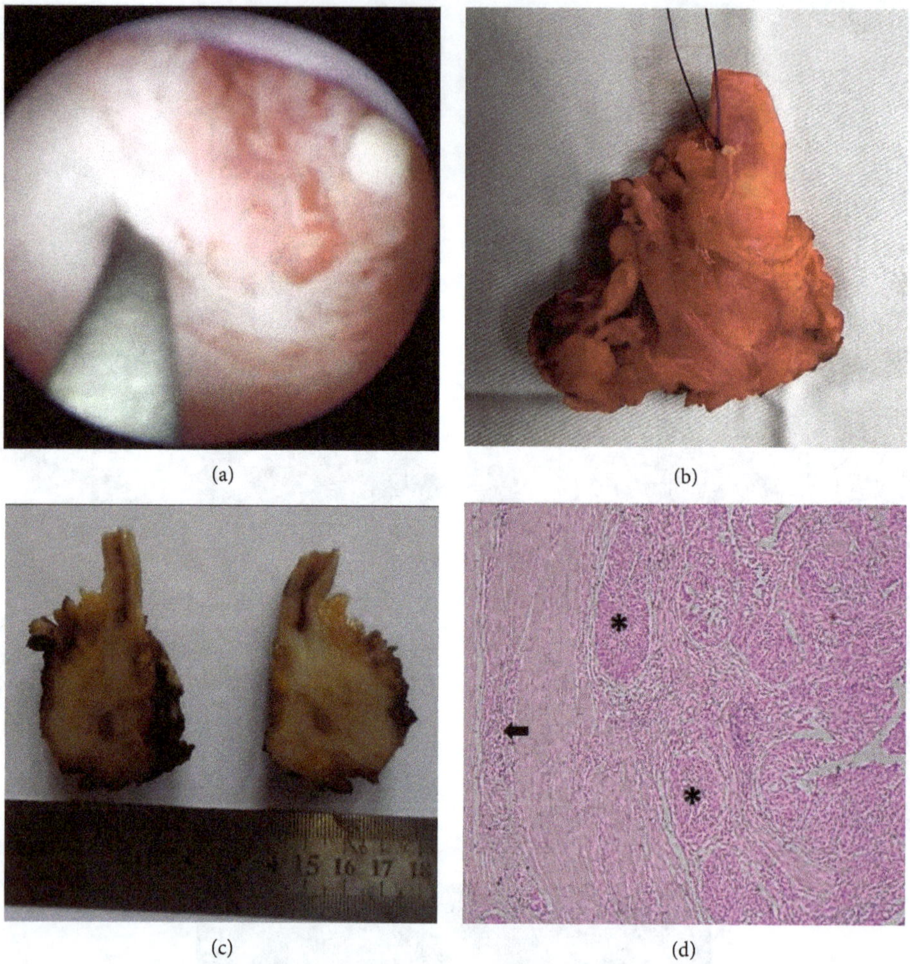

Figure 2: Right ureteric tumour. (a) Ureteroscopic view of the tumour completely obstructing the lumen of the ureter. (b) Macroscopic view of the separately resected tumour with a bladder cuff. (c) Cut surface appearance of the tumour. (d) ×10 view illustrating the nests of malignant (∗) cells invading the muscularis propria of the ureter (arrow).

lower ureter, resulting in moderate hydronephrosis of the right kidney with a cortical thickness of 12 mm. In the left kidney, there was an enhancing, exophytic mass, measuring 43 × 38 mm involving the lower pole (Nephrometry/RENAL score 5a) (Figure 1). There was no abdominal lymphadenopathy or evidence of metastasis. The differential function of the two kidneys was right—35% and left—65%. Flexible cystoscopy revealed no synchronous bladder lesions. The ureteroscopic biopsy of the lesion in the right lower ureter revealed a high-grade urothelial carcinoma with focal nested pattern, and the image-guided biopsy of the left renal mass confirmed a clear cell renal cell carcinoma (ccRCC). Following multidisciplinary discussion, right nephroureterectomy with removal of a bladder cuff was performed initially. A single bladder instillation of mitomycin C was also offered the same day. Histology of the specimen confirmed a high-grade UTUC with extensive lymphovascular and perineural invasion. All resection margins and three local lymph nodes were negative for malignancy. However, there was evidence of invasion of periureteric fat ($pT_3N_0M_0$) (Figure 2).

Left open partial nephrectomy was performed six weeks later. Histology of which revealed a low-grade (ISUP grade 2) ccRCC without sinus fat or capsular involvement, and the resection margins were negative ($pT_{1b}N_xM_0$) (Figure 3). Following the partial nephrectomy, the patient went into a status of acute kidney injury (AKI) where S.Cr raised to 4.5 mg/dl. Despite the biochemical derangement, he maintained a good urine output throughout and recovered from AKI in two weeks without requiring any renal replacement therapy and S.Cr came down to 1.1 mg/dl. The patient was given six cycles of cisplatin-based combination chemotherapy without detectable toxicity. No recurrence of either malignancy was detected at one-year follow-up. He is scheduled for annual CT imaging and three monthly clinic follow-up.

## 3. Discussion

Many reported cases of SPUC involve the bladder and the prostate gland [4]. 23% to 54% of patients who undergo radical cystoprostatectomy for bladder cancer were found to have synchronous prostate cancer [5]. Several cases of bladder cancers associated with RCC are reported [6, 7]. Two sporadic urological cancers involving the upper GUS are very rare. A case of a RCC and an ipsilateral TCC in the renal pelvis was reported by Lu et al. [8]. In this case, both malignancies were found in the same kidney which makes

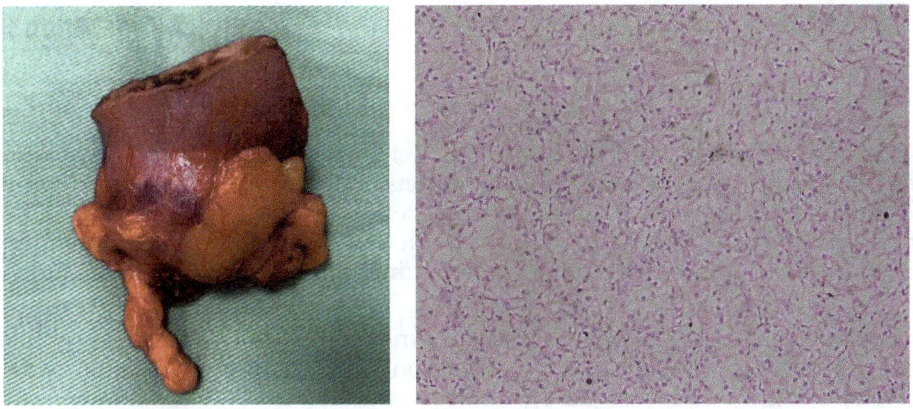

(a) (b)

FIGURE 3: Left renal cell carcinoma. (a) Macroscopic appearance of the resected tumour. (b) Histology showing typical clear cell carcinoma.

it less complex to management. To the best of our knowledge, this is the first case to be reported with a UTUC with a contralateral RCC.

Clinical guidelines recommend nephroureterectomy for a high-risk UTUC as the right-sided malignancy the index patient had [9]. However, the management of the index case was complicated due to the presence of the contralateral RCC, which again requires partial nephrectomy with a clear margin. A surgeon should be satisfied with the renal remnant to maintain the excretory function when planning this type of cases. Transient impairment of the renal function should be expected in a case like this because of the surgical trauma to the remnant kidney. However, there needs to be a contingency plan if an unexpected intra/postoperative complication makes the patient anephric. Preoperative planning, counseling, and consenting for such potential unfortunate events are mandatory in the management of rare cases of bilateral SPUC like the index case. Also, the involvement of specialties such as oncology, pathology, nephrology, and anesthesia is critical in tailor mating the treatment for puzzling cases like the index case.

Long-term follow-up of patients with SPUC is also pivotal because of high risk of recurrence due to higher stage and grade of individual malignancies. Recurrence from both malignancies was reported in the above discussed case by Lu et al. [8], emphasizing the requirement of special follow-up protocols for the long-term management of patients with SPUCs.

## 4. Conclusion

A UTUC when associated with a contralateral RCC poses several challenges in patient management. Staged ipsilateral nephroureterectomy and contralateral partial nephrectomy can be performed safely while preserving renal excretory functions.

## Consent

Informed, written consent was obtained for the publication of this article from the patient involved.

## References

[1] T. Billroth, "General Surgical Pathology and Therapeutics," in *51 Vorlesungen: A Textbook for Students and Physicians in Fifty-one Lectures*, p. 908, G. Rerimer, Berlin, 14th edition, 1889.

[2] C. G. Moertel, M. B. Dockerty, and A. H. Baggenstoss, "Multiple primary malignant neoplasms. I. Introduction and presentation of data," *Cancer*, vol. 14, no. 2, pp. 221–230, 1961.

[3] J. Qin, B. Fan, X. Chen et al., "Clinicopathologic insight of synchronous primary urologic cancers," *International Journal of Clinical and Experimental Medicine*, vol. 9, no. 6, pp. 11458–11466, 2016.

[4] T. Y. Chun, "Coincidence of bladder and prostate cancer," *The Journal of Urology*, vol. 157, no. 1, pp. 65–67, 1997.

[5] J. A. Pettus, H. al-Ahmadie, A. Barocas et al., "Risk Assessment of Prostatic Pathology in Patients Undergoing Radical Cystoprostatectomy," *European Urology*, vol. 53, no. 2, pp. 370–375, 2008.

[6] M. T. Smith, F. D. Taylor, W. P. Gianakopoulus, and R. R. Brown, "Two separate synchronous primary genitourinary tumors," *Revista de Urología*, vol. 14, no. 3-4, pp. 104–107, 2012.

[7] R. Espinosa Bravo, J. C. Morales Concepción, and O. M. Lemourt, "Simultaneous renal cell carcinoma and transitional cell carcinoma of bladder: a case report," *Archivos Españoles de Urología*, vol. 47, pp. 1028–1030, 2000.

[8] Q. Lu, J. Zhuang, and H. Guo, "Renal cell carcinoma with synchronous ipsilateral urothelial carcinoma of the renal pelvis," *Oncology Letters*, vol. 13, no. 6, pp. 4521–4525, 2017.

[9] M. Rouprêt, M. Babjuk, M. Burger et al., "EAU guidelines on upper urinary tract urothelial carcinoma 2018," in *Vol presented at the EAU Annual Congress Copenhagen 2018 Arnhem*, vol. 73-pp. 111–122, European Association of Urology Guidelines Office, The Netherlands, 2018 edition, 2018.

# Permissions

All chapters in this book were first published by Hindawi Publishing Corporation; hereby published with permission under the Creative Commons Attribution License or equivalent. Every chapter published in this book has been scrutinized by our experts. Their significance has been extensively debated. The topics covered herein carry significant findings which will fuel the growth of the discipline. They may even be implemented as practical applications or may be referred to as a beginning point for another development.

The contributors of this book come from diverse backgrounds, making this book a truly international effort. This book will bring forth new frontiers with its revolutionizing research information and detailed analysis of the nascent developments around the world.

We would like to thank all the contributing authors for lending their expertise to make the book truly unique. They have played a crucial role in the development of this book. Without their invaluable contributions this book wouldn't have been possible. They have made vital efforts to compile up to date information on the varied aspects of this subject to make this book a valuable addition to the collection of many professionals and students.

This book was conceptualized with the vision of imparting up-to-date information and advanced data in this field. To ensure the same, a matchless editorial board was set up. Every individual on the board went through rigorous rounds of assessment to prove their worth. After which they invested a large part of their time researching and compiling the most relevant data for our readers.

The editorial board has been involved in producing this book since its inception. They have spent rigorous hours researching and exploring the diverse topics which have resulted in the successful publishing of this book. They have passed on their knowledge of decades through this book. To expedite this challenging task, the publisher supported the team at every step. A small team of assistant editors was also appointed to further simplify the editing procedure and attain best results for the readers.

Apart from the editorial board, the designing team has also invested a significant amount of their time in understanding the subject and creating the most relevant covers. They scrutinized every image to scout for the most suitable representation of the subject and create an appropriate cover for the book.

The publishing team has been an ardent support to the editorial, designing and production team. Their endless efforts to recruit the best for this project, has resulted in the accomplishment of this book. They are a veteran in the field of academics and their pool of knowledge is as vast as their experience in printing. Their expertise and guidance has proved useful at every step. Their uncompromising quality standards have made this book an exceptional effort. Their encouragement from time to time has been an inspiration for everyone.

The publisher and the editorial board hope that this book will prove to be a valuable piece of knowledge for researchers, students, practitioners and scholars across the globe.

# List of Contributors


**Tyler J. Maiers, Daniel C. Wang, Ali H. Houjaij and Oussama M. Darwish**
Western New York Healthcare System-Buffalo Veterans Affairs Medical Center, 3495 Bailey Ave, Buffalo, NY 14215, USA
Department of Urology, Jacobs School of Medicine and Biomedical Sciences, University at Buffalo, Buffalo General Medical Center, Suite B280, 100 High Street, Buffalo, NY 14203, USA

**Yasukiyo Murakami, Tetsuo Fujita, Yoji Wakatabe and Masatsugu Iwamura**
Department of Urology, Kitasato University School of Medicine, Japan

**Henry Atawurah and Patrick Opoku Manu Maison**
Department of Surgery, School of Medical Sciences, College of Health and Allied Sciences, University of Cape Coast, Cape Coast, Ghana

**Mohammed Owusu-Ansah**
Department of Radiology, Cape Coast Teaching Hospital, Cape Coast, Ghana

**Alvin Asante-Asamani**
Department of Surgery, Cape Coast Teaching Hospital, Cape Coast, Ghana

**João Pádua Manzano**
Surgery Department at Federal University of São Paulo, São Paulo, Brazil
São Paulo's Military Hospital, Brazilian Army, São Paulo, Brazil

**Fábio da Silva Crochik, Felipe Guimarães Pugliesi and Renato Vasconcelos Souza de Almeida**
Division of Urology, Men's Health Centre, Hospital Brigadeiro, Sao Paulo, SP, Brazil

**Petronio Augusto de Souza Melo**
São Paulo's Military Hospital, Brazilian Army, São Paulo, Brazil

**Ricardo Luís Vita Nunes**

Benign Prostate Hyperplasia Department in Brazilian Urology Society, Urology Department in Sao Paulo's Military Hospital, Brazilian Army, São Paulo, Brazil

**Jacob D. McFadden**
Department of Urology, Walter Reed National Military Medical Center, 8901 Wisconsin Avenue, Bethesda, MD, USA

**Isabell A. Sesterhenn**
Joint Pathology Center, 606 Stephen Sitter Ave, Silver Spring, MD, USA

**Sean Q. Kern**
Department of Urology, Fort Belvoir Army Medical Center, 9300 DeWitt Loop, Fort Belvoir, VA, USA

**Takao Natsuyama**
Department of Urology, Chiba-Nishi General Hospital, 270-2251 Chiba, Japan
Department of Urology, Japan Community Health Care Organization, Tokyo Shinjuku Medical Center, Tokyo, Japan

**Yozo Mitsui**
Department of Urology, Chiba-Nishi General Hospital, 270-2251 Chiba, Japan
Department of Urology, Toho University Faculty of Medicine, 143-8540 Tokyo, Japan

**Masato Uetani and Shigeyuki Ohta**
Department of Urology, Chiba-Nishi General Hospital, 270-2251 Chiba, Japan

**Masafumi Inoue**
Department of Pathology, Japan Community Health Care Organization, Tokyo Shinjuku Medical Center, Tokyo, Japan

**Koichiro Akakura**
Department of Urology, Japan Community Health Care Organization, Tokyo Shinjuku Medical Center, Tokyo, Japan

**Fabian Brüning, Axel Hegele and Rainer Hofmann**
Department of Urology and Pediatric Urology, University Hospital, Philipps-University Marburg, Baldingerstr. 1, 35043 Marburg, Germany

**Günter Klaus**
KfH Pediatric Kidney Center and Department of Pediatrics, University Hospital, Philipps-University Marburg, Baldingerstr. 1, 35043 Marburg, Germany

**Rolf F. Maier**
Children's Hospital, Philipps-University Marburg, Baldingerstr. 1, 35043 Marburg, Germany

**Jonathan Kopel**
Texas Tech University Health Sciences Center, School of Medicine, Lubbock, TX, USA

**Pranav Sharma**
Department of Urology, Texas Tech University Health Sciences Center, Lubbock, TX, USA

**Irfan Warriach**
Department of Pathology, Texas Tech University Health Sciences Center, Lubbock, TX, USA

**Sriman Swarup**
Department of Hematology and Oncology, Texas Tech University Health Sciences Center, Lubbock, TX, USA

**Sarah Prattley, Timothy Bryant and Rowland Rees**
University Hospital Southampton, Tremona Road, Southampton, Hampshire SO166YD, UK

**Aikaterini Tsionga, Anastasios Anastasiadis, Wilbert Fana Mutomba, Dimitrios Memmos, Ioannis Vakalopoulos and Georgios Dimitriadis**
1st Department of Urology, Aristotle University of Thessaloniki, Ethnikis Aminis 41, 54635 Thessaloniki, Greece

**S. Venkat Ramanan, P. Velmurugan, A. R. Bhaskar Prakash, Anuj Arora and LeelaKrishna Karri**
Department of Urology, Sri Ramachandra Medical College and Research Institute, Chennai, India

**Seif Mokadem, Mohamed Ali Nouioui, Tarek Taktak, Houssem Mediouni, Ramzi Khiari and Samir Ghozzi**
Department of Urology, Military Hospital of First Instruction of Tunis, Tunisia

**Salma Kalai**
Department of Microbiology, Military Hospital of First Instruction of Tunis, Tunisia

**Rawad Abou Zahr, Khalil Chalhoub, Imad Matta, Imad Ghantous and Michel Jabbour**
Department of Urology, University of Balamand, Saint George Hospital University Medical Center, Beirut 1100 2807, Lebanon

**Sawsan Horani**
University of Balamand, Faculty of Medicine and Medical Sciences, Beirut 1100 2807, Lebanon

**Zarouhie Bedoyan**
Department of Pathology, University of Balamand, Saint George Hospital University Medical Center, Beirut 1100 2807, Lebanon

**Georges El Hachem**
Department of Hematology-Oncology, University of Balamand, Saint George Hospital University Medical Center, Beirut 1100 2807, Lebanon

**Raymond A. Stemrich**
Geisinger Health System, 100 N. Academy Avenue, Danville, PA 17822, USA

**Neel Hasmukh Patel, Jacob A. Baber and Mark J. Ferretti**
Geisinger, Urology Associate, 1000 E. Mountain Boulevard, Wilkes-Barre, PA 18702, USA

**Mohamed Jalloh, Oumar Gaye, Medina Ndoye, Mouhamadou Moustapha Mbodji, Ayun Cassell, Lamine Niang and Serigne Magueye Gueye**
Service d'Urologie, Hopital General Idrissa Pouye, 134 Rue GY, 530 Dakar, Senegal

**Jennifer Heibig, William Ghaul and Gabrielle Yankelevich**
Philadelphia College of Osteopathic Medicine (PCOM), 4170 City Ave, Philadelphia, PA 19131, USA

**Alejandra Perez, Adam Carl Nolte, Spencer Steve Liem, Jorge Francisco Pereira, Alan Scott Polackwich and Rafael Yanes**
Mount Sinai Medical Center, Department of Urology, 4302 Alton Road, MSOP Suite 540, Miami Beach, FL 33140, USA

**Giuseppe Maurici**
Olympus Medical Systems Corp., 4302 Alton Road, MSOP Suite 540, Miami Beach, FL 33140, USA

**Alexander Charles Small**
Montefiore Medical Center, 1250 Waters Place, Bronx, NY 10461, USA

**Ojas Shah**
Columbia University Irving Medical Center, Department of Urology, 161 Fort Washington Ave., New York, NY 10032, USA

**Nobuhiko Shimizu, Nao Katsumi, Kazuhiro Kanemoto and Hidetoshi Akita**
Department of Urology, Anjo Kosei Hospital, Anjo, Japan

**Yoshinobu Moritoki**
Department of Urology, Anjo Kosei Hospital, Anjo, Japan
Department of Urology, Toyokawa City Hospital, Toyokawa, Japan

**Takahiro Yanase, Teruaki Sugino and Takahiro Yasui**
Department of Nephro-Urology, Nagoya City University Graduate School of Medical Sciences, Nagoya, Japan

**Justin E. Dupey and Richard Y. Ball**
Norfolk and Waveney Cellular Pathology Service, Norfolk and Norwich University Hospitals NHS Foundation Trust, Colney Lane, Norwich, Norfolk NR4 7UY, UK

**Sarah J. Wood**
Department of Urology, Norfolk and Norwich University Hospitals NHS Foundation Trust, Colney Lane, Norwich, Norfolk NR4 7UY, UK

**Masresha S. Dino, Alemayehu Tegegn Tefera, Kaleab Hebtemichael Gebreselassie, Sena Sefera Akkasa and Ferid Ousman Mummed**
St. Paul's Hospital Millennium Medical College, Department of Surgery, Urology Unit, Addis Ababa, Ethiopia

**Jean Sossa, Lionelle Fanou, Yao Felicien Hounto and Felix Atadokpede**
Service d'Urologie, Hopital d'Instruction des Armees Centre Hospitalier Universitaire (HIA-CHU), Cotonou, Benin

**Dedjinnin Josue Georges Avakoudjo, Dodji Magloire Ines Yevi, Gilles Natchagande Michel Michael Agounkpe and Fred Hodonou**
Clinique Universitaire d'Urologie-Andrologie, Centre National Hospitalier et Universitaire Hubert Koutoucou Maga (CNHUHKM), Cotonou, Benin

**Kevin Krughoff, Bing Ren and Vernon M. Pais Jr.**
Department of Surgery/Section of Urology, Dartmouth-Hitchcock Medical Center, Lebanon, NH, USA

**Alan Schned**
VA Medical Center, White River Junction, VT, USA

**Nikolaos Grivas, Esther Wit and Henk G. van der Poel**
Department of Urology, The Netherlands Cancer Institute-Antoni van Leeuwenhoek Hospital, Amsterdam, Netherlands

**Alexander D. Horsch and Annemarie Bruining**
Department of Radiology, The Netherlands Cancer Institute-Antoni van Leeuwenhoek Hospital, Amsterdam, Netherlands

**Johanna van Sandick**
Department of Surgery, The Netherlands Cancer Institute-Antoni van Leeuwenhoek Hospital, Amsterdam, Netherlands

**Rawad Abou Zahr, Valentin Colinet, Aurore Mattlet and Romain Diamand**
Urology Department, Jules Bordet Institute, Université Libre de Bruxelles, Boulevard de Waterloo 121, 1000 Brussels, Belgium

**Teddy Jabbour**
Urology Department, Saint George Hospital University Medical Center, University of Balamand, Beirut 1100 2807, Lebanon

**Max J. Roehmholdt and Dennis F. Bentley**
Cleveland Clinic Foundation – Akron General Medical Center, 1 Akron General Avenue, Akron, OH, USA 44307

**Klaus-Peter Dieckmann and Christian Wülfing**
Asklepios Klinik Altona, Abteilung Urologie/ Hodentumorzentrum, Hamburg, Germany

**Julia Bertolini**
MVZ Hanse Histologikum, Hamburg, Germany

**V. Kalyvas, N. Kalinderis, K. Moysidis and K. Hatzimouratidis**
2nd Department of Urology, Aristotle University of Thessaloniki, Greece

**C. Gkekas, D. Papadopoulos, M. Papathanasiou and A. Malioris**
Department of Urology, 424 General Military Hospital of Thessaloniki, Greece

**S. Milias**
Department of Pathology, 424 General Military Hospital of Thessaloniki, Greece

**Yasuyuki Onishi, Yusaku Moribata, Yuji Nakamoto and Hironori Shimizu**
Department of Diagnostic Imaging and Nuclear Medicine, Kyoto University Graduate School of Medicine, Japan

**Kosuke Shimizu, Takeshi Sano and Takashi Kobayashi**
Department of Urology, Kyoto University Graduate School of Medicine, Japan

**Harshima Disvini Wijesinghe**
Department of Pathology, Faculty of Medicine, University of Colombo, Sri Lanka

**Ajith Malalasekera**
Department of Anatomy, Faculty of Medicine, University of Colombo, Sri Lanka

**Makoto Kawase, Keita Nakane, Sanae Namiki, Yasumichi Takeuchi, Shota Ueda, Kota Kawase, Chie Nakai, Shinichi Takeuchi, Daiki Kato, Manabu Takai, Koji Iinuma and Takuya Koie**
Department of Urology, Gifu University Graduate School of Medicine, Japan

**Masayuki Fuwa and Hiroyuki Morita**
Department of General Internal Medicine, Gifu University Graduate School of Medicine, Japan

**Chiemi Saigo and Tatsuhiko Miyazaki**
Department of Pathology, Gifu University Graduate School of Medicine, Japan

**A. Haffar**
West Virginia University School of Medicine, West Virginia, USA

**T. Trump, A. A. Elbakry, M. W. Salkini and A. Luchey**
Department of Urology, West Virginia University, West Virginia, USA
Department of Interventional Radiology, West Virginia University, West Virginia, USA

**K. McCluskey**
Department of Interventional Radiology, West Virginia University, West Virginia, USA

**Aykut Colakerol, Mustafa Zafer Temiz, Engin Kandirali and Ahmet Yaser Muslumanoglu**
Department of Urology, Bagcilar Training and Research Hospital, Istanbul, Turkey

**Mubarek Bargicho Adem**
Department of General Surgery, Urology Unit, St. Paul's Hospital Millennium Medical College, Addis Ababa, Ethiopia

**Kamil Ozdogan and Fatih Celebi**
Department of General Surgery, Bagcilar Training and Research Hospital, Istanbul, Turkey

**C. Crigger**
Johns Hopkins Children's Center, Baltimore, USA

**M. Jessop**
Benefis Health System Foundation, Great Falls, USA

**Chirag P. Doshi and Marcus L. Quek**
Department of Urology, Loyola University Medical Center, Maywood, IL, USA

**Guliz A. Barkan**
Department of Pathology, Loyola University Medical Center, Maywood, IL, USA

**Mikael Abi Abdallah, Naim Yarak and Jean Paul Noujeim**
Division of Urology, Faculty of Medical Sciences, Lebanese University, Beirut, Lebanon
Department of Urology, Lebanese Geitaoui Hospital, Beirut, Lebanon

**Nehme Raad and Antoine Noujeim**
Department of Urology, Lebanese Geitaoui Hospital, Beirut, Lebanon

**Amr Elmoheen and Khalid Bashir**
Emergency Department, Hamad Medical Corporation, Qatar
QU Health, College of Medicine, Qatar University, Qatar

**Mahmoud Saqr and Waleed Salem**
Emergency Department, Hamad Medical Corporation, Qatar

**Ayman Hagras**
Urology Department, College of Medicine, Tanta University, Egypt

**Rami Halabi, Maher Abdessater, Johnny Boustany, Anthony Kanbar, Halim Akl, Joey El Khoury, Charbel El Hachem and Raghid El Khoury**
Department of Urology, Notre Dame des Secours University Hospital Center (CHUNDS), Byblos City, Lebanon
Faculty of Medicine and Medical Sciences, Holy Spirit University of Kaslik (USEK), Jounieh, Lebanon

**Christopher Ferari, Chad Crigger and Chad Morley**
Department of Urology, West Virginia University School of Medicine, Morgantown, WV 26505, USA

**Taylor C. Peak, Michael B. Rothberg and Ronald L. Davis**
Department of Urology, Wake Forest Baptist Medical Center, Winston-Salem, NC, USA

**Elena M. Fenu**
Department of Pathology, Wake Forest Baptist Medical Center, Winston-Salem NC, USA

**Christopher Y. Thomas**
Department of Medical Oncology and Hematology, Wake Forest Baptist Medical Center, Winston-Salem NC, USA

**Edward A. Levine**
Surgical Oncology Service, Department of General Surgery, Wake Forest Baptist Medical Center, Winston-Salem, NC, USA

**A. K. Paré, A. Ouattara, D. Yé, B. Kabré, A. Bako and T. Kambou**
Department of Urology, Souro Sanou University Teaching Hospital, Bobo-Dioulasso, Burkina Faso

**B. M. Abubakar**
Department of Surgery, Federal Medical Center, PMB 02, Nguru, Yobe State, Nigeria

**M. Sivashankar and A. C. N. Nandasena**
Department of Urology, Colombo North Teaching Hospital, Ragama, Sri Lanka

**Van Schloegel, Syed M. Alam, Katie Dennis, Jeffrey Holzbeierlein and John A. Taylor III**
Department of Urology, University of Kansas Health System, 3901 Rainbow Boulevard, Kansas City, KS 66160, USA

**Aamer Alghamlas**
Department of Pediatric Surgery, CHU Besançon, F-25000 Besançon, France

**Frédéric Auber and Yann Chaussy**
Department of Pediatric Surgery, CHU Besançon, F-25000 Besançon, France
Nanomédecine, Imagerie, Thérapeutique EA 4662, Université Bourgogne Franche-Comté, F-25000 Besançon, France

**Valeria Pereira Martinez, Marilin Nicholson and Trushar Patel**
USF Health Morsani College of Medicine, 560 Channelside Drive, Tampa, FL 33602, USA

**Reza Abbasion**
Department of Pediatric Urology, Faculty of Medicine, Akbar Hospital, Mashhad University of Medical Sciences, Mashhad, Iran

**Amir Jafarpisheh**
Department of Urology, Faculty of Medicine, Mashhad University of Medical Sciences, Mashhad, Iran

**Paria Dehghanian**
Pathology Department, Pediatric Pathologist, Akbar Children's Hospital, Iran

**Mahdi Mottaghi**
Students Research Committee, Faculty of Medicine, Mashhad University of Medical Sciences, Mashhad, Iran

**Kenichi Hata and Kazuhiro Takahashi**
Department of Urology, Atsugi City Hospital, 1-16-36, Mizuhiki, Atsugi City, Kanagawa-ken 243-8588, Japan

**Takahiro Kimura and Shin Egawa**
Department of Urology, Jikei University School of Medicine, 3-25-8, Nishi-Shinbashi, Minato-ku, Tokyo 105-8461, Japan

**Ahmed Ibrahimi, Idriss Ziani, Hachem El Sayegh, Lounis Benslimane and Yassine Nouini**
Department of Urology A, Ibn Sina University Hospital, Faculty of Medicine and Pharmacy, Mohammed V University in Rabat, Rabat, Morocco

**Adil Kallat**
Provincial Hospital Center of Azilal, Azilal, Morocco

**João Rebelo, Margarida Morgado and Ana Sofia Preto**
Radiology Department, Centro Hospitalar Universitário de São João, Porto, Portugal

**Francisco Moreira**
Pathology Department, Centro Hospitalar Universitário de São João, Porto, Portugal

**António Madureira**
Radiology Department, Centro Hospitalar Universitário de São João, Porto, Portugal
Faculdade de Medicina da Universidade do Porto, Porto, Portugal

**Bikash Bikram Thapa and Sanjay Yadav**
Department of Surgery, College of Medicine, Nepalese Army Institute of Health Sciences, Nepal

**Sujit Pant**
Department of Radio Diagnosis, College of Medicine, Nepalese Army Institute of Health Sciences, Nepal

**Pratik Rajkarnikar and Pankaj Mandal**
Department of Pathology, College of Medicine, Nepalese Army Institute of Health Sciences, Nepal

**Idriss Ziani, Ahmed Ibrahimi, Omar Bellouki, Youssef Zaoui, Hachem El Sayegh, Lounis Benslimane and Yassine Nouini**
Department of Urological Surgery "A", Ibn Sina University Hospital of Rabat, Rabat, Morocco
Department of Anatomopathology and Cytology, Ibn Sina University Hospital of Rabat, Rabat, Morocco

**Yasmine Laraqui Housseini and Fouad Zouidia**
Department of Urological Surgery "A", Ibn Sina University Hospital of Rabat, Rabat, Morocco
Department of Anatomopathology and Cytology, Ibn Sina University Hospital of Rabat, Rabat, Morocco
Faculty of Medicine of Rabat, Mohammed V University, Rabat, Morocco

**A. M. Mainwaring, H. Wells, T. Banks, T. Ellul and P. Bose**
Department of Urology, Morriston Hospital, Swansea, UK

**Ryo Kasahara**
Department of Urology, Fujisawa City Hospital, 2-6-1 Fujisawa, Fujisawa City, Kanagawa Prefecture, Japan
Department of Urology, Yokohama City University School of Medicine, 3-9 Fukuura, Kanazawa Ward, Yokohama City, Kanagawa Prefecture, Japan

**Ryosuke Tajiri**
Department of Pathology, Fujisawa City Hospital, 2-6-1 Fujisawa, Fujisawa City, Kanagawa Prefecture, Japan

**Kota Kobayashi and Kazuo Kitami**
Department of Urology, Fujisawa City Hospital, 2-6-1 Fujisawa, Fujisawa City, Kanagawa Prefecture, Japan

**Masahiro Yao**
Department of Urology, Yokohama City University School of Medicine, 3-9 Fukuura, Kanazawa Ward, Yokohama City, Kanagawa Prefecture, Japan

**Ali Hajiran, David Zekan, Tyler Trump and Adam Luchey**
Department of Urology, West Virginia University, Morgantown, WV 26505, USA

**Dylan Dangerfield**
Department of Urology, University of Tennessee Graduate School of Medicine, Knoxville, TN 37920, USA

**Taro Ikeda, Noboru Hara and Tsutomu Nishiyama**
Department of Urology, Uonuma Institute of Community Medicine, Niigata University Medical and Dental Hospital, Minamiuonuma, Niigata, Japan

**Go Hasegawa**
Department of Pathology, Uonuma Institute of Community Medicine, Niigata University Medical and Dental Hospital, Minamiuonuma, Niigata, Japan

**Gen Kawaguchi**
Department of Radiotherapy, Uonuma Institute of Community Medicine, Niigata University Medical and Dental Hospital, Minamiuonuma, Niigata, Japan

**Yohei Ikeda**
Department of Diagnostic Radiology, Uonuma Institute of Community Medicine, Niigata University Medical and Dental Hospital, Minamiuonuma, Niigata, Japan

**Ichiro Tsuboi, Nobuyoshi Ando, Yasuhiro Nishiyama, Ryoji Arata and Noriaki Ono**
Department of Urology, Kochi Health Sciences Center, 2125-1 Ike, Kochi city, Kochi 781-8555, Japan
Okayama Urological Research Group (OURG), 2-5-1, Shikata-cho, Kita-ku, Okayama 700-8558, Japan

**Yuki Maruyama and Motoo Araki**
Department of Urology, Okayama University Graduate School of Medicine, Dentistry and Pharmaceutical Sciences, 2-5-1 Shikatacho, Kita-ku, Okayama 700-8558, Japan

**Grant Johnson**
Franciscan Health Olympia Fields Hospital, Midwestern University, Downers Grove, IL, USA

**Kiran Thalody**
ROWAN SOM, Stratford, NJ, USA

**Umesh Kapur**
Comprehensive Pathology Services, Silvercross Hospital, New Lenox, IL, USA

**Thai T. Nguyen**
Advanced Urology Associates, Silvercross Hospital, New Lenox, IL, USA

**Tetsuya Danno, Shohei Iwata, Fusako Niimi, Sachi Honda and Takeshi Azuma**
Department of Urology, Tokyo Metropolitan Tama Medical Center, 2-8-29 Musashidai, Fuchu, Tokyo 183-0042, Japan

**Haruka Okada**
Department of Pathology, Tokyo Metropolitan Tama Medical Center, 2-8-29 Musashidai, Fuchu, Tokyo 183-0042, Japan

**Antonio Francesco Maria Giuliano, Francesca Passerini, Anna Belfiore and Vincenzo Ostilio Palmieri**
Department of Biomedical Sciences and Human Oncology, Clinica Medica "A. Murri", Università degli Studi di Bari Aldo Moro Facoltà di Medicina e Chirurgia, Piazza Giulio Cesare n°11, 70124 Bari, Bari, Italy

**Marco Vulpi, Antonio Vavallo, Saverio Forte and Pasquale Ditonno**
Department of Emergency and Organ Transplantation, Urology and Andrology Unit II, Università degli Studi di Bari Aldo Moro Facoltà di Medicina e Chirurgia, Piazza Giulio Cesare n°11, 70124 Bari, Bari, Italy

**W. S. L. De Silva**
Postgraduate Institute of Medicine, University of Colombo, Sri Lanka
District General Hospital, Nuwara Eliya, Sri Lanka

**S. R. De Almeida, G. D. B. J. Karunarathne, A. A. S. Samarathunga, K. M. C. S. Gannoruwa and J. A. S. B. Jayasundara**
District General Hospital, Nuwara Eliya, Sri Lanka

# Index

www.ingramcontent.com/pod-product-compliance
Lightning Source LLC
LaVergne TN
LVHW082123200926
848484LV00008B/1996